PRAISE FOR THE

Insider's Guide to Graduate Programs in Clinical and Counseling Psychology

"An excellent resource....The authors are faithful to the title; this is truly an 'insider's guide.'...★★★★"
                                        —*Doody's Annual*

"Imagine, for a moment, a growing crowd of people who are all attempting to get through doors that are passageways to the careers they desperately want. If you find yourself in this reality that students face in attempting to gain admission to graduate programs in clinical psychology, the *Insider's Guide* is a 'must read.'"
                                        —C. R. Snyder, Ph.D.,
        Director of Clinical Psychology, University of Kansas

"The process of applying for admission to graduate programs in clinical and counseling psychology can be daunting. This valuable resource guides individuals through the process....Recommended."
                                        —*Choice*

"I was lost and confused before I stumbled across this wonderful piece of literature! It answered every question I had, narrowed down my choices. The ranking system was great!"
                        —**Lisa Oldfield, clinical psychology applicant**

INSIDER'S GUIDE TO GRADUATE PROGRAMS IN CLINICAL AND COUNSELING PSYCHOLOGY

INSIDER'S GUIDE

to Graduate Programs in Clinical and Counseling Psychology

2006/2007 Edition

Tracy J. Mayne
John C. Norcross
Michael A. Sayette

THE GUILFORD PRESS
New York   London

© 2006 The Guilford Press
A Division of Guilford Publications, Inc.
72 Spring Street, New York, NY 10012
www.guilford.com

Printed in the United States of America

Last digit is print number: 9 8 7 6 5 4 3 2 1

ISBN-10: 1-59385-258-4
ISBN-13: 978-1-59385-258-0

ISSN 1086-2099

CONTENTS

TABLES AND FIGURES

Tables

Figures

ABOUT THE AUTHORS

Tracy J. Mayne received his baccalaureate from the State University of New York at Buffalo, where he graduated *magna cum laude* and *Phi Beta Kappa*. He received his Ph.D. as an Honors Fellow from Rutgers University and completed his internship and postdoctoral fellowship at the University of California at San Francisco Medical School and the Center for AIDS Prevention Studies. He spent 2 years as an international scholar at the Institut Nationale de la Santé et de la Recherche Médicale in France and 3 years as the Director of HIV Epidemiology and Surveillance at the New York City Department of Health, where he received the Commissioner's Award for Outstanding Community Research. Dr. Mayne spent 5 years conducting research in cardiovascular medicine at Pfizer Pharmaceuticals and currently works in Global Health Economics at Amgen Inc., conducting research in cancer-supportive therapies. Dr. Mayne has published numerous articles and chapters in the area of health psychology, health economics, and emotion, and is the coeditor of *Emotions: Current Issues and Future Directions,* published by The Guilford Press.

John C. Norcross received his baccalaureate *summa cum laude* from Rutgers University. He earned his master's and doctorate in clinical psychology from the University of Rhode Island and completed his internship at the Brown University School of Medicine. He is Professor of Psychology and Distinguished University Fellow at the University of Scranton, a clinical psychologist in independent practice, past-president of the APA Division of Psychotherapy, and past-president of the International Society of Clinical Psychology. Dr. Norcross has published more than 250 articles and has authored or edited 15 books, the most recent being *Evidence-Based Practice in Mental Health, Authoritative Guide to Self-Help Resources in Mental Health, Psychotherapy Relationships That Work,* and *Psychologists' Desk Reference.* He has served on the editorial boards of a dozen journals and is editor of *Journal of Clinical Psychology: In Session.* Among his awards are the Pennsylvania Professor of the Year from the Carnegie Foundation, Distinguished Practitioner from the National Academies of Practice, and the Distinguished Career Contribution to Education and Training Award from the American Psychological Association. Dr. Norcross has conducted workshops and research on graduate study in psychology for many years.

Michael A. Sayette received his baccalaureate *cum laude* from Dartmouth College. He earned his master's and doctorate in clinical psychology from Rutgers University and completed his internship at the Brown University School of Medicine. He is Professor of Psychology at the University of Pittsburgh, with a secondary appointment as Professor of Psychiatry at the Western Psychiatric Institute and Clinic, University of Pittsburgh School of Medicine. Dr. Sayette has published primarily in the area of substance abuse. His research, supported by the National Institute on Alcohol Abuse and Alcoholism and by the National Institute on Drug Abuse, concerns the development of psychological theories of alcohol and tobacco use. He has served on National Institutes of Health grant review study sections and is on the editorial boards of several journals. He also is an associate editor of *Journal of Abnormal Psychology* and a former associate editor of *Psychology of Addictive Behaviors.* Dr. Sayette has directed graduate admissions for the clinical psychology program at the University of Pittsburgh, and has presented seminars on applying to graduate school at several universities in North America and Europe.

ACKNOWLEDGMENTS

To paraphrase John Donne, no book is an island, entire of itself. This sentiment is particularly true of a collaborative venture such as ours: a coauthored volume in its ninth edition comprising the contributions of hundreds of psychologists and of reports on individual doctoral programs provided by training directors throughout North America. We are grateful to them all.

We are also indebted to the many friends, colleagues, and workshop participants for their assistance in improving this book over the years. Special thanks to Liz Whitmer, who helped collect and organize data on individual program reports, as well as Jill Oliver for providing data analysis for this edition. Seymour Weingarten and his associates at The Guilford Press have continued to provide interpersonal support and technical assistance on all aspects of the project. Special thanks to our families for their unflagging support and patience with late night work!

Finally, our efforts have been aided immeasurably by our students, graduate and undergraduate alike, who courageously shared their experiences with us about the application and admission process.

PREFACE

One of the benefits of applying to clinical and counseling psychology programs is that you earn the right to commiserate about it afterwards. It was a night of anecdotes and complaints (while doing laundry) that led us to review our travails and compare notes on the difficulties we each experienced during the admission process. We emerged from three diverse backgrounds: one of us (T.J.M.) graduated from a large state university, took time off, and then entered a doctoral program; one of us (M.A.S.) graduated from a private liberal arts college and immediately pursued a doctorate; and another one of us (J.C.N.) graduated from a liberal arts college within a major state university after 5 years and then pursued doctoral studies.

Although we approached graduate school in different ways, the process was much the same. We each attempted to locate specific information on clinical and counseling psychology admissions, looked to people around us for advice, took that which seemed to be sound, and worked with it. Not all the advice was good (one professor went so far as to suggest a career in the theater instead!), and it was difficult to decide what was best when advice conflicted.

All in all, there was too little factual information available and too much unnecessary anxiety involved. No clearly defined or organized system was available to guide us through this process. So we decided to write an insider's guide to graduate programs in clinical and counseling psychology.

The last dozen years have seen the entire process of choosing schools and applying become progressively more difficult. Approximately 75,000 bachelor's degrees are awarded every year in psychology, and about 20% of the recipients go on to earn a master's or doctoral degree in psychology. Clinical and counseling psychology programs continue to grow in number and to diversify in mission: 224 APA-accredited doctoral programs in clinical psychology, 68 APA-accredited doctoral programs in counseling psychology, 10 APA-accredited programs in combined professional–scientific psychology, dozens of non-APA-accredited doctoral programs, and hundreds of master's programs. Which should you apply to? And which type of program is best for you—counseling or clinical, practice-oriented Psy.D. or research-oriented Ph.D.?

We shall take you step by step through this confusing morass and help you make informed decisions suited to your needs and interests. In this new edition, we provide additional information on the percent of applicants accepted to each doctoral program and the recent changes in the GRE General Test. In addition, we describe how you can capitalize on the Internet revolution to ease the graduate school admissions process—locating compatible programs, communicating with potential faculty mentors, submitting application forms, and helping faculty send letters of recommendation electronically. We also provide specific advice for racial/ethnic minority and lesbian, gay, bisexual, and transgendered (LGBT) applicants. Throughout the book, we provide Web sites to access for additional information and direction.

We also explore crucial issues regarding admission criteria, acceptance rates, financial aid, and theoretical orientations to help you decide which program best fits your needs.

What we would most like to do, in clear and concise language, is to help *you* through this process, from the initial decision to apply through your final acceptance. In Chapter 1, we describe the predominant training models in clinical and counseling psychology and alternatives to these disciplines. In the next chapter, we discuss the essential preparation for graduate school—the course work, faculty mentoring, clinical experiences, research skills, entrance examinations, and extracurricular activities. From there, in Chapter 3, we get you started on the application process and assist you in understanding admission requirements. In Chapter 4, we show you how to systematically select schools on the basis of multiple considerations, especially research interests, clinical opportunities, theoretical orientations, financial assistance, and quality of life. Then in Chapter 5, we take you through the application procedure itself—forms, curricula vitae, personal statements, letters of recommendation, academic transcripts, and the like. In Chapter 6, we review the perils and promises of the interview, required by three-quarters of clinical and counseling psychology programs. Last, in Chapter 7, we walk you through the complexities of the final decisions. With multiple worksheets and concrete examples, we will help you feel less overwhelmed, better informed, and, in the end, more aware that *you* are the consumer of a program that best suits *your* needs.

We have conducted original studies on graduate psychology programs for this book in an effort to inform your decision making. These results provide information on the differences between clinical and counseling psychology programs (Chapter 1), the importance of various graduate school selection criteria (Chapter 2), acceptance rates (Chapter 3), the probability of financial assistance (Chapter 4), interview policies (Chapter 6), research areas (Appendix E), clinical and practica sites (Appendix F), and more. Indeed, we have extensively surveyed all APA-accredited programs in clinical, counseling, and combined psychology and present detailed information on each in the Reports on Individual Programs. A detailed Time Line (Appendix A) and multiple worksheets (Appendices B, C, and D) also provide assistance on the heretofore treacherous journey of applying to graduate programs in clinical and counseling psychology.

This volume will assist anyone seeking admission to graduate school in clinical and counseling psychology, both master's and doctoral degrees. However, the primary focus is on Ph.D. and Psy.D. applicants, as the doctorate is the entry-level qualification for professional psychology. Just as a master's degree in biology does not make one a physician, a master's in psychology does not, by state licensure and APA regulation, typically qualify one as a psychologist. Forty-eight states require the doctorate for licensure or certification as a psychologist; almost half the states grant legal recognition of psychological associates, assistants, or examiners with a master's degree (APA Practice Directorate, 1999). But the material presented here is relevant for master's (M.A. or M.S.) applicants as well.

With this practical manual, we wish you an application process less hectic and confusing than ours, but equally rewarding in the end result. Good luck!

CHAPTER 1

INTRODUCING CLINICAL AND COUNSELING PSYCHOLOGY

If you are reading this book for the first time, we are assuming you are either considering applying to graduate programs in clinical and counseling psychology or are in the process of doing so. For even the best-prepared applicant, this can precipitate a great deal of stress and confusion. The mythology surrounding this process is foreboding, and you may have heard some "horror" stories similar to these: "It's the hardest graduate program to get into in the country"; "You need a 3.8 grade point average and 700s on your GREs or they won't even look at you"; "If you haven't taken time off after your bachelor's degree and worked in a clinic, you don't have enough experience to apply."

Having endured the application process ourselves, we know how overwhelming the task appears at first glance. However, we have found that much of the anxiety is unwarranted. It does not take astronomical test scores or years of practical experience to get into clinical and counseling psychology programs. Although these qualifications certainly help, they are not sufficient. Equally important are a knowledge of how the system works and a willingness to put in extra effort during the application process. In other words, in this book, we will help you to work smarter and work harder in getting into graduate school.

Clinical and Counseling Psychology

Before dealing with the question of "how to apply," we would like to address "why" to apply and what clinical and counseling psychology are about. Reading through the next section may be useful by making you aware of other programs of study that may be more suitable to your needs.

Let us begin with clinical psychology, the largest specialty and the fastest growing sector in psychology. Two-thirds of the doctoral-level health service providers in the American Psychological Association (APA) identify with the specialty area of clinical psychology (VandenBos, Stapp, & Kilburg, 1981). A census of all psychological personnel residing in the United States likewise has revealed that the majority reported clinical psychology as their major field (Stapp, Tucker, & VandenBos, 1985).

A definition of clinical psychology was adopted jointly by the APA Division of Clinical Psychology and the Council of University Directors of Clinical Psychology (see Resnick, 1991). That definition states that the field of clinical psychology involves research, teaching, and services relevant to understanding, predicting, and alleviating intellectual, emotional, biological, psychological, social, and behavioral maladjustment, disability, and discomfort, applied to a wide range of client populations. The major skill areas essential for the field of clinical psychology are assessment; intervention; consultation; program development and evaluation, supervision, and administration; conduct of research; and application of ethical standards. Perhaps the safest observation about clinical psychology is that both the field and its practitioners continue to outgrow the classic definitions.

Indeed, the discipline has experienced a veritable explosion since World War II in numbers, activities, and knowledge. Since 1949, the year of the Boulder Conference (see below), there has been a large and significant increase in psychology doctoral graduates. Approximately 2,400 doctoral degrees are now awarded annually in clinical psychology—1,400 Ph.D. degrees

TABLE 1-1. Popularity and Doctorate Production of Psychology Subfields

Subfield	Percentage of doctoral-level psychologists[a]	Number of Ph.D.s awarded[b]			
		1976	1994	1998	2002
Clinical	44%	883	1329	1350[c]	1312
Cognitive	1%	—	76	113	121
Counseling	11%	267	464	448	536
Developmental/child	4%	190	158	267	173
Educational	6%	124	98	61	54
Experimental and physiological	3%	357	143	149	201
Industrial/organizational	6%	73	124	189	154
Psychometric/quantitative	2%	27	23	23	22
School	5%	143	81	106	89
Social and personality	4%	271	165	210	197
Other or general	12%	387	560	673	438
Total	100%	2,883	3,287	3,681	3,199[c]

[a]From Stapp, Tucker, & VandenBos (1985). © 1985 American Psychological Association. Reprinted by permission.

[b]National Research Council, *Summary Report of Doctoral Recipients from United States Universities* (selected years), Washington, DC: Author.

[c]Plus 1,000 Psy.D. degrees awarded annually.

and 1,000 Psy.D. degrees. All told, doctoral degrees in clinical psychology account for about 45% of all psychology doctorates. Table 1-1 demonstrates the continuing popularity of clinical psychology and the growing number of clinical doctorates awarded annually.

These trends should continue well into the new millennium. After a drop in the early 1980s, the percentage of psychology majors among college freshmen has continued to increase nationally to over 3%. In fact, the proportion of college freshmen who explicitly express an intention of becoming clinical psychologists has steadily risen to 1.3% (Astin, Green, & Korn, 1987). A nationwide survey of almost 2 million high school juniors, reported in the *Occupational Outlook Quarterly,* found that psychology was the sixth most frequent career choice. Indeed, according to data from the U.S. Department of Education, interest in psychology as a major has never been higher (Murray, 1996). So, if you are seriously considering clinical or counseling psychology for a career, you belong to a large, vibrant, and growing population.

Counseling psychology is the second largest specialty in psychology and another rapidly growing sector. As also shown in Table 1-1, counseling psychology has experienced sustained growth over the past three decades. We are referring here to counseling *psychology*,

the doctoral-level specialization in psychology, not to the master's-level profession of counseling. This is a critical distinction: our book and research studies pertain specifically and solely to counseling psychology programs, not counseling programs.

The distinctions between clinical psychology and counseling psychology have steadily faded. Graduates of counseling psychology programs are eligible for the same professional benefits as clinical psychology graduates, such as psychology licensure, independent practice, and insurance reimbursement. The APA ceased distinguishing many years ago between clinical and counseling psychology internships: there is one list of accredited internships for both clinical and counseling psychology students. Both types of programs prepare doctoral-level psychologists who provide health care services.

At the same time, five robust differences between clinical psychology and counseling psychology are still visible (Morgan & Cohen, 2003; Norcross et al., 1998). First, clinical psychology is larger than counseling psychology: in 2005, there were 224 APA-accredited and active doctoral programs in clinical psychology and 68 APA-accredited and active doctoral programs in counseling psychology (APA, 2004) currently accepting students. Table 1-1 reveals that these counseling psychology programs—in addition to some unaccredited programs—produce about 500 doctoral degrees per year. By contrast, clinical psychology programs produce approximately 2,400 doctoral degrees (1,400 Ph.D. and 1,000 Psy.D.) per year. Second, clinical psychology graduate programs are almost exclusively housed in departments or schools of psychology, whereas counseling psychology graduate programs are located in a variety of departments and divisions. Our research (Turkson & Norcross, 1996) shows that, in rough figures, one-quarter of doctoral programs in counseling psychology are located in psychology departments, one-quarter in departments of counseling psychology, one-quarter in departments or colleges of education, and one-quarter in assorted other departments. The historical placement of counseling psychology programs in education departments explains the occasional awarding of the Ed.D. (doctor of education) by counseling psychology programs.

A third difference is that clinical psychology graduates tend to work with more seriously disturbed patients and are more likely trained in projective assessment, whereas counseling graduates work with healthier, less pathological patients and conduct more career and vocational assessment. Fourth, counseling psychologists more frequently endorse a client-centered/Rogerian approach to psychotherapy, whereas clinical psychologists are more likely to embrace behavioral or psychodynamic orientations. And fifth, both APA figures (APA Research Office, 1997) and our research (Bechtoldt, Norcross, Wyckoff, Pokrywa, & Campbell, 2001) consistently reveal that 15% more clinical psychologists are employed in full-time private practice than are counseling psychologists, whereas 10% more counseling psychologists are employed in college counseling centers than are clinical psychologists. Studies on the roles and functions of clinical and counseling psychologists substantiate these differences, but the similarities are far more numerous (Brems & Johnson, 1997; Fitzgerald & Osipow, 1986; Tipton, 1983; Watkins, Lopez, Campbell, & Himmel, 1986a, 1986b).

In order to extend this previous research, we conducted a study of APA-accredited doctoral programs in counseling psychology (95% response rate) and clinical psychology (99% response rate) regarding their number of applications, characteristics of incoming students, and research areas of the faculty (Norcross, Sayette, Mayne, Karg, & Turkson, 1998). We found:

- The average acceptance rates of Ph.D. clinical (6%) and Ph.D. counseling (8%) psychology programs were quite similar despite the higher number of applications to clinical programs (270 vs. 130).

- The average grade point averages (GPAs) for incoming doctoral students were identical in Ph.D. clinical and Ph.D. counseling psychology programs (3.5 for both).
- The average GRE scores of accepted students were similar, with Ph.D. clinical students having slightly higher scores as a group.
- The counseling psychology programs accepted more ethnic minority students (25% vs. 18%) and master's students (67% vs. 21%) than the clinical psychology programs.
- The counseling psychology faculty were far more interested than clinical psychology faculty in research pertaining to minority/cross-cultural issues (69% vs. 32% of programs) and vocational/career testing (62% vs. 1% of programs).
- The clinical psychology faculty, in turn, were far more interested than the counseling psychology faculty in research pertaining to psychopathological populations (e.g., attention deficit disorders, depression, personality disorders) and activities traditionally associated with medical settings (e.g., neuropsychology, pain management, pediatric psychology).

Please bear in mind that these systematic comparisons reflect broad differences in the APA-accredited Ph.D. programs; they say nothing about Psy.D. programs (which we discuss later in this chapter) or nonaccredited programs. Also bear in mind that these data can be used as a rough guide in matching your interests to clinical or counseling psychology programs. The notion of discovering the best match between you and a graduate program is a recurrent theme of this *Insider's Guide*.

As shown in Table 1-2, clinical and counseling psychologists devote similar percentages of their day to the same professional activities. About one-half of their time is dedicated to psychotherapy and assessment and a quarter of their time to research and administration. A stunning finding was that over half of clinical and counseling psychologists were routinely involved in all seven activities—psychotherapy, assessment, teaching, research, supervision, consultation, and administration. Flexible career indeed!

The scope of clinical and counseling psychology is continually widening, as are the employment settings. Many people mistakenly view psychologists solely as practitioners who spend most of their time seeing patients. But in truth, clinical and counseling psychology are wonderfully diverse and pluralistic professions. Consider the employment settings of American clinical psychologists: 40% in private practices, 19% in

TABLE 1-2. Professional Activities of Clinical and Counseling Psychologists

Activity	Clinical psychologists		Counseling psychologists	
	% involved in	Average % of time	% involved in	Average % of time
Psychotherapy	80	34	74	28
Diagnosis/assessment	64	15	62	12
Teaching	50	10	60	18
Clinical supervision	50	6	54	6
Research/writing	51	14	50	8
Consultation	47	7	61	7
Administration	53	13	56	15

Note. Data from Norcross, Karpiak, & Santoro (2005) and Watkins, Campbell, & Himmell (1986a).

universities or colleges, 5% in psychiatric hospitals, 9% in medical schools, 4% in general hospitals, another 5% in community mental health centers, 4% in outpatient clinics, and 11% in "other" placements (Norcross, Karg, & Prochaska, 1997a, 1997b). This last category included, just to name a few, child and family services, correctional facilities, rehabilitation centers, school systems, health maintenance organizations, psychoanalytic institutes, and the federal government.

Although many psychologists choose careers as clinicians in private practice, hospitals, and clinics, a large number also pursue careers in research. For some, this translates into an academic position. Uncertainties in the health care system are increasing the allure of academic positions, where salaries are less tied to client fees than in a clinical position. Academics teach courses and conduct research, usually with a clinical population. They hope to find a "tenure-track" position, which means they start out as an assistant professor. After a certain amount of time (typically 5 or 6 years), a university committee reviews their research, teaching, and service, and decides whether they will be hired as a permanent faculty member and promoted to associate professor. Even though the tenure process can be a pressured one, the atmosphere surrounding assistant professors is very conducive to research activity. They are often given "seed" money to set up facilities and attract graduate students eager to share in the publication process. (For additional information on the career paths of psychology faculty, consult *The Psychologist's Guide to an Academic Career*, Rheingold, 1994, or *Career Paths in Psychology*, Sternberg, 1997.)

In addition, research-focused industries (like pharmaceutical and biomedical), as well as community-based organizations, are increasingly employing psychologists to design and conduct outcomes research. The field of outcomes research combines the use of psychometrics and assessment, program design and evaluation, along with cost-effectiveness analyses within contexts as varied as clinical trials and community interventions. Although lacking the job security of tenure, industry can offer greater monetary compensation and is an increasingly viable option for research-oriented PhDs.

But even this range of primary employment settings does not accurately capture the opportunities in the field. About half of all clinical and counseling psychologists hold more than one professional position (Norcross et al., 1997a; Watkins et al., 1986a). By and large, psychologists incorporate several pursuits into their work, often simultaneously. They combine activities in ways that can change over time to accommodate their evolving interests. Of those psychologists not in full-time private practice, over half engage in some part-time independent work (Norcross et al., 1997b). Without question, this flexibility is an asset.

As a university professor, for example, you might run a research group studying aspects of alcoholism, treat alcoholics and their families in private practice, and teach a course on alcohol abuse. Or, you could work for a company supervising marketing research, do private testing for a school system, and provide monthly seminars on relaxation. The possibilities are almost limitless.

This flexibility is also evident in clinical and counseling psychologists' "self-views." About 60% respond that they are primarily clinical practitioners, 20% are academicians, 7% administrators, 5% researchers, 5% consultants, and 2% supervisors (Norcross et al., 1997b; Watkins et al., 1986a).

Also comforting is the consistent finding of relatively high and stable satisfaction with graduate training and career choice. Over two-thirds of graduate students in clinical and counseling psychology express satisfaction with their post-baccalaureate preparation. Moreover, 87 to 91% are satisfied with their career choice (Norcross et al., 1997b; Tibbits- Kleber & Howell, 1987; Watkins et al., 1986a). The conclusion we draw is that clinical and counseling psychologists appreciate the diverse pursuits and take advantage of their professional flexibility, which plays a significant role in their high level of career satisfaction.

The diversity in professional choice has produced a diversity of training models in professional psychology. Without a firm understanding of the differences in these training models, many applicants will waste valuable time and needlessly experience disappointment. Let us now distinguish between the two prevalent training models in clinical psychology—the Boulder model and the Vail model. Counseling psychology has parallel differences in training emphases; however, it does not typically employ the same terms as clinical psychology and only three APA-accredited counseling psychology programs offer the Psy.D. degree.

The Boulder Model (Ph.D.)

The first national training conference on clinical psychology was held during 1949 in Boulder, Colorado (hence, the "Boulder model"). At this conference, equal weight was accorded to the development of research competencies and clinical skills. This dual emphasis resulted in the notion of the clinical psychologist as a *scientist–practitioner*. Clinical psychologists were considered first and foremost as psychologists and were to have a rigorous, broad-based education in psychology. Their training would encompass statistics, history and systems, and research, with core courses in development, biopsychology, learning, and the like. The emphasis was on psychology; clinical was the adjective.

The Boulder conference was a milestone for several reasons. First, it established the Ph.D. as the required degree, as in other academic research fields. To this day, all Boulder model, scientist–practitioner programs in clinical psychology award the Ph.D. degree. Second, the conference reinforced the idea that the appropriate location for training was within university departments, not separate schools or institutes as in medicine and law. And third, clinical psychologists were trained for simultaneous existence in two worlds: academic/scientific and clinical/professional.

The important implication for you, as an applicant, is to know that Boulder-model programs provide rigorous education as a researcher along with training as a clinician. Consider this dual thrust carefully before applying to Boulder-model programs. Some first-year graduate students undergo undue misery because they dislike research-oriented courses and the research projects that are part of the degree requirements. These, in turn, are preludes to the formal dissertation required by Boulder-model programs. Many applicants are specifically seeking this sort of training.

A recent movement toward a "bolder" Boulder model was crystalized by the 1995 creation of the Academy of Psychological Clinical Science (APCS). According to its Web site, APCS is "an alliance of leading, scientifically oriented, doctoral training programs in clinical and health psychology, committed to empirical approaches to advancing knowledge," which was established in response to rapid changes taking place in the field of clinical psychology. "The Academy seeks as members those programs that are strongly committed to research training and to the integration of such training with clinical training." APCS includes 42 clinical psychology Ph.D. programs. These programs are listed in Table 1-3. More information on APCS can be found on their Web site: http://w3.arizona.edu/~psych/apcs/apcs.html.

Based on the data from our previous editions of the *Insider's Guide* we found that, compared to nonmember programs, APCS programs admitted a slightly lower percentage of applicants (who had higher GRE scores) and were more likely to provide full financial support. APCS programs also subscribed more frequently to a cognitive-behavioral orientation, reported a stronger research emphasis, and engaged more frequently in research supported by funding agencies than did non-APCS programs (Sayette, Mayne, Norcross, & Giuffre, 1999). Students interested in a Boulder-model clinical Ph.D program may find these programs to be especially attractive in that they represent empirically based, research-focused training.

Other applicants are seeking training focused on clinical practice. For these applicants, there is an alternative to the Boulder model: the Vail model of training psychologists.

The Vail Model (Psy.D.)

Some dissension with the recommendations of the Boulder conference emerged at later meetings; however, there was a strong consensus that the scientist–practitioner model, Ph.D. degree, and university training should be retained. But in the late 1960s and early 1970s, change was in the wind. Training alternatives were entertained, and diversification was

TABLE 1-3. APA-Accredited Clinical Psychology Programs That Are Members of the Academy of Psychological Clinical Science (APCS)

University of Arizona	University of Missouri
Arizona State University	University of Nevada–Reno
Boston University	Ohio State University
University of California–Berkeley	University of Oregon
University of California–Los Angeles	University of Pennsylvania
University of California–San Diego and San Diego State University	Pennsylvania State University
University of Delaware	University of Pittsburgh
University of Denver (Department of Psychology)	Purdue University
Duke University	Rutgers University
Emory University	University of Southern California
Florida State University	University of South Florida
University of Hawaii	State University of New York–Binghamton
University of Illinois at Urbana Champaign	State University of New York–Stony Brook
Indiana University	University of Texas
University of Iowa	University of Toronto
University of Kentucky	Vanderbilt University
University of Maryland	Virginia Tech
McGill University	University of Virginia (Department of Psychology)
University of Memphis	University of Washington
University of Miami (Health Psychology)	Washington University–St. Louis
University of Minnesota	University of Wisconsin
	Yale University

encouraged. This sentiment culminated in a 1973 national training conference held in Vail, Colorado (hence, the "Vail model").

The Vail conferees endorsed different principles, leading to a diversity of training programs (Peterson, 1976, 1982). Psychological knowledge, it was argued, had matured enough to warrant creation of explicitly professional programs along the lines of professional programs in medicine, dentistry, and law. These "professional programs" were to be added to, not replace, Boulder-model programs. Further, it was proposed that different degrees should be used to designate the scientist role (Ph.D.—Doctor of Philosophy) from the practitioner role (Psy.D.—Doctor of Psychology). Graduates of Vail-model professional programs would be *scholar–professionals*: the focus would be primarily on clinical service and less on research.

This revolutionary conference led to the emergence of two distinct training models typically housed in different settings. Boulder-model programs are almost universally located in graduate departments of universities. However, Vail-model programs can be housed in three organizational settings: within a psychology department; within a university-affiliated psychology school (for instance, Rutgers and Adelphi); and within an independent, "freestanding" psychology school (e.g., Massachusetts School of Professional Psychology). These latter programs are not affiliated with universities but are independently developed and staffed. Table 1-4 lists APA-accredited clinical Psy.D. programs.

Clinical psychology now has two established and complementary training models. Ph.D. programs produce approximately 1.5 times as many doctoral-level psychologists per year as Psy.D. programs. Although Boulder-model programs still outnumber Vail-model programs, Vail-model programs enroll, as a rule, three to four times the number of incoming doctoral candidates (Mayne, Norcross, & Sayette, 1994). This creates almost a numerical parity in terms of psychologists produced.

The differences between Boulder-model and Vail-model programs are quantitative, not qualitative. The primary disparity is in the relative emphasis on research:

TABLE 1-4. APA-Accredited Psy.D. Programs in Clinical Psychology

Adler School of Professional Psychology

Alliant International University–San Diego (California School of Professional Psychology)[a]

Alliant International University–San Francisco (California School of Professional Psychology)[a]

Alliant International University–Los Angeles (California School of Professional Psychology)[a]

Alliant University, Fresno (California School of Professional Psychology)[a]

Antioch New England Graduate School

Argosy University, Atlanta Campus (Georgia School of Professional Psychology)

Argosy University, Chicago Campus (Illinois School of Professional Psychology)

Argosy University, Chicago Northwest Campus (Illinois School of Professional Psychology)

Argosy University, Honolulu Campus

Argosy University, Phoenix

Argosy University, San Francisco Bay

Argosy University, Tampa

Argosy University, Twin Cities (Minnesota School of Professional Psychology)

Argosy University, Washington, DC

Azusa Pacific University

Baylor University

Biola University[a]

California Institute for Integral Studies

Carlos Albizu University–Miami Campus

Carlos Albizu University–San Juan Campus[a]

Chicago School of Professional Psychology

University of Denver[a]

Florida Institute of Technology

Forest Institute of Professional Psychology

Fuller Theological Seminary[a]

George Fox University

George Washington University[a]

University of Hartford

Immaculata College

Indiana State University

Indiana University of Pennsylvania

University of Indianapolis

John F. Kennedy University

La Salle University

University of La Verne

Loma Linda University[a]

Long Island University/C.W. Post Campus

Loyola University in Maryland

Massachusetts School of Professional Psychology

Nova Southeastern University[a]

Pacific University

Pepperdine University

Philadelphia College of Osteopathic Medicine

Ponce School of Medicine

Regent University

Roosevelt University

Rutgers University[a]

Spalding University

Virginia Consortium Program in Clinical Psychology

Wheaton College

Widener University

The Wright Institute[a]

Wright State University

Xavier University

Yeshiva University

[a] These institutions also have APA-accredited Ph.D. programs in clinical psychology.

Boulder programs aspire to train producers of research; Vail programs train consumers of research. Even Vail programs require some research and statistics courses; you simply cannot avoid research sophistication in any accredited psychology program. The clinical opportunities are very similar for students in both types of programs.

As we discuss in subsequent chapters, there are trade-offs between Vail- and Boulder-model programs. Vail-model, Psy.D. programs provide slightly more clinical experience and courses but less research experience and courses than do Boulder-model programs (Tibbits-Kleber & Howell, 1987). The additional research and the large dissertation required in Boulder-model Ph.D. programs translate into an additional year of training, on average. Vail-model programs afford easier (but not easy) admission but less financial assistance than Boulder-model programs. As a rule, students in Psy.D. programs tend to be older and more likely to have master's degrees already than their Boulder-model counterparts (Farry, Norcross, Mayne, & Sayette, 1995; Mayne et al., 1994). Both Vail and Boulder programs have similar admission criteria, which favor grade point average, entrance examination scores, letters of recommendation, and so on. (All these topics are covered in detail in later chapters.)

Several studies have demonstrated that initial worries about stigmatization, employment difficulties, licensure uncertainty, and second-class citizenship for Psy.D.s have *not* materialized (see Hershey, Kopplin, & Cornell, 1991; Peterson, Eaton, Levine, & Snepp, 1982). There do not appear to be strong disparities in the pre-internship clinical skills of Ph.D. and Psy.D. students as evaluated by internship supervisors (Snepp & Peterson, 1988). Nor are there discernible differences in employment except, of course, that the more research-oriented, Boulder-model graduates are far more likely to be employed in academic positions and medical schools (Gaddy, Charlot-Swilley, Nelson, & Reich, 1995). While Vail-model graduates may be seen as second-class citizens by Boulder-model traditionalists, this is not the case among health care organizations or individual consumers.

An important caveat: if you desire to teach full time at a 4-year college or university, we strongly advise you *not* to seek the Psy.D. degree. The Psy.D. is an explicitly professional or practitioner degree; your training and expertise will be as a practitioner, not as a professor, researcher, or academician.

One disconcerting trend is that Vail-model graduates do not perform as well as Ph.D. graduates on the national licensing examination for psychologists (Kupfersmid & Fiola, 1991; Maher, 1999). That is, doctoral students who graduate with a professional degree (the Psy.D.) score lower, on average, than doctoral students who graduate from a traditional clinical psychology Ph.D. program on the Examination for Professional Practice in Psychology (EPPP), the national licensing test. Higher EPPP scores have been reliably associated with smaller-sized clinical programs and larger faculty-to-student ratios, in addition to traditional Ph.D. curricula.

Vail-model graduates are typically less rigorously trained than Boulder-model graduates in research, evaluation, and statistical skills. These skills are likely to be particularly valued in the future as master's-level psychotherapists increasingly become first-line providers of psychotherapy, whereas doctoral-level psychologists perform more supervision, research, and teaching. The Psy.D. degree is explicit in providing training for practice, and to the extent that doctoral-level psychologists may do less psychotherapy in the new health care systems, a broad training may prove advantageous. Regardless of whether training occurs in the context of a Psy.D. or Ph.D. program, it is wise to seek training in a variety of professional activities, not solely psychotherapy.

A final difference between Ph.D. and Psy.D. programs concerns the length of training. Students in Ph.D. programs take significantly longer, approximately 1 to 1.5 years longer, to complete their degrees than do Psy.D. students (Gaddy et al., 1995; Norcross, Castle, Sayette, & Mayne, 2004). Various interpretations are given to this robust difference, from "Psy.D. training is more focused and efficient" on one pole, to "Ph.D. training is more comprehensive and rigorous" on the other.

Which training model do clinical psychologists themselves prefer? In one of our studies (Norcross, Gallagher, & Prochaska, 1989), we found that 50% favored the Boulder model, 14% the Vail model, and the remaining 36% both models equally. However, preferences varied as a function of the psychologist's own doctoral program: 93% of the psychologists trained in a strong Boulder tradition preferred the Boulder model or both equally. Likewise, 90% of the psychologists trained in a strong Vail tradition preferred the Vail model or both equally.

The key task for you as a potential applicant is to recognize the diversity in training emphases. We describe this as the practice–research continuum. On one end of the continuum are the Psy.D. programs that are practice oriented. These account for roughly 30% of APA-accredited clinical doctoral programs. In the middle of the continuum are the equal-emphasis Ph.D. programs that, as the name implies, emphasize both research and practice. These programs account for about 40% of APA-accredited clinical programs. On the other end of the continuum are the research-oriented Ph.D. programs that account for approximately 30% of the accredited programs (Mayne et al., 1994). Since the Psy.D. programs accept and graduate far larger numbers of students than research-oriented programs, the proportion of new doctorates in clinical psychology is almost equally divided among the practice, equal emphasis, and research programs.

The bottom line for applicants to clinical psychology programs is one of choice, matching, and parity. You have the choice of two training models (and all the programs in between the two extremes). The choice should be matched to your strengths and interests. Parity has been achieved in that almost half of all doctorates in clinical psychology are awarded by Vail-model programs (Turkington, 1986). The choices are yours, but make informed decisions.

A Word on Accreditation

Accreditation comes in many guises, but the two primary types are institutional accreditation and program accreditation. Institutional applies to an entire institution. Seven regional accreditation bodies, such as the Commission on Higher Education of the Middle States Association of Colleges and Schools, oversee accreditation for the university or college itself. A school receives accreditation when it has been judged to have met minimum standards of quality for postsecondary education.

Beware of any institution that is not accredited by its regional accreditation body. A degree from this institution will probably not be recognized by licensing boards, certifying organizations, or insurance companies (Dattilio, 1992). It is necessary to be particularly careful about nontraditional or external degree programs that offer the option of obtaining a degree based on independent study, typically away from the institution itself. Some of these are reputable programs, but many are "diploma mills" (Stewart & Spille, 1988). Many diploma mills have names similar to legitimate universities, so you must be vigilant. Here are several diploma mills with potentially misleading titles: Columbia State University (Louisiana), La Salle University (Louisiana), Chadwick University (Alabama), American State University (Hawaii), American International University (Alabama). (For additional information about diploma mills, consult the fact sheets at the Council for Higher Education Accreditation at www.CHEA.org, www.degree-finders.com/diplomamills.html and www.web-miner.com/deun accredited.htm).

If you have any doubt, inquire thoroughly into whether the institution as a whole is recognized by professional associations. This can be accomplished by referring to the document, *Doctoral Psychology Programs Meeting Designation Criteria*, jointly published by the Association of State and Provincial Psychology Boards (ASPPB) and the National Register of Health Service Providers in Psychology (2005). You can access an updated list at www.nationalregister.org/designate.htm.

The second type of accreditation pertains to the clinical or counseling psychology program itself. Specialized accreditation of the discipline is performed by the American Psychological Association (APA). This accreditation is a voluntary procedure for the doctoral program itself, not the entire institution. Most programs that are capable of meeting the requirements of APA accreditation will choose to apply for accreditation. Accreditation of a clinical or counseling psychology program by the APA presumes regional accreditation of the entire institution.

The APA only accredits doctoral programs in the four specialty areas of clinical psychology, counseling psychology, school psychology, and combined psychology. The last category is for those programs that afford doctoral training in two or more of the specialties of clinical, counseling, and school psychology.

The "combined" doctoral programs represent a relatively new development in graduate psychology training, and thus are relatively small in number, about 3% of APA-accredited programs. In emphasizing the core research and practice competencies among the specialities, combined programs try to enlist their respective strengths and to capitalize on their overarching competencies. In doing so, the hope is that a combined program will be "greater than the sum of its parts" (Salzinger, 1998). For students undecided about a particular speciality in professional psychology and seeking broad clinical training, these accredited combined programs warrant a close look.

The chief reasons that students select combined doctoral programs are for increased breadth and flexibility of training and for more opportunity of integrative training across specializations. The emphasis on breadth of psychological knowledge ensures that combined training will address the multiplicity of interests that many students have and that many psychologists will need in practice (Beutler & Fisher, 1994). The chief disadvantages of combined programs are, first, their lack of depth and specialization and, second, the fact that other mental health professionals may not understand the combined model. Our research on combined training programs (Castle & Norcross, 2002) does, in fact, substantiate the broader training and more varied employment of their graduates. Consult the Reports of Combined Programs at the end of this book for details on these innovative schools.

As of 2005, APA had accredited 224 active clinical psychology programs (53 of these awarding the Psy.D. degree), 68 active counseling psychology programs (3 of these awarding the Psy.D. degree), and 10 active combined professional–scientific psychology programs (including 3 Psy.D. programs) that are currently accepting students (Accredited, 2005). The Reports on Individual Programs in this book provide detailed descriptions of these 300 clinical psychology, counseling psychology, and combined programs, respectively.

Take note that APA does *not* accredit master's programs. Accordingly, references to "accredited" master's psychology programs are to regional or state, not APA, accreditation.

The program accreditation criteria can be obtained from the APA Office of Accreditation (www.apa.org/ed/accred.html). The general areas assessed include institutional support, sensitivity to cultural and individual differences, training models and curricula, faculty, students, facilities, and practicum and internship training. These criteria are designed to insure at least a minimal level of clinical and research quality.

The APA (Accredited, 2005) recognizes three categories of accreditation. Accreditation is granted to programs that meet the criteria in a satisfactory manner. "Accredited, inactive" is the designation for programs that have not accepted students for 2 years. This indicates that the program is taking a hiatus as part of a restructuring process, or is phasing out the program (for example, New York University's Clinical Psychology program). "Accredited, probation" is the designation for programs that were previously accredited but are not currently in satisfactory compliance with the criteria.

Our Reports on Individual Programs, located in the back of this book, provide crucial descriptive and application information on each APA-accredited doctoral program in clinical, counseling, and combined psychology. The APA Education Directorate updates the listing of accredited programs annually in the December issue of the *American Psychologist* and bimonthly on their Web site, www.apa.org/ed.

How important is it to attend an APA-accredited program? The consensus ranges from slightly important to absolutely essential. APA accreditation ensures a modicum of program stability, quality assurance, and professional accountability. Graduates of APA-accredited programs are practically guaranteed to meet the educational requirements for state licensure. Students are in a more advantageous and competitive position coming from an APA-approved program in terms of their internship choices (Drummond, Rodolfa, & Smith, 1981) and their eventual employment prospects (Walfish & Sumprer, 1984). The federal government, the Veterans Administration, and most universities now insist on a doctorate and internship from APA-accredited programs. Graduates of APA programs also score significantly higher, on average, than do students of non-APA-accredited programs on the licensure exam (Kupfersmid & Fiola, 1991). Licensure and employment as a psychologist are not precluded by attending a non-APA-accredited program, but the situation is tightening. Five states now license only graduates from APA-accredited programs. All other things being equal, an accredited clinical or counseling psychology program is a definite advantage over a nonaccredited program.

Online Graduate Programs

Practically every institution of higher education now offers some online courses and distance education. Some institutions have gone further to create graduate programs that are almost entirely online, with all discussions being conducted electronically on bulletin boards and all assignments being submitted by computer. The only on-campus contact might be a couple of weeks or several weekends per year.

Several of these online institutions offer doctoral programs in clinical and counseling psychology, including Walden, Capella, and Fielding. Fielding Graduate Institute requires several weeks of in-person residency per year, making it the only distance program that is APA accredited. Capella and Walden are both regionally accredited.

We are frequently approached by students intrigued with these and other online programs and asked whether we think they are credible programs. Our answer is that they are credible but definitely not preferred for several reasons. First, we recommend that students favor APA-accredited programs, and only one of these programs has met the minimum educational criteria set forth by APA. Second, online programs lack quality control over their clinical supervisors, who are scattered around the country. Third, much of the learning in doctoral programs occurs in close, interpersonal relationships with faculty on a daily basis. Frequent computer contact is useful, but in our opinion, not equivalent. And fourth, without sounding too stodgy, we believe online programs are still too new and alternative to have developed a track record of producing quality psychologists. Most internship directors and potential employers feel likewise; graduates of non–APA-accredited online programs are experiencing difficulty in licensure and employment as psychologists.

Of course, each online program needs to be evaluated on its own merits, and each graduate student must be considered for his or her individual abilities. In the end, graduate students will get out of a program what they put in—whether through a traditional, bricks-and-mortar institution or an innovative, online program. The early research on distance and online education indicates that it produces comparable outcomes to traditional education, at least in acquiring knowledge and academic skills. Unfortunately, there is insufficient research on the online preparation of professional psychologists to render any conclusions.

Should you decide to apply to online doctoral programs in psychology, we would advise you to:

- complete your master's degree in a conventional program to secure one in-person degree and to meet the admission prerequisites of most online doctoral programs.
- obtain information on the program's track record of producing graduates who secure APA-accredited internships and eventually licensure as psychologists.
- determine the residency requirement (how much time per year is expected on campus).
- expect no financial assistance from the online institution itself (but loans are available).
- become very comfortable and savvy with computers, as most of your contact and assignments will be conducted online.
- be an organized, self-motivated individual who can meet deadlines without supervision.
- realize that the vast majority of interaction with fellow students and professors will occur online, not in a conventional classroom.
- be prepared for intensive research and writing on your own.

Clinical Alternatives

In addition to doctoral programs in clinical and counseling psychology, we would like to describe several alternative programs of study that should be considered. We have classified these programs along a practice–research continuum. The practice-oriented programs are outlined first. Portions are abstracted from APA's (1986) *Careers in Psychology*, which can be found online at www.apa.org/students/brochure/index.html. Additional details on helping professions can also be accessed online at www.lemoyne.edu/OTRP. *A Student Guide to Careers in the Helping Professions* by Melissa Himelein provides information on typical job duties, potential earnings, required degrees, and the like.

You are restricted neither to clinical/counseling psychology nor even to psychology in selecting a career in mental health. School psychology, as discussed below, is a viable alternative. Also note that psychology is only one of five nationally recognized mental health disciplines, the others being psychiatry (medicine), clinical social work, psychiatric nursing, and counseling.

We do not wish to dissuade you from considering clinical or counseling psychology, but a mature career choice should be predicated on sound information and contemplation of the alternatives. A primary consideration is what you want to do—your desired activities. Conducting psychotherapy is possible in any of the following fields. Prescribing medication is currently restricted to physicians and some nurses, although psychologists are steadily securing prescription privileges around the country. Psychological testing and empirical research are conducted by psychologists. As discussed previously, psychologists also enjoy a wide range and pleasurable integration of professional activities. Following is a sampling of alternatives to a doctorate in clinical and counseling psychology.

1. School Psychology. Some undergraduates have a particular interest in working clinically with children, adolescents, and their families. Admission into the Boulder-model programs with a child clinical specialty is particularly competitive. A doctorate in school psychology is much more accessible, with two or three times the acceptance rate of clinical psychology programs. The APA (Accredited, 2005) has accredited 56 of these programs, which provide doctoral-level training in clinical work with children in school settings.

One disadvantage of pursuing a career as a master's-level school psychologist lies in the fact that, unlike the other alternatives, one's professional work may be limited to the school. If this limitation is not a concern, then training as a school psychologist can be an excellent option for those interested in clinical work with children and families (Halgin, 1986).

At the doctoral level, school psychologists are credentialed to function in both school and nonschool settings. Research finds substantial overlap in the coursework and requirements of child clinical programs and school psychology programs (Minke & Brown, 1996). Some differences remain, of course—such as more courses in consultation and education in school programs and more courses in psychopathology in child clinical programs—but the core curricula are quite similar. School psychology training at the doctoral level is broadening to include experience outside of the school setting and with adolescents and families as well (Tryon, 2000).

For further information, check out the following Web sites:

- www.indiana.edu/~div16/
  (APA's Division of School Psychology)
- www.naspweb.org
  (National Association of School Psychologists)
- www.ispaweb.org/en/index.html
  (International School Psychology Association)

- www.schoolpsychology.net
  (comprehensive links to the field and graduate schools)

2. Community Psychology. This field shares with clinical and counseling psychology a concern with individual well-being and healthy psychological development. However, community psychology places considerable emphasis on preventing behavioral problems (as opposed to only treating existing problems), adopting a broader ecological or community perspective, and changing social policies.

Graduate training in community psychology occurs within clinical or clinical community psychology programs or within explicitly community psychology programs. The former are clinical psychology programs with an emphasis on or a specialization in community; these doctoral programs are listed in Appendix E (Research Areas) under "community psychology." Eighteen explicitly community doctoral programs are described in a Spring 1996 special supplement of *The Community Psychologist* (copies of the publication can be obtained from Dr. Jean Ann Linney, Editor, TCP, 251 Gambrell Hall, University of South Carolina, Columbia, SC 29208 for $3.00 made payable to "Society for Community Research and Action"). If your interests lean toward prevention and community-based interventions, then by all means check out a specialization or a program in community psychology. The Web sites at www.apa.org/divisions/div27 and www. communitypsychology.net provide further information about the field and training programs.

3. Clinical Social Work. A master's degree in social work (M.S.W.) is a popular clinical alternative these days. One big advantage of this option is a much higher rate of admission to M.S.W. programs, with about 65% of applicants being accepted to any given program, on average (O'Neill, 2001). Other advantages are GREs less often required for admission, fewer research requirements, an emphasis on professional training, and completion of the M.S.W. in less than half the time necessary to obtain a psychology Ph.D. With legal regulation in all 50 states and third-party vendor status (insurance reimbursement) in 48 states, social workers are increasingly achieving autonomy and respect, including increased opportunities for independent practice.

The major disadvantages lie in the less comprehensive nature of the training, which is reflected in a lower pay scale as compared to psychologists. Not becoming a "doctor" and not being able to conduct psychological testing also prove troublesome for some.

Students interested in clinical social work as a career should peruse an introductory text on the profession and should also contact the National Association of Social Workers (NASW). This organization provides detailed information on the emerging field, student membership, and accredited programs in clinical social work. NASW resources can be accessed via the Web (www.naswdc.org), the telephone (1-800-742-4089), or good old-fashioned mail (750 First Street, NE, Suite 7000, Washington, DC 20002-4241). Three other Web sites on social work programs are also handy: Petersons.com/graduate/select/socw.html; www. socialworksearch.com; and www.gradschools.com.

4. Psychiatry (Medicine). Students often dismiss the possibility of applying to medical schools, believing that medical school admission is so difficult that it is out of the question (Halgin, 1986). However, the student interested in neuroscience and the more severe forms of psychopathology may find this an attractive choice. Although the application process necessitates more rigorous training in the "hard" sciences than most psychology programs, the admission rate may also be higher than the most competitive doctoral programs in clinical and counseling psychology. Of the 35,000 people applying to medical school annually, about 48% are admitted, and half of them are women. The average GPA of applicants accepted to medical school is between 3.5 and 3.6 (see aamc.org for details).

Medical school thus remains an attractive option for many students headed toward a career in the mental health professions. For further information and demystification of this subject, refer to *Medical School Admissions: The Insider's Guide* (Zebala, Jones, & Jones, 1999) or *The Complete Medical School Preparation and Admissions Guide* (Goliszek, 2000). Prime Web sites include www.premedonline.com and www.aamc.org, the official Web site of the Association of American Medical Colleges.

The advantages of a medical degree should be recognized. First, an M.D. (allopath) or D.O. (osteopath) allows one to prescribe medication. Second, the average income for psychiatrists is higher than for psychologists. Third, a medical degree permits more work in inpatient (hospital) facilities. Applicants should not dismiss this possibility out of hand, and should explore medicine as a viable alternative, especially if their interests lie on a more biological level.

5. Psychiatric Nursing. Although sometimes regarded as the handmaiden of psychiatry, master's-level psychiatric nursing is an autonomous profession. The employment opportunities for nursing are excellent at this time, especially for psychiatric nurses who have the flexibility of working in hospitals, clinics, health centers, or private practice. Of course, psychiatric nurses are nurses first and are required to obtain a bachelor's degree (B.S.N.) and to become registered (R.N.) prior to obtaining their Master of Science in Nursing (M.S.N.). They do not conduct psychological testing and rarely perform research, but psychiatric nurses practice psychotherapy in both inpatient and outpatient settings. Further, certified nurse practitioners now have the authority to write medication prescriptions in 47 states. Consult a textbook on mental health nursing and visit the Web site of the American Psychiatric Nurses Association at www.apna.org/ to learn more about psychiatric/mental health nursing and its graduate programs.

6. Psychology and the Law. There is a great deal of interest in the burgeoning amalgam of psychology and law, as evidenced by an APA division, two energetic professional societies, and at least six scholarly journals (Bersoff et al., 1997; Otto & Heilbrun, 2002). Doctoral students must be trained in both fields, of course, increasing the length of graduate training. At least five programs now award law degrees and psychology doctorates together—joint J.D. and Ph.D./Psy.D. programs (Arizona, Drexel, Nebraska, Pacific, and Widener Universities). Graduates pursue both clinical and research careers—practicing law in mental health arenas, specializing in forensic psychology, working in public policy, and pursuing scholarship on the interface of law and psychology, for example. This is an exciting career, albeit one requiring extra commitment in terms of effort and knowledge during doctoral studies.

Another two dozen clinical programs offer Ph.D.s or Psy.D.s with specializations in forensic psychology or clinical forensic psychology. (Consult Appendix F and the following Web sites for a list of the programs.) These clinical psychologists specialize in the practice of forensic psychology. It's a growing and exciting specialization in psychology, but one that rarely involves the criminal profiling featured in television shows and *Silence of the Lambs!* Instead, forensic psychologists are far more likely to conduct child custody evaluations, assess a patient's psychological damage, evaluate a person's competence to stand trial, consult with lawyers on jury selection, and conduct disability evaluations.For additional information on forensic psychology and psychology of the law, peruse these Web links:

- www.unl.edu/ap-ls/
  (APA's American Law–Psychology Society)
- www.abfb.com
  (the American Board of Forensic Psychology)

- flash.lakeheadu.ca/~pals/forensics
  (a student-friendly collection of resources and links)

7. Other. Counselor education, art therapy, student guidance, occupational therapy, rehabilitation counseling, and a plethora of other human service programs can be attractive alternatives to clinical and counseling psychology. They are typically less competitive master's-level programs in which admission rates are quite high and in which the training is quite practical. Relative disadvantages of these programs, in addition to lack of a doctorate, include less prestige, lower salaries, diminished probability of an independent practice, and variable licensure status across the United States.

If one or more of these options seem more suited to your needs, discuss it with a psychology advisor, interview a professional in that field, peruse the Web sites, or write to the respective organizations for additional information.

Research Alternatives

Some graduate students enter clinical or counseling psychology to become researchers. They are less interested in working with patients than researching clinical phenomena. If you are most interested in research, here are some nonclinical alternatives that might appeal to you.

1. Social Psychology. Social psychology is concerned with the influence of social and environmental factors on behavior. Issues such as personality, attitude change, group processes, interpersonal attraction, and self-constructs are some of the research interests. Social psychologists are found in a wide variety of academic settings and, increasingly, in many nonacademic settings. These include positions in advertising agencies, personnel offices, corporations, and other business settings. Check out the official Web sites of the Society for Personality and Social Psychology (www.spsp.org) and the Social Psychology Network (www.socialpsychology.org) for additional resources.

2. Industrial/Organizational Psychology. This branch of psychology focuses on the individual in the workplace. Industrial/organizational psychologists frequently select and place employees, design jobs, train people, and help groups of workers to function more effectively. Master's programs generally prepare students for jobs in human resources and personnel departments, whereas doctoral programs are more geared to preparing students for academic positions and for management and consulting work on larger-scale projects. Industrial/organizational psychologists earn among the highest median salaries compared to other areas of psychology (Kohout & Wicherski, 1992). Academics find positions in both psychology departments and business schools.

The Society for Industrial and Organizational Psychology (2003) produces a useful list of *Graduate Training Programs in Industrial/Organizational Psychology and Related Fields*, which describes 195 graduate programs in "I/O" psychology and how to contact each. It is available free from the society's Web site (www.siop.org). Students interested in pursuing a career in I/O psychology should obtain, beyond psychology classes, courses in management, marketing, and organizational behavior as well as research experience.

3. Behavioral Neuroscience. For the student interested in biological research, the workings of the brain and hormonal systems, and the influence of the brain on behavior, programs in neuroscience may be a better match. By employing animal subjects, researchers can control the conditions of their studies to a level often elusive when using human participants. Research areas include learning, psychopharmacology, memory, and motivation. For example, recent investigations on memory have provided valuable insight into the etiology and course of Alzheimer's disease. Go to www.andp.org/training/usindex.htm for a splendid list of graduate programs in neuroscience.

Research demonstrates that neuroscience graduate programs expect entering students to possess course work and lab work beyond the standard psychology curriculum (Boitano, 1999). Essential courses would include biology, chemistry, calculus, and introduction to neuroscience, and desirable courses would sample from cell biology, biochemistry, and anatomy and physiology. These are all possible, with adequate planning, to incorporate into the psychology major, should you decide on this path relatively early in your undergraduate career. The Web site (www.undergraduateneuroscience.org/) of Faculty for Undergraduate Neuroscience (FUN) provides a bounty of useful information on preparing for a career in neuroscience.

4. Developmental Psychology. The developmental psychologist studies behavior change beginning at the prenatal stages and extending through the lifespan. Areas such as aging, identity, and development of problem-solving abilities are popular areas within developmental psychology. The characteristics of individuals at different age ranges, such as the work of Piaget on child cognition, are of particular interest to developmental psychologists.

Geropsychology, or the psychology of aging, has become a popular specialty of this area as the increasing elderly population in this country presents special needs that currently are being insufficiently addressed. Employment opportunities in geropsychology are sure to grow over the next several decades. Visit the Web sites of APA's Division of Adult Development and Aging (aging.ufl.edu/apadiv20/apadiv20.htm) and the friendly Geropsychology Central (www.premier.net/~gero/contents.html) for more.

5. Cognitive Psychology. Cognitive psychology may be an attractive option for students whose interests lie in the exploration of human thought processes. Major areas include language structure, memory, perception, attention, and problem solving. Research in cognitive psychology has gained insight into what in the past was considered inexplicable behavior and has led to significant gains in the understanding of mental disorders. For example, research into how moods affect the interpretation of ambiguous events has implications for the study of depression. Much research on the accuracy of eyewitness testimony has been conducted by cognitive psychologists. Cognitive programs emphasize artificial intelligence, cognitive neuroscience, and affective neuroscience. Indeed, interest in cognitive neuroscience and affective neuroscience has increased of late. It is also possible at some universities for clinical psychology students to receive explicit training in these areas.

6. Experimental Psychology. Often a student is interested in research but has not yet defined an area of interest. Or a student has a very specific area of interest in a certain psychopathology but does not desire to do clinical work. In both cases, a graduate program in experimental psychology might be the ticket. These programs allow a student to explore several research areas, such as animal learning or memory. Other programs focus on experimental psychopathology, which is geared more specifically for the researcher interested in clinical populations. Experimental programs offer excellent training in research methods, statistical analysis, and a great deal of hands-on research experience.

7. Sport Psychology. This emerging specialization typically entails both research and applied activities. Research focuses on all aspects of sports, whereas clinical services include psychological assessment, individual psychotherapy, and group consultation. Research and training encompass stress management, self-confidence, mental rehearsal, competitive strategies, and sensory-kinetic awareness. Consult the *Directory of Graduate Programs in Applied Sport Psychology* (Sachs, Burke, & Schrader, 2001) for information on specific psychology programs. Consult, too, the Web site of APA's Division of Exercise and Sport Psychology at www.psyc.unt.edu/apadiv47/ for information on career possibilities in this area.

8. Medicine. A medical degree (M.D., D.O.) earned concurrently or sequentially with a psychology doctorate (Ph.D.) may allow the greatest flexibility of all the aforementioned programs of study. This option allows one to practice medicine and psychology while also affording a basic education in research and statistics. For an extremely bright and motivated student, this can be a real possibility, but it is certainly the most challenging of all the alternatives. Earning two doctoral degrees will take longer than earning either alone. This choice is for someone interested in the biological aspects of behavior in addition to gaining a rigorous education in the scientific study of human behavior.

Once again, if your interest lies in research, there are many options available besides clinical and counseling psychology. Talking to a professional in the relevant discipline and consulting textbooks about the discipline will help you to explore that option more fully. An increasing number of Web sites also offer valuable career advice. Five of our favorites are:

- www.psychwww.com/careers/index.htm
- www.lemoyne.edu/~hevern/PsychSTAC/career.html
- www.apa.org/students/
- www.socialpsychology.org/career/htm
- www.gradschools.com

A Word on "Backdoor" Clinicians

The APA ethical guidelines outline two pathways to becoming a clinical or counseling psychologist. The first is to complete a doctoral program and formal internship in clinical or counseling psychology. The second is to obtain a nonclinical psychology doctorate and then to complete a formal respecialization program in clinical or counseling psychology, which includes the internship. Formal training and supervised experience, not simply the desire to become a clinical or counseling psychologist, are required according to the APA ethical code.

In the past, some psychologists obtained doctorates in developmental, experimental, social, or educational psychology or in a psychology-related discipline and managed to practice as "clinical psychologists" or "counseling psychologists." This was possible because of the paucity of clinical and counseling psychology doctoral programs and because of generic state licensure laws, which recognize only one broad (generic) type of psychologist. However, this educational and licensure process circumvents the established pathway, increases the prospects of inadequate training, and in some cases results in unethical representation. Hence the term "backdoor"—unable to enter through the front door, they sneak in through the back entrance. Major universities, the federal government, the Veterans Administration, and practically all universities now insist on the doctorate (or respecialization) in clinical or counseling psychology for employment as a clinical or counseling psychologist. Although individuals with non-clinical psychology doctorates may be eligible for state licensure, they will be increasingly unable to identify themselves as clinical or counseling psychologists.

Circuitous routes to becoming a clinical or counseling psychologist may still exist, but they have become far less common and ethical. We emphatically recommend against these "backdoor" practices on both clinical and ethical grounds.

To Reiterate Our Purpose

The purpose of this book is to help you navigate the heretofore unknown and frightening process of applying to clinical and counseling psychology graduate programs. But nothing can eradicate the fact that gaining admission to such competitive programs requires a good deal of time and energy. There are the matters of taking the appropriate undergraduate courses, gaining clinical experience, acquiring research competencies, requesting letters of recommendation, locating the appropriate schools to which to apply, succeeding on entrance examinations, completing the application, creating personal statements, traveling to interviews, and deciding which program actually to attend. We have known people who have quit jobs or taken months off just to invest all their time to the application process. However, with this book and a fair degree of organization, you can make such extremes unnecessary.

Emotional strain is an inherent part of the application process. This is unlike many job interviews, where you are marketing yourself merely as a provider of services. Here you are marketing yourself as a human being. This is a personal process. The application forms and interviews require self-exploration and even a certain amount of justification. Why do you like clinical work? What do you enjoy about spending time with people who are disturbed? Do you really like research? You may end up questioning your answers and may feel compelled to examine the beliefs that have led you to this point in your life.

With the help of this book, you ultimately become the consumer for a program best fitted to you. And 86% of students say that their sense of fit with a program is the single most important factor in choosing a graduate program (Kyle, 2000). By negotiating this process in an informed and systematic manner, you can become a consumer of psychology graduate programs. Many interviewers recommend that the final interview should be approached by the applicant in this way. With this approach to the admission process, much of the stress can be allayed.

Although the application process itself can appear intimidating, or the prospect of being rejected upsetting, we urge you *not* to allow fear to cause you to abandon the process altogether or to dismiss the option prematurely. Do not allow yourself to be one of the students who gets rejected unnecessarily. If you apply to the appropriate programs and present yourself with a certain savvy, your chances of getting in are vastly improved.

Our Approach

Having now counseled hundreds of clinical and counseling psychology aspirants and conducted scores of workshops on applying to graduate school, the three of us have gravitated toward a particular approach to the topic. It might be called *realistically encouraging*.

It is realistic in that we present the hard facts about the competition for entrance into doctoral psychology programs. We will not resort to the disservice of feeding you illusions ("Anyone can become a psychologist!"), even though the reality may leave you feeling discouraged at times.

Still, our approach is unabashedly encouraging in that we support people seeking their goals. With knowledge and perseverance, most of our students have made it. Consider the real-life story of Justin, a success story in the quest for a doctorate in clinical psychology.

Justin almost flunked out of college during his first 2 years, before discovering his abiding interest in clinical and counseling psychology. He took his GREs late in his senior year without adequate preparation but obtained combined verbal and quantitative scores of 1100. His applications to doctoral programs that year were hastily and poorly prepared. Justin was, to complicate matters, grossly unaware of typical admission requirements, acceptance rates, and application guidelines. He had no clinical experience whatsoever and had never engaged in research beyond course requirements. Not surprisingly, letters of recommendation about him were mildly positive but without detail or conviction (the deadly, two-paragraph "He/she's nice, but we haven't had much contact" letters). He received dismal rejections, not even a hint of a possible interview or finalist pool.

Well, as people are apt to do, Justin was about to give up and throw in the towel. But he then attended one of our workshops and began to understand that he had neglected virtually every guideline for sophisticated application to graduate school. The next year was devoted to preparing himself for the hunt: he took extra courses after receiving his degree in order to increase his GPA and to improve his GRE psychology score; he volunteered 10 hours a week at two supervised clinical placements; he worked 20 hours a week for a small stipend as a research assistant; and he copublished three articles. Not surprisingly, his letters of recommendation were now enthusiastic and detailed. That year, Justin obtained six acceptances into clinical doctoral programs with full financial support at three of them.

There *are* concrete steps you can take to improve your application. It is as much knowing how to apply as it is your actual credentials. And if you do get rejected once, many steps can enhance the probability of acceptance the next time around, as in Justin's case. Knowledge of the process can make a tremendous difference. The following chapters provide suggestions and strategies that will increase your attractiveness as an applicant.

CHAPTER 2

PREPARING FOR GRADUATE SCHOOL

People begin the graduate school application process at different stages in their lives. You may be a junior or a senior in college. Maybe you have a bachelor's degree in psychology and have worked for a year or two. Perhaps you are a master's-level counselor or social worker who has decided to return for a doctorate. Or maybe you were not a psychology major but have decided you want to make a career change. Depending on your perspective, your needs will be somewhat different. Therefore, each perspective is addressed separately throughout this chapter.

But whatever your current status, recognize this about becoming a clinical or counseling psychologist: *Do not wait until the year of your application to begin the preparation.* Securing admission into competitive doctoral programs necessitates preparation throughout your undergraduate career and any intervening years. Good grades, adequate test scores, clinical work, and research experience cannot be instantaneously acquired simply because you have made a decision to pursue psychology as your career.

Plan ahead of time using the knowledge and strategies presented in this chapter. Preparing for graduate study is *not* for seniors only (Fretz & Stang, 1980). Timeliness is everything, or, in the vernacular, "you snooze you lose" (Mitchell, 1996).

Much of the "advice" bandied about by fellow students and even some faculty is hopelessly general. Their well-intentioned comments are meant to be universal—one size fits all. However, this advice is akin to the bed of the legendary Greek innkeeper, Procrustes, who insisted on one size bed and who stretched or shortened his unfortunate guests to fit that bed! Do not fall prey to these Procrustean maneuvers; different applicants have different needs. Understanding your particular circumstances and needs will produce an individualized plan for applying to graduate school.

Different Status, Different Needs

Underclassmen

Some of you will be undergraduates, not yet in your senior year. By getting a head start, you can take the appropriate courses and attain the optimal clinical and research training possible at your institution. The more time invested in preparation, the better able you will be to meet the requirements of the application process with confidence, which puts you in a very desirable position. This book will provide you with information that can help guide your undergraduate experiences, academic as well as clinical. The "Time Line" presented in Appendix A outlines important steps to be taken during your freshman, sophomore, and junior years.

Seniors

Some of you are seniors, deciding whether to go directly on to graduate school. This is a difficult time, and you are likely to be given advice ranging from "everyone *must* take time off" to "if you take a year, you'll lose the momentum and study skills and never go back." Obviously, this decision is based on the needs and experiences of each individual. There are two guidelines, however, that can help you muddle through these decisions.

1. Are you primarily interested in becoming a practitioner and wish to have only a minimal amount of research training? If so, a practice-oriented psychology program will probably best suit your needs. These programs tend to put the emphasis on clinical experi-

ence (Piotrowski & Keller, 1996). They favor applicants who have a master's degree or have been involved in a clinical setting and who will come into a program with some clinical skills already in their repertoire. The average age of students admitted into these programs is slightly higher than that in research-oriented programs, reflecting time spent out of school in a work environment. Consequently, if you are interested in a practice-oriented program, you could take time off to gain relevant experience in clinical work and research.

2. Are you interested in a program that is primarily research oriented? If you have a solid grounding in research as an undergraduate, such a program is less likely to emphasize the need for postgraduation clinical experience. The necessary and sufficient research experience can certainly be attained during an undergraduate education without taking time off. Adding work experiences and clinical skills to an application, however, can only improve your chances of getting accepted to a research-oriented program.

The decision to postpone graduate school for a year or more can be influenced by the time constraints of the application process. Applications for doctoral programs in clinical and counseling psychology are typically due between early January and mid-February of the year before you plan to attend school. First-semester seniors just beginning an honors or research project may not be in a position to showcase their talents effectively by application time. The additional preparation for the Graduate Record Examination (GRE) (see Entrance Examinations) may lead a potential applicant to elect to wait a year before applying.

For all these reasons, first-semester seniors may not easily meet the requirements of the recommended Time Line presented in Appendix A. This is a frequent predicament, the solution to which is to wait another year to apply or to do what you can in the remaining time available. In either case, do not give up! Rather, review the Time Line carefully and check off what you have and have not accomplished before making the momentous decision to go for it this year, or to wait until next year. Some shortcuts may well be necessary to apply this year; the ideal time line will need to be modified to fit your reality (Keith-Spiegel, 1991). Some of the items will have to be sacrificed, some accomplished later or more hastily, and others with great energy.

Should you elect to wait a year after receiving your baccalaureate degree, you will begin the application process almost immediately after graduation. In addition to gaining research and clinical experience, the year away from school is spent applying to graduate school. This is not a year to relax or "goof off"; rather, it should be an intense year of preparation for graduate admission.

Our research on the admission statistics of APA-accredited clinical psychology programs demonstrates that, on average, approximately three-quarters of incoming doctoral students held bachelor's degrees only and one-quarter possessed a master's degree (Mayne et al., 1994; Norcross et al., 1998). However, this generalization is limited by significant differences among the types of programs: research-oriented Ph.D. programs enrolled a significantly higher percentage of baccalaureate-level students (85% on average; 15% master's), while Psy.D. programs enrolled more master's-level students (47% on average).

In summary, the advantages of taking time off depend on the type of psychology program you desire and the strength of your current credentials. If you desire to focus exclusively on clinical work and a Psy.D. degree, it may be advisable to take time off to gain some practical experience and to save some money. If you are more research oriented and already possess skills in this area, you may be in a position to apply at present. If your current credentials—grades, GRE scores, research—are marginal, then another year may also be required.

In using this book, you will be introduced to the admission criteria for graduate school. And by using the worksheets, you can determine how well prepared you are to apply to schools at this point. Following the steps in this book will help you assess how prepared you are to apply to graduate school successfully and whether some time out in the "real world" would be advised.

Previous College Graduates

Some of you are college graduates and have already taken time off, or you are a member of the working world contemplating a career change. A solid work record and a mature perspective on psychology are certainly advantageous. However, these alone will not compensate for a lack of course work or experience germane to clinical or counseling psychology. By reviewing the admissions criteria for graduate programs and using the worksheets provided, you will be able to evaluate the degree of your preparation in order to decide whether it is prudent to begin the application process immediately or to bolster some of your weaker areas before beginning. Pay particular attention to the steps listed under "application year" in the Time Line (Appendix A).

Returning Master's-Level Clinicians

Some of you will be master's-level clinicians interested in obtaining the doctorate in clinical or counseling psychology. Although your wealth of clinical experience gives you an immediate edge over undergraduates in the admissions race to practitioner-oriented programs, you cannot ignore the importance assigned to standardized test scores and research experience.

Psy.D. programs and practice-oriented Ph.D. programs tend to accept proportionally more incoming students with master's degrees than with baccalaureate degrees only. Interestingly, counseling psychology programs also seem to prefer master's-level students: Two-thirds of incoming students in APA-accredited counseling psychology programs already held their master's. Of course, these are merely averages that mask the huge differences between, for example, the one-third of counseling psychology programs which *only* accept master's recipients and the one-tenth of programs which primarily accept baccalaureate recipients (Turkson & Norcross, 1996).

Hines (1985) conducted a survey of clinical psychology doctoral programs regarding their policies and experiences in accepting students with master's degrees in psychology. Following are several of the salient findings.

The first question was "What effect (if any) will having a master's degree have on an applicant's chances for admission to your program?" Most responses indicated that having a master's per se made little or no difference, with some respondents suggesting that it was the student's performance in the master's program that was more important. However, 10% answered that having a master's degree had a definite positive effect. Only 3% indicated that having a master's would have a definite negative bias.

The second question requested that respondents rate the importance of seven criteria for admission to their programs. Each criterion was rated on a 5-point, Likert-type scale ranging from least important to most important. The three highest ratings were for GRE scores, letters of recommendation, and research experience. The rest, in descending order of importance, were undergraduate grades, graduate grades, quality of the master's program, and clinical practicum experience.

As you can see, GRE scores and research experience definitely do count in admissions decisions for master's-level applicants. The lower ratings given to graduate grades and to undergraduate grades reflect a difference among schools in whether graduate or undergraduate grades are considered more important. The standard deviation for graduate grades was particularly high, indicating wide variability in the importance placed on graduate grades among different programs. Comments suggested that some schools tended to downplay graduate grades "because they are universally high"; another suggested that "high grades don't help, but poor grades hurt."

Having a master's degree in and of itself, then, neither helps nor hinders your chances in most admission decisions. It is not possessing the graduate degree itself that matters, but the quality of performance in academic courses, clinical practica, and research experiences during master's training and thereafter that give a definite edge in the admission process. This is particularly true for Psy.D. and practice-oriented Ph.D. programs, which enroll a much higher percentage of master's-level students (Mayne et al., 1994).

Master's degree recipients with combined Verbal and Quantitative GRE scores below 1,000 can take hope from a study of similar students admitted to Ph.D. programs (Holmes & Beishline, 1996). Ten such applicants were admitted by virtue of "compensatory virtues," such as presentations or publications that helped mitigate the effect of low GRE scores. If you find yourself in this position, emphasize the other, positive elements of your application and, again, seriously consider Psy.D. clinical and Ph.D. counseling psychology programs that enroll a higher percentage of master's-level students (Norcross et al., 1998). Assuming other parts of your credentials are acceptable, master's recipients should not be discouraged from applying to doctoral programs on the basis of GRE scores alone.

While clinical experience is valued, for most doctoral programs this factor is a secondary consideration to research. The vast majority of clinical and counseling doctoral programs prefer a thesis or a journal article over a graduate internship or post-master's clinical experience (Keller, Beam, Maier, & Pietrowski, 1995). All programs expect evidence of conducting empirical research: Ph.D. programs favor it over clinical experience and Psy.D. programs weigh it equally with clinical experience.

A Master's Degree First?

A common question during our graduate school workshops is whether students should secure a master's degree before seeking the doctorate. Fortunately, our workshop participants and you realize that no simple answer is possible to such a complex question. Nonetheless, the following are some broad reasons for seeking a master's degree first.

- *Low grade-point average.* The vast majority of doctoral programs will not consider applicants with a GPA below 3.0.
- *Weak GRE scores.* Similarly, doctoral programs rarely accept bachelor's-level applicants whose combined Verbal and Quantitative scores fall below 1,000.
- *Scarce research or clinical experiences.* Doctoral admission committees understandably desire that you have had some direct experience with those activities you intend to pursue for a lifetime.
- *Uncertain career goal.* Indecision about your subfield in psychology, or outside of psychology, is a strong indicator for a master's program initially.
- *Late application.* Doctoral programs hold to earlier deadlines than do master's programs, so those students waiting too late to apply will be redirected to master's programs.
- *Terse letters of recommendation.* By virtue of late transfer into a university or into psychology, some students lack sufficient contact with faculty for them to write positive and detailed letters of recommendation expected by doctoral programs.
- *Inadequate coursework in psychology.* Doctoral programs require a minimum level of education in the discipline prior to acceptance, typically at least 15 to 18 credits of psychology course work.

Completing a rigorous master's program in psychology can correct many of the foregoing impediments to acceptance into a doctoral program. As we describe in Chapter 7, students typically strengthen their grade point average, acquire clinical and research experience, sharpen their career goals, and establish close relationships with faculty during the 2 years of a master's program. For these and other reasons, many students opt for a master's degree at one institution before seeking the doctorate at another.

Doctoral psychology faculty were surveyed in detail regarding the value of a clinical master's degree for gaining admission to their programs (Bonifzi, Crespy, & Rieker, 1997). Assuming a *good* undergraduate GPA and *good* GREs, the effect of having a master's degree on the applicant's chances for admission was negative for 7% of the programs, neutral for 48% of the programs, and positive for 45% of programs. However, assuming *mediocre* GPA and *mediocre* GREs, the effect of having a master's was more neutral than positive overall. Put another way, it is clearly the applicant's overall credentials—rather than possession of a master's degree—that carries the day.

This same study (Bonifzi et al., 1997) and our own research (Mayne et al., 1994; Norcross et al., 2004)

consistently demonstrate that Ph.D. clinical programs hold a positive bias toward baccalaureate-level applicants. By contrast, Psy.D. clinical, Ph.D. counseling, and Ph.D. school psychology programs view master's degree recipients more favorably and accept higher proportions of master's-level applicants. Keep these biases in mind as you consider the selection criteria of graduate schools.

Graduate School Selection Criteria

As an applicant, your perceptions of graduate admissions criteria probably differ from those of the admissions committee. Some of the things you may think are important are actually not so important (Collins, 2001). For two examples, your GRE Psychology Subject score is less important than your GRE Verbal and Quantitative scores, and your extracurricular accomplishments do not count as much as you might like (Cashin & Landrum, 1991). On the other hand, you probably underestimate the importance of other admissions criteria; two examples are letters of recommendation and research experience, which students routinely underestimate compared to admissions committees (Nauta, 2000).

In this section we acquaint you with the data-based practices of graduate admissions committees. Learn what they value in graduate applicants and then tailor your application to those criteria in order to maximize your success.

A number of studies have been conducted to determine the relative importance of selection criteria in psychology graduate programs. The findings of our most recent and largest study (Norcross, Kohout, & Wicherski, in press) are summarized in Table 2-1. This table presents the average ratings of various criteria for admission into 410 doctoral programs and 179 master's programs in psychology. A rating of 3 denotes high importance; 2, medium importance; and 1, low importance.

The top-rated variables for doctoral programs were letters of recommendation, personal statements, GPA, interview, research experience, and GRE scores. All received ratings of 2.50 and higher on the 3-point scale, indicative of high importance. Extracurricular activity and work experience were valued significantly lower.

The implications for enhancing your application are thus clear and embedded throughout this *Insider's Guide:* secure positive letters of recommendation, write compelling personal statements, maintain your GPA, ace the preadmission interview, secure research experience, and prepare thoroughly for the GREs. At the same time, being heavily involved in student organiza-

TABLE 2-1. Importance of Various Criteria in Psychology Admissions Decisions

Criteria	Master's programs		Doctoral programs	
	Mean[a]	SD	Mean[a]	SD
Letters of recommendation	2.74	.49	2.82	.42
Personal statement/goals	2.63	.55	2.81	.41
GPA	2.75	.43	2.74	.45
Interview	2.30	.76	2.62	.60
Research experience	2.04	.74	2.54	.65
GRE scores	2.36	.66	2.50	.55
Clinically related public service	1.94	.70	1.91	.69
Work experience	1.91	.65	1.87	.68
Extracurricular activity	1.46	.54	1.41	.55

Note. Data from Norcross, Kohout, & Wicherski (in press).

[a]Means are calculated on a coding scheme where 1 = low importance, 2 = medium importance, 3 = high importance.

tions and campus activities does not carry nearly as much weight as these other criteria.

Another study (Eddy, Lloyd, & Lubin, 1987) investigated the selection criteria of only APA-accredited doctoral programs in clinical psychology. Program directors rated the importance of each type of undergraduate preparation on a scale ranging from very low importance, 1, to very high importance, 5. Table 2-2 presents the mean ratings and standard deviations for clinical psychology programs.

Research experience emerged as the top-rated variable. The authors of the study concluded that there is simply no better way to increase one's chances for acceptance than research. Personal visit to a department

(on your own or on an invited interview), computer proficiency, and human service experience were also highly valued. However, as in the previous study, extracurricular activities, such as Psi Chi membership, were rated relatively unimportant.

To sum up, the results of these and other studies (e.g., Briihl & Wasielski, 2004; Mayne et al., 1994; Munoz-Dunbar & Stanton, 1999; Purdy, Reinehr, & Swartz, 1989) consistently indicate that the ideal applicant has high GRE scores, strong letters of recommendation, some research experience, clinical experience, and high overall GPA. The results also consistently demonstrate that the admission requirements for doctoral programs are more stringent than for master's programs.

TABLE 2-2. Importance Assigned by Clinical Psychology Doctoral Programs to Various Types of Undergraduate Preparation

Preparation	Mean	SD
Research methods	4.28	0.91
Personal visit to department	3.14	1.41
Computer knowledge and skills	3.00	0.85
Paid human service experience	2.90	1.07
Volunteer human service	2.85	1.13
Double major with basic science	2.78	1.10
Master's degree	2.16	0.99
Double major with social science	2.08	0.84
Psi Chi membership	2.00	0.94

Note. From Eddy, Lloyd, & Lubin (1987). © 1987 Lawrence Erlbaum Associates. Reprinted by permission.

TABLE 2-3. Undergraduate Courses Required or Recommended by APA-Accredited Clinical Psychology Programs

Psychology course	Percentage of programs		
	Required	Recommended	Either
Statistics	65	29	94
Experimental methods/research design	48	19	68
Abnormal/psychopathology	29	22	51
Physiological/biopsychology	10	23	33
Learning/cognition	10	19	30
Personality	15	13	28
Child/developmental	11	13	24
Social psychology	7	16	23
History and systems	6	9	16
Tests and measures/psych testing	6	8	15
Laboratory course	6	5	11
Sensation and perception	3	2	5
Computers	1	3	4
Clinical/psychotherapy	1	1	2
Comparative	1	1	2
Motivation and emotion	1	1	2
Neuropsychology	1	0	1

Note. Adapted from Mayne, Norcross, & Sayette (1994).

The remainder of this chapter highlights these pivotal criteria used by graduate admissions committees in selecting their students. We consider, in order, course work, faculty mentoring, clinical experience, research skills, entrance examinations, and extracurricular activities.

Course Work

Although graduate programs differ in the courses they prefer you to have taken prior to admission, there are some "core" courses that nearly all require (Smith, 1985). These include Introduction to Psychology, Statistics, Research Methods, Abnormal Psychology, Physiological Psychology/Biopsychology, and Learning/Cognition.

Our research on clinical doctoral programs in the United States and Canada reveals that both Vail- and Boulder-model programs hold similar expectations on desirable undergraduate courses (Mayne et al., 1994; Oliver et al., 2005). Approximately 60% of the programs require or recommend specific undergraduate courses, 15% require an undergraduate psychology major, 10% specify a minimum number of psychology credits (but

not specific courses), and the remainder have no set policy on the matter.

Table 2-3 presents the percentage of psychology courses required (first column), recommended (second column), and either required or recommended (third column) for entry into APA-accredited clinical programs. Bear in mind that these figures systematically *underestimate* the actual percentage of programs requiring these courses as they do not include those graduate programs requiring a psychology major as a prerequisite and thus probably requiring most of the courses listed in Table 2-3. Introduction to Psychology was presumed to be a prerequisite for these advanced psychology courses and was therefore omitted from the table. Courses you should complete, according to these results, are Statistics, Research Methods, Abnormal Psychology, Physiological Psychology, Learning/Cognition, Personality, and Child/Developmental Psychology.

Doctoral programs require more courses on average than do master's programs (Smith, 1985). Accordingly, both to meet admissions criteria and to improve your GRE Psychology Subject score, we heartily recommend that you complete Social Psychology, History and

Systems, Psychological Testing (or Tests and Measures), and at least one laboratory course. The safest plan, of course, is to complete a rigorous undergraduate major in psychology to satisfy all these courses, but a well-planned minor in psychology may suffice. The rule of thumb: the more competitive the graduate program, the more stringent the required undergraduate course work.

If you were not a psychology major, it is still important that you take the minimum of six core courses mentioned. In addition, you may have to invest additional time studying for the Psychology Subject test of the Graduate Record Examination (more about this later).

If you have been out of college for several years and feel deficient in this course work, you might consider taking a course or two as a part-time student at a local college or university. This will shore up your record and prepare you more fully for admission and the GRE. Those of you who are not psychology majors but have studied extensively for this test and have done well will often be considered favorably by admissions committees.

Beyond these classes, we recommend an introductory computer science course, particularly if you are interested in research-oriented programs. Not only will it accustom you to the workings of computers, which are standard research tools, but it will also serve as a springboard for learning the statistical software used for data analysis. Recall that computer proficiency is rated a moderately important admission variable by doctoral programs.

Graduate selection committees prefer a broad undergraduate background in a variety of arts and sciences (Fretz & Stang, 1980). Exposure to biological sciences, math competency, and verbal skills are generally valued. If you are anxious or phobic regarding oral presentations, then by all means complete a public speaking course. Composition and writing courses are also vital; you may well face three or four major papers each semester in graduate school.

At this point, you may want to glance at the Reports on Individual Programs following Chapter 7 to get a better idea of which courses particular programs recommend or require of applicants. You will find the specific courses that each accredited clinical and counseling psychology program recommends as well as requires applicants to have taken.

For students who have gotten an early start or who are seniors, we would like to suggest considering advanced course work. To allay any anxieties, we would emphasize that the vast majority of applicants do *not* take these courses as undergraduates. Your application can be very strong without taking the courses we

are about to mention. However, those fortunate enough to be in a position to add these to their academic transcripts should seriously consider taking advantage of the opportunity.

Consider an advanced or graduate statistics course. Statistical acumen is highly regarded, especially in research-oriented programs, and advanced knowledge may pave the way for funding as a graduate assistant or research assistant. Another suggestion would be to take a course specifically focused on one of the data analysis programs. Learning one of the major statistical packages—Statistical Analysis System (SAS) or Statistical Package for the Social Sciences (SPSS)—is a definite advantage. Such knowledge increases your employability and may catch the eye of a professor in need of a data analyst. Lastly, we suggest an advanced course in physiological psychology, biopsychology, or neuroscience. This is certainly helpful in increasing your understanding of the biological aspects of behavior, an increasingly important focus in psychology today. If you have the time and abilities, these courses can help distinguish a very good application from an outstanding one.

As mentioned earlier, your GPA is a very important criterion for admission. Three types of GPA may be considered by graduate programs: overall GPA, psychology GPA, and GPA during your junior and senior years. Schools vary in the importance they place on these different scores, with some programs only considering one or two of them. When receiving information from schools, determine which GPAs they evaluate and also how much importance they place on them. For example, if you have an overall GPA of 3.2 (on a 4-point scale where $A = 4$, $B = 3$, $C = 2$, and $D = 1$), a psychology GPA of 3.6, and a junior/senior GPA of 3.5, you might concentrate on schools that emphasize the latter two averages.

Our research has shed light on the average GPAs among incoming doctoral and master's students in psychology (Norcross et al., 1996). For doctoral programs, the mean and median GPA is 3.5 for all undergraduate courses, 3.6 for psychology courses, and 3.6 for the last 2 years of course work. For master's programs, the mean and median GPA is 3.3 for all undergraduate courses, 3.4 for psychology courses, and 3.4 for the last 2 years of course work. Please employ your statistical sagacity in interpreting these figures: half of the incoming students will possess GPAs above these medians, and half of the students will possess GPAs below these medians.

Although we do not want to discourage anyone, a GPA below 3.0 is considered unsatisfactory by most APA-accredited programs. Regardless of the prestige of the institution, admissions committees view a GPA under 3.0 as below the acceptable limits of quality course work. If your GPA is below 3.0, then consider the following steps:

- Take additional courses to bolster your GPA.
- Retake courses to improve it.
- Wait another year to apply in order for all of your senior-year grades to be factored into your GPA.
- Complete a master's program first to show doctoral admissions committees you can perform academically at a higher level.

Try to speak with an academic advisor about how best to improve your standing within the workings of your own institution. Academic performance in your junior and senior psychology courses is particularly vital. Regardless of the type of GPAs emphasized by a graduate program, these courses affect your overall, final 2 years, and psychology GPAs.

Your "academic" performance is not limited to exam grades in the classroom. Faculty members—several of whom may submit a letter of recommendation on your behalf—also assess your interpersonal skills, verbal ability, and professional commitment in the classroom, outside formal course work, and in everyday interactions. The direct implication is to avoid undesirable interpersonal behaviors—for instance, silliness, arrogance, and hostility—in any interactions with your professors (Keith-Spiegel, 1991). Although the wisdom of avoiding such undesirable behaviors may be obvious, students are frequently unaware of the importance faculty attach to good questions, genuine attentiveness, respectful disagreements, office visits, mature disposition, interpersonal responsibility, and so forth. These are the characteristics a student heading for graduate studies should manifest in and outside of the classroom.

Finally, there is a corpus of general knowledge regarding clinical and counseling psychology that may not have been covered in your courses. This body of information includes at least a cursory understanding of diagnosis, for example, the *Diagnostic and Statistical Manual,* 4th ed. (DSM-IV); various assessment devices, such as the Minnesota Multiphasic Personality Inventory-2 (MMPI-2) and the Wechsler Intelligence Scales (WAIS-Iv, WISC-III); and ordinary therapy practices, such as individual, group, and family therapy. You must have a passing familiarity with theoretical orientations, for example, cognitive-behavioral, psychodynamic, family systems, and eclectic, in order to understand program materials. If you are not already familiar with these concepts, it would be wise to review an introductory textbook in clinical psychology.

You should also be gaining knowledge specifically about psychology as a field and about the current issues within this field. Toward this end, we suggest you begin reading the *Monitor on Psychology,* a publication sent to all APA members and student affiliates, or the *APS Observer,* the newsletter distributed to all members of the American Psychological Society (APS). Both publications feature articles dealing with psychology in general and clinical/counseling psychology in particular. You can become an APA or APS affiliate and receive a subscription, peruse your library's copy, or ask to borrow a professor's old issues.

Faculty Mentoring

Learning about psychology and achieving good grades are important components of academic work. But classes are also important in that they provide you with the opportunity to become acquainted and form relationships with faculty. It is natural to feel shy around faculty, especially if you are part of a 300-person lecture class. Substantial courage is required to muster the nerve to ask a question or to stay after class and introduce yourself. Equally anxiety provoking is a visit alone to a professor's office during office hours. In the one case, you expose yourself in front of your peers; in the other, you are individually vulnerable and do not have a crowd of faces to blend into. *But find a way to become comfortable in approaching faculty members.*

The irony of student reticence to approach faculty is that professors generally would like more students to approach them. Many faculty sit alone during office hours wondering why students never come to see them. They love to have students come after class or during office hours with questions. Ideas for questions can include something mentioned in the lecture or something you encountered in the readings. You do not have to be a star pupil or ask brilliant questions to begin a conversation with a professor. If you want to continue developing a relationship, ask professors about their research or other courses they are teaching.

What is the importance of meeting faculty? Three compelling reasons spring to mind. First, having a mentor to advise you in your growth as a future psychologist is invaluable. There is no better way to learn about psychology than in a one-on-one, mentoring relationship. When you apply to graduate school, having a professor to guide you through the process is one of the biggest advantages you can have. Second, eventually you will need faculty to write letters of recommendation on your behalf. Whether you are applying to graduate school or for employment, everyone wants a few references regarding your performance and responsibility. Occasionally faculty members are asked to write a letter for a pupil who has taken a lecture course with 100 or more students—the professor may not even know the student until he or she requests a letter! It makes a huge difference if you have spent some office hours or time after class with a faculty member, and he or she knows you more personally.

And third, once you get to know professors, you may have the opportunity to work for them on a research project or as part of their clinical activities. You will be working closely with your major professor in graduate school, and you might as well begin as soon as possible as a colleague-in-training. Though more will be said about this later, we cannot overemphasize the need to cultivate such a relationship and obtain the rewards that can ensue.

To put it bluntly, the single largest contributor to preparedness for graduate school is students' interaction with faculty members at their undergraduate institution. That's what the research concludes and what graduate students report (Huss et al., 2002). Psychology students who had a mentor and who had high-quality interactions with faculty felt more prepared for graduate school. And the second largest contributor to graduate school preparedness is research activity—a point to which we shall return in a few pages.

Beyond meeting professors, read your textbooks with an eye toward graduate school. If you come across an interesting study, note the author and check in the back of the text for the reference. When you have time, you may want to go to the library or online and read the original article. If it is recent, note the author's university. You will be surprised at how much you can learn about the field just by doing your typical class work.

Clinical Experience

What is clinical experience? In its loosest sense, it involves spending time working in any number of human service or mental health agencies. Graduate programs in clinical and counseling psychology expect that you will have some experience working with emotionally, intellectually, or behaviorally disadvantaged people. Many students volunteer during their undergraduate years, whereas other people get paid as part of a summer job or during their time off. In research-oriented Ph.D. programs, you will be expected to have some clinical experience as a prelude to your clinical training and as an aid to researching clinically

relevant problems. Experience of this nature will be considered essential.

What kinds of clinical experience count? Largely two types—paid and volunteer—under individual supervision. Paid part-time work in a clinical setting may be available in your community (but your involvement should not be at the expense of your academic performance). Returning master's-level clinicians will obviously have a multitude of employment possibilities, whereas undergraduates will have to search vigilantly for part-time employment.

For college students, a prime opportunity is to complete an undergraduate practicum (or field experience) for academic credit. This is a great way to "kill two birds with one stone." One study (VandeCreek & Fleisher, 1984) found that over two-thirds of colleges and universities provided undergraduate practica in psychology. Further, students consistently rate fieldwork as one of the most rewarding experiences and relevant courses in their college career. The advantages in terms of your application credentials are many: clinical experience, academic credit, familiarity with human service agencies, professional supervision, and exposure to potential sources for research pursuits and letters of recommendation.

Check with your undergraduate advisor and the college catalogue to determine whether such an opportunity exists for you. To learn more about the specific placements, you should consult the Psychology Department or the faculty member responsible for fieldwork placements.

In selecting a place to work or volunteer, please consider several factors. Although it may be difficult to accomplish, it is ideal to gain clinical experience in a setting that complements a research interest. For example, if your research is in the area of alcohol abuse, you might seek experience in a college counseling center or a substance abuse prevention program. Find out exactly what your responsibilities will entail.

The optimal program is one that will train you in clinical skills (such as crisis counseling on a hot line), will allow you to deal directly with clients, and will provide regular supervision by an experienced clinician.

Supervision is probably the most important consideration in choosing a clinical setting. It is important that you be supervised by a professional, one with at least a master's degree, though preferably a doctorate. Determine the qualifications of the person who will be supervising your work. Aside from the valuable insight supervisors can offer, they may also be familiar with faculty at different graduate programs and assist you in selecting schools. In addition, you may eventually decide to request letters of recommendation from them. Letters from a clinical supervisor are particularly important for practice-oriented graduate programs. In a later section we offer suggestions regarding approaching professors for letters of recommendation. The same strategies apply here.

If you are volunteering, you should insist on receiving supervision. Learn not only who will supervise you, but also how often and for what length of time. You will need to be assertive when searching out and interviewing possible agencies. If this seems difficult for you, try to remember that you are a volunteer—giving your time and energy, without financial compensation, to an agency that is in need of people like yourself. You seek only experience and supervision. You are a valuable commodity, so do not sell yourself short!

Numerous settings are available to people seeking clinical experience. Here are several excellent sources of hands-on experience that can be found in most communities:

- *Crisis hot lines.* These typically provide training in counseling skills, suicide prevention, and outreach services. The clientele range from sexual assault victims to suicidal teens to lonely elderly who need to talk with someone. Volunteers usually provide telephone counseling, although opportunities to work with an emergency outreach team may also be available. This can be a great way to gain exposure to a multitude of psychopathologies and to acquire fundamental helping skills. One word of caution: new members of most crisis hot lines are expected to take a large share of the midnight to 8 A.M. shifts. Be prepared to pay your dues.

- *Centers for homeless or runaway adolescents.* Much of what is done in these settings is similar to case management, in that these teenagers need to be put in contact with the appropriate social service agencies. However, in-house counseling may also be provided to these youths, who frequently come from disadvantaged families. Be particularly careful about specifying the supervision arrangement before starting. The facilities are often understaffed and financially strapped, meaning you may have to be assertive to get the training you desire.

- *Schools for emotionally disturbed children and adolescents.* These placements offer exposure to both educational and clinical services. Educational activities might include tutoring, classroom management, and one-on-one homework supervision. Clinical activities typically entail recreational supervision, art therapy, and perhaps individual, group, and family therapy.

- *Supervised homes for the developmentally disabled or chronically mentally ill.* These are unlocked transitional facilities where clients live and work in a therapeutic milieu (an environment consisting of peers). Depending on your prior experience, you might be expected to conduct skills training, recreational counseling, and work/school supervision. The programs are often behavioral, affording you experience with reinforcement schedules, shaping techniques, and token economies. Often the goal is to graduate clients to the outside world.

- *Summer camps for the physically challenged, developmentally disabled, or emotionally disturbed.* These can be either day or overnight camps, where counselors are expected to supervise recreation and train campers in skills and vocational activities. The positions are usually paid, ideal for college students who want to gain field experience while working for the summer. They also tend to be full-time positions, while they last. They offer short-term but rather intensive training.

- *Community mental health centers.* These provide experience with patients suffering from serious mental disabilities, such as schizophrenia, biploar disorders, substance abuse, and anxiety disorders. The programs vary but are likely to include an outpatient department, partial (day) hospitalization, and an education/outreach wing. Duties may include helping out during recreational activities or assisting with individual and group therapy. Though supervising recreational activities allows contact with patients, you might not be observing any clinical techniques. Do not be shy about asking for greater responsibilities!

- *College peer programs.* These provide students with peer education and assistance on specific disorders, such as bulimia or substance abuse. Less common but still available is peer counseling on more general concerns, for example, "Need to Talk? Call Us." Both peer education and peer counseling programs are typically flexible in the number of hours you must work and usually provide training in listening and counseling skills. They may also provide an opportunity to begin learning about a specific clinical disorder.

- *Women's resource centers.* These are multiservice centers that offer or coordinate a plethora of human services for women—rape crisis counseling, domestic violence education, "safe homes" for victims of abuse, and so on. Possible activities likewise vary, but the training and *esprit de corps* are highly regarded. Students with abiding interest in women's issues and feminist therapy will find these placements particularly satisfying.

- *Drug and alcohol treatment facilities.* These offer a variety of detoxification and rehabilitation interventions designed to help patients cope with the physical and psychological components of addictions. Although not all "D & A" programs will afford undergraduate field placements, substance abuse is one of the most popular research areas in clinical and counseling psychology (see Appendix E). Students can gain exposure to several models of addiction, interact with a multidisciplinary treatment team, and observe clinical services with substance abusers across gender, racial, and socioeconomic lines.

A word of caution about initial clinical encounters. Be careful not to generalize from one experience. One of the authors worked with runaways at a crisis center for adolescents in the Times Square area of New York City. The rate of employee turnover at this facility was exceptionally high. The "success" rate for clients was low, and the population was difficult indeed. Although it was a rich experience, some of the volunteers became disillusioned with psychology as a result of working there. Settings vary considerably, depending on the populations they serve and the resources available. An unpleasant experience may only mean that the specific population you were working with was not ideally suited to you. Try something else, and you may feel quite differently.

Though clinical work is important (and often rewarding), remember it is only one of several experiences you must acquire for admission to graduate school. Some Ph.D. applicants make the mistake of accumulating a wealth of clinical experiences at the expense of gaining research background. By doing so, you may be inadvertently presenting yourself as being uninterested in research or perhaps better suited to a Psy.D. than a Ph.D. program. Clinical experience must be balanced with research competencies. This balance will be weighted toward clinical work or research depending on your desire to gain either a Psy.D. or Ph.D. or whether the Ph.D. program is practice or research oriented.

Research Skills

Research experience, as discussed earlier in this chapter, is one of the most important admission criteria to nearly all Ph.D. programs in clinical and counseling psychology. To a lesser but still significant degree, Psy.D. programs also value your research experience for what it communicates about your intellectual ability and professional commitment. Recall the conclusion of one study on graduate school admission: there is simply no single better way to enhance an application than by obtaining research experience (Eddy et al., 1987). The desired skills—to critique the literature, to apply methodological reasoning, to write in scientific language, among others—are essential. Even though all psychologists need not produce original research, all must intelligently consume and apply research.

The benefits of student research, according to recent research (Landrum & Nelsen, 2002), boil down to two dimensions. The first might be labeled specific skills and abilities. These skills include developing clear research ideas, conducting literature searches, choosing appropriate measures, analyzing data, using statistical procedures, preparing conference presentations, and improving writing ability. The second dimension might be called interpersonal goals. These tend to be overshadowed by the specific technical skills listed above, but they are critical benefits in preparing and mentoring psychologists-in-training. These entail influencing decisions about graduate school, meeting other students involved in research, getting to know faculty members better, improving teamwork, forming relationships for the basis of letters of recommendation, developing leadership, and improving interpersonal communication. You seek *both* types of benefits in securing a research experience or assistantship.

Gaining research experience is largely dependent on your own initiative. It can be an intimidating process, and a knowledge of the potential opportunities can help you to maximize your gains during the course of your research.

Common Paths

Let us begin by outlining six common avenues for students engaging in scholarly research. The first is probably the most frequent—volunteering to work with a faculty member on one of his or her research projects. A second avenue is to complete a student research program for a notation on your transcript but not academic credit. Students identify potential professors to work with from a faculty directory of research interests, jointly complete a learning contract, and then devote a minimum number of hours (say, 75) throughout a semester working directly with the faculty sponsor. A third option is to enroll in independent psychology research for academic credit. This entails individual study and research under the supervision of a faculty member and is ordinarily limited to junior and senior psychology majors.

A fourth and increasingly common approach is to work or volunteer for a researcher outside of your university—in a hospital, medical center, research institute, industry, or community-based organization for example. Especially in large cities, researchers with major grants depend upon individuals (both pre- and post-baccalaureate) for many elements of study management, data collection, and statistical analyses. Many industries, especially biomedical and pharmaceutical research, offer summer research internships. These positions can provide valuable experience, specifically in randomized controlled trial research. Conversely, community-based organizations commonly conduct outcomes research around clinical or community interventions and accept interns throughout the year. If you have taken a statistics or research methods course that included SPSS or SAS, you may have sufficient skills for an entry-level position on an active research team outside of a university.

A fifth alternative, restricted to matriculated undergraduates, is to complete an honors thesis in either a departmental or a university-wide honors program. As with additional courses and postcollege work, an honors thesis is a "feather in your cap." For students desiring to move straight into a Ph.D. program, it is one means of presenting evidence to graduate admissions committees that you are capable of performing graduate-level work. Many schools allow motivated students to complete an honors thesis, an original study that the student conceptualizes, conducts, analyzes, and has some hope of presenting at a regional conference or even publishing. An honors thesis shows a genuine commitment to psychology and is a palpable sign of ability in the applicant.

A sixth and final avenue toward acquiring research competencies is restricted to master's students. A comprehensive paper or a formal master's thesis, requiring original research, practically guarantees additional experience with research. For this reason, undergraduates denied admission directly into doctoral programs frequently enter master's programs to gain valuable research (and clinical) competencies. And remember: the majority of clinical psychology doctoral programs prefer master's-level applicants to have completed a thesis (Piotrowski & Keller, 1996).

Whatever avenue you eventually pursue, the procedures are quite similar. Following is a step-by-step guide to help you make the most of your research experience.

Determining Your Interests

The first step is finding a research area that interests you. If you are not interested in the work, it will diminish your energy and enthusiasm and probably your decision to apply to a graduate program. A good place to begin is to read through your department brochure or Web site describing faculty interests and current research. If you are out of school, check with a local university. Look for professors who have a proven track record of scholarly publications. If the program has a graduate psychology faculty, so much the better—look to those professors first.

Once you have a list of faculty interests, you may find someone interesting but not be sure exactly what the research is all about ("I've heard about autism and think I'd like to study it, but I don't really know much about it. . . ."). If specific publications are not provided in the Web site or brochure, or if reprints are not posted in the department, then you can go to *PsycLIT* or *PsycINFO* (found in most university libraries; ask at the reference desk) and read what that professor has published in the area over the last 5 to 7 years. This should make it easier to decide which professor you would like to approach to volunteer to do research with. *Do not narrow your choices too quickly!* Find at least two or three professors whose work initially interests you.

Selecting Professors

Next, find out more about that professor as a person. Do you know people who have taken a class with him or her? What did they think? Are there other undergraduate or graduate students working with this professor now? What do they do exactly, and what is it like working under this person? Is the professor easy to get along with? Is the professor helpful to students? Do not be afraid to approach people and ask questions.

Having narrowed the choice to two or three professors whose work interests you and with whom you think you might get along, you might consider the rank of the professor. There are tenured faculty (a *full* or *associate* professor) and untenured (an *assistant* professor), both with respective advantages and disadvantages.

Full or associate professors have been in the field longer and will probably have colleagues at other universities. If the professor is well known, it gives your letter of recommendation that much more weight. If your professor's reputation in the field is strong, with a long list of publications, you are also likely to learn more and increase your own attractiveness as a candidate. However, once a faculty member becomes tenured, he or she is no longer under the same pressure to produce research as when he or she was pursuing tenure. Certainly if these faculty members are still conducting grant-funded research, they are likely to be committed to maintaining their productivity. Regardless, you should establish that tenured faculty are actively engaged in research and are currently publishing their work.

Assistant professors are newer to the field, probably 1 to 6 years postdoctorate. They are often in more need of undergraduate help and will likely involve you to your full potential. The possibility of being included on a presentation or publication as a coauthor may also be increased. What they lack in terms of a reputation built on years of publications may be balanced by their energy and their motivation to produce.

One word of caution: some professors have large research facilities and employ vast numbers of undergraduates to help them with their data management. If there are 10 or 15 undergraduates working in a lab, the attention given to each individual tends to decrease, as well as the value of the research experience. On the other hand, some large laboratories provide unique research opportunities unavailable elsewhere. The key is to talk to students who have worked there to learn about their experiences and to determine if former students have had success applying to graduate school.

An optimal research context, then, is one in which there is a faculty member or research mentor who has an established reputation in his or her field of inquiry, a record of producing publishable research, similar interests to your own, a history of working successfully with students, a propensity to share authorship credit with students, and the ability to construct discrete research projects. Be guided by these general principles in selecting professors to approach, but do not expect all these qualities to be available to you.

Making Initial Contact

Having chosen a professor you would like to work with, it is now time to make yourself known to him or her. You need to schedule an appointment or approach the professor during posted office hours. It is natural for you to be nervous! However, the more familiar with his or her work you are, the more secure you are likely to feel. Once again, read what the professor has written. Additionally, it helps to remember that you are coming to the professor to offer your services.

A good opening line might be, "Hello, Dr. Jones, my name is Chris Smith. I've been doing some reading on autism and came across several articles you've written. I'm pretty interested and was wondering if I could help out with a project you're working on now." As the conversation progresses, let the professor know your long-term goals as well as your immediate desire both to contribute as a member of the research team and to acquire research skills. Let him or her know you

are seriously considering graduate study in clinical or counseling psychology—it will increase your appeal.

Negotiating Research Responsibilities

"Well Mr./Ms. Smith, I'd be very interested in speaking with you about helping out with my research. . . ." You have made the contact. If the professor does not need help, you have lost nothing and gained the experience. Ask if he or she knows of someone with similar interests who is looking for help, or simply approach the next person on your list.

After the initial contact, your next move is dictated by your professor's needs and your abilities. Regardless of all your wonderful qualities, be prepared to run some of the grunt work! Photocopying needs to be done, literature searches need to be conducted, and at times you might well be expected to do some lab cleanup. You are "low person on the totem pole," so approach this with humility. But if you have experience with test administration or statistical analysis, let the professor know, being aware that ultimately your activities will be dictated first by his or her needs. However, if grunt work is the full extent of your duties, your needs are not being addressed properly. Spending a year doing nothing but photocopying would be a waste of time.

Research experience is, above all, an opportunity to learn. Volunteer to be trained to be of more use. For example, learn the computer skills to input data and conduct statistical analyses. Learn to score and, more importantly, to *understand* a Minnesota Multiphasic Personality Inventory-2 (MMPI-2) or a Beck Depression Inventory (BDI-II). Learn how to calibrate and run psychophysiological equipment. Whatever equipment or tests, find out about them and their use. And always ask questions about what you do not understand. When it comes time to put your research on your curriculum vitae, these are the responsibilities you will want to list.

Some researchers have a weekly lab group or research meeting with graduate students, undergraduates, or both. These might entail a discussion of the project at hand, or a presentation on another area within the field, or a training session for new people. In any of these cases, it is an opportunity to learn more about your area of interest. If you have not been invited to these meetings, go ahead and ask about them. Optimize your contact with your professor! Convey your willingness and enthusiasm. Give your professor reason to write an outstanding letter of recommendation.

Finally, there are some instances where undergraduates are solely supervised by graduate students and have little contact with the professor in charge of the project. This can happen if faculty members have a large number of students working with them or if they are well known and are continually approached by masses of students. Being supervised exclusively by a graduate student is an undesirable situation for a potential applicant. Although there is much to be learned from graduate students—and they are fresh from the application process themselves—a letter of recommendation from a graduate student does not carry the same weight as one from a professor. Moreover, a lack of interaction with the professor means that he or she must depend solely on graduate students for feedback on your work, thus detracting from the value of his or her assessment.

This is *not* to say that you must avoid research opportunities that are primarily supervised by graduate students. Personal access to the faculty member is, however, one of several important factors to be considered in your decision on where to volunteer for research experience.

Arranging Credit and Semesters

Most colleges allow students to take a certain amount of research for academic credit. If the opportunity is available, take advantage of it. Some professors may even demand that you sign up for credit, because it institutes a contract between them and you as to the number of hours per week required and how long they can count on you to work with them. Generally speaking, multiply the number of course credits by 3, and this will give you the number of weekly hours that you should anticipate spending doing research.

Expect to spend at least two semesters on a project. This demonstrates your commitment and allows ample contact between you and your professor. Thus, it is a good idea to work with someone at least 1 year before you plan to apply to graduate school. For instance, begin research in fall 2005 if you are applying in fall 2006 for a fall 2007 entrance to graduate school.

In consultation with your faculty advisor, consider applying for a university or national grant to fund your research project. These grant monies may be used to purchase equipment, pay postage for surveys, reimburse research participants for their time, and send you to a convention to present your findings. In most colleges and universities, these small grants are called undergraduate research grants, summer research fellowships, or something similar. At the University of Scranton, for example, the summer grants allow students to live on campus free for the summer, provide a tidy stipend, and contribute up to $500 for supplies. At the national level, Psi Chi and several publishers provide small awards and grants for research. Go to www.psyichi.org/awards to access the list.

In terms of research, there is no such thing as too much for a Ph.D. applicant. The longer you have worked on a project and the greater your responsibilities, the more attractive you are as an applicant. Ideally, you would work with two professors over the course of your undergraduate education. This is not necessary, but when schools expect three letters of recommendation, having two letters summarizing two different research experiences is particularly strong. Although they will allocate less attention to research than Ph.D. applicants, Psy.D. applicants are reminded that research is still an important admission criterion.

One word of caution: do not overextend yourself. Be realistic about the amount of time you can commit. Some students juggle two or three research projects at once and end up performing poorly on them all. It is far more important to concentrate your energies and perform solidly on one project than it is to spread yourself too thin. Do as much research as your academic studies and other commitments allow.

An ideal time to begin research is during the summer, when you can balance it with a part- or full-time job. Since most undergraduates and some graduate students leave during the summer, professors may be short-staffed during this period. It is a prime opportunity to optimize your usefulness at the outset and increase your chances of picking up desirable skills.

The net result of your research experiences will be skill enhancement and professional identification. Depending on the nature of your project, you will probably have engaged in a literature search, hypothesis generation, experimental design, data collection, statistical analyses, and the write-up.

Presenting and Publishing Research

Presenting or publishing your research is a definite asset. Opportunities for presentation are numerous: a department or university colloquium, a local or regional undergraduate psychology conference, a state or national psychology convention. Participation in research conferences is viewed favorably as an index of your professional identification and commitment. Check with your advisor about these opportunities and other possibilities for your work to be seen by colleagues.

Publication of your research in a scholarly journal is held in very high regard by graduate admissions committees. As we discuss in Chapter 6, research experience leading to a coauthored publication is the most highly rated final selection criterion for Ph.D. (though not necessarily Psy.D.) admission decisions following the interview. The peer-review process by which journals accept papers for publication gives a seal of collegial affirmation that the research contributes to the scientific understanding of behavior. Although not common, undergraduate publication is slowly becoming more frequent.

If your research project is not quite up to the standards of a competitive, peer-reviewed journal, then by all means consider sending the paper to a journal publishing student research in psychology. One such publication is the *Psi Chi Journal of Undergraduate Research*, which has the twofold purpose of fostering the scholarly efforts of undergraduate psychology students and of providing them with a valuable learning experience. Other publications for student research in psychology are *Modern Psychological Studies, Journal of Psychology and Behavioral Sciences*, and *Journal of Psychological Inquiry*. All these journals publish research in psychology conducted and written by students. Look for their instructions to authors on the Web (www.Lemoyne.edu/OTRP/otpresources), on departmental bulletin boards, or in *Eye on Psi Chi* (the national newsletter of Psi Chi).

Of course, though submission to these journals can be instructive, publishing in them does not carry as much weight as publication in established peer-reviewed journals. In fact, recent research suggests that a student publication in an undergraduate journal may be judged neutral or even unfavorably by research-oriented professors in a doctoral programs (Ferrari & Hemovich, 2004). So, always aim to publish your research in peer-reviewed, scholarly journals.

Still impressive is a paper/poster presentation at a state, regional, or national meeting. Only between 10% and 20% of undergraduate psychology majors present their research at some type of research conference, whether local, regional, or national (Terry, 1996; Titus & Buxman, 1999).

Most regional and national meetings are listed in each issue of the *American Psychologist, APS Observer*, and *Eye on Psi Chi*. These meetings are also listed on the Psi Chi Web site. Psi Chi members who present papers can receive a certificate recognizing their excellence in research. This award should be duly noted on your curriculum vitae and application. Refer to *Eye on Psi Chi*, ask your local Psi Chi moderator or consult their Web site at www.psichi.org to receive the form entitled "Certificate Recognition Program for Paper Presentations by Psi Chi Members."

Different graduate programs will assess your research experience in different ways, of course. None-theless, as an aid to applicants, we reproduce below (with permission) two rating scales employed at different times by one clinical program (University of Rhode Island) over the past 10 years. The first rating scale emphasizes research activity. Examples of relevant activities might include producing honors theses, serving as a research assistant, conducting independent research, coauthoring scientific publications, and developing research skills, such as data analysis and interviewing.

Rating	Criteria
5	Senior author of one or more articles in significant journals in addition to experience that provided a basis for extensive mastery of one or more directly related research skills.
4	Coauthor of one or more articles in significant journals in addition to experiences providing considerable familiarity with one or more directly relevant research skills.
3	Project leadership or significant participation in research activity (beyond activities connected with course work) serving to provide for considerable development of mastery of one or more relevant research skills.
2	Experience that provides a basis for some familiarity with relevant research skills.
1	Little if any experience according to these criteria.

The second rating scale, now in use at the University of Rhode Island, favors four criteria in evaluating research experience.

1. *Demonstrated research productivity:* sole or co-authorship of research publications, presentation of papers at scientific meetings, other tangible indications of research achievement.
2. *Breadth and quality of experience:* development of one or more research skills, data collection with different populations, work on more than one project.
3. *Research interest:* the strength of interest in research can be inferred from research activity over a sustained period of time and recommendations from research supervisors documenting skills, motivation, participation, and accomplishments.
4. *Individual autonomy:* responsibility for planning, implementing and carrying out research tasks as a member of a research team or evidence of independent work.

Rankings are based on the aforementioned criteria and assigned as follows:

Rating	Criteria
5	Satisfies all four criteria
4	Satisfies three criteria
3	Satisfies two criteria
2	Satisfies one criterion
1	Evidence of some prior research involvement or interest

Research is an area of your application that will be considered important and, at most Ph.D. programs, weighted heavily. Balance is the key. On the one hand, an absence of research experience is usually seen as a serious drawback to an application. On the other hand, over committing yourself to multiple projects at one time can lead to poor performance and a neglect of clinical experience and GRE preparation. And do not forget, research also provides you with the opportunity to make professional contacts. The professors or graduate students with whom you collaborate are excellent sources of information about the field and about applying to graduate schools.

Entrance Examinations

About 90% of doctoral clinical psychology programs (Mayne et al., 1994; Steinpreis, Queen, & Tennen, 1992) and 80% of doctoral counseling psychology programs (Turkson & Norcross, 1996) require you to complete two exams: the Graduate Record Examination (GRE) General Test and the GRE Psychology Subject Test. The two GRE tests are often used to complement each other in admission decisions because the General Test is a measure of developed abilities and the Subject Test is an index of achievement in a specific field of study. The Miller Analogies Test (MAT) is required by fewer programs, about 3% of doctoral programs and 9% of master's programs in psychology (Murray & Williams, 1999; Norcross et al., in press).

Blanket statements about entrance exams are difficult because not all schools require all tests, and some schools require additional testing (e.g., in the past the University of Minnesota required clinical psychology applicants to take the MMPI—a personality inventory!). Moreover, not all schools weight these tests equally among the application criteria. Some schools clearly state a minimum score that all applicants must obtain, whereas others state that they have no such criteria. Interestingly, a study at Boston University (Rem, Oren, & Childrey, 1987) showed that even without an imposed cutoff, applicants admitted into its program had GRE scores of 600 or better. This suggests that even if a school does not emphasize standardized test scores, (1) scores can still play a major role in the selection of candidates, or (2) applicants with high exam scores are also the applicants considered most desirable on the other admissions criteria.

Consequently, the best assistance that can be offered is a brief description of each test, an overview of minimum and actual GRE scores of incoming graduate students, guidelines for deciding how much preparation will be needed, and some suggestions as to the available study aids for each test.

GRE General Test

Use of GRE scores for admission to clinical and counseling psychology programs continues to be the norm and continues to be controversial (Dollinger, 1989; Ingram, 1983; Sternberg, 1997). The traditional rationale—buttressed by some evidence—is that the GRE is ordinarily more valid than undergraduate GPA in predicting graduate school success (Boudreau et al., 1983; Goldberg & Alliger, 1992). Another rationale is that GRE performance is an "equalizer" among the diverse curriculum requirements and grading practices in thousands of undergraduate institutions. The entrance exam is probably the only standardized measure of all applicants that an admissions committee has. Does a 3.7 GPA and stellar letters of recommendation from Backwater College reflect more, the same, or less knowledge than a 3.3 GPA and strong letters of recommendation from Ivy League University? Since all students take the identical GRE test, the playing field is somewhat leveled.

The empirical research indicates that the GRE General Test has modest predictive validity for graduate school performance. In a meta-analysis of studies conducted in psychology and counseling departments, Goldberg and Alliger (1992) found that GRE scores predicted about 8% of the variance in graduate school GPA. In a later meta-analysis of two dozen studies encompassing more than 5,000 test takers, Morrison and Morrison (1995) similarly found that 6% of the variance in graduate-level academic achievement was accounted for by GRE scores. These and other studies (e.g., Chernyshenko & Ones, 1999; Kuncel, Hezlett, & Ones, 2001) indicate that GRE General Test scores are generalizably valid in a modest way for all sorts of measures of graduate performance, especially when selection/admission ratios are taken into account. At the same time, Subject Test scores tend to be better predictors than the General Test scores (Kuncel et al., 2001).

The Educational Testing Service (ETS), located in Princeton, New Jersey, provides a free booklet entitled

GRE Information & Registration Bulletin (Graduate Record Examinations, 2001), which describes the test and offers examples of the types of questions you can expect to encounter on each section. You can obtain the same information and register for the test by visiting GRE online at www.gre.org. In addition, at this Web site you can order (with a credit card) ETS test preparation books and download preparation software directly onto your home computer.

The test is very similar in format to the Scholastic Aptitude Test (SAT) that most of you took prior to college. The three GRE scales are Verbal Reasoning (V), Quantitative Reasoning (Q), and Analytical Writing (AW). The Verbal and Quantitative scales are multiple-choice in format, and scores on the test are based on the number of correct answers selected. Most graduate schools use only the Verbal and Quantitative scores in evaluating candidates.

The Analytical Writing section, in which you write two essays, is delivered on the computer, and you word-process your responses. For the "Present Your Perspective on an Issue" task, you will choose one of two essay topics selected by the computer from a larger pool of topics. For the "Analyze an Argument" task, you do not have a choice of topics; the computer will present you with a single topic. Your essays are read and scored by two trained raters using a holistic 6-point scale (scoring guidelines can be found at www .gre.org/pracmats .html). Your Analytical Writing (AW) score is reported on the 0–6 scale in half-point increments. Since the AW test is relatively recent, many graduate schools are not yet placing as much emphasis on it as the Verbal and Quantitative scores in admission decisions. But this will surely change in the near future, as graduate admissions committees seek an independent measure of your writing ability.

The GRE General Test is now available only on computer; the traditional paper-and-pencil version was phased out in 1999. This computer-based test always begins with the 75-minute Analytical Writing section: 45 minutes for the Issue essay and 30 minutes for Argument essay. Then follows the 30-minute Verbal section and the 45-minute Quantitative section.

In addition, a pretest section or research section may be included, but answers to these sections do not count toward your score. All told, you will probably spend about 4 hours at the testing center.

The GRE registration booklet and the free tutorial software (POWER PREP, available at www.ets/org/ cbtdemo.html) will familiarize you with the computer-based adaptive format of the Verbal and Quantitative sections. Briefly put, adaptive testing means that your responses to the early items determine the difficulty

level of subsequent items and your range of possible scores. As you answer each question, the computer immediately scores that question and your preceding answers to determine which question is presented next. Correct answers lead to increasingly difficult items (and eventually higher test scores); incorrect answers lead to less difficult items (and lower test scores). As a consequence, you may not skip any questions and you may not go back and change a previous answer. An equally important consequence is that you should be very familiar with the test format and computer functions before test day!

In deciding how much and what type of preparation you will need for this test, ask yourself several questions:

1. What were my SAT scores? These two tests are highly correlated in a positive direction, so this may be your first clue as to how much preparation is ahead of you.
2. How well have I done on multiple-choice tests in college? There is a certain savvy to taking standardized tests, and this is one way to assess yours.
3. How anxious do I become in a testing situation? A moderate amount of test anxiety is optimal: too little anxiety can breed indifference, but too much begets interference. If you tend to approach tests with more than moderate discomfort, you might benefit from additional preparation aimed at relaxing yourself and building your confidence.
4. Can I discipline myself to do the necessary studying? If you are in need of additional preparation, this question is important in deciding what the most appropriate form of preparation will be for you. Be honest with yourself. If you cannot imagine sitting down regularly and studying independently for the GREs, you might be better off taking a preparatory course offered privately in most cities.

Students typically spend an inordinate amount of time worrying about the GREs. The myth exists that clinical applicants need a score of 650 on each of their subscales to be considered seriously. This is simply not the case. Some Psy.D. programs do not even require the GREs. On the other hand, many APA-approved programs prefer GREs of 600 or above. The average GRE score (combined Verbal and Quantitative) of first-year graduate students in psychology master's programs is 1053; in doctoral psychology programs, 1183 (Norcross et al., in press).

However, even these averages mask considerable variation in preferred minimum GRE scores. In our study of the admission statistics of APA-accredited clini-

TABLE 2-4. Minimum GRE Scores Preferred by APA-Accredited Clinical Psychology Programs

Preferred minimum score	Psy.D. programs		Practice-oriented Ph.D.		Equal-emphasis Ph.D.		Research-oriented Ph.D.		All programs	
	M	SD	M	SD	M	SD	M	SD	M	SD
Quantitative scale	544	46	566	58	580	44	598	36	581	46
Verbal scale	533	50	566	58	583	46	598	36	580	48
Psychology subject test	542	49	601	17	581	48	605	43	587	47

Note. Adapted from Mayne, Norcross, & Sayette (1994).

cal doctoral programs (Mayne et al., 1994), we found that the preferred minimum scores differed consistently according to the type of program. As shown in Table 2-4, research-oriented clinical Ph.D. programs preferred the highest GRE minimum scores—about 600 each for the Quantitative and Verbal scales. Psy.D. programs were willing to accept lower (but still not low) minimum GRE scores—about 520 to 540 each on the two scales. In between these two poles is the remainder of clinical and counseling psychology doctoral programs, which expect a minimum score of 550 to 560 on each of the scales, on average (Turkson & Norcross, 1996).

Even if your scores are lower than 550, you can bolster other areas of your application to overcome low scores. But if your GREs are below 500, then most doctoral programs in clinical and counseling psychology will not seriously consider your application. In this case, it will probably be necessary to take them again after taking a preparatory course or after spending time with a study guide.

But here overconfidence can be disastrous. Even if you obtained 700 SATs, aced every multiple-choice exam in college, and are cool-headed in testing situations, you should still familiarize yourself with the test format and complete the practice test offered in the application booklet. It certainly would not hurt to prepare more, but this should be considered the bare minimum.

Many self-study manuals and software packages are sufficient for a disciplined applicant to ready him or herself for the GRE. The books provide helpful test-taking hints, vocabulary and math reviews, and sample tests that the student can self-administer. Many include actual questions given on past GREs that can provide a real flavor for the material likely to be seen on testing day. The software packages administer sample tests and give helpful hints. Sample questions, practice manuals, and downloadable practice software packages can also be found and ordered on the official GRE Web site at www.gre.org. In addition to the official ETS site, several comprehensive and commercial Internet sites provide valuable tips and full-length practice tests. Some of the material is offered for free; some offered for a price. Visit:

- www.princetonreview.com
- www.kaptest/com/gre
- www.testtuto.com/gre
- 800score.com/gre-index.html
- www.home.mastersites.com/greguide

We heartily recommend taking an online GRE practice test. A practice GRE serves as a diagnostic tool to assess your abilities, gauge your competitiveness for admission to graduate programs, and identify areas that need further improvement (Walfish, 2004). Our favorite is the practice GRE at www.kaplan.com. It is free and confidential; use it as a starting point.

Lastly, give yourself *at least* 6 weeks of study time if you decide to use a manual or 8 weeks if you do not have a lot of time to devote solely to studying.

Students feeling less confident, more anxious, or "out of the exam business" should contemplate private courses designed to help you prepare for the GRE. They offer a number of benefits beyond those of study guides:

- A structured time one or more times a week when the material is taught by an impartial instructor who can assess your strengths and weaknesses
- An abundance of study materials and the possibility of individual tutoring
- The chance to take tests under actual test-taking conditions (especially helpful for those with test anxiety)
- Specific work on test-taking skills and the short-cuts that can make problems easier
- Brief introduction to relaxation exercises to counter test anxiety

The imposed structure on studying and the conscious use of test-taking skills can be very useful. Although these classes cannot guarantee that they will improve your scores, they are undoubtedly the best course of action for some students. Having worked for one of these agencies, we have seen the benefits of this system for many students.

Many students attempt to strengthen their vocabulary for the GRE Verbal section by preparing flashcards or memorizing a vocabulary word each day. The early research on the word-a-day method suggests it can slightly enrich your vocabulary (Prevoznak & Bubka, 1999), but more importantly, it gets you into the swing of GRE preparation and the admissions process. If you are inclined to try this method, consider receiving a word a day from the Web site, www.wordsmith.org, which presents a word with its pronunciation and examples. Or try the vocabulary builders at www.bestvocab.com and www.number2.com. They require only a couple of minutes per day.

Scheduling *when* to take your general GRE should be carefully considered. If you do poorly on the test, you can retake it. Consequently, it is prudent to take it at least 6 months before the application deadline, which gives you time to study and prepare for a second administration. For undergraduates planning to apply to graduate school during their senior year, this means taking it during the summer following your junior year or early fall of the senior year. For graduates, this means taking it the spring before you plan to apply. Even if you improve your scores, the current ETS policy is to send to each institution scores from *all* your tests taken during the last 5 years.

We are frequently asked by students in our graduate school workshops if they should retake the GRE General Test if they are dissatisfied with their original scores. Our immediate answer is: it depends. If you studied diligently for the test and if you performed on the test similar to the practice tests, then no—do not retake the test. But if any of the following five factors apply to you, then retaking the test once seems like a good idea (Keith-Spiegel & Wiederman, 2000): (1) You were ill the day you took the GRE; (2) you were immobilized by test anxiety; (3) you did not prepare for the test content; (4) you were unfamiliar with the computer-based format and the adaptive design; (5) your SAT scores were much higher than your GRE scores.

Should you decide to retake the GRE General Test, please be aware of the probable effects of repeating it. The average score gain for repeaters is about 27 points on the Verbal scale and 30 points on the Quantitative scale. Increases of more than 100 points rarely occur, in only 1 or 2% of repeaters (ETS, 1984).

Your GRE score can partially determine where to apply. Low scores suggest applying only to institutions whose cutoffs you meet. In this way, your GREs can help you make realistic decisions as to your chances of being accepted at a given school and ultimately whether to apply there.

GRE Psychology Subject Test

The General Test measures knowledge acquired over a long period of time and not indigenous to any specific field of study. By contrast, the Subject Tests—such as the Psychology Subject Test—assume an undergraduate major or extensive background in the specific subject. Consequently, the test may be relatively difficult if you were not an undergraduate psychology major.

Another difference between the General Test and the Subject Test lies in the mode of administration. The General Test is a computer-based test available year-round at over 600 test centers. The Subject Test, by contrast, continues to be a paper-based test offered three times during the academic year.

Table 2-5 summarizes the differences between the GRE General Test and the GRE Subject Test. These profound test differences will lead to different preparation and test-taking strategies on your part.

The GRE Psychology Test consists of about 215 multiple-choice questions. Each item has five options, from which you select the correct or best response. The total time allotted for the test is 2 hours and 50 minutes.

The GRE Psychology Test yields a total score and two subscores. Virtually all programs, however, concentrate on the total score, not on the subscores. The preferred minimum score is 587 for clinical psychology doctoral programs and 541 for counseling psychology doctoral programs (Mayne et al., 1994; Turkson & Norcross, 1996). That is, most programs will be expecting you to secure a score at or above this number. But here again, as shown in Table 2-4, the preferred minimum ranges from a low of 542 in Psy.D. programs to a high of 605 in research-oriented Ph.D. programs.

The two subscales are an Experimental or natural science orientation and a Social or social science orientation. The Experimental subscore covers questions in learning, cognition, perception, comparative psychology, sensation, and physiological psychology. The Social subscore includes an equal number of questions in personality, clinical, abnormal, developmental, and social psychology.

Percentages of questions devoted to a subject area will vary somewhat from one test administration to

TABLE 2-5. Comparison of the GRE General Test and the GRE Psychology Subject Test

	General test	Subject test
Content assessed	Broad knowledge	Specific knowledge in psychology
Test format	Computer	Paper-and-pencil
Administration schedule	Throughout the year	Three times per year (Nov., Dec., & Apr.)
Recommended test date	Summer of junior year Early Fall of senior year	Fall of senior year for Ph.D./Psy.D. applicants December for master's applicants
Administration format	Individual	Group
Test cost (2005–2006)	$115	$140
Repeat policy	May repeat test once per calendar month up to 5 times per year	May repeat test as often as it is offered up to 5 times per year
Testing time	2 hours, 45 minutes	2 hours, 50 minutes
Scoring procedure	Adaptive: your early responses determine difficulty level of subsequent questions	Total items answered correctly minus one-fourth the number answered incorrectly
Skipping questions	Not permitted; computer administers one question at a time	Permitted
Scores provided	3 scores (Verbal Reasoning, Quantitative Reasoning, & Analytical Writing)	1 total score, 2 subscores
Scores range	200–800 for Verbal & Quantitative; 0–6 for Analytical Writing	200–990
Score mean (*SD*)	500 (100)	540 (100)
Recommended preparation	Intense	Moderate

another. Nonetheless, one set of investigators (Waters, Drew, & Ayers, 1988) found these approximate percentages on past tests:

Physiological/comparative psychology	14%
Developmental psychology	12%
Learning and motivation	12%
Sensation and perception	12%
Clinical/abnormal psychology	11%
Personality and social psychology	11%
Cognition and complex human learning	10%
Applied psychology	9%
Research methodology	9%

Scores on the GRE Psychology Test are best predicted by your GRE General Test scores and the number of basic psychology courses completed. The irony is that students can obtain excellent grades in all their psychology courses but still not perform adequately on

the Psychology Test if they have not taken the critical courses. A narrow focus on—and many courses in—clinical psychology will probably detract from your score since this one area only accounts for 10 to 12% of the test items. The questions are drawn from courses most commonly offered at the undergraduate level within psychology (ETS, 1995).

A maximum number of "traditional" courses in psychology, as represented in the foregoing list, and a minimum of special topics and "pop" psychology will prepare you best for the GRE Psychology Subject Test. Choose your elective courses for breadth and rigor, not merely your specialized interest.

The GRE Psychology Subject Test is designed to be challenging. Students accustomed to getting 90% correct on in-class exams often worry about the large number of items they miss. The average student answers about half the items correctly, misses about 30%, and omits 20% (Kalat & Matlin, 2000). Because your score is based on the number of questions answered correctly minus one-fourth of the questions answered incorrectly, guessing does *not* lower your score. You are not penalized for guessing; but you are rewarded for eliminating one or two possible answers.

Adequate preparation is essential for this test. We—and others—suggest four steps: (1) obtain the free ETS booklet *A Description of the Advanced Psychology Test;* (2) read a good introductory psychology textbook; (3) volunteer to be a TA (teaching assistant) for the Introduction to Psychology course; and (4) purchase one of the study guides with practice tests. Our favorite study guides are *Practicing to Take the GRE Psychology Test* (published by the GRE board, which can be ordered at the ETS Web site), *Graduate Record Examination—Psychology* (Raphael & Halpert, 1999; published by Prentice Hall), *Best Preparation for the GRE in Psychology* (Kellogg, 2000; published by Research & Education Association), and *Cracking the GRE Psychology* (Jay, 1999; published by Princeton Review). If these four steps do not suffice, then private courses in preparing for the psychology test are available.

The standard error of measurement for the GRE is quite small, and retaking the General Test in the absence of any *intense* remediation is unlikely to result in a significant change in your score. Your Psychology Test scores, however, may be significantly different if intervening study or additional courses occur between the test sessions.

A graduate school may adopt one or more policies in handling cases in which a candidate reports two sets of GRE scores: consider only the most recent one; consider the higher of the two scores; or average the scores. The latter is probably the best alternative, since it creates the least bias and is the most reliable.

Miller Analogies Test

A few clinical and counseling psychology doctoral programs request the MAT, a 50-minute test consisting of 100 word analogies. Your score is the total number correct; the mean for students intending to study psychology in graduate school is 50 to 51 (The Psychological Corporation, 1994). As with the GREs, booklets are available to help improve your scores on the test, and it is useful to take practice tests to familiarize and prepare yourself for the actual event. There are states in which the MAT cannot be administered (e.g., New York) because of test disclosure laws enacted in those states, so be sure to locate the testing center nearest you.

The MATs are less frequently required by graduate schools than either of the GRE tests. Because the tests can be scheduled at any time, through a network of over 600 testing centers nationwide, you might consider taking this test after you have received your GRE scores and after you have selected the schools you would like to apply to. You may save yourself some time and money if none of the schools that interest you require the test.

Part of the expense of applying to graduate school is the cost of sending test scores. One possible way to reduce costs is to make copies of the test results sent to you and mail them with your application. Any school that is interested in you will request that you have the scores "officially" sent to them. Any school not interested will not need your official scores, and you will have saved the expense of having them forwarded.

Two words of caution must accompany this possibility. First, only do this if you send in your application early. Unless you check with a school before the application deadline to make sure that this procedure will not exclude you as an applicant, you should not send copies. Second, some students send copies of test scores after altering the original document, for example, whiting out poor scores or past scores, putting scores in different columns, and even falsifying scores. *You must never resort to these practices!* These should immediately invalidate your application, and any school that accepts you will need official copies sent anyway.

Finally, low scores on entrance exams do not automatically preclude you from applying to clinical or counseling psychology graduate programs. Rather, low scores mean you must select and apply to programs that do not emphasize test scores or that accept scores in your range. You can partially compensate in other areas to help offset weak tests. As with each admission criterion, standardized test scores are only one part of the overall picture of a candidate. The best anyone can do is to make his or her overall application as attractive as possible.

Extracurricular Activities

Empirical research and personal experience alike indicate that an applicant's extracurricular pursuits are accorded less weight than GPAs, GRE scores, research competency, and clinical experience. The research reviewed earlier in this chapter clearly bears this point out. However, extracurricular activities, such as Psi Chi membership and campus involvement, are still considered in evaluating the "total person" of the applicant.

The admission implications are thus proscriptive and prescriptive. Strictly in terms of enhancing your candidacy (not in terms of other goals, such as life satisfaction), you should favor good grades and research experience over extracurricular activities.

Involvement in dozens of student organizations will not compensate for meager grades and research; doctoral programs will not accept you because you coached youth soccer. When confronted with time conflicts, recall that admissions committees place a premium on variables other than intense campus commitments.

Having stated the obvious but unpleasant facts, we would also urge you to routinely engage in *some* campus and community pursuits. The reasoning here is that clinical and counseling psychology programs seek well-rounded individuals with diverse interests. The "egghead" or "Mr. Peabody" image is to be avoided in the practice of psychology, where your interpersonal skills are as critical as your scientific preparation. Moderate involvement can also better acquaint you with faculty members, who may serve as sources of recommendations, and with the discipline of psychology itself. You can create professional opportunities by simply being involved in departmental activities. "Familiar faces" are frequently given first shots at clinical or research opportunities.

Applicants frequently learn too late that active involvement outside of the classroom is an indispensable education in and of itself. Consider the following student qualities contained in many standard letter of recommendation forms:

- Academic performance
- Organizational skills
- Interest/enthusiasm
- Interpersonal skills
- Emotional stability
- Communication skills
- Originality/resourcefulness
- Social judgment
- Responsibility/dependability
- Stress tolerance

Most of these dimensions refer to faculty–student interactions *outside* of the classroom, not to your course grades. Many a bright student has sabotaged his or her educational experience, recommendation letters, and career goal by not becoming involved outside of the classroom.

In your extracurricular activities, try to exhibit the chief personality trait which, interacting with intelligence, relates most to vocational success—namely, conscientiousness (Jensen, 1998). Be responsible, dependable, organized, and persistent. This trait applies to every kind of educational and job success; what's more, you want colleagues and friends to document in their letters of recommendation that you are extraordinarily conscientious.

Four specific suggestions come to mind regarding the type of extracurricular activities to pursue. First, join departmental student organizations, such as the Psychology Club, Psi Chi, and the American Psychological Society's Student Caucus. Second, we heartily recommend that you join the American Psychological Association (APA) and/or the American Psychological Society (APS) as a student affiliate. Your APA affiliation brings with it monthly issues of the *American Psychologist*, the flagship journal, and the *APA Monitor*, the association's newspaper. Similarly, APS membership includes subscriptions to the monthly journal *Psychological Science* and the *APS Observer*. Student membership in professional associations reflects favorably on your commitment to the discipline, and this affiliation should be recorded on your curriculum vitae. Your psychology advisor might have applications for student affiliation in his or her office; if not, go online to www.apa.org/membership/forstudents.html and www.psychobiologicalscience.org/join.

Third, additional campus and community commitments should be guided by your interests. But those associated with human services, social causes, and artistic endeavors seem to be differentially rewarded. These will obviously vary with the locale; examples include Hand-in-Hand, campus ministries, course tutoring, peer advising, homeless shelters, women's centers, BACHUSS, SADD, theater productions, creative writing, Amnesty International, and the like.

A fourth and invaluable extracurricular experience is to attend a regional or national psychology convention. The benefits are many: socializing you into the profession; learning about current research; discovering how students and professors present research; meeting and hearing nationally known psychologists; adding to your growing professional network; attending and perhaps participating in sessions designed for prospective graduate students (e.g., the Psi Chi sessions and workshops); experiencing the intellectual stimulation; and enjoying the interpersonal camaraderie of fellow students and psychologists (Lubin, 1993; Tryon, 1985). For all these reasons, we have never—and we mean *never*—heard a single graduate school applicant express disappointment about attending his or her first psychology convention.

The challenge for most prospective psychologists is to locate and afford travel to one of the regional or national psychology conferences. To locate upcoming conferences in your area, ask your psychology professors, consult the lists regularly published in *Eye on Psi Chi* and *American Psychologist*, and keep an eye open for announcements and posters on departmental bulletin boards. "Convention season" in psychology is from

March to May, when the regional psychological associations hold their annual conventions. These include the Eastern Psychological Association, Midwestern Psychological Association, Rocky Mountain Psychological Association, Western Psychological Association, and Southeastern Psychological Association. The national conventions of APA and APS are annually held in the late spring and summer months. To afford the travel and lodging, consider organizing a convention trip with your fellow students, requesting information on special hotel and registration rates for students, volunteering as a convention assistant, and holding fund-raisers with psychology student organizations to offset your expenses. By hook or crook, definitely plan on expanding your extracurricular horizons by attending a psychology convention.

Extracurricular activities should reflect your active and passionate pursuit of excellence. This is, after all, your chosen profession, your career, your future. Join honor societies, compete for awards, pursue honors, and consider applications for Truman, Rhodes, and Fulbright scholarships. You should be actively investigating undergraduate grants for your research, such as those administered nationally by Psi Chi or those awarded locally in your university. Passivity doesn't cut it in graduate school (or life).

Finally, as part of your preparation, discuss your graduate plans with those people who will be affected by those plans, such as partner, spouse, parents, children, and close friends. The sooner you start discussing your plans, the better. You may move hundreds of miles away and will probably be working 60 hours a week as a graduate student. Your absence—psychological and physical—will likely impact other people close to you. Begin the discussions now, not after you apply (Megargee, 2001).

In this chapter, we reviewed six admission criteria—course work, faculty mentoring, clinical experience, research skills, entrance examinations, and extracurricular activities—and suggested ways to improve in these areas. The material covered in this chapter is concerned with how you as the applicant can improve your credentials or marketability. But the application process goes both ways. In addition to selling yourself, you are also a consumer, evaluating the programs and deciding which ones are for you. The next two chapters help you evaluate characteristics of graduate programs.

CHAPTER 3

GETTING STARTED

Up to this point, we have focused on what you can do to enhance your credentials before beginning the application process. At some point, you must take realistic stock and evaluate where you stand as an applicant. Maybe you have taken your GREs. Perhaps you have signed up for some advanced psychology courses and have a satisfactory GPA. You have been supervised in a clinical setting and have begun research. You have reviewed your credentials and found that you have many strengths but also some weaknesses. You either shore up the deficient areas or make a decision to go ahead with what you have and hope to sell it well. In other words, you are ready to get started with the application process.

Process is an appropriate word to describe the endeavor that you are about to begin. The way you approach this task will greatly influence your chances of gaining admission. Sure, you can simply complete an application and passively wait for an interview. And this may work if your credentials are extremely strong. But for most individuals, an informed approach to the process can make all the difference!

Prospective graduate students frequently become nervous about the application process for several reasons. Perhaps the following remarks sound familiar: "Well, I have good recommendations and a 3.2 GPA, but my GREs are low"; "I have good GREs and spent a year working on a suicide hot line, but I don't have a lot of research experience"; "Although my credentials are excellent, all the schools that I applied to only accept 10 out of 300 applicants." Whichever of these situations applies, simply submitting an application minimizes your chances of acceptance. You can do a great deal to increase your admission probabilities and to decrease your anxiety as you compare yourself to exaggerated standards.

Common Misconceptions

We would like to begin by dispelling three common misconceptions about clinical and counseling psychology programs. The first misconception: there is a direct correlation between a university's undergraduate reputation and the status of its psychology graduate programs. In fact, there is no such correlation. Many of the best undergraduate institutions—Brown, Princeton, and the elite liberal arts colleges, for example—do not even have graduate studies in clinical or counseling psychology.

A second misconception is that you should apply to a graduate psychology program on the basis of that institution's sports performance. We have met a number of students who have used this selection criterion with unfortunate consequences. Please do not allow your application decisions to rest on whether a university has an excellent football team or whether their basketball team made it to the Final Four of the NCAA tournament! Do not scoff at the reality of this practice; careful research has demonstrated that winning a national championship in a visible college sport consistently translates into increased applications to the winning institution (Toma & Cross, 1998).

A third common misconception is that there is an authoritative list of the finest graduate programs in clinical psychology. In reality, unlike business or law schools, there is no definitive ranking of the "best" psychology graduate programs. The quality of a program depends on what *you* are looking to get out of it. The best school for someone seeking to become a

TABLE 3-1. Average Acceptance Rates for APA-Accredited Clinical Psychology Programs

	Freestanding Psy.D.	University-based Psy.D.	Practice-oriented Ph.D.	Equal-emphasis Ph.D.	Research-oriented Ph.D.
Number of applications	186	164	154	170	189
Number of acceptances	93	53	18	21	13
Acceptance rate	50%	41%	10%	10%	6%

Note. Data from Norcross, Castle, Sayette, & Mayne (2004); Norcross & Oliver (2005); and Norcross, Sayette, Mayne, Karg, & Turkson (1998).

psychologist conducting psychoanalytic psychotherapy in private practice is probably not going to be the program of choice for someone who has set his or her heart on becoming a psychophysiological researcher at a medical school. Each person could attend the "best" school for psychology in his or her area.

What we want to do is to shift the burden from you trying to meet a school's admissions demands to you finding a school that meets *your* needs. Graduate schools are looking for students with direction and passion. This does not mean you have made an irrevocable commitment to an area of research or type of clinical work. It means that you have an idea of what type of professional work you would like to do and toward which theoretical orientation(s) you seem to be leaning.

You are selecting an institution based on your belief that it will mold you in the direction *you* have chosen. Schools will look for this attitude in your statement of purpose. During your interviews, you will be asked about which professors you want to work with and what thoughts you have about their research projects. Even more likely, you will be directly asked, "Why are you applying here instead of someplace else?" By identifying your graduate training goals, you will impress interviewers at your selected programs with your direction and passion.

Acceptance Rates

The most pervasive myth about doctoral psychology programs is that "hardly anyone gets in—only 10%." Like most myths, this one does have a grain of truth. The average acceptance rate for *all* APA-accredited doctoral programs in clinical and counseling psychology is, in fact, 10% (Norcross et al., 2004; Turkson & Norcross, 1996). But in a very real way, the 10% figure is misleading and inaccurate on many counts.

Let's begin our foray into acceptance rates by defining the term. "Acceptance rate" refers to the percentage of applicants accepted for admission into a single graduate program, *not* the percentage of the

entire applicant pool to all programs accepted for admission in a given year. The clinical doctoral program at University X may accept only 15 of 150 applicants (10%), but many of the applicants to University X not accepted there will be admitted elsewhere. Although only 10% of the applicants to a single doctoral program might be accepted into that *particular* program, about half of the entire applicant pool will be accepted into *some* clinical or counseling doctoral program. And half a chance isn't that bad.

Note, too, that the 10% figure refers only to acceptance rates of APA-accredited doctoral programs in clinical or counseling psychology. The acceptance rates at *non*-APA-accredited doctoral programs are double that for APA-accredited programs: 20% for nonaccredited Ph.D. programs and 60% for nonaccredited Psy.D. programs (Norcross et al., in press). The acceptance rates for master's programs are also much higher than those for doctoral programs. The median acceptance rates for master's programs are 49% in clinical psychology and 67% in counseling psychology (Norcross et al., in press).

Most importantly, the acceptance rates vary tremendously from doctoral program to doctoral program as a function of the research–practice continuum. As shown in the Reports on Individual programs following Chapter 7, acceptance rates at research-oriented Ph.D. programs, such as Yale and Duke, are as low as 3%. The acceptance rates at freestanding Psy.D. programs are often over 50%.

Table 3-1 summarizes the findings of several of our studies on acceptance rates to APA-accredited doctoral programs as a function of the type of program. All types of program average between 150 and 200 applications per year. Research-oriented Ph.D. programs accept only 6% of their applicants, on average, whereas the corresponding figures are 10% for equal-emphasis Ph.D. and 12% for practice-oriented Ph.D. programs. University-based Psy.D. programs accept 41% of their applicants on average, and freestanding Psy.D. programs accept 50%. That's quite a range of acceptance rates—6% to 50%—all in APA-accredited doctoral programs in clinical psychology. And that's why we urge caution in tossing around the 10% acceptance rate.

Costs of Applying

Applying to graduate school is an expensive proposition—not only in terms of your valuable time but also in terms of hard money. Application fees average $50 per doctoral program and $35 per master's program (Norcross et al., 2004). Only 7% of graduate schools let you apply for free (Norcross et al., 1996). The fee (in 2006) for the GRE General Test is $115, with a $40 rescheduling fee, and the Psychology Subject Test costs another $140. ETS will electronically transmit your GRE scores free of charge to five graduate schools that you designate in advance; however, each additional score report costs $15. Throw in the costs of transcripts, photocopying, postage, and the innumerable telephone calls, and the investment can become quite costly. All told, we estimate that applying to 12 schools will run about $1,000 (and that number can increase depending on the cost of traveling to multiple interviews).

Several students challenged our estimate that the graduate application process would cost them $1,000. They protested that our figure was way too high. So, we encouraged them, like good psychologists, to collect data as they proceeded through the process. Here is the breakdown of costs from one typical applicant (Dennis Reidy) who applied to 13 doctoral programs in 2003:

Taking the GRE tests	$235
Sending GRE scores	$180
Requesting transcripts	$106
Application fees	$455
Mailing applications	$78

That's a total of $1,054 in 2003 dollars, before he traveled to three programs for personal interviews. He now believes the $1,000 estimate is on target.

The good news is that graduate schools are sensitive to financial hardship and that, for many students, the burdensome short-term cost is an excellent long-term investment. Schools build into the application process allowances for students who cannot afford the expense. Even the GRE has a fee waiver for students in dire financial circumstances. One of us was supporting himself on a meager social service salary and was able to keep the cost down to a few hundred dollars.

Moreover, think of the application cost as an investment in yourself and in your career. If you gain acceptance into a doctoral program with tuition remission and a stipend for 4 years, your $1,000 can be converted into a $60,000 to $100,000 payback over the course of your graduate school career.

The bottom line in getting started is this: anticipate the costs of applying to graduate school and plan to have the funds (or waivers) available before you begin completing applications.

Starting Early

Let's discuss timing up front. Applications are typically due from the last week in December to the second week in February. The sooner you begin preparing, the more advantage you can take of an aggressive, early start to the admission process. As mentioned in earlier chapters and in the Time Line (Appendix A), for undergraduates, ideally this would take place the summer of your junior year. For others, this would best occur the summer of the year before you actually plan to attend graduate school. If it is past that point, you are not too late. You can follow the steps we will describe as late as October of your application year.

Applying to graduate school is like planning a political campaign or a military operation. It is impossible to begin too soon or to be too thorough (Megargee, 1990). Recognize this about the application process and *start almost a year before you expect to begin graduate school*. Completing the application materials in the fall semester alone will consume as much time as a 3-credit course!

Virtually all APA-accredited clinical and counseling psychology programs only accept matriculating students for their fall semesters. As mentioned earlier, in order to be accepted for the fall of 2007, most doctoral programs have application deadlines anywhere from late December 2006 to February 2007. The typical deadline for doctoral programs in clinical and counseling psychology is January 15 (Norcross et al., 1996). Accordingly, you will need college transcripts, test scores, and letters of recommendation, not to mention time to prepare yourself before the application deadline. You should expect to begin no later than the fall of the year before you intend to attend graduate school. If you are willing to put in the maximum effort to get into a program, expect to begin the spring before that.

The APA has accredited 224 active doctoral programs in clinical psychology, 68 active doctoral programs in counseling psychology, and 10 active doctoral programs in combined psychology throughout the United States and Canada. Toss in nonaccredited doctoral programs and the mass of master's programs in clinical and counseling psychology and you wind up with roughly 600 graduate programs. How does one proceed in whittling this list to a manageable number?

To begin the selection process, ask yourself, "What kind of research or clinical work do I like? Is there some article I've read or presentation I've heard that really interests me?" There is a certain advantage if you have already conducted research or had some clinical experience as an undergraduate and know something about the field. And if you have completed an honors project or thesis, you may even have a certain amount of expertise. Or you may decide you would like to try something different now.

For example, suppose you have an interest in suicidology, but you are not sure that you want to do research in that area or exactly what that research would entail. Or you think you'd like to specialize in suicide prevention, but you're not sure how psychologists deal with the issue clinically. There are several approaches you can take to familiarize yourself with this area. Ask one of your professors for some readings. Check out a current textbook in the area. Go to a suicide prevention or crisis center and read through their literature. Then decide whether you like the questions being asked and the methods people are using to answer them.

In summary, have an idea of the field(s) in which you would like to work, either the ones with which you are already familiar or those you are willing to research. Familiarize yourself with the questions being asked and the techniques being used to answer them. Use as many sources as possible to gain information to help you narrow down your interests and educate yourself about them.

In addition to the resources in this book, a number of Internet sites will help you at this stage of the process. You can familiarize yourself with psychology graduate programs in the United States and Canada by accessing a large number of Web sites. Our favorites are:

- www.apa.org/students/
  (APA's site for students includes a list of accredited programs, relevant articles, and other useful materials)
- www.socialpsychology.org/clinical.htm
  (useful page features hyperlinks to 185 departments in the United States offering a Ph.D. in psychology)
- www.clas.ufl.edu/CLAS/american-universities.html#A
  (links for a a plethora of American universities)
- www.psychwww.com/resource/deptlist.htm
  (an impressive listing of over 1,000 psychology department Web sites)
- www.petersons.com/graduate/select/224010se.html
  (brief descriptions of programs offering graduate training in clinical psychology)

- www.petersons.com/graduate/select/224020se.html
  (as above, but for counseling psychology)
- www.gradschools.com/listings/menus/psych_clinic_menu.html and www.gradschools.com/listings/menus/psych_cmt_menu.html
  (for searching clinical and counseling psychology programs, respectively, with the added ability to search by geographic region)
- www.jobweb.org/catapult/gguides.htm
  (links to sites about applying to and financing graduate school, and about making the transition to graduate school)

All these—and other—sites enable you to take a virtual tour of graduate programs in professional psychology. Develop an early feel for various departments and begin to sharpen your interests.

Next is the task of putting this knowledge to use. You have ideas that interest you, and you now need to learn which graduate programs can provide these research or clinical opportunities. Though knowing how much you enjoy research or clinical work may not take a lot of reflection, deciding whether to select a research-oriented, a practice-oriented, or an equal-emphasis program is a question with far-reaching ramifications. This question tends to divide people into three groups: the research oriented (scientists); the clinically oriented (practitioners); and the dually committed (scientist–practitioners). The following sections are designed to lead each group in its appropriate direction. These groups tend to follow three rather distinctive career paths in the profession of clinical and counseling psychology (Bernstein & Kerr, 1993; Conway, 1988).

We have repeatedly surveyed the APA-accredited clinical and counseling psychology programs in the United States and Canada over the past 20 years. Their responses to our questionnaires (e.g., Farry et al., 1995; Mayne et al., 1994; Norcross et al., 1998; Norcross et al., 2004; Norcross, 2005; Oliver, et al., 2005; Sayette & Mayne, 1990; Sayette et al., 1999; Turkson & Norcross, 1996) can serve as the basis for your initial selection of schools. By using their responses, we will lead you through an exercise that will provide you with a list that ranks schools by how closely they meet your expectations and interests.

As you peruse the Reports on Individual Programs, bear in mind that the listings are alphabetical, not geographical. We list the programs alphabetically as they are on the APA (2006) materials, but sometimes the order is counterintuitive. For example, the University of Arkansas is not listed under "U," but between Arizona

State University and Auburn University. Thus, you might need to look under two letters to identify specific programs of interest.

For the Research Oriented and Dually Committed

This section gives guidance to those applicants who are more centrally focused on research and those with equal practice and research interest. We group these two sorts of applicants together because their initial selection of schools will place a bit more emphasis on the research available at each program and secondarily on the clinical work available. This will allow people with an equal emphasis to cast their nets as widely and as efficiently as possible.

One question we asked of each program in our studies was "In which areas of research are your faculty presently working? Do they presently have a grant in that area?" Appendix E offers a list of all the research areas provided by the graduate programs along with the number of faculty interested in these areas and an indication of whether they have a grant. This information provides you with an index of how intensively each program is pursuing this area of research. Thus, a program with three faculty members researching autism that has a grant supporting some of their work indicates serious involvement on the part of that faculty.

Find your areas of interest in the appendix; underneath them you will see a list of programs doing that type of research. In addition, you will know the number of professors with whom you could potentially work and whether there is grant money supporting this research.

A few words of caution in interpreting this appendix: not all programs were equally comprehensive in completing the survey. Some schools only included core faculty, whereas others included adjunct faculty. This accounts for what seems to be an overrepresentation of some institutions in the list. Also, some schools had research interests combining two different areas and listed a single grant under both.

Appendix B, entitled "Worksheet for Choosing Schools," is used to select the program to which you will eventually apply. Begin by writing your research interest in the far left-hand column. In the next column, marked "Schools," write the list of schools under that heading in Appendix B. In columns 3 and 4, write down the number of faculty in that area at each school and whether they are grant funded. In addition, some schools merely indicated the presence of grant funding and not the total number of grants. Thus, a "1" in the "Grants" column indicated *at least* one grant. A "0"

indicates no grants, and numbers greater than 1 indicate multiple grants.

There are two worksheets provided in Appendix B, allowing you to explore different areas of interest. If you have more than two main areas of interest, unless they are closely related, you may find the list becoming exceptionally long. In that case, you may wish either to narrow your areas of interest or to complete this worksheet with the aid of a trusted professor who can help you pare down the list of schools to a more manageable number. If you have more than one area of interest, put stars next to the schools that have faculty doing research in both of them.

If your interests lean toward research, then you want to pick a school highly regarded in the area of research you would like to pursue. How do you evaluate the clinical and counseling psychology programs on your list in terms of research? Refer to Table 3-2, which is adapted from the results of the *Social Sciences Citation Index* (SSCI) and *Science Citation Index* (SCI) databases. More than 225 psychology journals from 1998 to 2002 were analyzed to determine the institutions with the most citations. The goal was to identify the institutions employing faculty members who authored the most frequently referenced articles in psychology journals. The table lists, in rank order, the frequency with which articles written by members of a particular institution are cited. Only those institutions with an APA-accredited clinical or counseling program are included on this list. It should also be noted that the list only includes those institutions that produced at least 100 papers over the 5-year span; as a result, several smaller institutions with clinical or counseling psychology programs did not make the list.

Using Table 3-2, write the citation ranking for each school in column 5, labeled "Citation Rank." Be advised that this ranking reflects the psychology department in general, not just the clinical or counseling program. In fact, about 20% of the institutions on the original list of 75 were deleted because they do not have clinical or counseling psychology programs. Inclusion of these nonclinical influences will affect the ranking of the schools you have selected. Still, this will provide you with a rough idea of where each school stands in terms of its research. Our position is that a school that makes it onto this list is probably a strong research-oriented institution. If the school fails to appear on the table, then it may or may not emphasize psychological research. Recognize that only about 20% of APA-accredited programs appear on this list.

Table 3-2 also contains a column headed "Faculty Production Rank." This number represents the rank ordering of APA-accredited clinical psychology programs on the basis of the total number of clinical faculty members trained by that program (Ilardi, Rodriguez-Hanley, Roberts, & Seigel, 2000). Any program that received a ranking in the top 60 has an established track record of producing clinical psychologists who, themselves, later assumed clinical psychology faculty positions. Remember that these lists heavily favor older programs and that no single measure can ever capture the excellence of graduate education. And, again, only about 20% of APA-accredited clinical programs appear on the list. Still, the list does direct students interested in academic careers to programs that have historically excelled in this domain.

As mentioned, any APA-accredited program must provide both clinical and research training. Thus, it is important also to evaluate the clinical opportunities available. As already mentioned, Psy.D. programs by definition emphasize practice and train students to be practitioners. Although it is possible to obtain research training at a Psy.D. program, this is not the primary emphasis of such programs. Consequently, a student with a clear research orientation should probably choose a Ph.D. program. For the research oriented, this column will be used to cross schools off their application list. Look up each school on your list in the reports on individual programs. If any of these schools offer only Psy.D. programs (see Table 1-4), you can delete that program.

The first column under the "Clinical" section of Appendix B is marked "Orientation." Under each program listed in our reports on individual programs, you will see a list of five theoretical orientations:

- Psychodynamic/psychoanalytic
- Radical behavioral/applied behavioral analysis
- Systems/family systems
- Humanistic/existential
- Cognitive/cognitive-behavioral

If you are clearly committed to (or strongly leaning toward) one of these particular orientations, then it is important that some faculty share that orientation with you. Check each program on your list and see if a suitable percentage of the faculty shares your orientation. If so, mark the "Orientation" column with a "+" sign. If not, mark it with a "–" sign.

If you are unsure of an orientation, or see yourself as integrative or eclectic, then be sure there is a wide variety of faculty orientations. If there is representation among the faculty in four or more of these orientations, that's a good sign. If the total you get when adding up all the percentages in the different orientations is greater than 100%, this is also a plus. It means some (or most)

of the faculty bridge orientations and are integrative themselves. In other words, professors are listed under more than one category. In either case, mark the "Orientation" column with a "+" sign. If the faculty are of one or two orientations and without overlap, then mark this column with a "–" sign.

The second column under "Clinical" is "Res/Clin." Turn to Appendix F, "Specialty Clinics and Practica Sites." This is a list of specialty clinics and practica available at different schools. Specialty clinics focus on and have available to them a specific clientele, such as depressed or eating-disordered clients. Practica are placements where students will conduct clinical work in their second, third, and/or fourth years of study. Some practica also specialize in a certain clientele. If you have a research interest in a particular population, it is important that the population be available for you to study and that you have the chance to work with that population clinically in order to broaden your understanding of them. For this reason, it may be important for a researcher to have a specialty clinic or practicum in his or her area.

Look up your research area in Appendix F. If any of the schools on your list in Appendix B has a clinic or practicum in that area, mark the "Res/Clin" column with a plus.

Again, this is just one indicator and must be kept in perspective. Most programs will have their own psychological training clinic, where a wide range of clinical populations may be seen or made available for research. Additionally, a faculty member may have a research population readily available in the community. And last, a few programs did not include practica placements off campus in the community, thus underrepresenting their practica opportunities. Still, being informed about a clinic or practicum specializing in your population of interest is certainly an advantage in selecting potential graduate programs.

The third column under the "Clinical" section is marked "Rank." Here, we can refer to a program's production of students who go on to distinguished careers as clinicians, as measured by becoming ABPP Diplomates and by election as Fellows in APA's Division of Clinical Psychology or Division of Counseling Psychology. The "ABPP" refers to diplomate status awarded by the American Board of Professional Psychology (www.abpp.org), which certifies excellence in 13 fields of psychology, including clinical psychology and counseling psychology. Applicants for ABPP must have at least 5 years of postdoctoral experience, submit examples of their clinical work, and pass an oral examination. The entrance requirements and performance standards are more rigorous than those involved in licensure and

TABLE 3-2. Institutions with Most Citations, Most Papers, and Strongest Clinical Faculty Production in Psychology

Citation rank	Institution[a]	Citations	Papers	Faculty production rank
2	University of Michigan	3,999	816	3
4	University of Minnesota	3,231	741	4
5	University of California–Los Angeles	3,211	867	9
6	University of Wisconsin–Madison	2,901	652	5.5
7	University of Illinois at Urbana–Champaign	2,856	690	1
8	Yale University	2,816	585	18.5
9	University of Pittsburgh	2,555	542	10
10	University of Pennsylvania	2,514	582	29
11	Indiana University	2,387	667	7.5
12	University of Washington	2,362	619	13.5
13	Duke University	2,344	453	18.5
14	Pennsylvania State University	2,302	766	11.5
15	University of California–San Diego	2,220	504	—
16	Ohio State University	2,177	617	22
17	Columbia University	2,170	652	29
18	University of Texas at Austin	2,085	551	7.5
19	University of Missouri	2,019	625	26
20	University of Iowa	1,968	495	34.5
21	University of Arizona	1,950	412	—
22	Northwestern University	1,935	449	48.5
23	University of North Carolina at Chapel Hill	1,933	468	31.5
24	University of Maryland College Park	1,921	546	48.5
26	Rutgers State University	1,872	473	18.5
27	University of California–Berkeley	1,862	436	34.5
29	University of Colorado	1,846	476	53.5
30	University of Rochester	1,817	292	15.5
31	New York University	1,775	503	34.5
32	Arizona State University	1,701	526	53.5
33	Vanderbilt University	1,658	340	13.5
34	University of Virginia	1,612	332	—
35	Boston University	1,573	369	—
36	University of Florida	1,498	537	18.5

continued

represent excellence in applied psychology. Fellowship in APA is based on evidence of unusual and outstanding performance in psychology.

One study (Robyak & Goodyear, 1984) investigated the graduate school origins of ABPP Diplomates and APA Fellows in clinical and counseling psychology.

Although older and larger doctoral programs are obviously favored in such a historical study, the results nonetheless give some indication of institutional reputation and their graduates' accomplishments. Table 3-3 presents the top 25 institutional origins of clinical psychology diplomates and fellows as well as the top

TABLE 3-2. Continued

Citation rank	Institution[a]	Citations	Papers	Faculty production rank
38	Emory University	1,470	325	—
39	University of Southern California	1,446	447	34.5
40	Purdue University	1,436	521	22
42	University of Oregon	1,401	241	26
43	University of Georgia	1,362	462	5.5
44	Michigan State University	1,355	411	31.5
45	University of Connecticut	1,308	407	29
48	State University of New York at Buffalo	1,252	322	38
49	Texas A&M University	1,244	399	—
50	Florida State University	1,237	353	22
51	University of Illinois at Chicago	1,231	350	58
52	Washington University	1,224	279	42.5
53	University of Massachusetts at Amherst	1,146	314	42.5
54	City University of New York	1,131	434	48.5
55	University of Miami	1,122	317	58
56	State University of New York at Stony Brook	1,056	285	2
57	University of California–Santa Barbara	1,041	275	—
58	Iowa State University	970	238	—
59	University of Kentucky	970	261	—
60	University of Kansas	944	384	15.5
61	Case Western Reserve University	928	222	—
62	University of Utah	916	256	38
63	University of Alabama	912	381	48.5
67	University of Nebraska	822	354	58
68	Louisiana State University	814	287	42.5
69	Wayne State University	775	281	53.5
71	University of Delaware	669	189	—
72	University of New Mexico	635	173	—
74	Washington State University	626	211	—
75	Yeshiva University	619	158	—

Note. Adapted from 1998–2002 *Social Sciences Citation Index* (SSCI) and *Science Citation Index* (SCI) databases. Also adapted from Ilardi, Rodriguez-Hanley, Roberts, & Seigel (2000).

[a]Institutions without APA-accredited programs in clinical or counseling psychology have been omitted from this table.

12 institutional origins of counseling psychology diplomates and fellows. Clinical psychology diplomates graduated from 153 different universities; fellows from 92. Counseling psychology diplomates graduated from 55 universities; fellows from 46.

If a school is listed in Table 3-3, place a "+" in the "Rank" column in the "Clinical" section. Though many schools not listed on this table provide fine clinical training, this listing indicates that the program is outstanding in terms of its track record for producing excellent professional psychologists.

Finally, there is a column in Appendix B marked "Self-Rating." The first question we asked each program to answer was, "On a 7-point scale, how research or

TABLE 3-3. Institutional Origins of Clinical and Counseling Psychology Diplomates and Fellows

University	Rank order	
	Diplomates	Fellows
Clinical psychology		
New York University	1	2
Columbia University	2	1
University of Chicago	3	3
University of California–Los Angeles	4	14
University of Michigan	5.5	9
University of Iowa	5.5	5
University of Minnesota	7	6
Northwestern University	8	7.5
University of California–Berkeley	9	15.5
Harvard University	10	7.5
Pennsylvania State University	11	17.5
Purdue University	12.5	—
Boston University	12.5	17.5
Ohio State University	14	4
University of Washington	15	5.5
University of Southern California	16	11.5
Duke University	18	—
Stanford University	18	10
University of Texas	18	—
University of Pittsburgh	20	11.5
University of Kansas	21	—
Case Western Reserve University	23.5	—
University of Illinois at Urbana–Champaign	23.5	—
Yale University	23.5	13
University of Pennsylvania	23.5	—
Counseling psychology		
Columbia University	1	2
Ohio State University	2	3
University of Minnesota	3	1
New York University	4	4.5
University of Michigan	5	—
University of Chicago	6	8
Stanford University	7	7
University of Iowa	8	7
University of Texas	9.5	—
University of Wisconsin	9.5	—
Catholic University	11.5	—
Harvard University	11.5	4.5

Note. From Robyak & Goodyear (1984). © 1984 American Psychological Association. Reprinted by permission.

clinically oriented would you rate your program?" (1 = clinical emphasis; 4 = equal emphasis; and 7 = research emphasis). You will find the school's rating of itself under each individual listing in the reports on individual programs sections. Mark this number under the "Self-Rating" column.

What you now have before you is a list of programs that offer research in your area of interest. You also have the number of faculty in the area that you might work with and whether they presently have grant funding. Finally, you have an approximate rank of that school's research standing.

In clinical terms, you have some sense of whether that school will conform to your theoretical orientation, whether it has special clinical training in your area of interest, how it ranks in terms of producing outstanding clinicians, and whether it rates itself as emphasizing practice or research.

Given the information before you, you may already want to begin crossing programs off your list. If you're research oriented, and the program is a Psy.D. program or rates itself a 1, 2, or 3 (meaning it is practice oriented), you may choose to delete that school. Alternatively, if your interests reflect equal research and clinical emphasis and you lean toward a psychodynamic orientation, you may want to cross off a school that rates itself as a 7 (very research oriented) or whose faculty is 100% behavioral.

Your revised list of schools can probably satisfy your research and clinical interests. In addition, you have the start of a ranking system, which at this point gives you a rough idea of how well each school conforms to your interests and needs. Unfortunately, this provides you with only half of the information you need to begin writing to schools. The second part of this process asks, "How close do you come to the standards they specify?" This is covered in a later section entitled "Assessing School Criteria."

For the Practice Oriented

This section gives guidance to those applicants who are more centrally focused on psychological practice. These applicants will want to begin to choose their programs based on their theoretical orientation and the availability of clinical opportunities.

The first thing that you will want to do is turn to Table 1-4, which lists all the APA-accredited Psy.D. programs. With this list, turn to Appendix B, "Worksheet for Choosing Schools." Under the column marked "School," write the names of the programs found in Table 1-4.

In addition to these programs, you may have a specific population in mind that you are especially eager to work with. Perhaps you already have a sense that you want to work specifically with patients suffering from, say, anxiety disorders. In this case, turn to Appendix F. This appendix, "Specialty Clinics and Practica Sites," lists several sorts of specialty clinics or practica areas available at different schools. Specialty clinics focus on and have available to them a specific clientele, such as depressed or eating-disordered clients. As mentioned in the previous section, practica are placements where a student will conduct clinical work in his or her second, third, and/or fourth year of study, and some practica also specialize in treating a certain clientele. For a practice-oriented student, it would be especially desirable to be in a program with a specialty clinic in his or her particular area of treatment interest. Therefore, write down the names of programs with specialty clinics or practica in your area of interest on your list in Appendix B.

A word of caution is in order. Most programs will have their own psychology training clinic where a wide range of clinical populations may be seen or made available for research. Practica may also be available in a wide range of settings in the community, providing fertile ground for a rich clinical experience. Still, a clinic or practicum specializing in a population that is of special interest to you is a definite plus and an additional piece of information on which to base your decision. If a program both offers a Psy.D. and has a specialty clinic in your area, put a star next to it.

The next important column for the clinically oriented applicant is marked "Orientation." In the reports on individual programs, you will find each school listed, along with information pertaining to its program. Among that information, you will see a list of five theoretical orientations, followed by the percentage of the faculty that subscribes to that orientation:

- Psychodynamic/psychoanalytic
- Radical behavioral/applied behavioral analysis
- Systems/family systems
- Humanistic/existential
- Cognitive/cognitive-behavioral

If you are clearly committed to (or strongly leaning toward) one of these particular orientations, then it is important that some portion of the faculty share that orientation with you. Check each program on your list and determine if a suitable percentage of the faculty shares your orientation. If so, mark the "Orientation" column with a "+" sign; if not, mark it with a "−" sign.

If you are unsure of your orientation or see yourself as integrative or eclectic, then be sure there is a wide variety of faculty orientations. If there is representation among the faculty in four of these orientations, that's a good sign. If the total you obtain after adding up all the percentages in the different areas is greater than 100%, this is also advantageous. It means some (or most) of the faculty bridge orientations and are eclectic themselves. In either case, mark the "Orientation" column with a "+" sign. If you're eclectic and the faculty are of one or two orientations and do not overlap, then mark this column with a "−" sign.

The next column is marked "Res/Clin." As we mentioned previously, even if you are looking for a practice oriented program, you still will have to do research: a lengthy professional paper or a clinical dissertation at the very least! Consequently, it is important that someone in your program is conducting research in an area that interests you. With this in mind, look through Appendix E and find the area(s) of research that you find interesting. Under each area, you will find a list of schools that have researchers in that field. If any of the schools on your list in Appendix B is listed here, place a "+" in the column marked "Res/Clin."

The third column under "Clinical" is marked "Rank." Here, we can refer to a program's production of students who go on to distinguished careers as clinicians, as imperfectly measured by their becoming ABPP Diplomates and by their election as Fellows in APA's Division of Clinical Psychology and Division of Counseling Psychology. The "ABPP" refers to diplomate status awarded by the American Board of Professional Psychology (www.abpp.org), which certifies excellence in 13 fields of psychology, including clinical psychology and counseling psychology. Applicants for ABPP must have at least 5 years of postdoctoral experience, submit examples of their clinical work, and pass an oral examination. The entrance requirements and performance standards are more rigorous than those involved in licensing and represent excellence in applied psychology. The APA Fellowship is based on evidence of unusual and outstanding performance.

One study (Robyak & Goodyear, 1984) investigated the graduate school origins of ABPP Diplomates and APA Fellows in clinical and counseling psychology. Although older and larger doctoral programs are obviously favored in such a historical study, the results nonetheless give some indication of institutional reputation and their graduates' accomplishments. Table 3-3 presents the top 25 institutional origins of these diplomates and fellows as well as the top 12 institutional origins of counseling psychology diplomates and fel-

lows. Because this list indicates programs that have historically produced outstanding clinicians, place a "+" in this column for any program included in Table 3-3. Though many schools not listed in this table offer fine clinical training, the list provides an indication of the Ph.D. programs (Psy.D. programs are too new to be listed) that are likely to offer the sort of clinical training you seek.

Finally, there is a column in Appendix B marked "Self-Rating." In the reports on individual programs you will find each school's rating of itself (1 = clinical emphasis; 4 = equal emphasis; and 7 = research emphasis). Mark this number under the "Self-Rating" column. Though Psy.D. programs are practice oriented by definition, they vary on how much research they expect their students to conduct. Thus, their ratings will allow you to guide your expectations of what each program will expect of you. This self-rating will also help you avoid a Ph.D. program with a specialty clinic in your area that is clearly research oriented.

What you now have before you is a list of programs that are practice oriented and/or that offer a specialty clinic or practica in your area of interest. You have some sense of whether these schools will conform to your theoretical orientation and whether they have ongoing research in your area of clinical interest. You also have their self-rating of the program's emphasis on clinical work or research.

Given the information on your worksheet, you may already want to begin crossing programs off your list. If you're practice oriented and a Ph.D. program offers a specialty clinic in your area but rates itself with a 6 or 7 (very research oriented), you may choose to delete that school. Alternatively, if you're very behaviorally oriented, you may want to cross off a school where 100% of the faculty is psychodynamic/psychoanalytic.

Your revised list of schools can provide you with practice oriented training and possibly special clinical training in your population of choice. In addition, you have the start of a ranking system that at this point gives you a rough idea of how well each school conforms to your interests and needs. Unfortunately, this only provides you with half the information you need to begin writing to schools. The second half of this process is related to how closely you come to the specified standards of these programs. This is covered in the "Assessing School Criteria" section.

For the Racial/Ethnic Minority Applicant

Before continuing to the assessment of program criteria, it is important to discuss the special case of minority applications. "Minority" in this context primarily refers to racial or ethnic background, although with women comprising 70% of all doctoral students in psychology (Pate, 2001), a few graduate student programs are starting to treat men as minority applicants. Ethnic minority students now account for 21% of master's students in psychology and 27% of doctoral students in psychology (Norcross, Kohout, & Wicherski, in press).

Nearly every APA-accredited program makes special efforts to recruit minority applicants (Munoz-Dunbar & Stanton, 1999), recognizing the need in our society for well-trained minority professionals. Typical methods for recruiting underrepresented groups to clinical and counseling psychology programs are offers of financial aid, the use of personal contacts, visits to other schools, use of APA's Minority Undergraduate Students of Excellence (MUSE) program, special events, reimbursements of application fees, and preferential screening (Steinpreis et al., 1992). Programs often make an extra effort to review minority applications to ensure that qualified candidates are given appropriate consideration.

In fact, a study of Vail-model professional psychology programs revealed that 82% of them implemented formal minority admissions policies designed to improve racial representation (Young & VandeCreek, 1996). The study found that:

- 94% of the programs gave extra points on ratings of application materials to minority applicants;
- 69% of the programs waived or lowered GRE scores for minority applicants;
- 41% of the programs waived or lowered GPA cutoffs for minority applicants; and
- 21% of the programs interviewed all minority applicants, regardless of the quality of their application materials.

As a consequence, ethnic minorities in the applicant pool are significantly more likely than whites to receive offers of admission (Munoz-Dunbar & Stanton, 1999). The generic guidelines and the following worksheets in this *Insider's Guide* may thus not accurately reflect a minority applicant's enhanced chances of acceptance. We recommend that you carefully read program descriptions regarding their minority selection procedures and encourage you to apply to programs that are within reach of your credentials.

Several ethnic/racial minority students have written to us over the years and complained that they were neither actively recruited nor accepted for admission into the doctoral psychology programs to which they had applied. So let us be perfectly clear and honest: Most, but not all, doctoral programs have implemented

policies (as reviewed above) to recruit and admit underrepresented racial/ethnic minority students. However, that does not mean that all programs will be knocking down your door to interview you. Nor does that mean that most programs will finance your interview. Nor does that mean acceptance is a certainty. Doctoral programs will evaluate all candidates on their GPAs, GREs, letters of recommendation, research experiences, and so on. A modest advantage is just that—an advantage, never a guarantee.

Both the American Psychological Association and the American Psychological Society are committed to ensuring that the practice of psychology—and the production of psychologists—is in the vanguard of addressing the needs of culturally diverse populations. The APA's Commission on Ethnic Minority Recruitment, Retention, and Training in Psychology produces several valuable publications in this regard. Contact the APA to obtain copies of these informative publications, notably the free guidebook, *For College Students of Color Applying to Graduate & Professional Programs.* Also consult the Web site of *Project 1000,* a national program created to assist students of color applying to graduate school (mati.eas.asu.edu:8421/p1000).

Although the special consideration given minority applicants is advantageous, it also represents a special challenge. One well-qualified minority student we knew was advised by a university career counselor that he would have no problem getting into the school of his choice. He applied to several very competitive programs, and received acceptances and offers of financial aid across the board. Unfortunately, he skipped the process of matching his interests with the strengths of the program. After 1 year, he was looking to transfer to another program that had more faculty conducting research and psychotherapy in his areas of interest.

The moral of the story is: Don't let the potential advantage of being a minority candidate become a disadvantage. Just because you can get into a program doesn't mean that it is the best program for you. A rigorous approach to the application process is the best approach for everyone.

For the LGBT Applicant

Lesbian, gay, bisexual, and transgendered (LGBT) applicants to doctoral programs can face the same social and interpersonal hurdles (or potential advantages) as ethnic/racial minority applicants. There is, however, a key difference: There are limited federal protections for members of the LGBT community, and though some states offer equal access and protection, others do not. This fact may lead lesbian, gay, bisexual, and transgendered students to question whether to disclose their sexual orientation ("come out") in the application process, or even to inquire about the atmosphere of inclusivity toward sexual minorities within a particular program or school. In this section, we review some research and advice on LGBT applicants' selection of graduate programs and present potential strategies for those who elect to come out during the application process.

Qualitative research (e.g., Lark & Croteau, 1998; Rader, 2000) indicates that LGBT psychology students screen prospective graduate schools for their gay affirming (or at least, nonhomophobic) position. The typical criteria used for screening prospective programs were (Biaggio et al., 2003):

- Reports of other LGBT students
- Presence of faculty who were openly lesbian/gay or heterosexual allies
- Availability of specific training on LGBT issues and opportunity to work with LGBT clients
- Sensitivity to diversity issues on campus (including the presence of LGBT support and advocacy groups)
- Geographic location of the program (frequently avoiding programs in rural settings)
- Size of the educational institution (larger public institutions being relatively more liberal)

In addition, we recommend that LGBT students screen prospective programs by

- searching departmental or university homepages for the presence of an LGBT student union, faculty actively teaching and researching on sexuality, and specific housing policies for LGBT couples (remember, though legally married in one state, another state may not recognize your gay marriage or civil union, and the university may not be legally bound to provide equal access to "married" housing).
- seeking programs with curricula that explicitly integrate LGBT and other diversity issues.
- reviewing the APA's list of graduate faculty in psychology interested in lesbian and gay issues (available at www.apa.org/pi/lgbc/lgbsurvey/).
- examining the psychology department's contacts with the LGBT community in clinical and outreach services, including practica.
- evaluating the university's mission statement for a formal commitment to diversity of sexual orientation.
- considering the state laws concerning equitable treatment of LGBT, such as civil unions, domestic partnership, adoption, health insurance for partners, and the like.

Homophobia and heterosexism continue to exist in the United States and, unfortunately, also in institutions of higher education. Although the situation has improved considerably in recent decades, some institutions remain "tolerant" as opposed to "affirming" of sexual diversity, whereas other institutions may favor an LGBT student to maintain or expand program diversity. The question, then, is whether to come out during the application process. On one side, there is the risk of being rejected from a program where some level of discrimination may exist. On the other side, there is the potential advantage of being a member of a minority group in a program that actively pursues diversity. In either case, the alternative to not coming out during the application process is to come out later, or to try to hide your sexual orientation for 4 to 6 years.

If and when to disclose sexual orientation in the admissions process is ultimately a personal decision, and it can occur at different stages in the process: in the application, during the interview, upon acceptance to the program, or upon the decision to attend the program. As part of your application, you can indicate your sexual orientation in your research interests (e.g., lesbian health issues), clinical experiences (e.g., working with gay youth), and/or extracurricular activities (e.g., member of the LGBT alliance on campus). More directly, you can incorporate your sexual identity into your personal statement, especially if it has bearing on your choice of clinical or research work, or your decision to pursue clinical psychology as a career. If you do come out in your personal statement, be sure that this fact is integrated into the overall statement and not simply a dangling fact unconnected to the rest of what you've written.

One of the authors came out during the interview process with a simple but straightforward statement: "As a gay man, it's important to me to be in a gay-friendly environment. Would being gay be an issue in this program?" Though it would be a mistake to over-generalize, this statement was uniformly met with positive responses about program diversity and discussions of specific resources for LGBT students. Had it been met otherwise, it would have served as a key piece of information in the decision process. Another strategy is to raise sexual orientation at the point at which an offer of admission is tendered. As discussed in subsequent chapters, once an offer is made, an applicant has some latitude in negotiating issues around admission, tuition remission, funding, etc. This can be a point to indicate that having a gay-affirmative environment is one of the factors in your decision of which program to accept and to inquire about the atmosphere in that program. Still other LGBT students elect not to disclose until they are actually matriculated in the program and have begun coursework.

Whatever path you decide to take, your sexual orientation should not be the defining issue of your application; your composite strengths as a potential doctoral student remain the center of your application.

Assessing School Criteria

Assessing the criteria clinical and counseling psychology programs use to evaluate applicants is an important step in the process of applying to graduate school. To illuminate this point, we will relate the story of one applicant we knew several years ago. She was an Ivy League graduate, a 3.8 psychology major, who had conducted research with a prominent psychologist. She had fine letters of recommendation and some clinical experience with developmentally disabled children, but her GREs were in the low 500s. Thinking that her credentials were excellent, she applied to the most competitive research programs and one practice-oriented program. She was rejected across the board at these top research schools and just barely made it into what she had mistakenly considered her practice-oriented "safety school." Her mistake was to ignore the fact that all the research-oriented schools to which she applied specified minimum GRE scores of 600 or more. Her application was unsuccessful because she ignored one piece of information each school had indicated to be essential. She was nearly rejected in the more practice-oriented program she had felt was a "sure thing" because she did not have the clinical experience they were looking for. And she was lucky that that particular doctoral program did not have GRE requirements beyond her range!

The moral of the story is twofold: (1) Attend closely to the admission standards of each program. If a school sets standards you cannot realistically meet, you need to work very, very hard to get them to make an exception. In other words, think twice about applying there. (2) Apply to programs with a range of admission criteria, and consider a safety school as one that announces admission requirements that you exceed by a wide margin. This does not guarantee acceptance, but does dramatically increase the probability of making it into their finalist pool.

Now, turn your attention to Appendix C, "Worksheet for Assessing Program Criteria." In Appendix C,

you will rate yourself on how well you conform to each school's admission requirements. The aim is that you not waste time and money applying to programs that indicate in no uncertain terms that you do not meet their criteria. There is no reason to feel inadequate because you fall short of these specifications. There may be programs on your list with requirements you do meet or exceed. If you are unable to meet the minimum requirements of any schools on your list, you should seriously consider taking time off to better prepare yourself or applying to less competitive master's programs.

Begin by transferring the name of each school from Appendix B to the "School" column of Appendix C. Simply copy the list from one table to the other. Also copy the number in the "Self-Rating" column from one worksheet to the other. Next, look up the first school on your list in the reports on individual programs. Read through all the information provided just to start familiarizing yourself with that program.

As you begin filling out Appendix C and listing each school's admission criteria, remember that these are simply indications of your strength as an applicant to each school. These scales are not set in stone and do not guarantee that you will be accepted. You may not readily fall into any of the categories listed and will have to make some rough approximations for yourself. Or you may find that you fall between categories and have to add 0.5 point here or subtract 0.5 point there. If you think it is appropriate to modify the categories or scoring systems, by all means do so. *The most important result is not an absolute number but a relative sense of how well you meet each program's admission criteria.*

You may also find that a school does not require certain test scores, or gives no mean GRE scores, or doesn't have preferred or mandatory courses. In this case, simply score a "0" in the appropriate column. When it comes time to total each school's score, this will neither detract from nor add to your ability to meet their requirements.

Now, go to the respective Reports on Individual Programs and look at the prerequisite courses. You will see two questions pertaining to course preparation prior to applying: "What courses are required for incoming students to have completed prior to enrolling?" and "Are there courses you recommend that are not mandatory?" Underneath each question you will find a list of courses that the particular school assigned to each category. On your list in Appendix C, under the column marked "Courses," score yourself as follows (in this table, "M" indicates "mandatory" and "R" indicates "recommended"):

+2 You have taken all the M and R courses and earned B+ or better in them all.

+1 You have taken all the M courses and/or several of the R courses and earned B+ or better.

0 You have taken all the M courses, but none of the Rs, or earned B– or lower in some M courses.

1 You have not taken one or two of the M courses, or have earned B– or lower in several of them.

–2 You have not taken several or any of the M courses or have received C or lower in some of the M or R courses.

The next section on each "Program" page is marked GREs and GPA. This section gives mean scores for the GREs and GPAs for each program listed.

On your list, under the columns marked "GRE-V" (verbal), "GRE-Q" (quantitative), and "GRE-S" (psychology subject test), score yourself as follows:

+2 You exceed the school's M score by at least 100 points.

+1 You exceed the school's M score by more than 50 but less than 100 points.

0 You meet the school's M minimum or exceed it by less than 50 points.

1 You do not meet the school's M score, but are less than 100 points below it.

–2 You are below the M score by 100 points or more.

For GPA, we asked programs for the mean score of their incoming class and asked if that applied to more than one type of GPA. It is not uncommon for programs to look at cumulative or overall GPA (all undergraduate courses taken), psychology GPA (only psychology courses), and junior/ senior GPA (all courses taken in the last 2 years of college). Again, it is wise to review the average GPA of incoming students when you receive the information packets from the various schools. Under the column marked "GPA," score yourself as follows:

+2 You exceed the school's M GPA by 0.5 points or more.

+1 You exceed the school's M GPA by less than 0.5 points.

0 You meet the school's M GPA.

1 You do not meet the school's M GPA, but are less than 0.2 below it.

–2 You are below the school's M by more than 0.5 points.

Next, look back to the second column of Appendix C, "Self-Rating." This is how the program rates itself on the practice–research continuum. If a program emphasizes one more than the other, this gives some indication of what it would consider important in an applicant. A school that stresses research will probably desire an applicant to have some amount of research experience. Under the "Research" column in Appendix C, rate yourself as follows:

+2 The school rates itself as a 6 or a 7 and you will have completed an honors thesis or will have at least 2 years of experience in psychology research.

+1 The school rates itself as a 4, 5, 6, or 7 and you will have at least 1 year of experience in psychology research.

0 The school rates itself as a 1, 2, or 3.

1 The school rates itself as a 4 or 5, and you have no research experience.

–2 The school rates itself as a 6 or 7, and you have no research experience.

Similarly, a program emphasizing clinical work will prefer that an applicant enter with some practical experience in human services or health care. Under the "Clinical" column, rate yourself as follows:

+2 The school rates itself as a 1 or a 2, and you will have worked in a full-time (35+ hr./week) clinical position for at least 1 year.

+1 The school rates itself as a 1, 2, 3, or 4 and you will have volunteered part-time (8+ hr./week) at a clinical facility for at least 1 year.

0 The school rates itself as a 5, 6, or 7.

1 The school rates itself as a 3 or 4, and you have no clinical experience.

–2 The school rates itself as a 1 or 2, and you have no clinical experience.

At this point, you should have completed the first nine columns of Appendix C from "School" to "Clinical."

Additional information provided for each program in the Reports on Individual Programs are "How many applications were received in 2005?," "How many applicants were given an admission offer in 2005?," and "How many admitted students are incoming?" These give a rough estimate of the competitiveness of a program.

You may be amazed at how high this ratio can become. The average acceptance rates at freestanding Psy.D. programs is now 50% (Norcross et al., in press). In applying to programs, be realistic and reasonable. You may have a sterling application, but when Yale accepts roughly 1 in 50 applicants, you had best be applying to other places as well.

Bear in mind: Programs accept more applicants than actually end up attending. This makes programs appear more restrictive than they actually are. This is why we added the third item regarding the number of students who will enter the program—a number invariably smaller than the number of accepted students. For example, an applicant gaining acceptance to five places will ultimately reject four schools. A program planning on an incoming class of six students will accept more than six before gaining their new class. Nonetheless, apply to several schools with a range of competitiveness as a precautionary measure.

In the column marked "Compete" in Appendix C, record the ratio of applications to acceptances. It should be noted that competitiveness is difficult to quantify. Although we have selected the ratio of applicants to acceptances as our measure, other relevant criteria include test scores and GPA. Since we have already discussed these criteria, we are using this opportunity to highlight yet another area related to competitiveness.

The last column is marked "Total." Add the numbers under the "Courses," "GRE-V," "GRE-Q," "GRE-S," "GPA," "Research," and "Clinical" columns. This will provide you with a total somewhere between −14 and +14, which is a rough indication of how well you meet each school's admission requirements and expectations.

Now you have a grand list of programs that are performing research or clinical work in the areas you have specified. In addition, you have several indications of how well each school will address your needs and expectations as a graduate student. Finally, you have a rating of yourself as an applicant to each program.

The best way to begin your decision-making process is to select the programs that have admission requirements within your reach. As you look through the "school requirements" part of your list, note any −2s. Unless you can reasonably expect to change these to zeros or better before you complete your applications, you are better off dropping these programs from your list. After that, you will then have to decide for yourself what are reasonable places to apply.

Below is a rating system based on your "Total" column for each school. Although this system may help you decide where to write for information, it is by no means definitive. *These are rough approximations*, and ultimately you will have to decide where to apply based on this and any other information to which you are privy. From the "Total" column of Appendix C, evaluate each program as follows:

10 to 14 Your chances are very good. Apply to many of these schools, since your application may be especially strong here.

6 to 9 Your chances are good. These schools are within your reach, as you exceed several of the credentials they value.

4 to 5 Your chances are moderately good here, but be sure to apply to some schools where you rank more highly.

0 to 3 These schools are within your range of abilities. Your application may not be outstanding, but it is somewhere between "adequate" and "more than adequate." Be sure also to apply to several schools in a higher range.

1 to −4 These schools are a stretch for you. Go ahead and apply to a few, but the bulk of your applications should go to schools on which you achieved a higher score.

< −4 These schools are looking for something different from your experience or performance at this time. If you really wish to attend a school in this range, take time off or attend a master's program to bolster your research, clinical, and academic performance.

Although this worksheet embodies many of the relevant criteria used by admissions committees, it of course cannot integrate all possible criteria. If a professor has expressed interest in working with you, for example, the worksheet total may underestimate your chances for acceptance. Other useful resources when selecting your list of schools include specific professors, undergraduate psychology advisors, and bulletin boards in the psychology building that display postgraduate brochures. Graduate students at your local university can also be helpful, and a few large universities have even created notebooks on clinical and counseling psychology graduate programs (Todd & Farinato, 1992). Take advantage of all the information available to you to augment the data provided in the Reports on Individual Programs.

Using the system in Appendix C, delete some of the schools that have admission criteria outside of your present range. This will enable you to begin the next phase: selecting programs that match your expectations in terms of the training you desire.

678 Wilmington Drive
Derby, NY 14047

September 3, 2006

Director of Admissions
Department of Psychology
Bogus University
1234 Monument Square
Upstate, NY 14000

Dear Sir or Madam:

I am interested in applying to your Ph.D. (Psy.D.) program in clinical (counseling) psychology for the fall of 2007. Please send me an application and any information you have available concerning your program. Kindly include financial aid information as well.

Thank you for your time and consideration.

Sincerely yours,

Chris Smith

FIGURE 3-1. Sample letter (or e-mail) requesting application and information.

For the research-oriented applicant, these decisions may be easiest. Look at the schools remaining on your worksheet. Note the number of faculty interested in your research area(s) and whether any of them are funded. Grant funding is a rough indicator of the intensity of the program's commitment to a particular research area. The premise is that a grant-funded area may offer more opportunities to study the issue and may be more likely to generate research. In addition, grant funding has the potential of making assistantship money available. This by no means suggests that a program that does not have a grant in your area is not conducting current research or will not have money available to you. Additionally, a program with several faculty in an area may simply be "between" grants. Thus, the number of faculty alone also can indicate a school's commitment to this area of research.

Next, check the program's productivity ranking and their self-rating as being more practice or research oriented. Again, if you are more research oriented, you may well find yourself crossing those schools off your list that are low on productivity and that are clearly

clinically oriented. You are going to find that this shortens your list but that you still have a number of schools that cover a wide range of desirability. This is exactly where you want to be at this point! What you desire is a list of 15 to 30 schools for which you will secure additional information. Then, you can begin fine-tuning and selecting the 10 to 20 schools to which you will actually apply.

If you are more strongly oriented toward practice, you will find yourself crossing schools off your list that are research oriented, favor theoretical orientations different from your own, or are too restricted for your needs. The schools highlighting clinical work, and especially those sharing your orientation or providing a specialty clinic or practicum in your area, will be the most desirable.

The applicant who equally emphasizes practice and research training is the most challenged. You want a program that is research oriented, but not at the cost of clinical work. But you also want a program that will offer high-quality clinical training without sacrificing high standards in research. Using your list, find the programs that are moderate or high in productivity and that have a number of people interested in your area. Check to see that they rate themselves as a 4 or 5, indicating that they emphasize clinical and research work nearly equally. Then, check to see if their theoretical orientation conforms to your own and whether they have a specialty clinic or practicum in your area. Again, you are going to find a range of schools, some conforming to your needs better than others. This is exactly what you want at this point in the process.

You are now ready to gather the detailed information necessary to choose among the 15 to 30 programs you will use for your selection pool. If your number of schools does not fall within these parameters, you should consider modifying your list. The Web site, mailing address, and e-mail address of each program are listed with each entry in the Reports on Individual Programs. At this point, all you need is to spend a few hours on the Web. Research demonstrates that Web sites provide more information about graduate programs than direct mailings, especially in areas not directly related to graduate applications (Bartsch, Warren, Sharp, & Green, 2003), so feel comfortable in securing the requisite information online.

Instead, you could send a brief letter requesting information and an application. If you are requesting information by post or e-mail, the message or letter should be neat, typed, and focused. Figure 3-1 shows a sample letter or e-mail.

Congratulations! You have taken the first steps in your application process.

CHAPTER 4

SELECTING SCHOOLS

Between late summer and late fall you will spend time on the World Wide Web, or e-mail or "snail mail" a letter similar to the one displayed in Figure 3-1 to a number of graduate programs for information. You will scan Web sites, download files, or receive large envelopes stuffed with guides describing each program. You are ahead of the game if you begin during late summer, because most applicants will not be starting this process for another 2 to 3 months. This is an opportunity for you to take advantage of an early start to set yourself apart as an organized and optimal candidate.

In order to select programs that best suit your needs and interests, we again return to the questions: What is it I want for myself? What is it I'm interested in doing? And where do I want to do it? A firm commitment to a single clinical interest, research area, geographic location, or theoretical orientation is not required at this time; however, the more specific your interests, the more intelligent a choice you are going to make.

In the previous chapter we helped you to get started in narrowing down your choices of potential graduate programs. We did so by considering your credentials and interests and by searching for potential matches with the requirements and offerings of graduate programs. In this chapter we will help you by reviewing five critical variables to take into account in narrowing your choices: research interests, clinical opportunities, theoretical orientations, financial aid, and quality of life.

A Multitude of Considerations

Each graduate school applicant is undeniably unique in his or her reasons for applying to particular programs in clinical or counseling psychology. As we advise students and conduct workshops on graduate school admission, we hear a litany of specific restrictions: "I have to stay close to my spouse in Los Angeles," "It must be a Catholic school," "I can only attend if I receive full financial aid," "The program needs to be gay friendly, or have gay faculty mentors," "I am interested solely in cognitive-behavioral programs," "I would really like to be near the mountains," "The program must have lots of women faculty," and so on. There is obviously no single, definitive list of factors to consider in selecting potential schools. Although we will examine in some detail the five most common considerations, we will be unable to canvass the almost infinite range of reasons for selecting programs to which to apply.

In an ideal world, graduate student aspirants would have sufficient funds and freedom to consider any clinical or counseling psychology program in the country. In the real world, however, you may be limited in your choice by financial, family, and geographic considerations. Although we appreciate these very real constraints, we encourage you not to be prematurely limited by your own vision. Try to think broadly and boldly. It is, quite simply, your career at stake.

Geographic location will be a determining factor for some applicants. By this we mean both the area of the country and proximity to significant others in your life, such as parents, spouses/partners, siblings, or lovers. If you do not possess the mobility to relocate to another area of the country, then you might delay applying until your situation changes or apply only to regional schools, even if they are less desirable in some ways. Don't spend time, money, and energy on futile missions, in this case applying to programs you will be unable to attend.

At the same time, we heartily encourage you to "get out of town." Far too often students restrict themselves unnecessarily to schools close to their homes or to their undergraduate institution. Yet, graduate programs that better match their needs may be located across the country or four states south. Your future demands that you "look around" the entire country and Canada.

The gender, ethnicity, or sexual orientation makeup of programs may be an influential factor for other applicants. If this is the case for you, obtain updated resource directories from the American Psychological Association and apply accordingly. Three examples are APA's *Graduate Faculty Interested in the Psychology of Women*, *The Directory of Ethnic Minority Professionals in Psychology*, and *Graduate Faculty Interested in Gay and Lesbian Issues in Psychology* (available online at www.apa.org/pi/wpo/gradfac/html). The Reports on Individual Programs also present the percentage of ethnic minority, international, and women students in each clinical and counseling psychology program; these can be a useful source of direction in your choice.

Our general point is this: think through your personal criteria for applying to certain programs and then be proactive in securing information about those criteria. Even if your choice of programs is limited, make it an informed choice. Accept as you must the restrictions in the range of potential graduate schools, but do not leave your future to chance!

Research Interests

The Web site for most programs, or the materials contained in their information packets, should include a list of psychology faculty members in that department and their current research. You are looking to learn something from the faculty, so our advice is to find the professors who are experts in the areas of interest to you. If you are interested in family therapy, locate those psychologists active in training and research in that field. If you are interested in alcohol studies, find the alcohol researchers or clinicians. Download the faculty member's Web page, or the description provided by the department. Read their descriptions carefully with a highlighter. What kind of questions are they asking? Have you asked yourself those same questions? Is this the sort of thing you can envision yourself exploring? Have you read a sample of what they have written?

In selecting professors whose interests parallel your own, you are searching for a good *match*. You are looking for mentors—psychologists who will take you on as an apprentice and teach you about your chosen profession. The more similar your views are, the better the match. For example, if you are practice oriented,

psychodynamically disposed, and interested in private practice, you might choose to cross off your list a program with professors who operate exclusively from behavioral orientations and research perspectives. This does not mean your interest has to be pinpoint focused. Knowing you would rather investigate or treat psychodynamically may be enough to narrow your list of schools down to a sufficient range. But it is our experience that the more focused you are, the better fit you can find.

As you peruse the faculty list and other materials, you should begin to get a sense of whom you would like to work with, who is going to have the facilities to allow you to research or treat the population in which you are interested. You should eventually have a list of 10 to 20 programs that have faculty with whom you would like to work and a general idea of what each of them does.

Having created such a list of programs, we suggest that you review some of the articles or books that these professors have written. Most Web sites include a list of each faculty member's recent publications. So examine their bibliographies on the Web, inspect the program brochure, or search the *Psychological Abstracts* on *PsycLIT* for the last 5 to 7 years to locate some recent publications. Then go online and look them up. What methods do they use? What are the specifics of their psychotherapy or research that really hold your attention? If you find yourself quickly getting bored or saying, "So what? OK, so alcoholics tend to smoke more? Who cares?", then you have a very important piece of information. If you are finding these articles interesting, you are on the right track. This is a time to get excited about your field and where you want to attend graduate school!

Here are some additional bits of information you can gather to whittle down your number of applications. Consult (1) the data provided by the director of training in the Reports on Individual Programs in this book, (2) the program's Web page, (3) the information packet provided by the school, (4) correspondence with faculty, and (5) interviews with professors and/or graduate students at your own school about the programs in question. The important thing is to get the information and corroborate it, if possible.

When it comes to your research interests, discover if there is a medical school library or science facilities at your disposal. Library facilities in general should be a prime consideration, but we have found that medical libraries in particular contain journals and books not usually available elsewhere. Access to journals online through university computer facilities is also important. An associated medical school or hospital may also have facilities and populations available for your research. Determine if they are present, and then investigate their relationship to the Psychology Department. In addition, learn more about the research space specific to your area. For example, does someone have the equipment you need, lab or research space, funding? If you desire to conduct research in cardiovascular psychophysiology and you have found a professor who has published several articles, determine if he or she has equipment to monitor cardiac responses. If not, there should be equipment available somewhere in the department.

We realize that this process requires a great deal of time and energy. It may also provoke anxiety in an already exhausting application process. This is one reason why we advocate an early start. Again, we would like to emphasize that you can get into a program without doing this extra work. This preparation, however, will give you the edge to get into the program of your choice or to overcome any weaknesses in your application.

Clinical Opportunities

Having read articles by the professors with whom you would like to work, you know better which ones you find interesting. However, if your interest is primarily practice, it is possible you might find that the person you're most interested in working with does not have recent publications in your area(s) of interest. Or you know a program has an alcohol abuse clinic, but you can't figure out which professors treat clients there. Your first recourse should be to search the university's Web site to try to locate this information. If it is not on the psychology program's Web page, it may exist somewhere else within the university's Web site. If all else fails, call the department and ask to speak with the director of training. Simply ask this person for materials specific to the clinic you would like to work in, or ask to speak with the director of that clinic to determine which faculty are practicing there.

Now, we are going to suggest something that we have found to be a powerful way of making final decisions about where to apply and of increasing your chances of being accepted there. During early fall of the year you apply, contact a *few* of the professors you have been investigating. E-mail the ones whose interests seem most closely aligned to your own. Most program Web sites include faculty e-mail addresses.

There are many reasons to directly contact a faculty member. First, it gives you an opportunity to gain information you probably could not gather in any other way—information about the program, its facilities, and its faculty. Second, these e-mails give you a chance to get to know someone you are genuinely interested in

working with. It gives you an opportunity to evaluate how happy you would be in a mentorship with this faculty member. Of course, there must be aspects of this person's research or clinical work that attract you. If you do not know his or her interests or the literature well enough to demonstrate a working knowledge of the individual's contributions, do *not* write to him or her. Professors routinely receive letters from people looking to make contact, and unless you can pique their interest and demonstrate familiarity with their work, you are unlikely to receive a response.

Whether your interests are oriented toward research, practice, or both, you are not looking to take this person or his or her field by storm. You seek to make a contribution in this particular area, a contribution made *after* you have taken the time to learn and gain experience in the field under their mentorship. Or, you are looking to gain experience and clinical training with an experienced practitioner.

Take a moment to look at this relationship from the professor's perspective. If she is a researcher, then she is looking for students to help with that research, for students with the knowledge and drive to run studies. If she is a clinician, then she is looking for individuals eager for supervision who will be able to carry a client load. And that is what you have to offer. You are looking for the best fit of a program and faculty to your interests.

Contacting a professor is not a necessity. Many students are admitted to excellent programs and then take 1 or 2 years to explore, to figure out what they want and where they fit in. In fact, some programs require students to work with several professors during their initial year before selecting an adviser. Nonetheless, it is to your advantage to spend sufficient time deciding which professors would be best suited for you. Locate programs and professors who seem appropriate; then go ahead and contact a few of them to test the waters.

Figures 4-1 and 4-2 show sample e-mails of introduction, the former for research-oriented applicants and the latter for practice oriented. *These are not forms to copy in which you simply insert your own words where appropriate!* You may want to show your letter to a professor to preview how well it is likely to be received.

Some students have asked whether it is acceptable to send letters to more than one faculty member at the same program. Despite the fact that applicants may have multiple research and clinical interests, most faculty (ourselves included) have a negative reaction to learning that the same person has written to more than one faculty member. Remember, there is a certain amount of self-interest involved: We're looking for bright, motivated students to collaborate on research

246 Wood Street
Babylon, NY 14000

September 3, 2006

Pat Morris, Ph.D.
Department of Psychology
University of Southern States
13 Peachtree Drive
Wilkesville, VA 15000

Dear Dr. Morris:

I am a psychology senior at Babylon University, where I have been working with Dr. Frances Murrow, studying the effects of self-esteem on math performance anxiety. As I was searching the literature, I read several articles you had written concerning the use of relaxation techniques to improve self-esteem and test anxiety.

After reading your paper "The Uses of Relaxation in Schools" (December issue of *School Psychology*), I had some questions I hoped you could answer. We used several of the questionnaires that you used in that study. In looking at our data, we have found that participants respond quite differently to the Test Anxiety Questionnaire at various times in the semester. We found that the further into the semester students progressed, the more their anxiety affected their scores. Have you also found this to be true in your research? Secondly, I have begun to wonder if self-efficacy might not be a factor affecting both test anxiety and self-esteem. I noticed that you had done some early work involving self-efficacy and was wondering what ideas you might have on this subject.

On a related matter, I will soon be applying to clinical psychology doctoral programs that offer research training in performance anxiety. I would be very interested in learning whether you routinely supervise the research of doctoral students at the University of Southern States on this topic and, if so, whether you will be taking any new students in the next academic year.

Thank you for your time and consideration. I look forward to hearing from you.

Sincerely yours,

Chris Smith

FIGURE 4-1. Sample e-mail of introduction—research oriented.

and clinical work. It can be awkward when an admissions committee is discussing an applicant, and two faculty express a desire to work with him/her, only to find that the applicant has been actively expressing interest in *both* of them. Our advice: Don't write to more than one faculty member in any one program.

What if the person does not respond within a month? Absence of a response does not mean that you will not be able to work with that individual if you are accepted. Most likely the professor may receive too many queries to respond. Indeed, at some schools, professors are receiving dozens of e-mails during the months leading up to the application deadline. Later, when your application is reviewed, your e-mail may be read.

If the selected professor does write back, then it may be the beginning of a working relationship. Even if you are not accepted to his or her program or ultimately decide not to attend, you are making professional contacts in your field. There is no guideline as to exactly how to behave from here, since each professor is different. But you should begin getting a sense of whether this is the right person (and program) for you.

246 Wood Street
Babylon, NY 14000

September 3, 2006

Pat Morris, Ph.D.
Department of Psychology
University of Southern States
13 Peachtree Drive
Wilkesville, VA 15000

Dear Dr. Morris:

I am a psychology senior at Babylon University, where I recently completed an upper-level course in clinical/counseling psychology. My professor, Dr. Frances Ellis, discussed your social problem-solving program targeted to elementary school children. Dr. Ellis spoke highly about the manner in which you use your clinical findings to derive theoretical models of problem solving and use these models to guide your interventions.

I am interested in learning more about school-based social problem-solving programs. I have been involved in such a project with Dr. Ellis and wish to continue my education in this area. I am preparing applications for Psy.D. programs and would like to learn more about your particular program. Specifically, what opportunities exist for clinical Psy.D. students to work on your social problem-solving program? My interests are based primarily in the clinical aspects of your school-based program. I would like to help train teachers in imparting social problem-solving skills to students.

I would appreciate any materials that you could send me describing your problem-solving program in greater detail. I am especially interested in the role for Psy.D. students. Thank you for your time and consideration.

Sincerely yours,

Chris Smith

FIGURE 4-2. Sample e-mail of introduction—practice oriented.

If the task of introducing yourself to a professor "cold" seems overly daunting, consider alternatives. Local and regional conferences present prime opportunities for meeting potential mentors and gathering information about graduate programs. Numerous societies hold yearly conferences in which research is presented in specialty areas of psychology. For example, if one of your interests lies in health psychology or behavioral medicine, there is the Society for Behavioral Medicine, the American Psychosomatic Society, the Society for Psychophysiological Research, and many others. If, for another example, your interests lie in psychotherapy, there are the annual conferences of the Society for Psychotherapy Research, the APA Division of Psychotherapy, and the Society for the Exploration of Psychotherapy Integration. Your psychology advisor can probably suggest several societies in each area of psychology.

Student membership in a scientific society brings a number of benefits. For beginners, it will probably provide you with a directory of members (including contact information), which is an easy way of quickly ascertaining who is doing research in your area. Most scientific organizations will invite you to join their electronic listserve. With membership also typically comes a newsletter or a journal, which can give you a sense of the leaders in the field.

Attending a conference can provide a great deal more information, as we have already emphasized in Chapter 2. If you are interested in particular professors,

TABLE 4-1. Questions to Ask about Psy.D. Programs

Is the program freestanding or part of a university? (If freestanding:) Is it a for-profit school?

If the program also has a clinical Ph.D. program, are the "best" practicum opportunities available to Psy.D. students or Ph.D. students? Is it possible to take the Ph.D. courses as well? What is the relationship between the Psy.D. and Ph.D. students?

Will the internship be in the third or fourth year (i.e., do you complete an internship before or after your dissertation)?

What percentage of Psy.D. students receive financial support? What is the annual tuition?

Are practicum opportunities available outside the institution or only in the institution?

Are there opportunities for live supervision? Do the full-time faculty perform the clinical supervision?

Does the school offer exposure to a variety of theoretical orientations, or is it dominated by one orientation?

Is it possible to gain experience working with . . . ? With families? With groups?

What types of clinical populations are available?

How interested are the faculty in the students?

Do the faculty have independent practices? What percentage of the faculty are full-time?

What percentage of first-year students complete the program? How many years does it typically require to complete the program?

What is the size of the incoming class? How many students are in a typical graduate course?

you may have a chance to see them "in action" if they are presenting a poster or a paper. In this way, you can get acquainted with the person and the research without taking the risk of formally introducing yourself. Alternatively, you may approach the professor directly and express your interest in the research or ask your psychology advisor to make the introduction. Many graduate students first met their mentors in these ways.

After you have communicated with a professor, it may be appropriate to ask to tour this person's research lab or clinical facilities. This is a very important time, in that you will get a chance to gather all sorts of information if you visit a school ahead of time. Meeting this person face to face, getting a sense of his or her personal, clinical, and research style, and seeing how you might fit into an ongoing team can be indispensable information. If you do find yourself in the position of visiting a professor before interviews, use the advice in Chapter 6 to help guide you in gathering information during this phase.

During your visit try to determine if this department's psychological clinic serves the surrounding community or only the college community. College students are fine clients with whom to begin, but you will probably desire a greater diversity of populations and

disorders. Learn more about the school's affiliated or specialized departmental clinics. Who can work there and when? Who does the supervision? Do you have to be affiliated with a specific professor, or is there a competitive process toward earning that placement? If you're choosing a school in part based on the availability of this clinic, how available will this clinic really be to you?

Table 4-1, "Questions to Ask about Psy.D. Programs," contains questions more specific to Psy.D. and clinically oriented Ph.D. applicants. This list was compiled, in part, by surveying the clinical Psy.D. students at the Graduate School of Applied and Professional Psychology at Rutgers University and asking them what questions they had (or wish they had) asked when applying to Psy.D. programs.

Theoretical Orientations

A question related to clinical and research opportunities is whether the graduate program will provide you with training in the desired theoretical orientations. We are *not* recommending that you prematurely affiliate with any theoretical camp; rather, we suggest that you identify those orientations you are interested in learning

TABLE 4-2. Theoretical Orientations of Faculty in APA-Accredited Clinical and Counseling Psychology Programs

Orientations	% of clinical faculty	% of counseling faculty
Psychodynamic/Psychoanalytic	24	28
Applied behavioral analysis/Radical behavioral	7	4
Family systems/Systems	19	24
Existential/Phenomenological/Humanistic	10	28
Cognitive/Cognitive-behavioral	51	43

Note. Data from Oliver, Norcross, Sayette, Griffin, & Mayne (2005).

more about and those you are not. Several programs in the Northeast are strongly committed to a psychoanalytic approach and offer few, if any, training opportunities beyond that. The obvious implication is to avoid applying to programs that will not offer supervised experience in your theoretical approach(es). By the same token, you may scratch programs from your preliminary list that rigidly adhere to, say, a behavioral persuasion if you are disinclined toward behaviorism.

The Reports on Individual Programs provide the approximate percentage of faculty in each program who subscribe to the five most popular theoretical orientations—psychodynamic/psychoanalytic, behavioral analysis/radical behavioral, family systems/systems, existential/phenomenological/humanistic, and cognitive/cognitive-behavioral. Let these figures guide you in ruling out a few programs that fail to address your theoretical predilections or, if you are uncommitted, that neglect exposure to multiple or integrative approaches to clinical work.

Table 4-2 presents the average percentage of faculty endorsing these five theoretical orientations in APA-accredited clinical and counseling programs. In general, the cognitive/cognitive-behavioral tradition predominates, accounting for half of the faculty members. Radical behaviorism is relatively infrequent, with psychodynamic, systems, and humanistic theories falling in between these two extremes. These global figures do not specifically include the integrative/eclectic orientation, which is the most popular approach of contemporary mental health professionals (Norcross & Goldfried, 2005). The fact that the percentages add up to more than 100% indicates that faculty practice across orientations. Note too that the counseling psychology faculty endorse the humanistic/existential orientations much more frequently than do the clinical psychology faculty (28% versus 10%).

These average percentages mask significant differences among programs as a function of their placement along the practice–research continuum. Research-oriented programs, as a rule, have a higher percentage of cognitive-behavioral faculty, while practice-oriented programs have a higher percentage of psychodynamic faculty (Mayne et al., 1994). These differences are quite large: Fully 64% of faculty members in research-oriented Ph.D. programs are cognitive-behavioral versus 33% in practice-oriented Psy.D. programs; and only 12% of faculty in research-oriented Ph.D. programs are psychodynamic versus 29% in practice-oriented Psy.D. programs (Norcross et al., 2005).

The upshot is to investigate thoroughly the area of psychology (clinical, counseling) and the type of program (practice-oriented to research-oriented) that regularly provide training in your preferred theoretical orientation(s).

In addition to reviewing the listing of theoretical orientations in the Reports on Individual Programs, those of you with an intense hankering for training in a particular theoretical orientation may want to peruse specialty directories. A number of professional societies maintain or publish lists of graduate programs that offer training in their theory of choice. The Association for Advancement of Behavior Therapy (AABT), for example, publishes a directory of graduate programs in behavior therapy and experimental clinical psychology (www.aabt.org). The Society for the Exploration of Psychotherapy Integration (SEPI), for another example, has pulled together a list of integrative and eclectic training programs throughout North America (visit www.cyberpsych.org/sepi/sepinorc.htm, Norcross & Kaplan, 1995). The APA Division of Humanistic Psychology, for a final example, cosponsors a directory of graduate programs in humanistic and transpersonal psychology (visit www.westga.edu/~psydept/humanisticdirectory). Consult your advisors regarding the existence of speciality directories in your field of interest.

TABLE 4-3. Percentage of Students Recieving Financial Aid in APA-Accredited Clinical Psychology Programs

	Psy.D. programs	Equal-emphasis Ph.D.	Research-oriented Ph.D.
Tuition waiver only	8	5	2
Assistantship only	19	26	8
Waiver and assistantship	18	57	84

Note. Data from Norcross, Castle, Sayette, & Mayne (2004).

The popularity of theories, as with other professional fads, undergoes transformation over time. Extrapolating from historical trends and expert predictions (Norcross, Hedges, & Prochaska, 2002), cognitive-behavioral, eclectic/integrative, family systems, and multicultural theories will be in the ascendancy in the future. By contrast, classical psychoanalysis, humanistic theories, and existentialism are expected to decline. In an era of managed care, theoretical orientations that emphasize brief problem-focused treatments and document their effectiveness will probably thrive.

Financial Aid

The next question, and it is by no means premature, is the availability of financial aid. Unless you can afford to pay for graduate school on your own or you are prepared to take out substantial loans, you need to have some idea of the probability of support. This is not a suggestion to avoid schools with scarce financial aid. It is a suggestion not to apply only to schools with scarce financial aid.

Figuring the total cost of full-time graduate study must include both academic expenses and living expenses. The academic side includes tuition, fees, supplies, books, and journals. The living side includes rent, transportation, food, clothing, insurance, and entertainment. Not surprisingly, most graduate students are relatively poor; at least you will have company in your financial misery (Fretz & Stang, 1980). Find out which fellowships, teaching assistantships, and research assistantships are available. In particular, find out the percentage of first-year students who receive assistantships. Is it 100%, 50%, or 0%?

On average, 57% of full-time doctoral students in psychology receive some support from the program; the remaining 43% do not. The picture is less encouraging for full-time master's students in psychology: only 23% receive any support (Gehlman, Wicherski, & Kohout, 1995). As you can see, the probability of financial support from the program itself is a very salient issue in narrowing down choices.

The Reports on Individual Programs provide the percentages of incoming doctoral students who receive tuition waiver only, assistantship/fellowship only, and both tuition waiver *and* assistantship for each doctoral program. Table 4-3 summarizes these data across the practice–research continuum, from the practice-oriented Psy.D. programs on one end, through the equal-emphasis Ph.D. programs in the middle, to the research-oriented Ph.D. programs on the other end. As seen there, the probability of receiving financial assistance in graduate school is a direct function of the type of program (Norcross et al., 2004). Only 18% of Psy.D. students, on average, will receive both a tuition waiver and an assistantship, compared to 84% of students in research-oriented Ph.D. programs in clinical psychology. You don't need to perform a *t* test; that is a large, significant difference. The equal-emphasis programs tend to fall in between; about 57% of their students receive both a tuition waiver and an assistantship.

In other words, higher acceptance rates come at a (tuition and living) cost to the incoming student. More rigorous admission standards and acceptance odds translate into increased probability of substantial financial aid (Kohout, Wicherski, & Pion, 1991; Mayne et al., 1994). In the most extreme case (Psy.D. vs. research-oriented Ph.D. programs), students are five times more likely to gain acceptance but six times less likely to receive full funding (stipend plus tuition waiver). An awareness of these trade-offs among the different types of programs will better enable you to make informed choices regarding your applications and career trajectories.

There *is* financial aid available from graduate schools to students possessing sterling credentials, and we wish to reaffirm its existence. Nevertheless, the increasing number of acceptances into clinical and counseling psychology doctoral programs during a period of economic "downsizing" raises difficult questions about internal funding opportunities and federal financial assistance. Our findings (Mayne et al., 1994, Norcross et al., 2004) on financial aid portend a "pay as you go" expectation for up to half of all doctoral candidates in clinical and counseling psychology. This is particularly true, as we have seen, in Psy.D. programs. The explicit expectation, as is true in such other practice disciplines as medicine and law, is that graduates will be able to repay their debt after they are engaged in full-time practice. We should note, however, that uncertainties regarding health care—specifically changes in insurance coverage for mental health—in the United States make this expectation difficult to evaluate at the present time.

The debt may be substantial. Research (APA, 2003) demonstrates that 77% of recent graduates in clinical and counseling psychology have debt related to graduate studies (over and above any debt associated with their undergraduate education). Graduates of Vail-model Psy.D. programs report a median debt of $53,000 to $60,000. Recipients of Boulder-model clinical Ph.D.s, by contrast, report a median level of debt of $22,000 (Kohout & Wicherski, 1999). Twenty-six percent of pscyhology doctoral graduates report debt of $75,000 or more (APA, 2003). With a median starting salary of approximately $45,000 for new psychology doctorates (APA, 2003), this debt represents a significant financial burden for many years. (Go to the Loan Repayment Calculator at www.finaid.org for a sobering look at repayment schedules.) In large part, the difference in debt between Psy.D.s and Ph.D.s is attributable to the huge differences in financial aid between Vail-model and Boulder-model programs as pictured in Table 4-3. The APA researchers who compiled these data conclude, "It is important to disseminate this information to students who may be considering a career in psychology—so that their decisions can be fully informed" (Kohout & Wicherski, 1999, p. 10). We wholeheartedly agree.

In fact, we recently completed a study that looked specifically at the financial assistance offered by various types of Psy.D. programs (Norcross, 2004). You may recall from Chapter 1 that Psy.D. programs can be housed in three different settings: (1) in a university's Psychology Department; (2) as a separate school or institute in a university; (3) as a private, freestanding institution without a university affiliation. As you have already learned, Psy.D. programs give proportionally less financial assistance to students than Ph.D. programs. But it gets a bit more complicated because not all Psy.D. programs are created equally with regard to financial assistance. Only 6% of incoming Psy.D. stu-

dents to a freestanding program will receive a full boat (tuition remission plus assistantship), but 38% of incoming Psy.D. students to a Psychology Department program, on average, will receive a full boat. That's a whopping difference. If you desire considerable financial assistance directly from the school, then do not apply to freestanding Psy.D. programs. Your best bet, financially speaking, will be the university-affiliated Psy.D. programs.

Many universities provide specific Web pages on financial aid. In addition to general information, they often list school- or program-specific scholarships and fellowships available to incoming students. It is worth the added effort to examine the financial aid pages at each school to search for special scholarship programs for which you may be eligible.

In addition to aid provided by the school itself, financial assistance is available from external private and public organizations. This funding comes under various names—self-sought, external, independent—to distinguish it from financial aid provided internally by the university. A variety of scholarships and fellowships is offered annually, but you will need to research those that pertain to your circumstances.

Your local Office of Career Services and Office of Financial Assistance should be able to direct you to potential sources of external support for graduate studies. One very useful resource is *Financing Graduate School*, a compact paperback authored by Patricia McWade (1996). The subtitle captures the importance of the topic—*How to Get the Money for Your Master's or Ph.D.* The book transverses the entire geography of financial aid—grant applications, loan possibilities, federal and state support, and other sources of money for graduate study. A companion volume from the same publisher is *Peterson's Grants for Graduate and Post-doctoral Study* (1998), which details over 1,400 potential fellowships, scholarships, grants, and awards. Peterson also offers a free online cram course in financial aid at www.petersons.com/resources/finance.html. Be sure to check out the loads of advice and searchable databases on line at www.finaid.com and at www.ed.gov/prog_info/SFA/StudentGuide.

Federal funding is also available for pyschology graduate students, either in the form of training and research grants to institutions, which then fund graduate assistantships, or in the form of fellowships and dissertation grants awarded directly to students (Bullock, 1997). The National Science Foundation (NSF) funds separate competitions for Graduate Fellowships and for Minority Graduate Fellowships. Note that NSF does not support clinical or counseling research per se, only research directed at elucidating basic functioning, not focused on disease-related processes. The National Insitutes of Health (NIH) also funds psychology student awards through the National Institute of Mental Health, the National Institute on Drug Abuse, the National Institute on Alcohol Abuse and Alcoholism, and the Office of AIDS Research. Check out these programs through their Web pages: www.nsf.gov and www.nih.gov.

Several specialty directories are also available free of charge from philanthropic and professional organizations. Among the more prestigious (and therefore, more competitive) are the predoctoral fellowships sponsored by the Danforth Foundation, Ford Foundation, and Armed Forces Health Professions Scholarship. The American Psychological Association publishes an online *Directory of Selected Scholarship, Fellowship, and Other Financial Aid Opportunities for Women and Ethnic Minorities in Psychology*, which we highly recommend (www.apa.org/pi/financialaid). The APA Minority Fellowship Program is now online at www.apa.org/mtp. APA also offers an online list of resources for financial assistance at www.apa.org/ppo/fineduc.html.

As you can anticipate, the Web has literally exploded with interactive sites devoted to securing financial assistance for graduate school. Many of these are useful and recommended, but be wary of and avoid those that charge you for their services. In addition to the APA sites listed above, we would suggest you visit:

- www.gradview.com/finaid/
- www.scholarships.com
- www.petersons.com/resources/financ.html
- www.finaid.org/otheraid.grad.phtml
- collegeapps.about.com/cs/graduatestudents

Explore all these possibilities early and actively.

Student loans are also available for graduate students, but these are loans that must be repaid. The Federal Family Education Loan (FFEL) Program and the William D. Ford Federal Direct Loan (Direct Loan) Program, generally known as Stafford Loans, are available to assist graduate and professional students. Students may borrow up to $8,500 per academic year through the subsidized Stafford Loan. The interest on these loans is subsidized by the federal government and repayment at reasonable interest rates does not begin until 6 months after graduation, or following withdrawal from the program. In addition to this $8,500, up to an additional $10,000 per academic year can be borrowed through the unsubsidized Stafford Loans. The in-school interest on the unsubsidized Stafford Loans may be paid quarterly or deferred and repaid when principal repayments begin.

The total amount that can be borrowed, including both subsidized and unsubsidized portions, is currently $138,500. Some institutions also award Federal Perkins Loans, a long-term loan program with a 5% interest rate available to graduate students demonstrating financial need. Other state loan programs exist; check these out as well. The bottom line is that every full-time graduate student is eligible for loans to finance his or her education, if necessary.

Speaking of loans reminds us to mention loan repayment options and loan forgiveness programs. We recommend that you visit the U.S. Department of Education Web site, www.ed.gov, which describes student loan types and loan repayment options. Three options that can trim loan payments for graduate students are the graduated repayment plans, income-sensitive repayment plans, and the loan consolidation plans. See the Web site for details, but remember that most student loans only permit a single refinancing or consolidation. Clinical and counseling psychologists working in designated underserved areas as part of the National Health Services Corps (NHSC) are also eligible for loan forgiveness (up to $25,000 or $35,000 per year) while receiving a competitive salary. Go to nhsc.bhpr.hrsa.gov for details of the program.

Quality of Life

A fifth and final consideration in selecting schools is the quality of student life. It may be difficult to imagine, but occasionally you will want a break from graduate studies, to relax or engage in some nonpsychological pursuit!

You should have a handle on the specifics of your own needs. Can they be met by the university and surrounding community? Do you want museums, fine dining, and professional theater? Then you probably want to live in or near a large city. If not, do you have a car capable of regularly getting you to one? Or do you get away to the mountains, enjoy rock climbing and camping, or find the city distracting? Or do you prefer to work late at night and need a campus that's safe after dark? Then be sure to apply to some more rural places. Also, consider whether you have friends or family nearby. Having a place to escape to can be important, especially if you do not have the funds to *really* escape. You are not going to base your decisions exclusively on any of these factors. But you can increase the probability of having everything you want by applying to schools you know can provide it all.

The Web is an excellent resource for investigating locations, towns, and cities that are far away and that you may not have the time or finances to visit at this time. Most cities have their own Web pages, which include pictures, maps, lists of attractions, and so on, for potential visitors and residents. Take the time to "virtually" explore the towns and cities of programs on your list. You may find that it is far more (or less) desirable than you had imagined.

The weight accorded to the quality of life in application decisions varies considerably among people. At one extreme are those applicants who give little thought to program location and heavily value the research and clinical opportunities. In the words of one colleague, "I'd live in hell for 4 or 5 years [the time it ordinarily takes to complete a doctorate] to be trained by the best people in my field." At the other extreme are those who will only apply to programs situated near family, friends, or an attractive community. "Five years," they say, "is too long to be away from what I need as a person." We will not be so presumptuous as to advise which position you should adopt for yourself, except to remark that you should carefully weigh personal (location, fit) and professional (reputation, opportunities) considerations.

Putting It All Together

Having seriously reflected on your own interests and having carefully examined the clinical opportunities, research training, theoretical orientations, financial aid, and quality of life of various programs, you are very close to completing applications. Now is the time to put together all the information you have obtained about yourself and graduate programs in the form of a final list of schools—anywhere from 10 to 20, depending on the specificity of your interests and the strength of your credentials. As you make a final list of the applications you are about to complete, make one last check to insure that you are applying to the programs that best fit your needs. You may do this informally by mentally reviewing the program information you have obtained or you may do this systematically by completing Appendix D.

To complete Appendix D, write the name of each school in the first column. In column 2, "School Criteria," write the total you computed for each school in Appendix C. This is an index of your strength as an applicant and should range from about 5 to 15. For each of the next five columns, you can rate your impressions about each program on a 5-point scale. Create these scales yourself in ways that are personally relevant to

you. The important thing is to know where each school rates in these areas in terms of your needs and desires. Below are some examples of rating systems you might model your own after.

In the column marked "Research," rate how strongly you feel toward the professors you have singled out as wanting to work with:

1	I do not know enough about them, but their research is in my area.
3	I like the specifics of their research but do not know enough about their lab or their personalities.
5	I have been in contact with these professors and am impressed by their facilities and by them personally. I would like to work with them.

In the column marked "Clinical," rate each school according to how its opportunities suit your needs.

1	The school has only a psychological training clinic that treats students, and I want more experience.
3	The school has a good psychological training clinic, but it has no practica in the community, and getting various populations may be difficult.
5	The school has many excellent clinical opportunities, including a specialty (e.g., eating disorders) clinic in the area that most interests me.

Or, possibly:

1	The school requires students to find their own clinical placements in the community, and I don't like that system.
3	The school has a college counseling center, but I'm not interested in working only with college students.
5	The school has a good psychological services clinic, and that's all I need.

"Theoretical Orientation" is the following column:

1	The program avers strict adherence to, and training in, a theoretical orientation that is in contrast to mine.
3	The program offers some courses and supervision in my preferred theoretical orientation.

5 The program provides considerable training in my preferred theoretical orientation plus other opportunities.

Next, consider "Financial Aid":

1 There is no funding for first-year students and no mention of outside means of support, and I need it.

3 I am likely to get at least tuition remission and have the possibility of working part-time for the university. It is likely that I could be a resident advisor and get free housing.

5 For the last 5 years, all first-year students have gotten full stipends and full tuition remission.

Or, possibly:

1 There is no funding for first-year students and no mention of outside means of support.

3 I am likely to get at least tuition remission, though only for the first 2 years.

5 The school guarantees tuition remission for 4 years, and that's all I need.

And last, rate the "Quality of Life":

1 This program is located in an unattractive area and seems bereft of culture.

3 I am indifferent to the location, and there is culture within the college community.

5 The area is ideal for me, and there are museums, concert halls, and theaters nearby.

Or, possibly:

1 This university is located in an unsafe section of a large city where I don't know anyone.

3 This university is located in a small city, and a friend of mine also attends.

5 This university is located in a small college town, and I have several close relatives and friends there.

Now look at your list. Are you applying to programs within a realistic range of admission criteria? Are you applying to at least some programs where you like the faculty, where the clinical facilities are suitable, where the theoretical orientation is compatible, where financial aid is available, and where you will feel comfortable living? If the answer to all of these is "No," then go back a step. Find at least a few schools where these qualities are present, possibly in abundance, and add them to your list of applications.

Before moving on to the next chapter of this *Insider's Guide* and the next step in the application process, take one final moment to celebrate. You deserve it! You have learned much about graduate training in clinical and counseling psychology, investigated potential graduate programs, assessed your match with those programs, and whittled down your final list. You have already mastered challenges more intense than those associated with many college courses. So, after weeks of arduous and sometimes anxious work, you deserve some affirmation and reward. Give them to yourself or, at least, allow us to affirm and reward you from afar.

CHAPTER 5

APPLYING TO PROGRAMS

You are ready to start completing the applications. You have assessed your interests and have located programs that provide the training and mentorship you desire. You have evaluated your own credentials and have chosen programs that will consider you seriously. You have received applications from these programs either by mail or by downloading materials from the 90% of clinical programs with Web pages (Corcoran, Michels, & Ahina, 1999). You have carefully looked at their research offerings, clinical opportunities, theoretical orientations, financial aid, quality of life, and other variables of importance to you. Your task now is to actually apply to these schools.

You should attack this application process with all the drive and commitment you can muster. Try to emulate the manic zeal of successful medical school applicants. As they will readily inform you, the application itself reflects directly on your potential as a graduate student. In a real sense, your professional future is at stake.

A completed application will typically consist of the following elements: application form, curriculum vitae, personal statement, letters of recommendation, transcripts, entrance examination scores, and an application fee. This chapter traces the requisite steps of compiling, completing, and transmitting these materials in a coordinated fashion. But before we address the nuts and bolts of doing so, let us touch upon the crucial question of how many programs to apply to.

How Many?

The average number of applications made by students to clinical and counseling psychology programs is about 13. The precise number to which you should apply depends on the strength of your credentials and the competitiveness of the programs to which you are applying; more applications are indicated for weaker credentials and more competitive programs.

Our rule of thumb is to apply to *at least* 10 to 12 programs: five "safe" or "insurance" programs (you clearly meet or exceed their standards); five "target" or "ambitious" programs (your credentials just make or miss their requirements); and perhaps one or two "reach" or "stretch" programs (where you do not approximate their standards but you have a particular hunch, research compatibility, or personal relationship that has a chance of sweeping you into the finalist pool). We have met industrious students who have applied to over 40 programs and confident students who have applied to just four or five.

But "don't pull a Missar," as we say at the University of Scranton. David Missar was an exceptional undergraduate and good-humored fellow (who gave us permission to use his story as a lesson for others to learn). He had a sky-high GPA, impressive GREs, a practicum to his credit, and even a coauthored publication. He was feeling a bit too confident in applying to only four doctoral programs, all located around his home town of Washington, D.C., which happens to have some of the most competitive programs in the country. Despite his stellar academic credentials, Dave did not receive any acceptances his first year simply because his research interests and strengths did not "match" those of the clinical faculty and institutions to which he applied. Had he applied to a greater number or larger variety of programs, he surely would have been accepted somewhere, as he was easily the next year when he corrected his miscalculations.

Application Form

You have a list of 10 to 20 programs in front of you. The deadlines range from mid-December to mid-February. You have used the late summer and fall months to investigate potential programs—the professors, the orientations, the locations, and the costs. It is now time to actually start writing.

One of the easiest parts is filling out the application itself. When you download an application from the Web, be sure it is on clean, white, high-quality paper. Some students have found it useful to make a copy of the application and complete a first draft on the photocopy. The completed application reflects on you; keep it as professional and neat as possible.

Slightly more than half of all programs allow you to submit an application through e-mail or the World Wide Web (Norcross, et al., in press). If you have the choice, we advise against doing this. Taking the time to carefully consider (and often change) portions of your application is an important part of the process. Your personal statement requires a great deal of thought and will go through many revisions. By completing the application and reading it over several times before mailing it, you are likely to catch and correct errors or poor choices. This is one of the places where we recommend against taking full advantage of technological advances!

Online applications can be an Internet nightmare. You don't know what your completed application will look like. You don't know where it goes—or where it does not go. You can easily fail to indicate essential information, such as faculty members with whom you desire to work. On the other hand, online applications are quick, potentially less expensive, and the software improving rapidly. So, if you elect to submit an application online, please be careful. Proofread the document several times and try to cut and paste a fully formed personal statement from a word processing file.

Begin the applications at least 1 month before the earliest deadline. Some applicants, particularly undergraduates in their senior year, wait until the end of the fall semester on the holiday break. *This is too late*—do not wait, lest you be rushed, unprepared, and working on a tight deadline.

Unlike the medical school process, which uses an identical application form for each school, practically every graduate program in psychology has its own, unique application. Providing the same information over and over again in slightly different formats can become frustrating and time consuming. Several years ago a committee recommended a standardized graduate application form to reduce the paperwork, but comparatively few programs have instituted it. Nonetheless, it provides a good idea of the information that will be requested of you:

- Full name
- Previous and maiden names
- Citizenship status
- Semester of entrance
- Current mailing address
- Permanent home address
- Educational history
- Degree sought
- Field of study
- Relevant courses taken
- Grade point averages
- Academic honors
- Clinical experience
- Special qualifications
- Employment history
- Teaching/research experience
- Career objectives
- References

Submitting applications is worse than filling out income tax returns (Fretz & Stang, 1980). Allow yourself enough uninterrupted time to do it carefully and completely. Illegible handwriting, incorrect spelling, and poor grammar will hurt your chances.

Some additional tips (Fretz & Stang, 1980):

- Keep the application forms for each school separated. Individual file folders might help. Since the forms are often poorly marked, you may not otherwise know which forms belong to what school.
- Enclose with each application a self-addressed, stamped postcard that the school can return to verify receipt of your application. On the back of the card simply type: "Please send to verify receipt of application to _____ University."
- Make a photocopy of each application before mailing it. Graduate schools and the postal service have been known to lose—or misplace—entire forms. A photocopy will enable you to quickly resubmit if necessary.
- Submit the application materials in a new legal size envelope on which you have typed the correct designation and your return address.

On a side note, completing application forms for graduate school marks a good time to critically examine the impression that your voice- and e-mail are communicating to others. A Dave Matthews tune on your answering machine may entertain fellow students, but probably not the director of clinical training. Cute e-mail addresses, such as studmuffin@email.com or hotchick@aol.com, may delight romantic partners, but certainly not the dean of the graduate school. So now may be the time to alter those messages and convey a more professional demeanor.

Curriculum Vitae

Curriculum vitae means, literally, "the course of your life." The vitae or CV summarizes your academic and employment history in a structured form, similar to a resume. Figures 5-1 and 5-2 present two possible formats for a CV; you will need to adapt these samples to your individual needs. Although the samples are single-spaced and occupy only one page, CVs are *double-spaced* between entries and occupy several pages.

As a general comment, keep the CV honest, terse, and positive. Never fabricate, but perhaps "embellish" appropriately. The line to be drawn here is demarcated by whether you can look an interviewer directly in the eye and factually defend an entry that could subsequently be corroborated by a supervisor, professor, or another person. Structured brevity is the key; lengthy expositions of experiences are best left to personal statements or job descriptions.

And this "academic resume" should be positive, upbeat in tone. Avoid any negative features that might red-flag your application. Save confessions and excruciating honesty for the clergy and psychotherapist. Omit sections that do not apply to you, such as "Presentations" or "Publications" if you have had none at this point in your career.

Let's proceed through the different sections of a CV and offer some additional hints. List your legal name, including any suffixes such as "Jr." Distinguish between a current address and a permanent home address, if this applies to your living circumstances. Note any anticipated changes in your address. Include telephone numbers and e-mail addresses at which program directors or professors can easily reach you. If you share voice mail or a telephone answering machine with other people, insure that they will graciously take a message for you and reliably transmit that message to you. As you draft your CV also take a moment to review your voice-mail message. Does it readily create the desired impression as a serious, doctoral-bound student?

Information on your marital status and dependents is definitely optional. Opinions differ widely on whether you should include this material on your CV:

the probable positives are that you are being honest and sharing information about yourself; the likely downsides are that the information may be used against you or lead to illegal considerations in admission decisions. The marital status question is now almost moot since approximately half of all graduate students in psychology are married (Pate, 2001).

Regarding education, list degrees as "anticipated" if they have not yet been awarded. Impressive grade point averages may also be listed here. Honors are listed in chronological order, usually excluding those obtained in high school. If you received an honor specific to a university (e.g., the Lawrence Lennon Memorial Award), then record what it is for. Similarly, specify the disciplines of honor societies. Clinical experiences and research experiences can be listed together or separately, depending on what will strengthen your CV, but in either case indicate position title, relevant dates, number of hours, duties performed, and the supervisor. Include any presentations or publications in APA style, thereby demonstrating your familiarity with the psychologist's publication manual. The names of references should be listed only after you have obtained their permission to do so. *Never list a reference on a CV or application form unless you have secured that person's agreement to write a letter in support of your application.*

Here is an idea to enhance the CV for students who have developed specific research or computer competencies. List them on your vitae as a separate section. Computer skills might include proficiency with SPSS, SAS, Pascal, Harvard Graphics, Chartmaster, SigmaScan, SigmaPlot, CricketGraph, and Aldus Pagemaker. Research skills might include performing computerized library searching on *PsycLIT* or *Medline*, administering the Wisconsin Card Sorting Test (or another psychological test), or operating an electroencephalograph (EEG). Also include here any special skills, such as fluency in foreign languages or proficiency in American Sign Language. A faculty member screening applications may realize that these competencies are exactly what he or she is looking for in a new graduate assistant or research assistant. So use your CV to highlight your abilities! Omit this optional section if you have none or only one specific competency; in the latter case, describe the special qualification in your personal statement.

What should *not* be put on the CV? Hayes and Hayes (1989) recommend eliminating listings of religion, hobbies, pets, favorite books, and items of that kind. They are unnecessary; save them for a resume. Nor is a photograph customary.

Padding of all varieties must be avoided. Padding occurs when a reader reacts to the CV as more form

November 2005

CURRICULUM VITAE

Name: Ted E. Bear
Address: 15 Easy Street
Babylon, NY 12345
Telephone: (516) 555-1212
E-mail: bear@babu.edu
Date of Birth: March 15, 1984
Place of Birth: Scranton, Pennsylvania
Citizenship: United States of America

Education:

H.S. Diploma: Cherry Hill High School, City, State, June 2002
B.S. (anticipated): Psychology, Babylon University, May 2006

Honors and Awards:

New York State Regents Scholarship, 2002–2006
Dean's List, Babylon University, 2005–2006
Psi Chi, 2006
Babylon University Honors Program, 2004–2006
Who's Who Among Students in American Colleges & Universities, 2006

Clinical Experience:

Mental Health Technician, Friendship House, Jackson, Wyoming, June 2004–August 2005. Duties: recreational counseling and supervision of 20 behaviorally and emotionally disturbed children. Supervisor: Doris Day, M.S. 40 hours weekly.

Telephone Counselor, Mesopotamia County Community Crisis Center, Babylon, New York, 2003–2004. Duties: used a crisis intervention model to counsel a wide range of callers. Supervisor: Randal Kaplan, M.A. 4 hours weekly.

Research Experience:

Research Assistant, Babylon University, Department of Psychology, September 2004–June 2006. Duties: word processing, manuscript preparation, and data analyses for Chris Demanding, Ph.D. 15 hours weekly.

Honors Research, Babylon University with Rita Murrow, Ph.D., 2005–2006. Duties: proposed and conducted an original project; data input and analysis using SPSSx; write-up and oral defense.

Professional and Honor Societies:

Psi Chi, National Honor Society in Psychology
American Psychological Association (student affiliate)
Alpha Gamma Epsilon Omega (National Honor Society in Ergonomics)

Presentations and Publications:

Bear, T. E., & Murrow, F. A. (2005, April). *Self-esteem and math performance: Another look.* Paper presented at the meeting of the Babylon Psychological Association, New York.

Murrow, F. A., & Bear, T. E. (2005). The effects of self-esteem on math test performance. *Journal of Psychology, 46,* 113–117.

Campus Activities and Leadership:

Psychology Club, member (2003–2006) and president (2005–2006)
University Singers, Babylon University, 2003–2005
Hand-in-Hand, participant (2003–2006) and campus coordinator (2005)

References:

Frances Murrow, Ph.D., Associate Professor, Department of Psychology, Babylon University, Babylon, NY 12345. Voice: 516-555-1212; e-mail: murrow@babu.edu

Chris Demanding, Ph.D., Professor and Chair, Department of Psychology, Babylon University, Babylon, NY 12345. Voice: 516-555-1212; e-mail: les@babu.edu

Doris Day, M.S., Senior Therapist, Horror House, 78 Oak Street, Jackson, WY 12345. Voice: 307-555-1212

FIGURE 5-1. One format for curriculum vitae.

Ted E. Bear   November 2005

Personal History:

Business Address: Department of Psychology
                           Babylon University
                           Babylon, New York 12345
Phone: (516) 555-1212
Home Address: 1017 Jefferson Avenue
                           Cherry Hill, NJ 08002
Phone: (609) 555-1212
E-mail: bear@babu.edu
Birthdate: March 15, 1984
Citizenship: United States of America

Educational History:

Babylon University, Babylon, New York
Major: Psychology
Degree: B.S. (anticipated), May 2006
Dean's List, 2005–2006
Who's Who Among Students in American Colleges & Universities, 2006
Honors Thesis: Investigation of the relationship between self-esteem and math performance (Chair-person: Rita Murrow, Ph.D.)

Professional Positions:

1. Telephone Counselor, Mesopotamia County Community Crisis Center, Babylon, New York. Part-time position, 2003–2005. Duties: used a crisis intervention model to counsel a wide range of callers. Supervisor: Randal Kaplan, M.A.
2. Mental Health Technician, Friendship House, Jackson, Wyoming. Full-time summer position, 2004. Duties: recreational counseling and supervision of 20 behaviorally and emotionally disturbed children. Supervisor: Doris Day, M.S.
3. Research Assistant, Babylon University. Half-time position, 2004–2005. Duties: word processing, manuscript preparation, and data analysis. Supervisor: Chris Demanding, Ph.D.

Membership in Professional Associations:

Psi Chi (National Honor Society in Psychology)
American Psychological Association (student affiliate)
Alpha Gamma Epsilon Omega (National Honor Society in Ergonomics)

Professional Activities:

President, Babylon University Chapter of Psi Chi, 2003–2004
Member of Program Committee, Babylon University Psychology Conference, 2004

Papers Presented:

Bear, T. E., & Murrow, F. A. (2005, April). *Self-esteem and math performance: Another look.* Paper presented at the meeting of the Babylon Psychological Association, New York.

Publications:

Murrow, F. A., & Bear, T. E. (2005). The effects of self-esteem on math test performance. *Journal of Psychology, 46,* 113–117.

Campus Activities:

Psychology Club, member (2003-2006) and president (2005–2006)
University Singers, Babylon University, 2003–2005
Hand-in-Hand, participant (2003–2006) and campus coordinator (2005)

References:

Frances Murrow, Ph.D., Associate Professor, Department of Psychology, Babylon University, Babylon, NY 12345. Voice: 516-555-1212; e-mail: murrow@babu.edu
Chris Demanding, Ph.D., Professor and Chair, Department of Psychology, Babylon University, Babylon, NY 12345. Voice: 516-555-1212; e-mail: les@babu.edu
Doris Day, M.S., Senior Therapist, Horror House, 78 Oak Street, Jackson, WY 12345. Voice: 307-555-1212

Note. Adapted from Hayes & Hayes (1989) with the permission of the authors.

FIGURE 5-2. Another format for curriculum vitae.

than substance ("Who are they trying to fool?!"). Potentially risky is listing professional projects under way—one or two legitimate research projects may pass but any more will probably be considered suspect. Other signs of padding, and therefore sections to exclude, are conventions attended, journals read, and projects you worked on in a nonprofessional capacity.

Pumping up your past on CVs and application forms is common but inadvisable. A recent survey of 2.6 million job applications discovered that 44% of them contained lies (Kluger, 2002); do not be among the 44%. Once you are caught fibbing on a graduate school application, it is practically impossible to restore your integrity and character at that program. While some of your friends may exhort you to exaggerate your previous positions and to inflate your GPA, we strongly advise honesty.

Although much of the information contained in the CV is requested on the application form itself, we believe the inclusion of a CV enhances your application—providing it is properly prepared. A CV denotes a scholarly demeanor, highlights your accomplishments, and communicates familiarity with the workings of academia.

Specific comments on the form and style of the CV might prove useful. Place the date (month and year) on the upper right-hand corner of the CV. In this way, you can submit an addendum if your credentials significantly improve by, say, having a paper accepted for publication or receiving your department's "student of the year" award. Lay out the information in an attractive and organized manner. Use a consistent format both within each section and between sections. For example, if you opt to list your clinical experiences from the most recent to the past, then maintain this format in all the other sections. Proofread the document carefully; review it with an advisor before you print it. It ideally would be produced on a laser printer with a few fonts, but any letter-quality printer will suffice. Staple the pages together when finished (Hayes & Hayes, 1989).

The CV, like personal statements (below), should be printed on standard-sized white or cream stock. Purchase good quality bond paper for these documents. Avoid onionskin paper, goldenrod color, odd-sized papers, memo pads, green or red ink, and other unconventional or "cheap" materials.

Personal Statements

Another bridge you must cross is writing the statement of purpose. Every program will want to know why you chose clinical or counseling psychology and the area within it that you plan to study. Admissions committees will also want to know how you came to this decision and what sorts of goals you have in mind. Each application will ask this question in a slightly different way because each program has slightly different expectations and approaches to training. *Read the instructions carefully.* Do not just word process one statement and submit it to everyone.

Do not misinterpret the meaning of personal in *personal statement.* This essay is not the place to espouse your philosophy of life, to describe your first romance, or to tell the story about your being bitten by the neighbor's dog and subsequently developing an anxiety disorder. Instead, think of the essay as a *professional statement.* Write about your activities and experiences as an aspiring psychologist (Bottoms & Nysse, 1999).

An analysis of 360 essays required as part of the graduate application process demonstrated wide variability in the content requested (Keith-Spiegel, 1991). The most frequent requests were to articulate:

- Career plans
- Clinical experiences
- Interest areas
- Specific faculty of interest
- Research experiences
- Autobiographical statement
- Academic objectives
- Reasons for applying to that particular program
- Educational background

To reiterate: carefully read the question, individualize your response to each program, and respond to all parts of the question posed to you.

Be attentive to what the program requests. If they stress research, highlight your research interests and experience. If they stress clinical work, highlight the development of these interests and your training experiences to date. Show how you started with a question or a clinical observation, how you pursued that question, and how it developed into a greater understanding of the issues at hand and a need to know more. Then demonstrate how this led you to pursue psychology and how this program meets your needs and is ideal to your continuing to pursue knowledge in this area. State the goals you wish to attain with this knowledge, the sort of career path you hope to work toward. If you are committed to the Boulder model, indicate how research is useful and how it is clinically applicable.

If you can make this connection in your personal statement, you will impress on the admission committee the integration APA sets forth as its ideal.

Graduate selection committees value clarity, focus, and "passion" in personal statements (Keith-Spiegel,

1991). Clarity and focus are typically construed as indicators of lucid thought, realistic planning, and self-direction, all valuable assets in a graduate student. At the same time, try to communicate a heartfelt commitment to your chosen career. "Passion" is not too strong a term—even relentless, obsessed, committed, fascinated; in short, what we call "catching the fever!" Your statement might well include such assertions as "I love college and the academic environment," "I am fascinated by counseling psychology and its potential to empower people and change communities," or "Research is a passion, not only a course requirement." Graduate faculty seek students who find it difficult to distinguish between work and pleasure when it comes to academic tasks (Kieth-Spiegel & Wiederman, 2000).

The personal statement is a prime opportunity to induce a match with the research and clinical interests of a faculty member. Many programs, as we have said, attempt to match faculty with incoming graduate students on the basis of mutual interest, for example, family therapy, women's issues, or neuropsychological assessment. This matching strategy is more often employed by research-oriented than practice-oriented programs, but attempt it in all of your personal statements.

To illustrate, consider the clinical admissions process of the University of Ottawa, a program with an equal emphasis on research and practice. Like many programs, they create a finalist pool by eliminating applications with inadequate GPAs and GRE scores. Then each of the clinical faculty members reviews all the finalist applications in order to locate several possible matches. These applicants then receive interviews. As you can see, and as we have repeated throughout this book, gaining admission into competitive doctoral programs is not limited simply to one's credentials but also includes a match in research and clinical interests.

Here, then, are a few general guidelines for writing personal statements that increase the probability of a match:

- Mention at least two and perhaps up to four of your interests. This obviously covers a wider range than a single interest.
- Cast your interests in fairly broad terms—not administering the Wisconsin Card Sorting Test, but neuropsychological assessment; not a mail survey of counseling psychologists, but the characteristics and practices of psychotherapists.
- Nominate at least two professors with whom you would like to work at that particular graduate program. This, too, enhances the chance of a successful match.

A commonly asked question is, "How personal should I get in my personal statement?" Although there is no universally correct answer, some suggestions can be offered. A personal detail, such as describing how growing up with a handicapped or disturbed sibling has affected your life and decision to enter psychology, is appropriate. However, depicting the situation in intimate detail without relating it to its contribution to your own growth may lead an admissions committee to question your judgment. A rule of thumb is to be introspective and self-revealing without sounding exhibitionistic. For example, it is appropriate for an applicant to state how personal life experiences have contributed to better self-understanding, but it sounds peculiar when the applicant goes into great detail about particular relationships or early life events (Halgin, 1986). Although allusions to integrating psychotherapy in personal statements does not appear to overly stigmatize candidates or lead disproportionately to their rejections (Schaefer, 1995), we recommend against including your personal therapy in written materials. Better to save such intimate disclosures for the personal interview, if appropriate.

Many personal statements are ineffective because, first, the student fails to spend time preparing them and, second, the student fails to be "personal" (Osborne, 1996). Therefore, as an applicant you should devote a substantial amount of time thinking, writing, rethinking, and rewriting the personal statement. Your statement should include personal details that relate to your ability to be a successful graduate student and that demonstrate maturity, adaptation, and motivation—the very characteristics sought by admissions committees.

Another question we are frequently asked, usually in private, is, "Should I disclose my disability in my personal statement or on the application form?" When and how to disclose a disability is a complex and personal decision, a decision that you must make after sorting through the choices and perhaps discussing them with a knowledgeable mentor. There are eight different occasions during the admissions process when you might choose to disclose (Khubchandani, 2002):

- In your CV or application form
- When a prospective graduate school contacts you for an interview
- During the interview
- After the interview but before an offer
- After the offer but before an acceptance
- After you start the graduate program
- After a problem on the job
- Never (disclose)

There are pros and cons for each timing of disclosure, but ultimately your decision will be based on what you know about your own needs and what you have learned about the specific graduate program (Khubchandani, 2002). If and when you do disclose a disability, be straightforward and factual about it only as it affects your specific job functions, as defined by the Americans with Disabilities Act. Specify the type of accommodation that you will require or the work restrictions that are involved. Don't dwell on your disability; rather, be enthusiastic about your skills and resources. Stress that your disability did not interfere with previous performance or attendance. It is your multiple abilities, not select dis-abilities, that count in graduate school.

A good idea is to show some humility. Even if you have golden research and clinical experiences and 1400 GRE scores, you are still entering as a student. You are coming to learn. Show some awareness of the areas you hope to develop during your graduate school experience.

Be prepared to back up the claims you make in your personal statements. If you profess a working knowledge of, say, experiential psychotherapy, then be prepared for questions on the work of Carl Whitaker, Leslie Greenberg, and Alvin Mahrer. Similarly, if you claim fluency in Spanish, then expect one of the interviews to be conducted entirely in Spanish (Megargee, 1990).

The "to do's" of personal statements are process suggestions and thus difficult to pinpoint, but the "not to do's" are content oriented and easier to delineate (Whitbourne, 1999). We characterize three such "nots" as the three H's: Humor, Hyperbole, and Hard luck stories. Humor rarely works in a formal written statement; so unless you are an unusually gifted satirist, we recommend you avoid jokes and funny stories about your life. Similarly, hyperbole rarely impresses the admissions committee. References to your "overwhelming childhood trauma" and "triumph over undiagnosed learning disabilities" in personal statements cast doubt on the veracity and accuracy of your judgment. And hard luck stories typically come off feebly. Many students financed their undergraduate educations, many survived disastrous relationship choices, and many muddled through three academic majors before finding their niche in psychology. Avoid making adversity the theme of your statement.

Our advice is supported by a recent study on the "kisses of death" in the graduate school application process (Appleby & Appleby, 2004). Eighty-eight chairs of graduate admissions committees provided examples of application materials that caused the admissions committee to draw negative conclusions about the applicant. A prevalent theme among these kisses of death was damaging personal statements that were (a) overly altruistic, (b) excessively disclosing, or (c) professionally inappropriate. Examples of the overly altruistic statements were "I want to help all people live happy lives" and "I want to help people because of how very much I have been helped." Examples of excessive self-disclosure were "being a recovering drug addict daughter of a sexually deviant and alcoholic mother" and excruciating details of an applicant's year-long struggle with painful hemorrhoids! Our favorite example of professional inappropriateness was the applicant who submitted a statement of purpose titled "Statement of Porpoise" that contained drawings of the sea mammal and a description of the applicant frolicking in the ocean with a porpoise on a visit to Florida. As we said, avoid humor, hyperbole, and hard luck in your personal statement.

One way to make your personal statement sparkle is to describe any teaching assistantships or experiences. Talk about how you learned leadership skills and teamwork in this role. Specific examples of how you responsibly handled challenging courses or teaching activities will lead the reader to infer you possess the "right stuff."

Your personal statement should tell a compelling, integrative story of a reflective individual who explicates accomplishments without joking or bragging or sobbing. As our colleague Sue Krauss Whitbourne (1999) puts it: Don't say it softly or loudly, just say it clearly!

You will be asked in practically every personal statement and personal interview why you chose to apply to *this* particular graduate program in clinical or counseling psychology. Figure 5-3 presents a *portion* of a sample statement, addressing this ubiquitous question, written by one of our undergraduate students in his successful bid for entry into a clinical psychology doctoral program committed to the scientist–practitioner model. His reasons for applying to "Bogus University" are presented only as a single example; your statements will need to be tailored to your interests and credentials as well as the application instructions. Remember that this is just one part of an entire autobiographical statement.

Nonetheless, his why-I-applied-to-your-program statement illustrates several important points. First, he advances multiple reasons for applying to that particular program. Five reasons sound much more convincing than one or two. Second, his reasons for applying to Bogus U. primarily address his professional match with the program (their reputation, faculty members, clinical opportunities) but nicely concludes with a

It is my strong desire to attend a doctoral program in clinical psychology. I am seeking a program committed to the Boulder model, training scientist–practitioners able to serve society in a variety of capacities. The program I attend should stress the importance of understanding and integrating the broad field of psychology, as well as providing the knowledge and training specific to clinical psychology.

After a thorough review of more than 50 programs in clinical psychology, I have chosen to apply to Bogus University for a number of reasons. First, your program is known for producing stellar graduates, and has been repeatedly recommended to me by several psychology faculty. Second, Bogus University allows students to immerse themselves in research early in their graduate careers. Third, I am drawn toward several of your faculty members, including Dr. Babe Ruth for her work in substance abuse and cognitive therapy, and Dr. Ty Cobb for his work in sexual health, stress, and coping. I would be pleased to have either of these faculty members as my mentor. Fourth, the available clinical experiences would allow me to work with a population I find of particular interest, such as adults and families at the Psychological Services Center. And fifth, I am looking to attend school in a scenic area of the country where both my fiance and I think we would be comfortable.

FIGURE 5-3. Portion of a sample autobiographical statement.

personal touch (geographic location). Third, he mentions two specific faculty and several potential research interests in an attempt to maximize the chances of a match. Fourth, the statement reflects his careful reading and incorporation of the program's self-description; for example, he cites the opportunity to immerse himself early into research and names the Psychological Services Center. Fifth, the statement is systematically organized and clearly written—indicators of an organized and clear-thinking graduate student!

Compose your personal statement as carefully as you would an important term paper. Write several rough drafts and then set it aside for a few days. Avoid slang words on the one hand, and overly technical or elaborate words on the other. Stick to the information requested; avoid too many "ruffles" and lengthy expositions of your own philosophy (Fretz & Stang, 1980). Write as many drafts as necessary until the statement sounds right to you.

Before you finish your personal statement, have friends read it for grammar, spelling, and typos. Regardless of the content, technical accuracy really makes a difference. Once it is error free, have one or more faculty members read it and make suggestions. Let them know where the statement is going, and they should be able to guide you on form and appropriateness.

For further tips on writing your personal statement, visit the following Web sites:

- www.essayedge.com
- www.psywww.com/careers/perstmt.htm
- www.accepted.com

- www.english.uiuc.edu/cws/wworkshop/tips/ writtechperstate.htm
- www.indiana.edu/~wts/wts/perstate.html

We hope that the suggestions in this section are helpful in guiding you in writing your personal statement. It is also our hope that they are not too constraining. This is the part of the application where a committee gets to see you in a more personal light, an area where "you can be you."

Letters of Recommendation

What do admission committees gain from letters of recommendation? The answer is a personal but objective evaluation of your work from someone experienced in the field. Admission committees desire a more objective sense of your abilities and experience than what you provide about yourself. Consequently, it is best to have at least two of the people writing your letters be at the doctoral level in psychology or psychology-related disciplines. One fine letter from a master's-level clinician is usually acceptable, but he or she will not be in a position to attest to your ability to complete doctoral studies. By the same token, bachelor's degree recipients, friends, and relatives should never write letters of recommendation to doctoral programs—they simply do not have the experience or knowledge of what it takes to earn a doctorate. Letters from politicians and your psychotherapists typically are inappropriate as well—they tend to write personal and psychological testimonies instead of academic letters of reference.

TABLE 5-1. Professors' Pet Peeves: Avoiding Neutral Letters of Recommendation

Students sometimes are unaware of how some of the seemingly innocuous things they do and say can annoy their professors. In turn, the professors provide students with less than enthusiastic letters of recommendation. Here are some examples suggested by William W. Nish of Georgia College, reprinted with his kind permission.

Be quick to apply such concise labels as "busy work," "irrelevant," and "boring" to anything you do not like or understand. Not only is this a convenient way of putting the professor down, but also you will not be bothered with the inconvenience of understanding something before you judge it.

Always be ready with reasons why you are an exception to the rules established for the class, such as the dates for submitting written assignments.

Avoid taking examinations at the same time as the rest of the class. Be certain to take it for granted that the professor will give you a make-up exam at your convenience, regardless of your reason for missing the exam.

Be very casual about class attendance. When you see your professor be sure to ask, "Did I miss anything important in class today?" This will do wonders for his or her ego. By all means expect the professor to give a recital of all of the things you missed instead of taking the responsibility for getting the information from another member of the class.

Be consistently late to class and other appointments. This shows other people how much busier you are than they are.

Do not read your assignments in advance of class lecture and discussion. This actually allows you to study more efficiently, for you can take up class time asking about things that are explained in the reading.

Avoid using the professor's office hours or making an appointment. Instead, show up when he or she is frantically trying to finish a lecture before the next class hour and explain that you must see him or her right that minute.

Do not participate in such mundane activities as departmental advising appointments. Instead, wait until the last minute for approval of your schedule, and then expect the professor to be available at your convenience.

Choose people with whom you have worked for a long enough period, preferably for a year or more. That typically excludes professor you have taken a single class with, even if you did get an A. If you wrote a particularly strong paper in the class and the professor knows you a bit better, then he or she could serve as a reference, but this reference is still not the most desirable. At best this person can say, "This student was always on time, participated in discussions, attended office hours, and tested very well. On this basis I consider him/her an intelligent student and a good candidate for graduate school."

By contrast, admissions committees want to hear something more detailed, like: "This student has worked with me for 1 year. During that time she scored MMPIs, tested participants using a Grass Model 7 polygraph, analyzed data, and conducted her own honors thesis. She was dependable and worked be-yond what was required by the department. Given this student's intelligence, motivation, and responsibility, I think she would make an outstanding graduate student." Though the above is a strong example, the point is that you want someone to attest to your ability and responsibility.

Table 5-1 lists some of the self-sabotaging things students do to receive neutral letters of recommendation. Although presented for its humorous nature, it also provides sage warnings about interpersonal behaviors that annoy professors.

Other students receive neutral letters of recommendation through no fault of their own. They experience difficulty in securing detailed letters of recommendation because they:

- Transferred from one college to another college before graduating (which occurs, according to the

U.S. Department of Education, to almost one-third of all students);

- Attended a mammoth state university where they only took huge lecture classes and never had the same psychology professor twice; or
- Switched majors relatively late in their college career and did not get to know their psychology professors well.

We are sympathetic to these plights. If you fall into one of these categories, then you need to double your efforts to get involved in clinical experiences, research activities, and departmental matters—and do so quickly.

Most graduate programs request three or four letters of recommendation. Try to secure letters that will give the admissions committee the information it desires. At a practice-oriented program, two letters from clinical supervisors and one from a research advisor might be prudent. At a research-oriented school, two letters from research advisors and one from a clinical supervisor would probably be more appropriate. All things being equal, it is preferable to have your "research" letters come from faculty. However, if you believe that a letter from an employer would be significantly more helpful than that of a professor with whom you are not well acquainted, then it is probably a good idea to use the employer.

Our general advice was recently confirmed in an interesting study (Keith-Spiegel & Wiederman, 2000) that asked members of admissions committees to rank sources of recommendation letters. Raters were asked to assume that the letters from these different sources were equally positive so that rating variations were due solely to the referee's characteristics. The most valuable sources of letters of recommendation were (in order): (1) A mentor with whom the applicant has done considerable work; (2) the applicant's professor, who is also a well-known and highly respected psychologist; (3) an employer in a job related to the applicant's professional goals; (4) the chair of the academic department in which the applicant is majoring; (5) a professor from another department from whom the applicant has taken a relevant upper-division course. By contrast, a letter from a graduate teaching assistant was rated, essentially, as no help. And a letter from one's personal therapist was actually rated negatively!

Very important: First ask the person writing the letters whether he or she can write you a good one. Ask this direct and specific question: "Can you write a good letter of recommendation for me?" If the person is hesitant or gives any indication of having reserva-

tions, *ask someone else!* A bad letter of recommendation is deadly. Better to have one brief letter from a professor who gave you an "A" than from someone who might express reservations about your abilities. "I don't know" is better than "I know, but I have reservations."

The way you approach professors for a recommendation is an underappreciated topic. You will ask specifically, "Can you write a good recommendation for me?" If the person responds in the affirmative, we strongly recommend that you provide that person with a letter similar to that shown in Figure 5-4. The person writing a letter of recommendation needs adequate information in order to produce a credible and informative letter. You can be powerful in shaping a professor's letter of recommendation!

This letter—and the attendant course listing and CV—will promote accuracy and detail. These are essential characteristics of strong letters of recommendation in that the admissions committee looks for positive tone *and* detail. A two-paragraph laudatory letter on the order of "Great student, fine person" simply doesn't make the detailed case for your admission into competitive doctoral programs.

What admissions committees also find useless in letters are duplicate and irrelevant information. One set of researchers (Elam et al., 1998) queried members of admissions committees and discovered the five least helpful aspects of letters of recommendation:

- Repetition of information from the application (e.g., repeating grades, honors, and scores available elsewhere on the application)
- Unsubstantiated superlatives or vague generalities
- Detailed descriptions of grades in one particular course
- Lack of strong relationship between applicant and letter writer
- Inclusion of irrelevant information, such as religious beliefs or hearsay

Put another way, give your referees sufficient data to render informed and positive letters about your personal characteristics, academic strengths, and interpersonal skills so that they do not resort to filling your recommendations with irrelevant content.

Here's how one doctoral program (University of Rhode Island) attempts to translate the content of recommendation letters into numerical categories.

1   Summary recommendations in all three letters are neutral or negative. Positive and

246 Wood Street
Babylon, NY 14000

November 2006

Leslie Jones, Ph.D.
Department of Psychology
East Coast University
1200 Faculty Building
Hausman, MD 43707

Dear Dr. Jones:

Thank you for agreeing to write a letter of recommendation on my behalf. I hereby waive (or do not waive) my right to inspect the letter of recommendation written for me and sent to the designated schools of my choice. I am applying to (master's, doctoral) programs in clinical (counseling) psychology. My earliest deadline is ____ _____.

Here are the courses I have taken from you.

Fall 2004	Abnormal Psychology	A–
Spring 2005	Clinical Psychology	B+
Fall 2006	Undergraduate Research	

Here are other activities in which I have participated.

| September 2005–January 2006 | Research Assistant |
| 2004–2005 | Vice President of Psi Chi |

My latest GRE scores were 600 Verbal, 590 Quantitative, and 580 Analytical Writing. My Psychology Subject Test score was 610.

Finally, I attach a copy of my current vitae and a list of psychology courses for any additional information that might prove useful. Please feel free to call me at 555-1212 or to e-mail me at Chris_smith@phonyemail.com. Thanks again.

Sincerely yours,

Chris Smith

Encls.

FIGURE 5-4. Sample letter to request a letter of recommendation.

negative assessments are listed. Overall evaluation in all three is neutral.

2 Letters meet criteria between anchor points 1 and 3.

3 Summary recommendations in all three letters are positive and general. Positive state-

ments from all three letters. Statements are general in nature.

4 Letters meet criteria between anchor points 3 and 5.

5 Summary recommendations in all three letters are excellent and detailed. Positive statements from all three letters are very favorable and very detailed in their support.

Note, again, that the emphasis is on positive tone *and* supportive detail. This is the desired result of your extra work in providing references with factual information and assertive requests for letters of recommendation. A "liability letter" is one that communicates limited knowledge of the applicant, leading an admissions committee to conclude that the person was only minimally connected to professors in his or her undergraduate or master's department (Halgin, 1986).

Many universities provide their own form for recommendations as part of the application package. Your institution will probably have one of two ways of handling these forms. One way is to provide your professor with these forms and stamped envelopes addressed to the schools to which the forms are to be sent. This is a small but crucial precaution—do not take the chance that postage will delay return of the letter. It is also courteous: Your professor is doing you a favor taking considerable time and contemplation to write a good letter. Another way is to provide your professor with these forms; he or she will then complete them and return them to the Office of Career Services/Planning for processing and mailing. Ask your reference which method he or she prefers.

A small but growing proportion of graduate schools are requesting that letters of recommendation be submitted electronically through their homepages or admission portals. In this case, you list the names, positions, and e-mail addresses of people writing you letters of recommendation on your application. The graduate schools then directly contact your referees via e-mail and provide them with the URL and a password to electronically submit their letters of recommendation to your application file. Online submission of recommendations will streamline the entire process and will become the rule in the near future.

The recommendation forms from graduate schools may appear to be quite different at first glance; however, closer inspection will reveal that they request essentially the same information. The forms typically ask the people writing the letters to note the length of time they have known you and in what capacities. Then the referees are asked to rate your research ability, originality, writing skills, organizational ability, maturity, interpersonal skills, persistence, and similar qualities on a structured grid. Typical forms request an appraisal of the applicant in terms of 10 qualities in comparison with others applying for graduate study whom the referees have known in the applicant's proposed field of study. The rating grid offers responses of top 3%, next 10%, next 20%, middle third, lowest third, and unable to judge. On most forms, an open space is then presented for a narrative description of your strengths and weaknesses. The forms usually conclude with a request for a summary rating: a check mark on a continuum from "not recommended" to "highly recommended" or a numerical value representing an overall ranking of this student to others taught in the past or some similar estimate.

A recent study identified and categorized the most frequent characteristics of applicants that recommenders were requested to rate on the forms (Appleby, Keenan, & Mauer, 1999). The resulting list—based on the analysis of 143 recommendation forms—describes the characteristics that psychology graduate programs value in their applicants. In descending order of frequency, the top dozen are as follows:

- Motivated and hardworking
- High intellectual/scholarly ability
- Research skills
- Emotionally stable and mature
- Writing skills
- Speaking skills
- Teaching skills/potential
- Works well with others
- Creative and original
- Strong knowledge of area of study
- Character or integrity
- Special skills, such as computer or lab

One important lesson to be learned from the results of this study is that graduate school aspirants should make a concerted effort to behave in ways that allow them to acquire relevant skills (research, writing, speaking, computer) and to be perceived by at least three of their professors as motivated, bright, emotionally stable, capable of working well with others, and possessing integrity (Appleby et al., 1999).

These forms, by law, will contain a waiver statement asking whether you do or do not waive your right to inspect the completed letter of reference. The Family Education Rights and Privacy Act of 1974 (the so-called Buckley Amendment) mandated that students over age 18 be given access to school records unless they waive this right. This is a complicated topic, but we advise applicants to waive their right of access *providing*, as previously discussed, the person writing the letter knows the student well and has unhesitantly agreed to serve as a reference. Do not waive access—or better yet, do not request letters—from persons you do not trust or do not know.

A confidential letter carries more weight. By waiving your right to access, you communicate a confidence that the letters will be supportive, and you express trust in your reference. In fact, over 90% of health professional schools prefer letters of recommendation that are waived by the student (Chapman & Lane, 1997). Our experiences and naturalistic studies (e.g., Ceci & Peters, 1984; Shaffer & Tomarelli, 1981) suggest that professors' honest evaluations will be compromised when you have access to what they have written. By waiving the right, you are communicating an intent to have the "truth" told. Otherwise, admissions committees may lump the letter with all the other polite and positive testimonials (Halgin, 1986).

In making your choice of whether to waive or not to waive, be clear about the law. Most students correctly know that if they waive their rights they may never see the letter. However, many students erroneously think that choosing not to waive their rights means that they can see their letter if they do not get accepted or that they have a right to preview the letter before it is sent (Ault, 1993). These are common fallacies, but fallacies nonetheless.

The relevant laws do not dictate that professors must show students the completed letter. One study (Keith-Spiegel, 1991) of college faculty found that 17% never show students their letters of recommendation, 46% usually do not, 8% only to students they know well, 15% only if students ask, and 14% routinely show students their letters. Nor does the law guarantee a student access to letters if the student is rejected from a graduate program; in fact, students may inspect their files at a graduate school only after they have been accepted at and enrolled in that graduate school (Ault, 1993).

Going one step further, contrary to some students' beliefs, faculty do *not* have to write letters of recommendation for students.

Letters are a common and voluntary courtesy, not a job requirement. Why might faculty members decline to write a letter for a student? The single most common reason is that they don't know the student well enough (Keith-Spiegel, 1991). Other frequent reasons given by faculty are that they question the student's motivation level, emotional stability, academic credentials, or professional standards. If faculty defer on your request for a letter, politely inquire about their reasoning and graciously thank them for their candor.

One creative study asked psychologists how they would handle requests for a letter of recommendation from a student exhibiting specific problems (Grote, Robiner, & Haut, 2001). The majority indicated that they would *not* write a letter for a student who was abusing substances or who had shown unethical behavior. For most of the other student problems—interpersonal problems, lack of motivation, paucity of responsibility, marginal clinical skills—psychologists routinely would tell the student about their reservations, then write the letter including the negative information. If faculty members tell you that they have reservations about your behavior, then they will probably include the negative evaluation in the letter of recommendation. Politely inquire if their reservation will in fact appear in the letter. If so, graciously thank them for their candor and withdraw your request for a letter.

Play it safe and provide the reference form at least 6 weeks before the deadline. Completing your recommendation may not be the top priority of the person you have asked to write it, or he or she may be out of town prior to the deadline. Do not take any chances that a letter will be late. Allow 2 weeks and ask if the letter has been sent. Be politic: do not pester, but do follow up.

If you seek additional information on requesting letters of recommendation, then we suggest the pointers offered by the following Web sites:

- gradschool.about.com
  (click on All About Recommendation Letters)
- www.uwm.edu/People/ccp2/work/recletter.html
- www.psychwww.com/careers/lettrec.htm

Transcripts and GRE Scores

An application file will not be complete—and probably not even considered by the admissions committee—unless the required academic transcripts and entrance examination scores have been received. Your task here consists of requesting the appropriate organizations to transmit official copies of these materials to the graduate schools of your choice and then ensuring that the schools have received them.

With respect to transcripts, you must request that the Registrar's Office of all attended colleges and universities mail an *official* copy of your transcript directly to the graduate school. An official copy will contain the seal, stamp, and authorized signature of the institution. The cost of transcripts varies from place to place, but it averages $3 to $5 per copy. Submit transcript requests at least 1 month before the application deadline. Many universities take 2 weeks during the semester to process these requests. The form requesting a transcript or the cover address will most likely accompany the transcript itself and thereby enter your graduate application file. Accordingly, this request form or mailing address should be typed or printed neatly.

A reminder: request an unofficial copy of your own transcript in September or October prior to applying. Inspect it closely for errors and omissions. Horror stories abound regarding erroneous transcript entries misleading admissions committees—an initial grade of I (incomplete) becoming an F (failure), honors credits not registered, unpaid term bills delaying transcripts, and so on. Don't leave it to chance; check it out yourself.

One creative researcher (Landrum, 2003) surveyed graduate admissions directors about the impact of transcripts and withdrawals in the admissions process. Results show that your transcript will get a careful review in practically all programs and will be reviewed by more than one member of the admissions committee in about 87% of the programs. With respect to the effects of course withdrawals (dropping a course after mid-semester) on transcripts, less than 4% of programs indicated that a withdrawal from a single course would hurt an applicant's chance of admission into the graduate program. But more than 20% of the programs indicated that two or more withdrawals hurt a student's entry into their graduate program. Thus, our advice to students contemplating a course withdrawal is that one is probably not hurtful, but that two or more withdrawals, especially from required courses such as statistics and research methods, may well have a negative impact.

With respect to GREs, score reports will automatically be mailed to you and electronically submitted to the four graduate schools you listed on your GRE registration form. The mailing date for the score reports is approximately 6 weeks after the test date for paper-based testing (Psychology Subject Test) and 2 weeks for computer-based testing (General Test). Your copy of the score report is intended only for your information; official reports are sent directly by ETS to the score recipients you designate. This procedure—as with the registrar transmitting an official transcript—"is intended to ensure that no questions are raised about the authenticity of a score report" (GRE, 2001, p. 16).

You will probably be applying to more than the four schools you initially designated for score reports. Toward this end, you can use the "Phone Service for Additional Score Reports" by dialing 1-888-GRE-SCORE. The charge is $10.00 per call plus $15.00 for each report requested, charged to your credit card. Your scores will be mailed within 5 working days. Or, you can submit an "Additional Score Report Request Form," published by ETS and obtainable at your Career Services Office, and remit your payment of $15.00 for *each* score recipient listed. The ETS pledges in writing to "make every effort to send your score reports within 10 working days after receipt of your request" (GRE, 2001), but you should allow for at least 1 month. You may have your GRE scores transmitted at any time during the 5-year period after they are initially reported.

Remember: only send unofficial copies of your GRE scores if you are applying well before the deadline, and telephone to be sure that this does not impede your application.

Unsolicited Documents

A frequently asked question is, "What if a program doesn't ask for something that I'd like to send?" Some examples are the curriculum vitae, a research paper, and job descriptions. If a program does not want additional documents, it will state so clearly on the application. In that case, do as the program requests. But even then, you may be able to make additinal documents a part of your application if you have come to know a professor at the school and have shared any of these documents with him or her. In general, it is a good idea to send a curriculum vitae, research paper, and/or job descriptions if they are applicable.

If you have relevant work and clinical experiences but can only use one for a letter of reference, then include a curriculum vitae or job description. One benefit is that these allow you to spend less time focusing on the details of these work experiences in your personal statement. You can relate how the experiences influenced you without wasting space explaining exactly what you did.

As a professional, you will need a CV eventually, and we recommend you begin one even if you do not use it in every application. Start a vitae file and toss notes and memos into it regarding assistantship duties, noteworthy activities, committee assignments, professional associations—in short, everything you need to update your vitae (Hayes & Hayes, 1989).

A job description details your specific duties and responsibilities. When asking a supervisor to write a job description, ask him or her to focus on your specific tasks and how well you performed them rather than asserting how well suited you are to graduate school. This allows you to spend less time describing what you did and how well you did it when writing your personal statement. For example, prior to graduate school, one of us worked with a psychotherapist conducting a social skills group for preadolescents. In his personal statement he was simply able to speak about how that experience had affected him. By referring to the "enclosed job description," the personal statement did not get bogged down in the details of this experience. Further, if you performed well at this job, having a supervisor's positive assessment allows you to be more modest in your personal statement.

If you have a large number of work experiences, be careful not to overwhelm admissions committees with paperwork. Choose two, or at the most three, experiences that showcase your diversity and that highlight characteristics not likely tapped by those writing your letters of recommendation. If you send more job descriptions than this, you may weaken their impact and increase the chances that the most laudatory ones will not be read (or at least not carefully).

If you have written a thesis or a research paper and have received feedback that it is well written, then include it. If there is someone whose research corresponds with your own, this may open a door for you. However, if there is a question as to your paper's quality, then do not to send it. A questionable paper may do more harm than good.

Application Fees

Last but unfortunately not least, most schools require application fees. These fees range from $0 to $100 per school, and average $50 for doctoral programs and $35 for master's programs (Norcross et al., in press). Send a personal check or a cashier's check (never cash). Attach the check securely and prominently on the front of the application with a paper clip.

If you are in financial need or are experiencing trouble meeting application expenses, read the application instructions carefully. There is usually a statement allowing fees to be waived because of financial hardship. Go to the school's application Web site, or call and ask how to have the application fee waived. That some students cannot afford the fees is the reason schools make the allowance in the first place. Graduate schools are sensitive to the impoverished status of many applicants, so please feel no compunction about requesting a fee waiver if it applies to you.

Check and Recheck

At this point, you have completed the application forms, requested letters of recommendation (and seen to it they were sent), written your personal statement, asked to have transcripts and GREs transmitted, and copied the unsolicited documents you plan to include in your applications. Once again, before you actually submit the material, have one of your professors check that it is accurate and well written. Have friends review it for typos and spelling. All material should be typed or word processed: it should look neat, error-free, and professional. It represents you in a very real way. Anything handwritten or tattered can convey the message that you are careless and unprofessional. Submission of materials should reflect a meticulous attention to detail. Finally, make sure your statement is not among those we see each year that carelessly includes the name of a different university when explaining why it is a perfect match!

After all this effort, make certain your application is sent on time. We suggest (if you can afford the extra expense) that you send your application via FedEx, UPS, Express, or certified mail. Each of these systems will allow you to track your materials to ensure they have arrived and to have the name of the person to whom they were delivered. However, our suggestion does not imply that you should wait until the last minute to express mail your application, implying procrastination (not a positive quality in a graduate student). Do express mail, but do it well ahead of the deadline.

One of the most frustrating experiences in the graduate application process is ascertaining that the respective programs have in fact, received all of your materials. Your application, transcripts, GREs, letters of recommendation—all need to be received, processed, and filed correctly by the graduate admissions office. Horror stories abound about application materials being lost or misfiled or sent to the wrong department. It happened to one of us! Recently, one of our students shared a similar story. The ETS claimed that her GRE scores were electronically transmitted to and downloaded at a major Midwest university. The university, which required two official sets of GRE scores, claimed that they never received either set. The student was caught in the middle between two opposing claims. She telephoned ETS again and the university's graduate admissions office repeatedly. The GREs had to be resent, at the student's expense.

We estimate that 50% of graduate programs will send a letter or e-mail apprising you of the application materials they have received on your behalf. Another 20% to 25% of graduate programs will post an application status page on their Web site where you can check yourself. That leaves 25% of the graduate programs that you can either blindly trust (which we *do not* recommend) or that you can contact (which we *do* recommend).

Call or e-mail the admissions office and verify that the material has been received. Some students prefer to include a self-addressed postcard to verify receipt, as discussed earlier, whereas others prefer the telephone. In either case, you have invested too much sweat, time, and money to leave the application to chance. Do not rely on graduate schools to keep you apprised; take personal responsibility.

CHAPTER 6

MASTERING THE INTERVIEW

The applications have been electronically submitted or mailed and are now out of your hands. Following the short-lived relief of finishing the applications, this period can be a nerve-wracking time. You have sold yourself on paper, and now it is up to the programs to decide which applicants to contact for further consideration and probable interviews.

The doctoral admissions process has been characterized as "multiple hurdles," with some of the hurdles applied sequentially (King, Beehr, & King, 1986). The initial hurdle in most programs is the GRE and GPA score minimums. The second hurdle is rating of applications on such criteria as clinical experience, research skills, letters of recommendation, and the like. Being invited for an interview means you have successfully leaped these early hurdles, and this is a great compliment in and of itself. The final and determining hurdle for many, but not all, programs is the personal interview.

Not all programs have interviews, and they will most likely state in the application if they do not. Make a note of this so that you do not become distressed when you are not invited. We wonder which is worse: the disappointment of not being asked to interview or the stress of being asked!

Our research on APA-accredited clinical, counseling, and combined psychology programs found that 93% of them required some type of preadmission interview (Oliver et al., 2005). As shown in Figure 6-1, 62% of APA-accredited programs strongly preferred an interview in person but were willing to accept a telephone interview. Another 27% of the programs absolutely required a face-to-face interview. Four percent required only a telephone interview. All told, only 7% of programs did not require an interview before admission into the program.

Nearly all clinical and counseling psychology programs, then, require some type of personal interview, be it by phone or in person, prior to acceptance. Since some programs absolutely insist on interviews in person, do *not* apply to distant programs requiring an in-person interview unless you can afford it. Only in very rare instances will programs reimburse the applicant for all interview costs, and only 10% of the programs reimburse for some of the costs (Kohout et al., 1991). In other words, 90% of the programs expect you to absorb all the interview expenses personally.

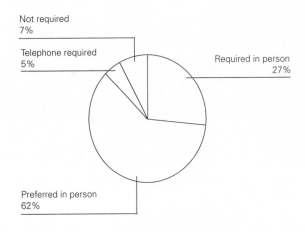

FIGURE 6-1. Preadmission interview policies of APA-accredited programs. Data from Oliver, Norcross, Sayette, Griffin, & Mayne (2005).

Expect to hear from interested doctoral programs that require interviews from mid-January through early March. Programs rarely contact students in the finalist pool after March 30 because the first round of offers usually goes out on April 1. It is still possible to be contacted, however, if you are on the alternate or waiting list.

If you have not received an interview request or a rejection letter by the middle of March, then calmly e-mail or telephone the doctoral program and inquire about the status of your application. If you have been rejected, politely thank the person. You never know, you may apply there again or have professional contact with the people from that program in the future. If your application is still being considered, it is permissible to ask when you might expect a decision. Just be careful not to be rigid or demanding.

Talented applicants are occasionally offered a personal interview at two doctoral programs on the very same day. Not to worry. Should you be so blessed, we recommend that you (1) inquire if the programs have alternative interview days (and schedule one program on the alternative day). If not, then (2) ask if you can complete a videoconference interview or telephone interview at the less-preferred program. Remember that approximately two-thirds of programs will accept a telephone interview. If you value both programs equally, then (3) accept the interview at the least expensive program or the program with the highest likelihood of acceptance.

The Dual Purpose

The interview is a critical opportunity for information gathering, not only for the program but also for you. That is, the dual purpose of an interview is for the program to check you out and for you to check the program out. Perhaps right now it seems outrageous to contemplate evaluating a doctoral program—you're probably delighted just to be asked! But a few interviews and an acceptance or two will reorient your perspective.

If you go on more than one interview, these interactions will give you information that will be the deciding factor in choosing which school to attend. You will find out about clinical training, student life, program fit, research facilities, and the like. Interviewers will be looking at your social skills, your emotional stability, your professional maturity, your focus, and your goals. The interviewers may want to see the development of your pursuits, the connection between your research and clinical work, or perhaps your adherence to the Boulder or Vail model. You may be asked pointed questions and will be expected to ask probing questions about the program.

Although the interview often generates anxiety for an applicant, it need not. As with anything else in the application process, the more you prepare, the more confident and less nervous you will feel.

A few basic observations about the interview process will contribute to your preparation. The interview is highly charged for the applicants and programs alike. *Both* wish to be evaluated positively and to achieve the best match. You are not alone in trying to put your best foot forward! Interview styles, moreover, vary tremendously—from a conversational tone to grueling questions, from casual to formal, from mundane content to intrusively personal content. Be prepared for all styles, and remember that all count equally in the final analysis.

That final analysis is the program's unenviable task of deciding which of the interviewees they will eventually select for admission. Programs ordinarily interview two to three times as many students as they can admit. The pool must be whittled down from, say, 200 applicants, from which 25 are selected for interviews, and from which 10 to 15 will be tendered an offer to obtain 7 confirmed acceptances.

Rehearsal and Mock Interviews

Rehearse the interview beforehand with a professor, a career counselor, or a knowledgeable friend. Although the research-oriented schools are usually less personal and invasive in their interviews, it may behoove you to get accustomed to being asked personal questions without being thrown. Such practice is invaluable, especially for preparing you to think on your feet. Rehearsing also will desensitize you to some degree, take the edge off of your anxiety, and add to your comfort with the process. During the interview you are on stage, selling yourself, and knowing what the interview is all about can only help you.

Moreover, in keeping with the dual purpose of the interview, rehearsing will afford you practice in the interview style you seek to convey. A respectful and curious tone—"I am wondering about the chances of receiving an assistantship if I am fortunate enough to be accepted?"—is preferable to a blunt and forceful disposition—"How much will you pay me if I come?" How you phrase a question is important. The interviewer will be more impressed with your eagerness to learn if you ask how many courses in an area are *offered* as opposed to how many are *required* (Megargee, 1990).

Rehearsing should also entail preparation for frequently asked questions of applicants. Table 6-1 pre-

TABLE 6-1. Common Interview Questions to Anticipate

1. Why do you want to be a psychologist?

2. What qualifications do you have that will make you a successful psychologist?

3. What attracts you to *our* program?

4. Will you tell me a little about yourself as a person?

5. Do you think your grades (or GRE scores) are valid indicators of your academic abilities?

6. What do you see as your strengths and weaknesses?

7. What do you bring into the program? What are your special attributes?

8. Have you ever had personal therapy? If yes, what sort of issues did you work on? If no, why not?

9. What are your research interests? Tell me about your research project/honors thesis.

10. What is your theoretical orientation?

11. Which of our faculty members do you think you would work with?

12. Where else have you applied or interviewed?

13. Can you tell me about a recent clinical encounter? How did you conceptualize or treat your last client?

14. What are your hobbies, avocations, favorite books, and interests outside of psychology?

15. What are your future plans and goals as a psychologist?

16. What questions do you have for me?

sents common interview questions to anticipate and prepare for. *We strongly recommend that you have a concise and thoughtful response ready for each of these.* An "I haven't really given that question much thought" answer hurts. Role-play these questions with a professor or, better yet, undergo a "mock interview" at your career services center. During this pretend experience, request that the interviewer ask several of the questions in Table 6-1 and videotape the encounter.

Of course, you cannot anticipate all possible questions. Some interviewers pride themselves on avoiding these stock questions and instead asking novel questions, thus precluding rehearsed and polished replies. The rationale behind these queries, such as "Who are your heroes?" and "What was the best day in your life?", is that they give a glimpse into your natural response style and tap into spontaneous information processing. One method to handle novel queries is to delay thoughtfully, remark that it is one you have not been asked before, request a moment of contemplation, and then respond forthrightly.

Similar to novel questions are behavior-based interview questions. These are increasingly being used to assess an applicant's behavioral repertoire and actual experiences. The behavioral questions rely on the familiar psychological dictum, "Past behavior is the best predictor of future behavior," to glean something about your future behavior in their doctoral program. Four examples are:

- Tell me about an instance when someone asked you to do something that you considered ethically or morally wrong. How did you respond?
- Describe the biggest challenges you faced in the past year and how you handled it.
- Tell me about a work or school situation where you had to do creative problem solving.
- Relate a recent situation in which you had to persuade someone to accept your idea or proposal.

Your answers will enable you to concretely demonstrate integrity, resilience, creativity, and persuasion as opposed to simply saying you possess the traits. Insure that your responses communicate a successful ending, both for you and the other party involved in the situation.

Interview Attire

Your interview rehearsal should direct attention to your physical attire, which will be an influential factor in attributions made about you. For men, we recommend a conservative two-piece suit or a jacket and slacks, white or light shirt, and contrasting tie. Three-piece suits and "funeral outfits" are out. Wear shined brown or black shoes that are well maintained; as your parents have probably told you, the way you take care of your shoes communicates a lot about you. Dark socks only; save your white socks for work-outs. Hair should be trimmed and neatly groomed. For women, we recommend a pant suit or a suit with a skirt, dark in color or muted plaid, polished pumps or medium heels in matching color. Wear a simple style blouse, white or soft color. Interview professionals suggest a "no distraction" hairstyle, tasteful makeup, and clear or light nail polish. One pair of small earrings should suffice. For both men and women, plan your interview clothes, try them on, and lay them out well before the interview to assure that they fit, are clean, and are in good repair.

Attire should err on the side of conservative and formal; better to be overdressed and loosen a tie or remove a scarf than to be underdressed for the occasion. Avoid flashy colors and loud fashions. Jewelry should be conservative and understated; go light on the perfume and cologne. Leave the piercings at home.

Some applicants complain to us that many faculty interviewers are wearing business casual, and thus ask why they (the applicants) can't wear business casual as well. Our answer is clear: You are an applicant trying to make a stellar impression as a serious, motivated candidate for a competitive graduate program. You are trying to distinguish yourself as one of the premier students, not one of the underdressed herd. We urge you to "dress for success" in interviews, not in business casual. You can wear casual clothes after you are admitted to the program for most of your graduate life. But during the interview, you never have a second chance to make a first impression.

Questions about the program and other written material should be held in a professional attaché or briefcase. The location and weather will influence your choice of clothing. Reliable answers about expected attire can be provided by graduate students with whom you are staying prior to the interview itself.

Travel Arrangements

While preparing and rehearsing for the interviews, you will simultaneously be making arrangements to travel to the interviews. The costs of travel vary wildly—from a few bucks for parking at a local university on interview day to more than $750 for a 3-day jaunt across the nation involving air travel, rental car, and hotel. Our intent in the following paragraphs is to save you hassle and money in getting to the interviews.

As a general rule, you can save a great deal of money by booking early and paying promptly for air travel, but you must pay a stiff penalty if you make any changes in your reservation. So begin early to find those bargains. Start by calling the airlines on their toll-free numbers to ask for their best rates. Then use your computer and go online to seek the best fares through that airline's Web site. Airlines typically post special discounted fares on their Web sites. Before booking, take a quick look at expedia.com, travelocity.com, and other commercial sites that promise the lowest possible fares. Compare the schedules and fares from all three sources—the airline booking agents, the airlines' Web site, and commercial Web sites—and then make a decision.

Being flexible in your travel schedule will probably save you money. It may save you money to leave from a different city than the one closest to you. We have saved hundreds of dollars on airfare by simply driving an extra hour to another airport. Or it may save you money to fly to a different city and then drive an hour or two to the interview. Try inserting nearby alternative cities in your computer search and see what fare comes up. One applicant flew out of Washington, D.C. instead of his home airport of Norfolk, Virginia, and reduced his ticket price from over $1,000 to $278 (Megargee, 2001).

Another way of being flexible is changing when you fly. As most business travelers return home on the weekend, airlines typically offer deep discounts on trips that extend over a Saturday night. The cost of another night at the hotel might save you hundreds in airfare. And consider flying on the "red eye" or "night owl" flights that criss-cross the country overnight. In order to fill otherwise empty seats, airlines frequently offer reduced fares at unpopular (and ungodly) hours (Megargee, 2001).

Some doctoral programs may coordinate rides from the airport to the university for applicants, but most do not. You are on your own. In advance of your arrival, check out bus and train routes. The university's homepage will typically have public transportation routes and driving directions from the local airport to the campus. If public transportation is unavailable, you will need to rent a car at the airport. You will find, again, that the rental costs vary widely. And you will, again, investigate the costs early and aggressively to locate the best fare. Rely on the three traditional sources—the rental company's toll free number, its Web site, and the commercial travel Web sites—for two or three rental companies.

Renting a car on your own will require at least three things: a valid driver's license; a major credit card in your name; and a chronological age over the minimum, typically 25 years of age. The latter can be a huge hassle if you are still an undergraduate; be aware of the company's age policy in advance. Most doctoral programs will extend you an invitation to room with a graduate student in the program the night before the interview. If possible, take advantage of this opportunity. It will allow you to save money, acquire masses of information, and gain a sense of student life and the campus community from people in a position to know. If you reside with a graduate student, ask for a tour the day or night before the interview. Ask to see the psychology building, the training clinic, the library, and some of the labs. If possible, get comfortable with the rooms where the interviews will be held.

Unfortunately, not all programs offer or provide a free place to sleep. In these cases, unless you have a large extended family, you will spend an evening or two in a hotel. Your task here is to secure a safe, convenient location at a reasonable rate. Use the AAA tour book and the Web for preliminary reconnaissance. If you have wheels, you can often save money by staying at one of the less expensive places on the edge of town or near an Interstate exit. In particular, if you are on a tight budget, be sure to check out places with the code word "Inn" in their names, as in Comfort Inn, Days Inn, Fairfield Inn, Hampton Inn, Hobo Inn, and Red Roof Inn (Megargee, 2001).

Even these inns may have negotiated rates. Ask the person scheduling your interview if the university has negotiated special rates with any local hotels. When booking your room, ask what discounts are available—for students, AAA members, government employees, and so on.

Whether you spend the night in a hotel or with a graduate student, you may well be invited to dinner. Be sociable and friendly, but do not drink heavily or party hearty the night before (even though you may be invited!). Get a solid night's sleep, arise on time, and eat a sensible breakfast.

Although we discussed attire and appearance in the previous section, it is worth a few more sentences as applied to travel. You may well experience some delays in your flight itinerary or in your driving time to the interview. As a consequence, you may not have that expected hour or two to clean up and change before the interview. Or you may well meet other applicants en route and faculty members at the airport. The moral: do not travel in cutoffs, warm-up suits, or t-shirts unless you are prepared to interview in that outfit. Dress and travel like a professional.

Interview Style

The objective of your interview style is to present yourself as a confident, knowledgeable, and genuine person—an imperfect human, to be sure, but one without major interpersonal deficits or gross psychopathology. Even if you are anxious, try to appear relaxed, calm, confident. Any anxiety you may be experiencing is understandable and should be dealt with maturely. Strive to be as genuine, mature, and natural as possible.

The interview is designed for the interviewer to get to know you as a person—your interpersonal skills, career goals, and clinical acumen. One of the few empirical studies on the role of the personal interview in the psychology admission process found that the rating of an applicant's clinical potential was the most highly weighted measure among all the interview data. Ratings of verbal skills and research skills also contributed to the prediction equation, but ratings of clinical potential contributed most to discriminating among groups of accepted applicants, alternates, and rejected applicants beyond that which could be accounted for by such objective measures as GRE scores and GPAs (Nevid & Gildea, 1984). In one way or another, you must impress the interviewers as someone they would be comfortable sending a member of their own family to for professional treatment.

The following factors, according to Fretz (1976), have been found to lead to rejection of an applicant during interviews:

- Poor personal appearance
- Overbearing, overaggressive, know-it-all style
- Inability to express yourself clearly—poor voice, diction, grammar
- Inadequate interest and enthusiasm—passive, indifferent
- Lack of confidence and poise—nervousness, appearing ill at ease
- Making excuses, evasiveness, hedging on unfavorable factors in record
- Lack of tact and maturity
- Condemnation of past professors
- Little sense of humor
- Emphasis on whom you know
- Inability to take criticism
- Failure to ask questions about the program

The last point is worth emphasizing. Each interviewer will want to get to know you as a person and will expect you to ask questions. Nothing is tougher on an interviewer than the person who does not ask questions or simply responds "Yes" or "No."

So even if it has been a long day, when the fifth interviewer asks you if you have any questions, don't reply, "No, all my questions have already been answered." And respond to the questions of the fifth interviewer with the same enthusiasm as you showed to the first interviewer (Megargee, 1990).

At the same time that you are conveying clinical potential and a mature interpersonal presence, you want to acquire the factual program information necessary to make informed decisions. Table 6-2 is a list of questions that you can have answered when you interview (or if you correspond with a professor and have an earlier chance to tour the facilities). You should ask some of these questions during the interview, others before, and others after. Some should be asked of professors, because they are best suited to answer them and asking can make you look prepared and informed. Some questions should be asked of first-year students because they have recently been through the process and are closest to your situation. Some questions are better asked of fourth-year students because they are about to leave and may have less investment in hiding the program's shortcomings.

The best questions to ask are those that indicate initiative, curiosity, and responsibility (Hersh & Poey, 1984). Try to communicate motivation to learn and eagerness to participate in many activities; avoid questions that promote a speculation that you are demanding, complaining, or single-minded.

A caveat: never ask for information that is available in the program description or the graduate catalog. These questions make you appear unprepared for the interview and uninterested in the program.

Alternatively, link your specific question to general information sent to you. Examples might include: "I read that all of your first-year students receive an assistantship and tuition remission. Is this also true of second-year students?" "Your graduate catalogue lists a Couples Therapy course, a special interest of mine, but it does not indicate if clinical supervision in that area is available." "While reading about your impressive Psychological Services Clinic, I wondered how many of the full-time clinical faculty provide supervision there." And so on.

The intent is to get beyond the gloss and formality of the published program descriptions to the lived and personal experiences of the program participants. Virtually all descriptions of clinical and counseling psychology programs, for example, will allude to ample opportunities for practical experience in off-campus placements. But when you directly ask students, "What is your clinical placement like?" their answers may diverge substantially from the published information. Their responses may indeed be positive, but it is not uncommon to learn that some of the placements are 50 miles away, do not offer any stipend, and are very competitive. To be sure, be tactful in your questioning, but also be assertive in securing crucial data.

Program directors (e.g., Hersh & Poey, 1984) have nominated certain questions to *avoid* asking. These unwittingly annoy interviewers or communicate an undesirable impression: questions regarding the typical length of a graduate-student week, which may indicate fear of hard work or a long week; persistent inquiries regarding an area of interest that the graduate program only minimally provides; questions reflecting resistance to learning the major theoretical orientation offered by that program; and antagonistic questions concentrating on the perceived limitations of the program, be they financial, faculty, or geographical.

Bring your list of questions with you to the interview, but do not constantly have it in plain sight to check off. Your task is to ask the questions of the most appropriate individuals in a respectful manner. On a similar note, many people have "palm pilots" to help organize personal information. Though you might use one to make an important note at the *end* of an interview, keep them away during the interview itself. And on that note, cell phones and beepers should be left at home, or turned off during the interview. Having one beep or buzz will be disruptive, and actually checking a pager or taking a call would be seen as *extremely* unprofessional and rude.

Extreme ideologies—religious, sociopolitical, or clinical—do not bode well in interviews. One interesting study (Gartner, 1986) mailed mock graduate school applications to professors of clinical psychology. The results showed that professors were more likely to admit an applicant who made no mention of religion than they were to admit an otherwise identical applicant who was identified as a fundamentalist Christian. Do not deny your beliefs, of course, but try to avoid expressions of rigid extremes. Academics favor informed pluralism and critical open-mindedness.

Bernard Lubin (1993), a former national president of Psi Chi and a veteran of conducting admission interviews, enjoins applicants to present themselves as *knowledgeable* and *collaborative* during the interview. Being familiar with the research interests and productivity of the program faculty can go a long way. Carefully reading the program's guide and identifying faculty publications through *PsycLIT* are direct evidence of a

TABLE 6-2. Interview Questions an Applicant Might Ask

Clinical

Is training available in different theoretical orientations?

Is the supervision individual or group?

Do the full-time faculty conduct the supervision?

What type of supervision will I receive?

When do I actually begin clinical work?

How many practica are offered?

What are your off-campus clinical practica like? Where are they located?

What types of patient populations are available?

Are specialty clinics available?

Do the faculty have active private practices?

Do faculty serve as clinicians or consultants at local mental health facilities?

Research

What is the student–faculty ratio?

About how many dissertations and master's theses are chaired by each faculty member?

When and how am I assigned an advisor?

Does this person have weekly research meetings?

Could I sit in on a lab meeting?

How many of the core faculty are actively involved in research projects (e.g., regularly publishing)?

Do any research grants finance graduate students?

If I wanted to change my mentor or advisor, is that allowed?

How many lab computers are available to graduate students?

Are computers readily available? Is photocopying free?

Is SAS or SPSS available?

What is the relationship with the medical or law school?

Finances

What percentage of students receive full financial support (assistantship plus tuition waiver)?

What types of fellowships are available?

What types of research and teaching assistantships are available?

What is the average amount of a 9-month assistantship?

Who gets tuition remission? What are my chances?

Do the stipends cover the costs of living in this area? How are the rents?

What percentage of students receive funding during the summer?

Do any of the assistantships include health insurance?

Quality of Life

What is it like to live around campus? Is it safe? Expensive?

What is the surrounding city/town like?

Is graduate housing available? Do most students live on campus?

What is the off-campus housing situation like? The neighborhoods?

Where can I go to get a housing application today?

Are there theaters, movies, decent restaurants nearby?

Is there public transportation, or do I need a car?

What are some of the campus events and clubs?

Is the Graduate Student Association active?

Do the students socialize frequently?

How is the student cohesion?

Do students and faculty attend the colloquia?

Department and Politics

Do students and faculty have good relationships with each other?

Do graduate students have a role in departmental policy and admission decisions?

Are there regular department meetings?

What is the standing of the psychology department within the university?

How do the different branches of psychology interact?

What are the professional goals of the current students?

How many fifth-, sixth-, seventh- . . . year students are there?

Is there a sense of competition or cooperation among the students?

How much emphasis is put on course work and grades?

How common are grades of C?

Do professors tend to collaborate on projects?

Do I get a master's degree along the way? When is this usually done?

Can the program be undertaken on a part-time basis? What percentage of the student body is part-time?

When do I take the qualifying exams? What are they like? How many people fail? Can they be retaken?

Could I see a course schedule for next (or last) year?

Are teaching opportunities available for graduate students?

For applicants who already have a master's: Once accepted, how are transcripts evaluated regarding credits?

Outcomes

Where do your students complete their internships?

What percentage of your students obtains an APA-accredited internship?

What is the average length of the program (including internship)?

What percentage of your incoming students eventually earn their doctorates here?

Do dissertations usually get published?

In what type of settings do most of your graduates eventually find employment—academic, private practice, clinics?

mature and scholarly attitude. This leads to presenting yourself as a potential collaborator: welcoming opportunities to work with faculty members and fellow students, displaying an affirming and positive attitude toward interdependent activities.

A final piece of advice on interview style concerns your nonverbal behavior. Some applicants are so preoccupied with asking questions and trying to impress the interviewer that they neglect the way they present themselves nonverbally. But interviewer impressions of candidate personality are heavily dependent upon nonverbal behaviors (Anderson & Shackleton, 1990). Maintaining eye contact, making changes in posture, and varying facial expressions strongly contribute to an image as a mature and enthusiastic person. The research consistently advises interviewees to keep high levels of eye contact with the interviewer and to display frequent positive facial expressions to maximize their chances of success. Your mock and actual interviews should strive for an interpersonally engaging style that creates personal liking and that cultivates an impression of interpersonal and intellectual skill.

Literally hundreds of Web sites offer advice on interviewing skills. Although they are no substitute for live rehearsals and mock interviews, they are a source of considerable information and examples. Some even offer virtual interviews. Our favorite sites are:

- www.quintcareers.com
- www.quintcareers.com/behavioral_interviewing.html
  (specifically on behavioral interviewing)
- www.content.monstor.com/jobinfo/interview/
- www.careercity.com
- www.nextstep.org

Stressful Questions

This brings us to consider a prominent fear, namely, being placed on the spot with intensely personal questions. You may have heard stories about applicants being asked intimate questions about their families of origin, romantic relationships, and personal history they would prefer not to share. You should be prepared to answer personal questions about such relationships and self-perceptions. Answering these questions in a straightforward manner contributes to the interviewer's positive evaluation of an applicant.

The nature of these questions varies with the interviewer's style as well as the program's theoretical orientation. Applying to a research-oriented behavioral program, however, is no guarantee that you will not be interviewed by a psychodynamic member of their faculty. Questions pertaining to family conflict or to your personal therapy could arise. Anticipating such questions can help you to determine how to handle them most comfortably and to decide how much information you are willing to disclose. Knowing where to set your boundaries can lead to a smoother interview.

Speaking of boundaries, the APA Ethics Code (APA, 2002, p. 1068) does not require students to disclose sensitive information regarding their "sexual history, history of abuse and neglect, psychological treatment, and relationships with parents, peers, and spouses or significant others" unless the training program has clearly identified this requirement ahead of time. Thus, unless the program sent you a specific notice of such a requirement for the interview, you are not ethically obliged to reveal such personal information. Our advice is to balance your need for privacy with the program's need for information about your personal history and psychological dynamics.

One stressful but popular question concerns your personal weaknesses. Applicants naturally wonder how honest to be about their deficits and try to balance the need for honesty with the need to leave a favorable impression of themselves. We have found three strategies useful in approaching this question. One is to minimize an existing limitation: showing your awareness of it but not articulating the full severity or manifestation. If being taken advantage of frequently is your perceived weakness, for example, you might reply on the order of "Occasionally I find myself being taken advantage of by others in small but consistent ways." A second strategy is to turn the weakness into a possible strength. Following the same example, you might remark that "I give to a fault on occasion and find some people will take advantage of my tendency to find the best in people." A third possible strategy is to express your awareness of the weakness and your efforts to remediate it; this reply demonstrates both introspective and corrective attitudes. "I've been working to become more conscious of how people, especially personality-disordered clients, can take advantage of me. My over-trusting nature is slowly giving way as I attend more closely to this relationship pattern." Whatever strategy—or combination of strategies—you elect, the response must be consistent with who you are. A phony or inauthentic response can immediately strike an applicant from further consideration.

One stressful situation necessitates your careful preparation. A few programs and faculty use what is called a "stress interview." In this interview, the faculty member intentionally acts inappropriately and tries to intimidate applicants, simply to see how they handle the stress of the situation. This can come in many forms:

long silences after you answer questions; asking overly intimate questions; disagreeing violently with your position or answer; feigning disinterest in you as an applicant; or even giving you coffee in one hand, a powdered donut without a napkin in the other, and then handing you an article to browse! Knowing ahead of time that this can happen is crucial, because you can remind yourself that it is not personal but simply part of the process. In a few programs, the professors place all the applicants in an empty room and suggest they speak with each other while the professors observe the interpersonal process: no other directions, no other structure. This all serves to compound the students' anxiety.

Stress interviews are designed to assess how comfortably you behave under such interpersonally challenging conditions. The interviewers deliberately arrange situations or ask questions that you cannot predict, for examples, "How would you redesign a giraffe?" or "Where is Oregon?" The particular answer you give is not as important as the manner in which you answer. Here your interpersonal savvy and presence can triumph. The interviewer is testing your reaction to stress: do you react to stress with humor, anxiety, self-denigration, anger? The stress interview is an ambiguous, semiprojective device.

Our advice is to remain calm and polite, yet assertive. Generally, it is not wise to become entangled in a verbal battle or retreat into an apologetic or defensive stance. In the face of an inappropriately personal question, a "I wonder how that question relates to my admission here?" will demonstrate both your personal boundaries and your willingness to broach a difficult topic. In the face of continuing conflict, a polite "we respectfully disagree" can suffice, and leave it at that (Heppner & Downing, 1982).

Practicing stress interviews with professors or peers may sufficiently desensitize you to keep your head and field the situation without too much ego bruising. Another way to prepare yourself is to stay overnight before the interview and take the opportunity to ask graduate students which professors might conduct such an interview, allowing you to know ahead of time that this person is likely to intentionally try to stress you. Foreknowledge and preparation are the best defenses.

Group Interviews

Admission interviews in clinical and counseling psychology differ markedly from one program to another. At one extreme, a few programs invite you for a single, 2-hour interview with a senior faculty member. That's it—no tour, no group interview, no program orientation, and no interaction with current graduate students.

At the other extreme, a number of programs invite selected applicants for an entire admissions weekend. At the University of Pittsburgh, for example, invitees to the clinical psychology program's weekend spend a full day (about 7 hours) interviewing with faculty and graduate students. In addition, there are clinical and research information sessions, laboratory tours, evening parties, and a poster session featuring research projects. Many of the applicants arrive on Friday and leave Sunday morning. In between these two approaches are intensive 1-day sessions. For instance, at Fordham University's counseling psychology program (Kopala et al., 1995), the interview process entails a brief orientation to the program, individual interviews with a faculty member and a graduate student, a videotaped group experience, a 30-minute writing sample, an open session with graduate students, and then a closing session with the director of training.

Virtually all programs will arrange for at least one individual interview with a faculty member and for some interactions with current doctoral students. A healthy proportion of programs will also include admission interviews featuring multiple candidates in the same room at the same time. This group interview may be conducted in the interest of sheer efficiency, of observing your interpersonal style, or both.

Our advice on your interview style and objectives in these group interviews remains essentially the same as for the individual interviews, but there are a couple of twists. First of all, strive to be pleasant and honest with the other interviewees. Share your experiences, never denigrate their credentials, and treat them like future colleagues (which they may very well be). A negativistic or superior attitude is likely to be held against you in the final deliberations of the admission committee.

Second of all, since it is a group situation, try to present yourself as an admirable facilitator. Don't be a group psychotherapist or a control maniac, but a respectful cofacilitator of the interview process. If you have already asked a few questions about the program, for instance, you might say that you have additional questions but would first like other people to have an opportunity to have their questions answered. As they say in the social psychology literature, try to manifest both a high task orientation and a high social orientation.

Additional Tips

Whether it is an individual interview or a group interview, here are additional tips regarding the interview.

- Arrive at least 15 minutes early on interview day. Find the offices, acclimate to the building, and get settled.
- Be compulsive and double-check your interview schedule. Being late or missing an interview (even when it is not your fault) can reflect poorly on you.
- Greet each interviewer in a friendly, open manner. Your handshake should be firm and your eye contact frequent.
- Demonstrate your active listening skills: wait to answer until the interviewer has completed asking the question and give complete answers to the question posed to you.
- Keep your answers to 1.5 to 2 minutes long. Use good grammar and diction. Say "No," not "nah."
- Avoid all irritating hiccups in your answers. On the short list are the irritating "you know," "like," and "okay."
- Always bring extra copies of your CV. Every interviewer may have not received a copy or may have not yet reviewed it, so bring along copies to present and leave with people (Megargee, 1990).
- Take cash along in case you are invited to lunch or dinner with graduate students.
- Conclude each interview by thanking the interviewer for her time and information. Wrap it up with a cordial and pleasant tone.

Our collective experience in conducting interviews also generates a list of *don'ts*:

- Don't call faculty members by their first names until (or if) they offer. The default option is to call them "Dr." or "Professor."
- Don't whine or complain about the interview arrangements. Accept the free housing with gratitude; be agreeable about the food; act flexibly about interview dates. Nobody, including admissions committees, likes a fussbudget.
- Don't accept offers of coffee or other beverages during the interview itself. It tends to be messy, distracting, and awkward for you as the interviewee. Wait until after the interviews are complete and then graciously accept the offer.
- Don't ask about or negotiate financial assistance before receiving an offer of admission. The nitty-gritty of finances can wait until later.
- And don't ask questions during the interview that are answered in the materials sent to you or posted on the program Web site. We have already made this point earlier in the chapter, but it is important enough to reiterate it here.

If you follow these steps, you will find it easier to relax during the interview. The more prepared you are, the more confident and at ease you will feel.

Telephone Interviews

Two situations may dictate a telephone interview. In the first, you are asked to visit the school for an interview, but you cannot afford to do so. This is no reason to be embarrassed, and the more straightforward you are about it the better. You can request a phone interview in advance if you do not have the resources for an actual visit. In the second situation, you receive the dreaded, unannounced phone interview. At least one of the programs you apply to will probably call without prior notice and ask to speak with you on the spot.

Luckily, if you anticipate telephone interviews, you have nothing to worry about. One strategy is to rarely or never take a phone interview "cold." Consider telling the caller, "I'm sorry, but I was just leaving for an appointment. Could you leave a number and arrange for me to call you back?" This buys you time to review your information on that program and to prepare for the interview. However, you do not want to communicate disinterest in the program.

Another strategy is to prepare phone cards, palm pilot notes, or computer files. These are 3 × 5 index cards or short files that you make for each program to which you applied. On it, record a few specific reasons for your interest in that school and the name(s) of the professor(s) you are interested in working with, a little about their research areas, and questions you may have about clinical training or facilities (many of the questions in Table 6-2). Figure 6-2 is an example of such a card. Keep a stack of these by the phone, or on a computer by the phone and in moments you will find the card for a particular school and not be caught unaware! This little extra effort can prevent a serious detraction from your application. If you receive one of these telephone calls and cannot remember which professors are at that school, their areas of research, or the kind of facilities they have, it tells the interviewer that you are not serious about his or her program. This could place you lower than someone who has this information off the top of his or her head.

A Note of Thanks

Once you have completed an interview, whether by telephone or in person, a brief note of thanks to the interviewer is in order. This gesture serves multiple

University of Alexandria

Reasons for my interest: Great reputation in child psychopathology and psychotherapy; specific professors (Smith, Adams); geographic location; has speciality clinic in behavioral medicine.

Key professors:

Dr. Smith: child psychopathology; substance abuse

I read your May [2003] article in *Journal of Bogus Psychology*, in which you found offspring of alcoholics to be more receptive to the anxiety-reducing effects of alcohol than control subjects. Do you expect to continue this line of research next year? Is an assistantship available?

Dr. Adams: behavioral medicine; psychotherapy

I was impressed that you have a separate clinic in behavioral medicine. What type of clients do you most often treat? What opportunities are there for clinical experience?

Other professors with potential interest:

Dr. Jones: prevention

Dr. Watson: forensic psychology

Program questions: [Refer to Table 6-2 for representative listing]

When do I begin seeing clients in the training clinic?

What percentage of incoming students are financially supported?

What are the research opportunities in child psychopathology?

FIGURE 6-2. Sample telephone card.

purposes: it demonstrates your social skills, communicates your gratitude to the faculty and students involved, reaffirms your interest in the program, and keeps your name alive in the admission process. Seldom will such a brief note do so much for you.

The "who" and "what" of these thank-you letters are almost entirely dependent on your interview experiences. The "who" should certainly include anyone who has shown you special attention, such as a graduate student you roomed with the night before or after the interview, a professor who personally escorted you around a lab or clinic, or a faculty member who offered an unscheduled interview. Letters to several people are often called for. If the interview was less personal, then at a minimum send the Director of Training a letter of appreciation. A sample letter is displayed in Figure 6-3. An e-mail note of appreciation may suffice, but we definitely prefer an ordinary letter by mail, because it will probably be placed in your application file for all to see and appreciate.

The "what" of the letter must be individualized to your particular experiences, but will probably contain at least three components: an expression of gratitude for the interview, an enumeration of your favorable impressions of the program, and a reiteration of your

interest in attending that program. Try to personalize each letter by referring to specific topics or experiences; for instance, recall your discussion of potential research studies or mention the friendliness of the graduate students. There is no definitive list of do's and don't's, but don't send a generic, impersonal letter and don't promote your candidacy. Do sound appreciative and personal. As with all written materials, insure that your letter communicates an image of sincerity and professionalism. Most of the letters should probably be word-processed, but a neat, handwritten note is appropriate if an interview was relatively informal and personal.

The Wait

Once you have finished the interviews and mailed the thank-you letters, it is a waiting game. But not for the programs, which still have a finalist pool of students much larger than they are able to accept! The interview process has probably weeded out a few, but the faculty are left with too many finalists, all of whom have very acceptable GPAs, GREs, and letters of recommendation.

What, then, are the *final* selection criteria? This pivotal question was addressed in a study by Keith-Spiegel, Tabachnick, & Spiegel (1994), who had 113

246 Wood Street
Babylon, NY 14000

March 16, 2006

Barry Bonds, Ph.D.
Director of Clinical Training
Department of Psychology
University of Western States
13 Orangegrove Drive
Wilksville, CA 98765

Dear Dr. Bonds:

I want to thank you for interviewing me for a position in your clinical psychology doctoral program. I enjoyed meeting with your faculty and staff and learning more about the program. My enthusiasm for the program was particularly strengthened as a result of my interactions with Drs. Timothy Hogan, Elizabeth Cannon, and Carole Buchanan.

I want to reiterate my strong interest in attending your program; the University of Western States offers a great deal that appeals to me. Please feel free to call me at (123) 456-7890 or e-mail me at csmith@uofs.edu if I can provide you with any additional information.

Again, thank you for the interview and your consideration.

Sincerely yours,

Chris Smith

FIGURE 6-3. Sample letter of appreciation to an interviewer.

faculty members actively involved in selecting psychology Ph.D. students rate criteria used in making the last cuts in admission decisions. (Results of this study should *not* be generalized to Psy.D. programs.) The faculty members were asked to imagine that they were left with a pool of finalists, three times the size of the number they can accept, all of whom had strong undergraduate GPAs, GRE scores, and letters of recommendation. They then rated 31 final variables in terms of importance on a 5-point Likert scale (5 = very important; 3 = somewhat important; 1 = not important).

Congruent with this book's advice and earlier studies, the top-rated criteria in clinical programs pertained to student match with the program and its faculty, research experience resulting in a journal article or a paper presentation, and the clarity and focus of the applicant's statement of purpose. Considered to be somewhat to generally important in assisting selection committees with their final admission decisions were research assistant experience; reputation of the student's referees; relevant clinical experience; membership in an underrepresented ethnic minority group; knowledge and interest in the program; number of statistics, methodology, and hard science courses completed; prestige of the psychology faculty in the student's undergraduate department; reputation of the undergraduate institution itself; and honors bestowed on the student by that undergraduate institution. Rated as not important or minimally important were such variables as the student's geographic residence, Psi Chi membership, and a close relationship between the student and former graduates of that program.

Demand always exceeds supply in competitive clinical and counseling psychology programs. The three primary criteria used to evaluate applicants by doctoral selection committees—grade point averages, GREs, and letters of recommendation—typically fail to narrow the applicant pool to the small number of slots available. At that point, research skills, clinical experiences, "good match" factors, and writing skills come to the fore (Keith-Spiegel et al., 1994). Bear these considerations in mind as you approach your interview—just as we have in preparing this book.

And now you wait until contacted with the final decision of the admissions committee. Until the week before April 1, it is probably not a good idea to contact a program and ask where you stand. Applicants who make repeated calls or e-mails may appear overly anxious and irritate the staff (Mitchell, 1996). The one exception is if you have received other offers, and the program you would most like to attend has not contacted you—a situation covered in Chapter 7.

This brings us to the last step in the application process and the final chapter of the *Insider's Guide*.

CHAPTER 7

MAKING FINAL DECISIONS

As with any realm of human affairs, good decisions regarding graduate school require time, preparation, and knowledge (Scott & Silka, 1974).

By April 1, all APA-accredited clinical and counseling psychology programs will make their first round of acceptance offers. At this point you will have 2 weeks to make your final decision as to where you want to go to school. By APA regulations, you have the right to consider offers until April 15, at which time an offer may be withdrawn. So you must be thoughtful but decisive in these 2 weeks.

To protect applicants from making hasty, premature decisions, all APA-accredited programs and most others have agreed to allow candidates until April 15 for a final decision (or the first Monday after April 15, if April 15 falls on a weekend). This is in accordance with a resolution adopted by the Council of Graduate Schools in the United States in 1965, approved by 317 universities and colleges, and further modified by the Council of Graduate Departments of Psychology (COGDOP) in 1981. As presented in the *Graduate Study in Psychology,* this resolution reads as follows:

> Acceptance of an offer of financial aid (such as graduate scholarship, fellowship, traineeship, or assistantship) for the next academic year by an actual or prospective graduate student completes an agreement which both student and graduate school expect to honor. In those instances in which the student accepts the offer before April 15, and subsequently desires to withdraw, the student may submit in writing a resignation of the appointment at any time through April 15. However, an acceptance given or left in force after April 15 commits the student not to accept another offer without first obtaining a written release from the institution to which the commitment has been made. Similarly, an offer by an institution after April 15 is conditional on presentation by the student of the written release from any previously accepted offer. It is further agreed by the institutions and organizations subscribing to the above Resolution that a copy of this Resolution should accompany every scholarship, fellowship, traineeship, and assistantship offer.

Acceptances and Rejections

What do you do when one program makes you an offer and you are still waiting to hear from another program you would prefer to accept? To begin with, *don't say yes to any school until you are certain that this is where you want to go!* Once you say "yes," that is it. You are committed. Saying yes to another school can endanger your acceptance at both places. If you have any reservations, do not feel pressured to say yes. Thank the person and say that you have been made other offers and you need a few days to consider this crucial decision.

If you have received offers but have not heard from the programs that most interest you, telephone or e-mail them. Explain that you are considering offers but that you do not want to act on them until you know what your status is there. It's OK to say, "I've been accepted at University X and Y, but I am most interested in your program. Can you give me an indication where my application stands, or at least whether it is still being considered?"

The "Guidelines for Graduate School Offers and Acceptances," adopted by the Council of University Directors of Clinical Psychology (1993), specifically

TABLE 7-1. Student Reasons for Choosing a Clinical Psychology Doctoral Program

Reason	Mean rating	Rank
Reputation of the program	4.29	1
Amount of clinical supervision	4.27	2
Training facilities available	4.21	3
Appropriate mentors available	4.19	4.5
Emotional atmosphere of the program	4.19	4.5
Tuition waiver available	4.10	6
Amount of stipend offered	4.07	7
Theoretical orientation	4.04	8
Diversity of program	4.00	9
Specific specialty training available	3.89	10
Research experience available	3.85	11
Expected length of program	3.82	12
Amount of research supervision	3.80	13
Success of previous graduates	3.79	14
Specificity of the training program	3.66	15
Geographic location	3.60	16
Specific professor to work with	3.57	17
Family/significant others in area	3.00	18
Recreational activities available	2.69	19
Number of minority members in program	2.48	20
Break required during program	2.30	21

Note. From Walfish, Stenmark, Shealy, & Shealy (1989). © 1989 American Psychological Association. Reprinted by permission.

encourage directors of training (or admissions) to apprise students of their position on the alternate list. Typically this entails a placement of high, middle, or low on the alternate list. If such a designation is used, the operational definition of "high on the alternate list" is that, in a normal year, the student would receive an offer of admission (but not necessarily funding) prior to the April 15 decision date.

Earlier, we emphasized the point that you should not accept an offer until you are certain that is the program you want to attend. On the other hand, if you have been accepted at three programs, and one of them is obviously less suited to your needs, be considerate of other applicants and decline that offer. The program can then make their offer to someone else who may very much want to attend that school. *Only keep two offers alive at any one time.* Otherwise, a huge "logjam" or "bottleneck effect" will occur across the country, with each program waiting for a few students to decide.

As long as there is a possibility that you may attend a certain program, be careful not to decline prematurely. As other students decline at these schools, you may be offered a better financial package if you have not yet made a formal commitment.

When all is said and done, how will you decide on which offer to accept? This is a difficult question to answer because of the multiple factors involved and because the final determinant will be how you, as an individual, weigh those various factors.

One study (Walfish, Stenmark, Shealy, & Shealy, 1989) had 201 first-year graduate students rate the reasons for their final selection of a doctoral clinical program. Their average ratings are shown in Table 7-1, where a rating of 1 was "very unimportant" and 5 was "very important." As seen there, the most important factors were the reputation of the program, the amount of clinical supervision, the training facilities, availability of mentors, and the emotional atmosphere of the program. We have emphasized throughout the preceding chapters the importance of the first four factors, but not the last.

The emotional and interpersonal ambience of a program should not be underestimated. You should seriously consider interactions with faculty and graduate students. The faculty–student relationship may be the single most important factor in your intellectual and professional development, and this relationship may be formal or informal, distant or close. Concurrently, the vast majority of graduate student time is spent with other students rather than with faculty members. You are likely to retain these personal contacts and professional relationships over the years. Moreover, fellow students are essential sources of encouragement, companionship, and inspiration. You want a good, lasting "fit" with the program (Scott & Silka, 1974).

In choosing a graduate program to attend, all students place a premium on general factors such as program quality, training opportunities, emotional atmosphere, and financial aid. At the same time, however, ethnic minority applicants rate the relevance of multicultural factors higher than do white students (Bernal et al., 1999; Toia, Herron, Primavera, & Javier, 1997). These considerations include minority students in the program, presence of minority faculty, research on minority topics, and opportunity to work with multicultural clients. Be particularly attentive to the program's diversity as it relates to your interests and goals.

The expected length of the doctoral program is a fairly important reason for choosing a particular program, as seen in the middle of Table 7-1. You may recall from Chapter 1 that clinical Ph.D. students take an average of 6.2 years to complete their doctorates, including the 1-year internship. Psy.D. students take an average of 5.1 years, a consistent difference of 1 to 1.5 years less. On the one hand, the shorter training period favors the Psy.D. programs. But, on the other hand, the financial aid favors the Ph.D. programs. As you have learned, far more Ph.D. students are receiving tuition waivers and assistantship stipends than Psy.D. students, most of whom are footing the entire bill for their doctoral education. Use the Reports on Individual programs to consider the expected length of the program in the context of probable financial aid from the program.

The reasons for choosing a clinical psychology program, as shown in Table 7-1, are largely self-evident, but two reasons *not* listed in that table deserve some consideration. *Attrition rates* refers to the percentage of students not completing the program. Attrition has been characterized as a "hidden crisis in graduate education" (Lovitts & Nelson, 2000). Between 20 and 24% of full-time psychology students, on average, formally leave programs without completing their doctorates (Fennell & Kohout, 2002). Attrition in graduate programs is not solely related to academic ability; life problems, financial difficulties, interpersonal conflicts,

and program dissatisfaction enter into the equation. Programs in which more than 25% of the doctoral candidates fail to graduate should be carefully screened when you make your final decision.

Preliminary or qualifying examinations, a second consideration in the complexities of your choice, are a series of structured tests that some programs require at the end of their first or second year. These examinations assume many forms, but generally they all test a candidate's knowledge of a wide range of areas in psychology—research methodology, learning, development, motivation, history, social, and personality. In some programs, only one attempt may be permitted to pass this examination (Scott & Silka, 1974). You should learn if the program requires "prelims" or "quals," whether multiple attempts are provided, and what percentage of students pass, before you make your final decision.

You should now be well acquainted with the importance of the decision criteria presented in Table 7-1 in your own life and well informed about the program's attractiveness on these criteria. If not, immediately request additional information on any of these for which you lack knowledge prior to making an informed choice of the program to attend.

The Financial Package

Note in Table 7-1 that the sixth and seventh most important selection factors are financial (tuition waiver and stipend amount). For many applicants, the financial aid offered by the school will probably assume an even higher priority in making final decisions. When an offer is made, establish if the program is offering financial assistance. If so, does it cover tuition remission? Is it guaranteed for 4 years? Is it considered taxable at that institution? Does it provide health insurance? If you have a teaching or research assistantship, how many hours per week will it entail? Are you allowed to earn additional outside income?

On average, private universities are more expensive than public or state universities. Typically, the "in-state" versus "out-of-state" cost difference that operates in undergraduate education is not as salient in graduate education. That is because (1) once you begin study, you can establish residency there and pay in-state tuition after the first year, and (2) many financial aid packages include a tuition remission.

But graduate training is expensive, and external sources of financial support are slowly drying up. Consider, for instance, the average stipends and accumulated loans for Ph.D. psychology students over the years (Golding, Lang, Eymard, & Shadish, 1988). Back

TABLE 7-2. Median Tuition Costs in Psychology by Institution Type and Degree Level

	Institution type		Degree level	
	Public	Private	Doctoral	Master's
State residents	$3,178	$16,596	$5,362	$2,776
Nonstate residents	$8,416	$16,596	$11,824	$7,217

Note. Adapted from Pate (2001).

in the 1960s and 1970s the average graduate stipend was higher, and the typical student's accumulated loan lower, than in the 1990s, adjusted for inflation. In fact, the average stipend amount decreased 36% (controlled for inflation) over the past 20 years. About three-quarters of psychology doctoral candidates carry loans. Support is still available but not to the degree it once was—which accounts, in part, for your professors' fond memories of their "good ol' graduate days."

Federal support for graduate training has been eroding in all fields, including psychology. In 1972, for instance, almost 7% of all full-time graduate students in psychology held federally funded research assistantships. Twenty years later, federal sources supported only 4% of full-time graduate students in psychology (Wicherski & Kohout, 1992). Similarly, almost 30% of Ph.D. recipients in clinical psychology back in the 1970s reported that federal fellowships and traineeships provided the major support for their graduate training. Twenty years later, that figure was down to 6% (Coyle & Bae, 1987).

Research supports the conclusion that today's graduate students are being asked to shoulder a larger share of their education costs. This is particularly true in Psy.D. programs, which fund proportionally fewer graduate students than Boulder-model Ph.D. programs. Refer to the Reports on Individual Programs for the percentage of a program's students who receive partial or full funding.

Table 7-2 shows the median tuition costs for psychology graduate students. The numbers demonstrate that tuition is largely a function of three variables: institution type, state residence, and degree level. Private universities uniformly charge higher graduate tuition than public institutions, just as is the case on the undergraduate level. Tuition at private institutions per academic year is five times higher than state tuition at public institutions. Freestanding Psy.D. programs, routinely charge between $15,000 and $25,000 per year for tuition. Although your state residence does not influence tuition at private universities, it definitely reduces your tuition at public universities—from a median of $8,416 for non-state residents to $3,178 for state residents per year. Predictably, too, tuition is higher for doctoral programs than for master's programs. So, your annual tuition can range from $0 if you secure tuition remission, to $3,000 if you are a resident attending your state university, to $16,000 if you attend a Ph.D. program at a private university with no financial assistance, all the way up to $25,000 if you attend a freestanding Psy.D. program.

Table 7-3 presents the assistantship stipends for psychology graduate students in 2004. As seen there, the median 9-month stipends for teaching and research

TABLE 7-3. Median Assistantship Stipends in Psychology

	Doctoral students	Master's students
Teaching assistantship	$10,617	$5,000
Research assistantship	$10,065	$5,000
Fellowship/scholarship	$11,500	$2,000
Traineeship	$13,658	$6,000

Note. Data from Norcross, Kohout, & Wicherski (in press).

assistantships averaged $5,000 for master's students and $10,000 for doctoral students (Norcross, et al., in press). The typical hours worked per week for an assistantship are 15 to 16. Stipends for doctoral students are consistently higher than those for master's students. (Fennell & Kohout, 2002).

Financial considerations include the tuition cost, available stipend, and living costs. The latter cannot be ignored: although tuition costs may be equivalent in New York City and Kansas, the living costs are certainly not.

Once accepted into a doctoral program, you will naturally be eager to learn about the status of your financial assistance, but you will hear from institutions at different times depending on the form of the financial assistance. If it is department-controlled financial assistance, then you will ordinarily hear when you are accepted or shortly thereafter. If it is university financial assistance, not directly controlled by the psychology department or school, then it may well be weeks after you are accepted. Examples in this category are fellowships from the Graduate School, resident assistantships from Student Affairs, or a Graduate Assistantship in the Admission Office. If it is financial assistance from a government agency, such as the National Science Foundation (NSF) or National Institutes of Health (NIH), then you will hear on or before their published notification dates. Finally, if it is financial assistance in the form of loans, then you will hear from the bank, Sally Mae, or the lending institution on their (painfully slow) schedule.

The Alternate List

Your fervent hope is to receive an e-mail or telephone call early in April from the director of admissions offering you acceptance into your top-rated program with generous financial aid. But this glorious dream may not happen; instead, the sobering reality is that many applicants will be rejected from several programs, will secure offers from programs lower on their list, or will receive offers without financial assistance. Many will also receive calls informing them that they have been "wait listed"—that is, placed on the alternate list.

As mentioned previously, ask the director of admissions where you stand on the alternate list—high, middle, or low. For your planning purposes, be politely assertive in probing further: "In typical years, what percentage of students with this position on the alternate list receive an admission offer? What percentage of the students admitted from the alternate list receive funding?" Without answers to these questions, you cannot render an informed decision on your other offers.

The admissions directors will, in all likelihood, arrange for you to be kept abreast of your admissions status until April 15th. They may telephone you or you may telephone them on occasion to determine the probability of admission.

When speaking with the program representative try to impress upon him or her three key ideas. First, you are keenly interested in attending that program. Second, express your availability by stating you have not accepted another offer of admission. And third, if you have received another offer, inform the program accordingly; most schools desire people who are attractive to others. Enthusiasm, availability, and attractiveness frequently move students up the alternate list.

The tricky part of this process is how frequently an alternate should contact (by telephone or e-mail) the program representative. Too much contact will appear aggressive or desperate; too little, passive or complacent. Strike a balance by asking the program representative how often you may contact him or her without being irritating.

Decision Making

The choice of which offer to accept and which program to attend is a momentous one indeed. You, like 86% of students enrolling in graduate programs, will quickly discover that the decision-making process boils down to your sense of fit with a program (Kyle, 2000). A few fortunate souls may receive an early offer with excellent financial aid from their number one program. But most graduate school applicants will ultimately select the program that makes the "best" offer—an offer that needs to be seriously weighed on a host of the aforementioned and often conflicting considerations.

The "April madness" abounds with such quandaries as: "Should I take the program with the best training but with no financial aid or the program with solid training and half tuition remission for 4 years?"; "Two programs have offered the same money, but the one that I prefer is 600 miles from my partner. What should I do?"; "My top program guaranteed me a teaching assistantship that requires 15 hours a week. My fourth choice is offering tuition remission and a fellowship. Any advice?"

Our advice centers on using systematic decision making. Begin by gathering all the salient data by interviewing program faculty and students, consulting published materials, and speaking with your mentors. Prioritize your primary reasons for selecting one program over another. Then develop a decision-making grid that will assist you in ranking your choices.

Two practical articles describe in detail how to apply decision-making techniques to choosing psychology programs and internships. Jacob's (1987) decision grid asks candidates to evaluate training programs along criteria that are important to them. You weigh those criteria that are more important to you correspondingly higher. You then tally the ratings for each training program to make the final decision. While it may sound a bit overintellectual, in practice we have found that the decision grid forces students to identify the criteria that they value most highly.

Stewart and Stewart (1996) describe a paired-comparison ranking technique, a method originally traced back to psychophysiological methods developed by Gustav Fechner. The first step of this technique is to select the relevant personal, professional, and practical criteria that you will use in comparing programs to one another. Consult the preceding pages to identify these criteria; more importantly, conduct an honest self-evaluation to determine which of these lie in your heart. The second step involves prioritizing these selection criteria. Do this by writing the name of each criterion on a single index card or piece of paper, and then forcing yourself to rank them in order. The third step entails generating a list of programs that will be compared to one another. We suggest that you use those programs that have accepted you or which have placed you on their waiting list.

The fourth step of the technique involves the actual pairwise comparison of the programs. Write the names of the graduate programs along one side of a large piece of paper and the selection criteria on the other side. Which of the training programs most clearly satisfies your criteria? Make a choice and allow no ties. For each criterion, put a hash mark across from the program that wins. The hash marks will be counted to determine your choice.

Although the final result will generally agree with what you expected, the more productive outcome of these two decision-making techniques may be that they force you to view your selection decision from multiple perspectives and to prioritize numerous criteria. To be sure, this is a complex method for a complex decision, but one that we and our students have repeatedly found surprisingly effective for making "impossible" choices more thoughtfully and systematically.

Finalizing Arrangements

An offer must eventually be formalized and specified in writing. Verbal offers and verbal acceptances are binding, but your acceptance of the offer should be in writing at the end of the process. Likewise, assistantships, tuition waivers, and stipends should be guaranteed in the written offer; respectfully insist that the financial arrangements be specified so that misunderstandings do not ensue. Should the offer be "contingent on expected funding," determine the odds of the funding coming through. No position is absolutely certain in life, but some are more certain than others.

Weighing offers, negotiating financial aid, and dealing with rejections make this a heady period. Be careful not to get caught up in the experience and forget the most important point: accept one offer and confirm it in writing!

One of our students (the affable Jean Willi) was offered admission to a prestigious doctoral program, with financial assistance. He carefully considered alternative offers, negotiated with other programs, leading to predictable delays. He awoke one morning in a cold sweat, realizing that he had turned down all other offers but had not formally accepted the offer of admission and financial package from his school of choice. He was in graduate school purgatory! Although the school was understanding and everything eventually worked out for Jean, because he missed the deadline, the school had the option of changing the financial aid package, or even revoking the offer of admission. The moral of the story: don't pull a Willi! Be clear and decisive and put it in writing.

Figure 7-1 presents a representative letter of acceptance. Note that the letter should explicitly mention any conditions of your acceptance, including financial assistance.

Once you have formally accepted an offer of admission in writing, two small matters of etiquette remain: (1) informing other programs who have accepted you, and (2) expressing your appreciation to those mentors who wrote letters of recommendation on your behalf and on their own time. Figure 7-2 offers a sample letter declining an offer of admission. It should be succinct yet polite. Thereafter, send a brief e-mail or thank-you note to those who have assisted you through your graduate application journey. They will be interested in the outcome of your application process and may well join the ensuing celebration!

If Not Accepted

What happens if you are not accepted anywhere? The grim truth is that one-third to one-half of the entire applicant pool to APA-accredited clinical and counseling psychology programs will *not* make it in a given year (Korn, 1984). There are at least five alternatives:

246 Wood Street
Babylon, NY 14000

March 25, 2006

Annika Sorenstam, Ph.D.
Director, Admissions Committee
Department of Psychology
University of Western States
13 Orangegrove Drive
Wilksville, CA 98765

Dear Dr. Sorenstam:

I am pleased to accept your offer of admission to the University of Western State's Ph.D. program in counseling psychology as a full-time matriculated student beginning in the Fall 2007 term. My acceptance is predicated on the conditions outlined in your letter of March 20th (attached), including full tuition remission for three years. I appreciate your confidence in me and very much look forward to joining the counseling psychology program.

Sincerely yours,

Chris Smith

FIGURE 7-1. Sample letter of acceptance.

1. *Contact the APA Education Directorate in early May and request a copy of the "Graduate School Openings List."* This document contains a list of graduate programs in psychology that still have openings for students in the fall. Although there are no clinical or counseling doctoral programs and only a few nonclinical doctoral programs on the list, you may find other programs of interest to you. To obtain a copy, call 202-336-5710, or go to the APA Web site in May at www.apa.org/ed.

2. *Apply to master's programs in clinical or counseling psychology.* Master's degrees are frequent stepping stones to the doctorate in psychology. Although taking your master's at one institution and transferring to another for the doctorate is not as efficient as being admitted directly into a doctoral program, there are advantages nonetheless. One is that the acceptance odds are more favorable—49% for master's programs in clinical psychology and 67% for master's in counseling psychology on average (Norcross, Kohout, & Wicherski, in press). A second advantage is that a few years of graduate training in psychology can improve your grade point average, GRE Psychology Test score, clinical acumen, and research skills. A third plus is an opportunity to confirm that psychology is the career for you. A cruel irony of baccalaureate recipients admitted directly into doctoral programs is that they have little direct contact with the field they claim as their lifelong career! A fourth advantage is exposure to twice the number of faculty supervisors and theoretical orientations. A fifth and final advantage is the flexible course offerings—part-time study and, frequently, night courses are available in master's programs (Actkinson, 2000).

Selecting a *quality* master's program in psychology may be a key to eventual admission into a doctoral clinical program. By all means try to avoid master's programs that have come to be pejoratively called "money mills." These programs exhibit most or all of the following features: accepting a very high percentage (80% plus) of applicants; offering courses only in the evening or largely by part-time faculty; providing no funded graduate assistantships; being reluctant or un-

246 Wood Street
Babylon, NY 14000

March 25, 2006

Annika Sorenstam, Ph.D.
Director, Admissions Committee
Department of Psychology
University of Western States
13 Orangegrove Drive
Wilksville, CA 98765

Dear Dr. Sorenstam:

I was pleased to receive your March 19th letter offering me admission to the Psy.D. program in clinical psychology at the University of Western States. I thoroughly enjoyed speaking with you and your colleagues and appreciated your generous offer of financial assistance. Unfortunately, I can only accept one admission offer, and I must regrettably decline your attractive offer. Please extend my genuine thanks and best wishes to the entire admissions committee.

Sincerely yours,

Chris Smith

FIGURE 7-2. Sample letter declining an admission offer.

willing to state what percentage of their graduates go on to doctoral programs; declaring openly their disinterest in research; requiring little undergraduate preparation in psychology; and communicating greater interest in filling classroom seats than in attracting qualified students.

By contrast, quality terminal master's programs in psychology can be roughly assessed by three criteria: exhibiting few of the aforementioned characteristics of "money mills"; holding a favorable reputation among the psychological community; and faculty producing published research. Gordon (1990) lists 20 American master's programs ranked highest in productivity in 15 APA journals; interested students are directed to that article.

In addition to the foregoing research-based article, we heartily recommend that you consult an extensive compilation of master's programs in psychology. The classic is APA's (2005) *Graduate Study in Psychology,* which lists hundreds of master's (and doctoral) programs in psychology throughout the United States and Canada. To order, call 1-800-374-2721 or order directly

from APA's Web site. A more recent source, consisting of over 260 master's programs, is *Master's Programs in Psychology and Counseling Psychology* (Buskist & Mixon, 1998). To order, call 1-800-278-3525 or e-mail ablongwood@aol.com.

3. *Apply to doctoral programs that are not accredited by APA.* In general these programs fit into one of two categories. They may be very credible institutions that simply have not been around long enough to gain APA approval. Programs cannot apply for accreditation until they have graduated students, which takes several years. Usually these programs are planning on applying for accreditation as soon as they are eligible. However, there is a second category of institution not accredited by APA. These programs usually do not conform to APA standards and often do not even attempt to gain accreditation. The quality of these programs is often considerably lower than those of the APA-accredited programs. Because of their status, non-APA-accredited programs typically provide greater probabilities for acceptance. If you do apply to such programs, by all means determine

why they are not accredited, and whether their students are able to gain admission into credible internships and, later, to become licensed psychologists. You should refer to the most recent edition of APA's *Graduate Study in Psychology* to explore these and other programs.

4. *Decide against a doctorate in clinical or counseling psychology.* If your goal is to become a researcher or a psychotherapist, psychology is not your only option. Reexamine the other choices listed in Chapter 1 and consult your advisors to see if one of these options is suited to your needs.

5. *Apply again in a year or two to APA-accredited programs.* Knowing the criteria used by graduate schools, take a realistic look at what seem to be the limitations in your application. Many students continue to resubmit the same rejected application year after year to no avail; "doing more of the same" typically results in more of the same misery.

Another year can be an opportunity to remediate your weaknesses. Were your GREs low? Take a professional preparation course and retake the test. Was your GPA a bit low? Then take some additional courses or retake some old courses in which you did not perform your best to improve it. Take some graduate courses in psychology on a nonmatriculating basis to demonstrate your ability. Were you short on research skills? Then take 1 or 2 years and acquire a research position, paid or volunteer, in a psychology or psychiatry department. Did you lack significant clinical experience? Then spend a night or two a week working for a suicide hot line or find a job at a women's shelter. Were your letters of recommendation tepid or brief? Then acquaint yourself better with potential referees so they can write a positive and detailed letter.

Another year can also provide an opportunity to enhance your interview style or to acquire better matches with graduate faculty members. Some applicants find themselves in the position of perennial "bridesmaids" or "best men," not because their credentials were inadequate, but because their interview style or matching potential was a tad weak. Spend the extra months improving your interpersonal presentation and investigating programs that promise to be better fits with your interests.

The so-called gap year is not intended as a vacation or a "year off." Instead, it is a year dedicated to improving your credentials and working hard at what interests you. When friends or parents ask what you are doing on your purported "year off," we believe the appropriate response is to proudly reply, "Preparing for my career in clinical/counseling psychology!"

In summary, reread this text and conduct a rigorous self-assessment of where you are and where you want to be. If you're still set on a career in clinical or counseling psychology, be prepared to take the time and energy to make yourself a better applicant. Especially if you are still in college and had planned to go straight on to graduate school, take time to gain some life experiences. Age and experience can work in your favor, and they will certainly help you better define your goals next time through the application process.

Two Final Words

Realism and persistence. Be realistic about your credentials, capacities, and acceptance odds. There are those applicants who refuse to accept the hard facts of the admission process and tragically resubmit the identically flawed application year after year to no avail. An honest evaluation of your credentials, perhaps with the assistance of an experienced professor, will enable you to strengthen your application, select more appropriate programs, or reevaluate your career decisions. This is not to dissuade or discourage you; it is realistic encouragement.

And be persistent! Many successful psychologists have required two or three tries to get into a doctoral program. Thousands of clinical and counseling psychologists have earned a master's degree at one institution before moving on to receive a doctorate at a different university. There is no shame in reaching for the stars; the real loss is not to reach at all.

We hope the information and suggestions contained in this *Insider's Guide* have been helpful to you. We wish you the best success in the application process and in graduate school.

REPORTS ON COMBINED PROFESSIONAL–SCIENTIFIC PSYCHOLOGY PROGRAMS

University at Buffalo/State University of New York

(counseling/school)
Department of Counseling, School, and Educational Psychology
Buffalo, NY 14260
phone#: (716) 645-2484
e-mail: stmeier@acsu.buffalo.edu
Web address: http://www.gse.buffalo.edu/DC/CEP/CP.html

1	2	**3**	4	5	6	7
Clinically oriented		Equal emphasis			Research oriented	

What percentage of your faculty subscribes to or practices in each of the following orientations?

Psychodynamic/Psychoanalytic	0%
Applied behavioral analysis/Radical behavioral	50%
Family systems/Systems	25%
Existential/Phenomenological/Humanistic	5%
Cognitive/Cognitive-behavioral	25%

What percentage of students applying for internship last year was accepted into APPIC-member internships? 82%

What courses are required for incoming students to have completed prior to enrolling?
Most students have a B.S. in psychology.

Are there courses you recommend that are not mandatory?
None

GRE mean
Verbal 602   Quantitative 618   Analytical Writing 5.0

GPA mean
Overall GPA 3.7

Number of applications/admission offers/incoming students in 2005
74 applied/12 admission offers/10 incoming

% of students receiving:
Tuition waiver only: 0%
Assistantship/fellowship only: 0%
Both tuition waiver & assistantship/fellowship: 100%

Approximate percentage of students who are
Women: 85%   **Ethnic Minority:** 20%   **International:** 0%

Average years to complete the doctoral program (including internship): 5 years

Personal interview
Required in person

Research areas	# Faculty	# Grants
assessment	4	0
family therapy	1	0
grief counseling	1	0
health psychology	4	0
multicultural psychology	1	0
rehabilitation psychology	2	0
vocational psychology	1	0

Clinical opportunities
Very diverse, including schools, community agencies, and hospitals in urban, suburban, and rural areas.

University of California–Santa Barbara

(counseling/clinical/school)
Department of Education
Santa Barbara, CA 93106
phone#: (805) 893-3375
e-mail: cosden@education.ucsb.edu
Web address: http://education.ucsb.edu/ccsp/

1	2	3	4	5	**6**	7
Clinically oriented		Equal emphasis			Research oriented	

What percentage of your faculty subscribes to or practices in each of the following orientations?

Psychodynamic/Psychoanalytic	20%
Applied behavioral analysis/Radical behavioral	10%
Family systems/Systems	50%
Existential/Phenomenological/Humanistic	40%
Cognitive/Cognitive-behavioral	60%
Developmental	50%
Feminist	10%
Eclectic	100%

What percentage of students applying for internship last year was accepted into APPIC-member internships? 100%

What courses are required for incoming students to have completed prior to enrolling?
None

Are there courses you recommend that are not mandatory?
Human development, personality or abnormal psychology, research design or statistics, physiological psychology

GRE mean
Verbal 600   Quantitative 645

GPA mean
Psychology GPA 3.8
Junior/Senior GPA 3.76

Number of applications/admission offers/incoming students in 2005
365 applied/27 admission offers/12 incoming

% of students receiving:
Tuition waiver only: 5%
Assistantship/fellowship only: 35%
Both tuition waiver & assistantship/fellowship: 60%

Approximate percentage of incoming students who entered with a B.A./B.S. only: 60%   **Master's:** 40%

Approximate percentage of students who are
Women: 85%   **Ethnic Minority:** 52%   **International:** 2%

Average years to complete the doctoral program (including internship): 6 years

Personal interview
Preferred in person but telephone acceptable

Research areas	# Faculty	# Grants
autism	1	2
career counseling	2	1
counseling LGBT clients	1	1
cross-cultural counseling	3	1
high-risk families, children	4	4
learning disabilities	3	3
multicultural counseling	4	1
school risk	5	3
school violence	3	2
substance abuse	3	4

Clinical opportunities
autism
career counseling
child abuse
community mental health
eating disorders
family therapy
school interventions
university counseling

Florida State University

(counseling/school)
Psychological Services in Education Program
Department of Educational Psychology and Learning Systems
307 Stone Building
Tallahassee, FL 32306-4453
phone#: (904) 644-1781
e-mail: gpeterso@admin.fsu.edu
Web address: http://www.epls.fsu.edu/general/programs.htm

1	2	3	4	**5**	6	7
Clinically oriented		Equal emphasis			Research oriented	

What percentage of your faculty subscribes to or practices in each of the following orientations?
Psychodynamic/Psychoanalytic 15%
Applied behavioral analysis/Radical behavioral 15%
Family systems/Systems 75%
Existential/Phenomenological/Humanistic 15%
Cognitive/Cognitive-behavioral 100%

What percentage of students applying for internship last year was accepted into APPIC-member internships? 75%

What courses are required for incoming students to have completed prior to enrolling?
Requirements for a master's degree in counseling or a related discipline

Are there courses you recommend that are not mandatory?
Not specifically

GRE mean
Verbal 550   Quantitative 550
Analytical Writing   Data not available

GPA mean
Junior/Senior GPA   Data not available

Number of applications/admission offers/incoming students in 2005
40 applied/11 admission offers/9 incoming

% of students receiving:
Tuition waiver only: 0%
Assistantship/fellowship only: 50%
Both tuition waiver & assistantship/fellowship: 50%

Approximate percentage of incoming students who entered with a B.A./B.S. only: 5%   **Master's:** 95%

Approximate percentage of students who are Women: 62%   **Ethnic Minority:** 20%
International: Data not available

Average years to complete the doctoral program (including internship): 5.9 years

Personal interview
Preferred in person but telephone acceptable

Research areas	# Faculty	# Grants
career development	3	2
counseling youth/prevention	2	3
school/community interventions	3	2

Clinical opportunities
adult learning and evaluation center (diagnose learning disabilities and prescribe treatments to adults)
full-service career center
human services center (general psychological services to 5-county area)

Hofstra University

(clinical/school)
Department of Psychology
Hempstead, NY 11550
phone#: (516) 463-5662
e-mail: Psyjtc@hofstra.edu
Web address: http://www.hofstra.edu/Academics/Graduate/Programs/GP_PSY/index_GP_PSY.cfm

1	2	3	**4**	5	6	7
Clinically oriented		Equal emphasis			Research oriented	

What percentage of your faculty subscribes to or practices in each of the following orientations?
Psychodynamic/Psychoanalytic 2%
Applied behavioral analysis/Radical behavioral 45%
Family systems/Systems 3%
Existential/Phenomenological/Humanistic 0%
Cognitive/Cognitive-behavioral 50%

What percentage of students applying for internship last year was accepted into APPIC-member internships? 0%
Not used by program

What courses are required for incoming students to have completed prior to enrolling?
Statistics, research design

Are there courses you recommend that are not mandatory?
Yes

GRE mean
Verbal 603   Quantitative 683
Advanced Psychology 654
Analytical Writing 5.0

GPA mean
Overall GPA 3.76

Number of applications/admission offers/incoming students in 2005
221 applied/22 admission offers/15 incoming

% of students receiving:
Tuition waiver only: 19%
Assistantship/fellowship only: 81%
Both tuition waiver & assistantship/fellowship: 0%

Approximate percentage of incoming students who entered with a B.A./B.S.only: 75%   **Master's:** 25%

Approximate percentage of students who are
Women: 70%   **Ethnic Minority:** 20%   **International:** 10%

Average years to complete the doctoral program (including internship): 5.5 years

Personal interview
Required in person

Research areas	# Faculty	# Grants
addictive behaviors (smoking, obesity, etc.)	3	1
anger disorders	2	0
attitudes and attitude change	1	0
behavior analysis	3	0
behavior modification (in industry, professional sports, depression, anxiety, social skills)	2	0
biofeedback	1	0
body image	2	0
communication of emotions	1	0
cross-cultural psychology	2	0
depression	1	0
family process/therapy	1	0
human error	1	0
infant/toddler development	1	0
normal and abnormal personalities	2	0
prevention of childhood disorders	2	0
psychotherapy for anger, guilt, fear, and anxiety	1	2
quantitative research methods	2	0
rational-emotive/behavior therapy for marital therapy	1	0
schizophrenia	2	1
self-report validity	1	0
sexual dysfunctions	1	0
verbal behavior	1	0
work attitudes and scholarly activities	1	0

Clinical opportunities
Professional services are offered to the community and to Hofstra University students. Placement throughout the New York city metro area.

James Madison University (Psy.D.)
(clinical/school/counseling)
Department of Psychology/School of Psychology
Harrisonburg, VA 22807-7401
phone#: (540) 568-2556
e-mail: shealycn@jmu.edu
Web address: http://www.psyc.jmu.edu/gradpsyc/

1	2	**3**	4	5	6	7

Clinically oriented   Equal emphasis   Research oriented

What percentage of your faculty subscribes to or practices in each of the following orientations?

Psychodynamic/Psychoanalytic	20%
Applied behavioral analysis/Radical behavioral	0%
Family systems/Systems	40%
Existential/Phenomenological/Humanistic	20%
Cognitive/Cognitive-behavioral	20%

What percentage of students applying for internship last year was accepted into APPIC-member internships? 100%

What courses are required for incoming students to have completed prior to enrolling?
Students are required to have a master's degree in a psychology-related field.

Are there courses you recommend that are not mandatory?
—

GRE mean
Verbal 530   Quantitative 620
Advanced Psychology 600
Analytical Writing 4.5

GPA mean
Master's GPA 3.8

Number of applications/admission offers/incoming students in 2005
55 applied*/7 admission offers/5 incoming
*applicants must have master's degree and professional experience

% of students receiving:
Tuition waiver only: 0%
Assistantship/fellowship only: 0%
Both tuition waiver & assistantship/fellowship: 100%

Approximate percentage of incoming students who entered with a B.A./B.S.only: 0%   **Master's:** 100%

Approximate percentage of students who are
Women: 86%   **Ethnic Minority:** 33%   **International:** 15%

Average years to complete the doctoral program (including internship): 3.8 years

Personal interview
Required in person

Research areas	# Faculty	# Grants
attachment theory	1	0
beliefs and values	3	0
clinical training processes	3	0
depression and suicide	1	0
family processes	2	0
international/cultural issues	4	1
parent–child interaction	2	0
social motivation and affect	1	0
social/skill development	4	0
suicide	1	1
supervision and leadership	1	0
theoretical unification	1	0
traumatic brain injury	1	0
treatment outcomes	1	0
worldview/cultural issues	2	0

Clinical opportunities
child/family therapy
counseling and psychological clinic
forensic assessment
inpatient/hospital practice
learning disabilities
multidisciplinary assessment
neuropsychology
outpatient private practice
school assessment
supervision/leadership

Northeastern University

(counseling/school)
Department of Counseling and Applied Educational Psychology
Bouve College of Health Sciences
203 Lake Hall
Boston, MA 02115
phone#: (617) 373-2708
e-mail: w.purnell@neu.edu
Web address: http://www.bouve.neu.edu/programs/combined/index.php

1	2	**3**	4	5	6	7
Clinically oriented		Equal emphasis			Research oriented	

What percentage of your faculty subscribes to or practices in each of the following orientations?

Psychodynamic/Psychoanalytic	10%
Applied behavioral analysis/Radical behavioral	10%
Family systems/Systems	30%
Existential/Phenomenological/Humanistic	20%
Cognitive/Cognitive-behavioral	30%

What percentage of students applying for internship last year was accepted into APPIC-member internships? 100%

What courses are required for incoming students to have completed prior to enrolling?
We require a master's degree in a field (applied preferred) of psychology

Are there courses you recommend that are not mandatory?
—

GRE mean
Verbal 500   Quantitative 500
Analytic Writing   Data not available

GPA mean
Overall GPA 3.0   Psychology GPA 3.0

Number of applications/admission offers/incoming students in 2005
501 applied/240 admission offers/135 incoming

% of students receiving:
Tuition waiver only: 25%
Assistantship/fellowship only: 25%
Both tuition waiver & assistantship/fellowship: 25%

Approximate percentage of incoming students who entered with a B.A./B.S. only: 0%   **Master's:** 100%

Approximate percentage of students who are Women: 85%   **Ethnic Minority:** 25%
International: Data not available

Average years to complete the doctoral program (including internship): 5.5 years

Personal interview
No preference given

Research areas	# Faculty	# Grants
consultation with telecommunication	1	1
counseling needs of minorities	1	1
early intervention	1	1
eating disorders	1	1
forensics in juvenile crime	1	1
impact of managed care on clinical training	1	0
leadership development	3	1
neuropsychological function	1	0
spatial ability and cognitive transfer	2	0

Clinical opportunities
Students have the opportunity to work with families, women, men, psychotics, chronically ill, autistic, etc. Training settings in the Boston area include all manners of ethnic and cultural diversity, medical, mental health, and private care facilities. Virtually everything and every kind of experience is available to students in a supervised setting.

Ontario Institute for Studies in Education

(clinical/school)
Department of Human Development and Applied Psychology
OISE/University of Toronto
252 Bloor Street West
Toronto, Ontario M5S 1V6 Canada
phone#: (416) 923-6641, ext. 2492
e-mail: jwiener@oise.utoronto.ca

Web address:
http://www.oise.utoronto.ca/depts/aecdcp/cp.html

1	2	3	4	5	**6**	7
Clinically oriented		Equal emphasis			Research oriented	

What percentage of your faculty subscribes to or practices in each of the following orientations?

Psychodynamic/Psychoanalytic	11%
Applied behavioral analysis/Radical behavioral	11%
Family systems/Systems	22%
Existential/Phenomenological/Humanistic	0%
Cognitive/Cognitive-behavioral	11%
Other-Psychoeducational	45%

What percentage of students applying for internship last year was accepted into APPIC-member internships? 25%

What courses are required for incoming students to have completed prior to enrolling?
6 six credit courses (or its equivalent) in psychology, 3 of which must be at a senior level; at least 3 credit courses in research methods

Are there courses you recommend that are not mandatory?
History and systems in psychology, developmental psychology, biological, social, and cognitive/affective bases of behavior.

GRE mean
We do not require GRE scores.

GPA mean
Students must have the equivalent of at least an A– (3.7) at the University of Toronto to be considered for the program, but most have an A average.

Number of applications/admission offers/incoming students in 2005
142 applied/19 admission offers/16 incoming
Admission numbers include the 8 students who are proceeding from the M.A. to the Ph.D. This year we accepted 8 new M.A. students and 1 new Ph.D. student. The remaining 7 Ph.D. students moved up from our own M.A. program.

% of students receiving:
Tuition waiver only: 0%
Assistantship/fellowship only: 0%
Both tuition waiver & assistantship/fellowship: 100%

Approximate percentage of incoming students who entered with a B.A./B.S. only: 62% **Master's:** 38%

Approximate percentage of students who are Women: 91% **Ethnic Minority:** 33% **International:** 10%

Average years to complete the doctoral program (including internship): 5 years

Personal interview
Preferred in person but telephone acceptable.

Research areas	# Faculty	# Grants
ADHD	4	9
anxiety disorders	2	2
behavioral/cognitive behavioural intervention	2	2
child epilepsy	1	1
child maltreatment	2	1
cognition (critical thinking, intentional learning)	2	2
cross-cultural psychology	3	3
developmental psychopathology	4	5
emotions	3	3
fetal alcohol disorder	1	1
gender identity disorder	1	1
hypothyroidism	1	1
learning disabilities	4	4
math and technology	2	1
parenting	3	3
peer relations	2	2
reading/literacy	5	7
social cognition (theory of mind, moral development)	3	2
young offenders/children's rights	2	1

Clinical opportunities
ADHD
anxiety/mood
autism
Bloorview-MacMillan Centre for Addiction and Mental Health (CAMH)
developmental
family
family life center
fire setting
gender identity
Hospital for Sick Children (HSC)
learning disabilities
mental retardation
OISE/University of Toronto, Integra
physical disabilities
psychoeducational
Surrey Place
traumatic brain injury
TREADD

Pace University (Psy.D.)

(school/clinical)
Department of Psychology
New York, NY 10038
phone#: (212) 346-1506
Web address: http://www.pace.edu/dyson/psychology/psydgi.html

1	**2**	3	4	5	6	7
Clinically oriented		Equal emphasis			Research oriented	

What percentage of your faculty subscribes to or practices in each of the following orientations?

Psychodynamic/Psychoanalytic	36%
Applied behavioral analysis/Radical behavioral	0%
Family systems/Systems	14%
Existential/Phenomenological/Humanistic	14%
Cognitive/Cognitive-behavioral	36%

What percentage of students applying for internship last year was accepted into APPIC-member internships? 75%

What courses are required for incoming students to have completed prior to enrolling?
General psychology, experimental psychology, statistics, developmental psychology, learning, personality, psychopathology

Are there courses you recommend that are not mandatory?
—

GRE mean
Verbal + Quantitative 1200
Analytical Writing   Data not available

GPA mean
Overall GPA 3.6

Number of applications/admission offers/incoming students in 2005
280 applied/41 admission offers/19 incoming

% of students receiving:
Partial tuition scholarship: 25%
Assistantship/fellowship only: 25%
Both tuition waiver & assistantship/fellowship: 0%

Approximate percentage of incoming students who entered with a B.A./B.S. only: 88%   **Master's:** 12%

Approximate percentage of students who are
Women: 85%   **Ethnic Minority:** 17%   **International:** 5%

Average years to complete the doctoral program (including internship): 5.7 years (varies from year to year)

Personal interview
Required in person (on occasion grant telephone interviews)

Research areas	# Faculty	# Grants
community psychology	1	0
gender	2	0
infant and early childhood	3	0
learning disabilities	1	0
learning	1	0
multicultural	2	0
posttraumatic stress disorder	1	0
psychometric	3	0

Clinical opportunities
early childhood
psychotherapy
neuropsychological assessment
many, varied opportunities available

Utah State University
(clinical/counseling/school)
Department of Psychology
Logan, UT 84322-2810
phone#: (435) 797-1460
e-mail:PsyDept@cc.usu.edu
Web address: http://www.coe.usu.edu/psyc/programs/phd_combined/index.html

1	2	**3**	4	5	6	7
Clinically oriented		Equal emphasis			Research oriented	

What percentage of your faculty subscribes to or practices in each of the following orientations?

Psychodynamic/Psychoanalytic	15%
Applied behavioral analysis/Radical behavioral	10%
Family systems/Systems	10%
Existential/Phenomenological/Humanistic	15%
Cognitive/Cognitive-behavioral	50%

What percentage of students applying for internship last year was accepted into APPIC-member internships? 100%

What courses are required for incoming students to have completed prior to enrolling?
General psychology, developmental psychology, learning, elementary statistics, personality, physiological, abnormal

Are there courses you recommend that are not mandatory?
Introduction to counseling, cognitive psychology, social psychology

GRE mean
Verbal 590   Quantitative 590
Verbal + Quantitative 1182
Analytical Writing   Data not available

GPA mean
Junior/Senior GPA 3.64

Number of applications/admission offers/incoming students in 2005
78 applied/14 admission offers/7 incoming

% of students receiving:
Tuition waiver only: 0%
Assistantship/fellowship only: 0%
Both tuition waiver & assistantship/fellowship: 100%

Approximate percentage of incoming students who entered with a B.A./B.S. only: 40%   **Master's:** 60%

Approximate percentage of students who are
Women: 70%   **Ethnic Minority:** 20%   **International:** 10%

Average years to complete the doctoral program (including internship): 6 years

Personal interview
Preferred in person but telephone acceptable

Research areas	# Faculty	# Grants
addiction/substance abuse	1	1
ADHD	1	0
behavioral medicine/health psychology	2	1
child behavior problems	1	1
childhood/adolescent depression	2	1
Native American mental health	1	0
rural mental health	2	1
school behavioral assessment	1	0

Clinical opportunities
behavioral medicine
cardiac rehabilitation
chronic mental health
community mental health

disabilities
early intervention
eating disorders
Head Start
minority mental health
neuropsychology
pediatric psychology
student counseling center
student wellness center

Yeshiva University (Psy.D.)

(school/clinical)
Ferkauf Graduate School of Psychology
Bronx, NY 10461
phone#: (718) 430-3945
e-mail: givner@aecom.yu.edu
Web address: http://www.yu.edu/ferkauf/
index_sub.asp?504

1	**2**	3	4	5	6	7
Clinically oriented		Equal emphasis			Research oriented	

What percentage of your faculty subscribes to or practices in each of the following orientations?

Psychodynamic/Psychoanalytic	50%
Applied behavioral analysis/Radical behavioral	10%
Family systems/Systems	20%
Existential/Phenomenological/Humanistic	0%
Cognitive/Cognitive-behavioral	40%

What percentage of students applying for internship last year was accepted into APPIC-member internships? 100%

What courses are required for incoming students to have completed prior to enrolling?
Statistics, abnormal psychology, child development

Are there courses you recommend that are not mandatory?
—

GRE mean
Verbal 560   Quantitative 610
Analytical Writing 5.0

GPA mean
Overall GPA 3.4

Number of applications/admission offers/incoming students in 2005
210 applied/33 admission offers/24 incoming

% of students receiving:
Tuition waiver only: 5%
Assistantship/fellowship only: 50%
Both tuition waiver & assistantship/fellowship: 0%

Approximate percentage of incoming students who entered with a B.A./B.S. only: 75%   **Master's:** 25%

**Approximate percentage of students who are
Women:** 86%   **Ethnic Minority:** 8%   **International:** 4%

Average years to complete the doctoral program (including internship): 5.0 years

Personal interview
Required in person

Research areas	# Faculty	# Grants
ADHD	2	0
adolescence	2	0
assessment	2	0
attachment	3	0
behavioral interventions	2	0
early childhood	1	0
fathering	2	0
learning disabilities	3	0
multicultural issues	3	0
nontraditional families	2	0
professional issues	3	0
symbolic play	1	0

Clinical opportunities
adolescence
bilingual/multicultural
early childhood
family–school collaboration
parent training
school age

Combined Professional–Scientific Psychology Programs That Have Been Discontinued

University of Pennsylvania (counseling/school) (accredited, inactive)

REPORTS ON INDIVIDUAL CLINICAL PSYCHOLOGY PROGRAMS

Adelphi University

Institute of Advanced Psychological Studies
Garden City, NY 11530
phone#: (516) 877-4800
fax#: (516) 877-4805
Web address: http://derner.adelphi.edu/doctoral

	1	**2**	3	4	5	6	7
	Clinically oriented		Equal emphasis			Research oriented	

What percentage of your faculty subscribes to or practices in each of the following orientations?

Psychodynamic/Psychoanalytic	100%
Applied behavioral analysis/Radical behavioral	15%
Family systems/Systems	10%
Existential/Phenomenological/Humanistic	10%
Cognitive/Cognitive-behavioral	20%

What percentage of students applying for internship last year was accepted into APPIC-member internships? 90%

What courses are required for incoming students to have completed prior to enrolling?
General Psychology, statistics, experimental psychology, developmental psychology, abnormal psychology

Are there courses you recommend that are not mandatory?
No

GRE mean
Verbal 620
Quantitative 660
Advanced Psychology 660
Analytical Writing N/A

GPA mean
Overall GPA 3.50   Psychology GPA 3.6

Number of applications/admission offers/incoming students in 2005
215 applied/35 admission offers/19 incoming

% of students receiving:
(Partial) tuition waiver only: 60%
Assistantship/fellowship only: 0%
Both tuition waiver & assistantship/fellowship: 0%

Approximate percentage of incoming students who entered with a B.A./B.S. only: 67%   **Master's:** 33%

**Approximate percentage of students who are
Women:** 80%   **Ethnic Minority:** 15%   **International:** 10%

Personal interview
Required in person

Research areas	# Faculty	# Grants
change processes	2	0
creativity	1	1
developmental	1	1
developmental (lifespan)	1	1
equity in personal relationships	1	1
group process	2	0
health psychology	1	1
marriage	1	1
psychoanalysis	8	1
psychotherapy process	3	2
unconscious processes and motivation	1	0

Clinical opportunities
addiction
child, adolescent, and family
group therapy
psychotherapy integration
short-term psychotherapy

Adler School of Professional Psychology (Psy.D.)

65 East Wacker Place, #2100
Chicago, IL 60601-7203
phone#: (312) 201-5900
admissions: (312) 201-5900 ext 222
e-mail: information@adler.edu
Web address:
http://www.adler.edu/content.aspx?ntopicid=1154

	1	**2**	3	4	5	6	7
	Clinically oriented		Equal emphasis			Research oriented	

What percentage of your faculty subscribes to or practices in each of the following orientations?

Psychodynamic/Psychoanalytic	10%
Applied behavioral analysis/Radical behavioral	0%
Family systems/Systems	10%
Existential/Phenomenological/Humanistic	40%
Cognitive/Cognitive-behavioral	40%

What percentage of students applying for internship last year was accepted into APPIC-member internships? 95%

What courses are required for incoming students to have completed prior to enrolling?
Advanced abnormal psychology, general psychology, psychometrics, theories of personality, and others to total 18 credits

Are there courses you recommend that are not mandatory?
No

GRE mean
N/A

GPA mean
Data not available

Number of applications/admission offers/incoming students in 2005
197 applied/58 admission offers/44 incoming

% of students receiving:
Tuition waiver only: 0%
Assistantship/fellowship only: 10%
Both tuition waiver & assistantship/fellowship: 0%

Approximate percentage of incoming students who entered with a B.A./B.S. only: 50%   **Master's:** 50%

Approximate percentage of students who are Women: 65%   **Ethnic Minority:** 20%   **International:** 25%

Average years to complete the doctoral program (including internship): 5.1 years

Personal interview
Required in person

Research areas	# Faculty	# Grants
adult human development	1	0
disabled children and coping	2	0
neuropsychology of offenders	4	1

Clinical opportunities
Department of Corrections
developmental disabilities
halfway release programs for sex offenders
schools

University of Alabama

Department of Psychology
P. O. Box 870348
Tuscaloosa, AL 35487-5083
phone#: (205) 348-1919
e-mail: mbhubbard@as.ua.edu
Web address: http://psychology.ua.edu/clinical.html

1	2	3	4	**5**	6	7
Clinically oriented		Equal emphasis			Research oriented	

What percentage of your faculty subscribes to or practices in each of the following orientations?

Psychodynamic/Psychoanalytic	0%
Applied behavioral analysis/Radical behavioral	10%
Family systems/Systems	10%
Existential/Phenomenological/Humanistic	10%
Cognitive/Cognitive-behavioral	80%

What percentage of students applying for internship last year was accepted into APPIC-member internships? 100%

What courses are required for incoming students to have completed prior to enrolling?
Undergrad statistics, research methods, abnormal psychology

Are there courses you recommend that are not mandatory?
No

GRE mean
Verbal 610   Quantitative 660
Advanced Psychology 650
Analytical Writing 5.0

GPA mean
Overall GPA 3.6   Psychology GPA 3.7
Junior/Senior GPA 3.7

Number of applications/admission offers/incoming students in 2005
177 applied/17 admission offers/12 incoming

% of students receiving:
Tuition waiver only: 0%
Assistantship/fellowship only: 90%
Both tuition waiver & assistantship/fellowship: 80%

Approximate percentage of incoming students who entered with a B.A./B.S. only: 90%   **Master's:** 10%

Approximate percentage of students who are Women: 75%   **Ethnic Minority:** 17%   **International:** 0%

Average years to complete the doctoral program (including internship): 6 years

Personal interview
Preferred in person but telephone acceptable

Research areas	# Faculty	# Grants
adult psychopathology	2	0
affective disorders/depression	1	1
aging	3	3
assessment	1	0
behavioral medicine	3	1
biofeedback	0	0
child clinical	3	1
clinical judgment	1	0
cross-cultural psychology	1	0
forensic	3	0
pain management	1	1
professional issues	2	0
psychotherapy process and outcome	2	0
social skills	2	0
violence/abuse	3	1

Clinical opportunities
autism
conduct disorder
factitious disorder
forensic psychology
gerontology
health promotion behavior
pain management
parent–child interaction

University of Alabama at Birmingham

Department of Psychology
CH 415
1530 3rd Avenue South
Birmingham, AL 35294-1170
phone#: (205) 934-8723
e-mail: medpsych@uab.edu
Web address: http://www.psy.uab.edu/medpsych.htm

1	2	3	**4**	5	6	7
Clinically oriented		Equal emphasis			Research oriented	

What percentage of your faculty subscribes to or practices in each of the following orientations?

Psychodynamic/Psychoanalytic	30%
Applied behavioral analysis/Radical behavioral	0%
Family systems/Systems	0%
Existential/Phenomenological/Humanistic	0%
Cognitive/Cognitive-behavioral	70%
Health psychology	100%

What percentage of students applying for internship last year was accepted into APPIC-member internships? 100%

What courses are required for incoming students to have completed prior to enrolling?
At least 18 credit hours of psychology, including statistics; at least 18 credit hours of life sciences (the number of hours are recommended, not required)

Are there courses you recommend that are not mandatory?
Psychopathology, learning, cognitive psychology, social psychology

GRE mean
Verbal 560   Quantitative 708
Analytical Writing & Subject Test not required for admission

GPA mean
Overall GPA 3.85

Number of applications/admission offers/incoming students in 2005
72 applied/15 admission offers/6 incoming

% of students receiving:
Tuition waiver only: 0%
Assistantship/fellowship only: 100%
Both tuition waiver & assistantship/fellowship: 100%

Approximate percentage of incoming students who entered with a B.A./B.S. only: 80%   Master's: 20%

Approximate percentage of students who are Women: 64%   Ethnic Minority: 11%   International: 11%

Average years to complete the doctoral program (including internship): 6 years

Personal interview
Preferred in person but telephone acceptable

Research areas	# Faculty	# Grants
aging	3	6
behavioral medicine	2	2
developmental disabilities	6	16
eating disorders	1	1
neuropsychology	3	2
psychophysiology	1	1
substance abuse	3	5

Clinical opportunities
behavioral medicine
neuropsychology

University at Albany/
State University of New York

Department of Psychology
1400 Washington Avenue
Albany, NY 12222
phone#: (518) 442-4820
e-mail: lhalpern@albany.edu
Web address: http://www.albany.edu/psy/
gradclinical.html

1	2	3	4	5	**6**	7

Clinically oriented   Equal emphasis   Research oriented

What percentage of your faculty subscribes to or practices in each of the following orientations?

Psychodynamic/Psychoanalytic	0%
Applied behavioral analysis/Radical behavioral	30%
Family systems/Systems	0%
Existential/Phenomenological/Humanistic	0%
Cognitive/Cognitive-behavioral	70%

What percentage of students applying for internship last year was accepted into APPIC-member internships? 100%

What courses are required for incoming students to have completed prior to enrolling?
18 semester hours in psychology, including classes in statistics and experimental design

Are there courses you recommend that are not mandatory?
No

GRE mean
Verbal 621   Quantitative 659
Advanced Psychology 675   Analytical Writing 5.2

GPA mean
Overall GPA 3.2   Psychology GPA 3.4

Number of applications/admission offers/incoming students in 2005
168 applied/14 admission offers/8 incoming

% of students receiving:
Tuition waiver only: 0%
Assistantship/fellowship only: 0%
Both tuition waiver & assistantship/fellowship: 100%

Approximate percentage of incoming students who entered with a B.A./B.S. only: 90%   Master's: 10%

Approximate percentage of students who are Women: 75%   Ethnic Minority: 22%   International: 12%

Average years to complete the doctoral program (including internship): 6.2 years

Personal interview
Preferred in person but telephone acceptable

Research areas	# Faculty	# Grants
anxiety disorders	1	0
autism/developmental disabilities	1	1

behavioral medicine	2	0
children	4	2
eating disorders	1	0
neuropsychology	1	1
psychopathology	1	0
substance abuse/addiction	2	1

Clinical opportunities
addictive disorders
adolescents
anxiety disorders
autism/developmental disabilities
behavioral medicine/health psychology
children
cross-cultural issues
eating disorders
neuropsychology

Alliant International University–Fresno (Ph.D.)

5130 East Clinton Way
Fresno, CA 93727
phone#: (559) 456-2777 ext. 2255
e-mail: dhernandez@alliant.edu
Web address: http://www.alliant.edu/wps/wcm/connect/
website/Home/About+Alliant/Schools+%26+Colleges/
California+School+of+Professional+Psychology/
About+CSPP+Programs/PhD+Clinical+Psychology+
Programs/Fresno+Clinical+PhD

1	2	3	4	**5**	6	7
Clinically oriented		Equal emphasis			Research oriented	

What percentage of your faculty subscribes to or practices in each of the following orientations?
Psychodynamic/Psychoanalytic	10%
Applied behavioral analysis/Radical behavioral	10%
Family systems/Systems	40%
Existential/Phenomenological/Humanistic	10%
Cognitive/Cognitive-behavioral	30%

What percentage of students applying for internship last year was accepted into APPIC-member internships? 11%

What courses are required for incoming students to have completed prior to enrolling?
Psychology undergraduate degree or coursework with a "C" or better in the following: abnormal psychology, statistics, experimental or physiological psychology, learning theory, tests and measurement or 80th percentile Psychology GRE

Are there courses you recommend that are not mandatory?
Please refer to above.

GRE mean
GRE not required

GPA mean
Overall GPA 3.5   Psychology GPA 3.5

Number of applications/admission offers/incoming students in 2005
10 applied/3 admission offers/2 incoming

% of students receiving:
Tuition waiver only: 75%
Assistantship/fellowship only: 25%

Approximate percentage of incoming students who entered with a B.A./B.S. only: 50%   **Master's:** 50%

Approximate percentage of students who are Women: 100%   **Ethnic Minority:** 1%
International: Data not available

Average years to complete the doctoral program (including internship): 5 years

Personal interview
No preference given

Research areas	# Faculty	# Grants
attachment behavior	1	0
epidemiology of neurological disorders	1	0
infant studies	1	1
Latino mental health	1	1

Clinical opportunities
behavioral medicine
children/families
domestic violence
sex offenders

Alliant International University–Fresno (Psy.D.)

5130 East Clinton Way
Fresno, CA 93727
phone#: (559) 456-2777 ext. 2255
e-mail: jkirkpatrick@alliant.edu
Web address: http://www.alliant.edu/wps/wcm/connect/
website/Home/About+Alliant/Schools+%26+Colleges/
California+School+of+Professional+Psychology/
About+CSPP+Programs/PsyD+Clinical+Psychology+
Programs/Fresno+-+Sacramento+Clinical+PsyD

1	**2**	3	4	5	6	7
Clinically oriented		Equal emphasis			Research oriented	

What percentage of your faculty subscribes to or practices in each of the following orientations?
Psychodynamic/Psychoanalytic	10%
Applied behavioral analysis/Radical behavioral	10%
Family systems/Systems	20%
Existential/Phenomenological/Humanistic	10%
Cognitive/Cognitive-behavioral	50%

What percentage of students applying for internship last year was accepted into APPIC-member internships? 50%

What courses are required for incoming students to have completed prior to enrolling?
Psychology undergraduate degree or coursework with a "C" or better in the following: abnormal psychology, statistics, experimental or physiological psychology, learning theory, tests and measurement or 80th percentile Psychology GRE

Are there courses you recommend that are not mandatory?
Please refer to above.

GRE mean
GRE not required

GPA mean
Overall GPA 3.5   Psychology GPA 3.5

Number of applications/admission offers/incoming students in 2005
39 applied/20 admission offers/12 incoming

% of students receiving:
Tuition waiver only: 91%
Assistantship/fellowship only: 18%

Approximate percentage of incoming students who entered with a B.A./B.S. only: 100%   **Master's:** 0%

Approximate percentage of students who are Women: 67%   **Ethnic Minority:** 25%   **International:** 1%

Average years to complete the doctoral program (including internship): 4 years

Personal interview
No preference given

Research areas	# Faculty	# Grants
health	1	0
high risk adolescents	1	2
Latino mental health	1	1
women's issues	1	0

Clinical opportunities
behavioral medicine
children/families
domestic violence
sex offenders

Alliant International University– Los Angeles (Ph.D.)

Admissions Office
1000 South Fremont Avenue, Unit 5
Alhambra, CA 91803-1360
Phone: 626-284-2777 X3026
e-mail: gbone@alliant.edu
Stephanie Byers-Bell, Director of Admissions
Web address: http://www.alliant.edu/wps/wcm/connect/
website/Home/About+Alliant/Schools+%26+Colleges/
California+School+of+Professional+Psychology/
About+CSPP+Programs/PhD+Clinical+Psychology+
Programs/Los+Angeles+Clinical+PhD/

1	2	3	**4**	5	6	7
Clinically oriented		Equal emphasis			Research oriented	

What percentage of your faculty subscribes to or practices in each of the following orientations?

Psychodynamic/Psychoanalytic	15%
Applied behavioral analysis/Radical behavioral	0%
Family systems/Systems	15%
Existential/Phenomenological/Humanistic	0%
Cognitive/Cognitive-behavioral	15%
Research	50%

What percentage of students applying for internship last year was accepted into APPIC-member internships? 38%

What courses are required for incoming students to have completed prior to enrolling?
If no BA in psychology or score is below the 80th percentile on the Advanced Psychology GRE then the following are required: statistics, tests & measurements, abnormal and one of the following: experimental or physiological or learning theory.

Are there courses you recommend that are not mandatory?
No

GRE mean
GRE scores are not used as part of the standard admissions process

GPA mean
Data not available

Number of applications/admission offers/incoming students in 2005
106 applied/40 admission offers/28 incoming

% of students receiving:
Tuition waiver only: 0%
Assistantship/fellowship only: 0%
Both tuition waiver & assistantship/fellowship: 0%

Approximate percentage of incoming students who entered with a B.A./B.S. only: 80%   **Master's:** 20%

Approximate percentage of students who are Women: 80%   **Ethnic Minority:** 39%   **International:** 0%

Average years to complete the doctoral program (including internship): 6 years

Personal interview
Preferred in person but telephone acceptable

Research areas	# Faculty	# Grants
acculturation	1	0
alternative and complimentary medicine	1	0
child assessment	2	0
ethnic minorities: health and mental health	5	0
gay and lesbian health and interpersonal functioning	1	0
infant mental health	1	1
interpersonal violence	1	0

traumatic stress	1	0
women's issues: minority populations	1	0

Clinical opportunities
behavioral medicine
child abuse
children and adolescents in school settings
chronic mental illness
college students
elderly
forensic populations
HIV/AIDS
neurological impairment
substance abuse

Alliant International University– Los Angeles (Psy.D.)

1000 South Fremont Avenue, Unit 5
Alhambra, CA 91803
Phone: 626-284-2777 X 3026
e-mail: gbone@alliant.edu
Web address: http://www.alliant.edu/wps/wcm/connect/
website/Home/About+Alliant/Schools+%26+Colleges/
California+School+of+Professional+Psychology/
About+CSPP+Programs/PsyD+Clinical+Psychology+
Programs/Los+Angeles+Clinical+PsyD

1	**2**	3	4	5	6	7
Clinically oriented		Equal emphasis			Research oriented	

What percentage of your faculty subscribes to or practices in each of the following orientations?

Psychodynamic/Psychoanalytic	50%
Applied behavioral analysis/Radical behavioral	0%
Family systems/Systems	30%
Existential/Phenomenological/Humanistic	10%
Cognitive/Cognitive-behavioral	10%

What percentage of students applying for internship last year was accepted into APPIC-member internships? Data not available

What courses are required for incoming students to have completed prior to enrolling?
If no B.A. in psychology or score is below the 80th percentile on the Advanced Psychology GRE then the following are required: statistics, tests and measurements, abnormal and one of the following: experimental or physiological or learning theory.

Are there courses you recommend that are not mandatory?
No

GRE mean
GRE scores are not used as a part of the standard admissions process.

GPA mean
Data not available

Number of applications/admission offers/incoming students in 2005
210 applied/104 admission offers/82 incoming

% of students receiving:
Tuition waiver only: 0%
Assistantship/fellowship only: 0%
Both tuition waiver & assistantship/fellowship: 0%

Approximate percentage of incoming students who entered with a B.A./B.S. only: 76%   **Master's:** 24%

Approximate percentage of students who are Women: 82%   **Ethnic Minority:** 27%   **International:** Data not available

Average years to complete the doctoral program (including internship): 5 years

Personal interview
Preferred in person but telephone acceptable

Research areas	# Faculty	# Grants
abuse issues	2	0
acculturation issues	2	0
cognitive processes	1	0
family relations	1	0
interpersonal conflict resolution	1	0
interpersonal processes	1	0
health issues	3	1
multicultural issues	6	0
psychotherapy integration	1	0
women's health	1	0

Clinical opportunities
behavioral medicine
child abuse
children and adolescents in school settings
chronic mental illness
college students
elderly
forensic populations
HIV/AIDS
neurological impairment
substance abuse

Alliant International University– San Diego (Ph.D.)

10455 Pomerado Road
San Diego, CA 92131-1799
phone#: (858) 635-4772
e-mail: admissions@alliant.edu
Web address: http://www.alliant.edu/wps/wcm/connect/
website/Home/About+Alliant/Schools+%26+Colleges/
California+School+of+Professional+Psychology/
About+CSPP+Programs/PhD+Clinical+Psychology+
Programs/San+Diego+Clinical+PhD

1	2	3	**4**	5	6	7
Clinically oriented		Equal emphasis			Research oriented	

What percentage of your faculty subscribes to or practices in each of the following orientations?

Psychodynamic/Psychoanalytic	15%
Applied behavioral analysis/Radical behavioral	31%
Family systems/Systems	38%
Existential/Phenomenological/Humanistic	0%
Cognitive/Cognitive-behavioral	16%

What percentage of students applying for internship last year was accepted into APPIC-member internships? 0%

What courses are required for incoming students to have completed prior to enrolling?
Bachelor's degree in psychology; or statistics, tests and measurement, abnormal psychology and one of the following: experimental psychology, physiological psychology or learning theory

Are there courses you recommend that are not mandatory?
No

GRE mean
GREs not required

GPA mean
Overall GPA 3.5

Number of applications/admission offers/incoming students in 2005
136 applied/56 admission offers/39 incoming

% of students receiving:
Tuition waiver only: 0% (scholarships)
Assistantship/fellowship only: 0%
Both tuition waiver & assistantship/fellowship: 10%

Approximate percentage of incoming students who entered with a B.A./B.S. only: 94% **Master's:** 6%

Approximate percentage of students who are Women: 84% **Ethnic Minority:** 45% **International:** 5%

Average years to complete the doctoral program (including internship): 5.6 years

Personal interview
Required in person (telephone interviews may be considered)

Research areas	# Faculty	# Grants
adolescent psychopathology	3	0
childhood psychopathology	3	0
developmental psychopathology	3	0
forensic psychology	2	0
health psychology	4	1
malingering	1	0
mood disorders	2	0
multicultural	3	0
severe psychopathology	1	0

Clinical opportunities
behavioral medicine
child custody evaluation
cognitive therapy
health
pain management
psychotherapy
trauma

Alliant International University– San Diego (Psy.D.)

10455 Pomerado Road
San Diego, CA 92131
Phone: (858) 635-4641
Web address: http://www.alliant.edu/wps/wcm/connect/
website/Home/About+Alliant/Schools+%26+Colleges/
California+School+of+Professional+Psychology/
About+CSPP+Programs/PsyD+Clinical+Psychology+
Programs/San+Diego+Clinical+PsyD/

1	**2**	3	4	5	6	7
Clinically oriented		Equal emphasis			Research oriented	

What percentage of your faculty subscribes to or practices in each of the following orientations?

Psychodynamic/Psychoanalytic	35%
Applied behavioral analysis/Radical behavioral	10%
Family systems/Systems	25%
Existential/Phenomenological/Humanistic	5%
Cognitive/Cognitive-behavioral	25%

What percentage of students applying for internship last year was accepted into APPIC-member internships? 0%

What courses are required for incoming students to have completed prior to enrolling?
Bachelor's degree in psychology; or statistics, tests and measurement, abnormal psychology and one of the following: experimental psychology, physiological psychology or learning theory

Are there courses you recommend that are not mandatory?
No

GRE mean
GRE not required

GPA mean
Overall GPA 3.45

Number of applications/admission offers/incoming students in 2005
185 applied/77 admission offers/49 incoming

% of students receiving:
Partial tuition waiver only: 0% (scholarships)
Assistantship/fellowship only: 0%
Both tuition waiver & assistantship/fellowship: 0%

Approximate percentage of incoming students who entered with a B.A./B.S. only: 84% **Master's:** 16%

Approximate percentage of students who are Women: 79% **Ethnic Minority:** 41% **International:** 7%

Average years to complete the doctoral program (including internship): 5.8 years

Personal interview
Required in person

Research areas	# Faculty	# Grants
adolescent psychopathology	2	0
alcoholism	1	0
assessment	1	0

127

childhood psychopathology	3	3
forensic psychology	3	0
health psychology	4	2
malingering	1	0
mood disorders	3	0
multicultural psychopathology	3	2
rehabilitation psych (deafness)	2	1
reproductive trauma	1	0

Clinical opportunities
assessment
autism clinic
biofeedback clinic
custody evaluation clinic
domestic violence
forensic assessment
health
media and psychology

Alliant International University– San Francisco Campus (Ph.D.)

Formerly Alameda Campus
Jennifer Kulbeck, Director of Admissions and Marketing
Admissions Office
One Beach Street, Suite 100
San Francisco, CA 94133
phone#: (415) 955-2146
e-mail: jkulbeck@alliant.edu
Web address: http://www.alliant.edu/wps/wcm/connect/
website/Home/About+Alliant/Schools+%26+Colleges/
California+School+of+Professional+Psychology/
About+CSPP+Programs/PhD+Clinical+Psychology+
Programs/San+Francisco+Clinical+PhD/

1	**2**	3	4	5	6	7
Clinically oriented		Equal emphasis			Research oriented	

What percentage of your faculty subscribes to or practices in each of the following orientations?

Psychodynamic/Psychoanalytic	30%
Applied behavioral analysis/Radical behavioral	0%
Family systems/Systems	60%
Existential/Phenomenological/Humanistic	20%
Cognitive/Cognitive-behavioral	50%

What percentage of students applying for internship last year was accepted into APPIC-member internships? 1%; 83% were accepted into CAPIC-member internships

What courses are required for incoming students to have completed prior to enrolling?
A bachelor's degree in psychology or courses on the following: statistics, tests and measurements, abnormal psychology, and one of the following: learning, physiological psychology, or experimental psychology.

Are there courses you recommend that are not mandatory?
—

GRE mean
GREs not required. If applicants do not have a bachelor's in psychology, GRE Advanced Psychology score in the 80th percentile may be considered in lieu of prerequisite coursework.

GPA mean
Applicants with score below 3.0 must submit statement of explanation.

Number of applications/admission offers in 2005
114 applied/44 admission offers

% of students receiving:
Tuition waiver only: 0%
Assistantship/fellowship only: 0%
Both tuition waiver & assistantship/fellowship: 0%

Approximate percentage of incoming students who entered with a B.A./B.S. only: 64%   **Master's:** 36%

**Approximate percentage of students who are
Women:** 80%   **Ethnic Minority:** 40%   **International:** 6%

Average years to complete the doctoral program (including pre-doc internship): 6 years

Personal interview
Preferred in person but telephone acceptable

Research areas	# Faculty	# Grants
development	2	0
family/child	6	0
gender studies	6	0
health psychology	5	2
multicultural/community	6	2
psychology of women	3	0

Clinical opportunities
We have over 125 practicum sites that specialize in almost all areas of psychology including inpatient, outpatient, and residential treatment programs for children, adolescents, and adults, hospitals specializing in behavioral health and neuropsychological populations, college counseling centers, mental health centers, forensic sites, and placements specializing in the treatment of specific ethnic minority populations, women, gay/lesbians, and the disabled.

Alliant International University– San Francisco Campus (Psy.D.)

Formerly Alameda Campus
Jennifer Kulbeck, Director of Admissions and Marketing
Admissions Office
One Beach Street, Suite 100
San Francisco, CA 94133
phone#: (415) 955-2146
e-mail: jkulbeck@alliant.edu
Web address: http://www.alliant.edu/wps/wcm/connect/
website/Home/About+Alliant/Schools+%26+Colleges/
California+School+of+Professional+Psychology/
About+CSPP+Programs/PsyD+Clinical+Psychology+
Programs/San+Francisco+Clinical+PsyD/

1	**2**	3	4	5	6	7

Clinically oriented   Equal emphasis   Research oriented

What percentage of your faculty subscribes to or practices in each of the following orientations?

Psychodynamic/Psychoanalytic	26%
Applied behavioral analysis/Radical behavioral	0%
Family systems/Systems	21%
Existential/Phenomenological/Humanistic	15%
Cognitive/Cognitive-behavioral	5%

What percentage of students applying for internship last year was accepted into APPIC-member internships? 11%; 74% were accepted into CAPIC-member internships

What courses are required for incoming students to have completed prior to enrolling?
Psychology courses: statistics, tests and measurements, abnormal psychology, and one of the following: learning, physiological psychology, or experimental psychology

Are there courses you recommend that are not mandatory?
No

GRE mean
GREs not required
If applicants do not have a bachelor's in psychology, GRE Advanced Psychology score in the 80th percentile may be considered in lieu of pre-requisite coursework.

GPA mean
Applicants with GPA below 3.0 must submit statement of explanation

Number of applications/admission offers in 2004
209 applied/120 admission offers

% of students receiving:
Tuition waiver only: 0%
Assistantship/fellowship only: 0%
Both tuition waiver & assistantship/fellowship: 0%

Approximate percentage of incoming students who entered with a B.A./B.S. only: 79% **Master's:** 21%

Approximate percentage of students who are Women: 77.6% **Ethnic Minority:** 24.7% **International:** 5%

Average years to complete the doctoral program (including internship): 5 years

Personal interview
Preferred in person but telephone acceptable

Research areas	# Faculty	# Grants
family/child	5	2
gender studies	3	0
health psychology	4	0
multicultural/community	5	0
psychodynamics	5	0

Clinical opportunities
We have over 125 practicum sites that specialize in almost all areas of psychology including inpatient, outpatient, and residential treatment programs for children, adolescents, and adults, hospitals specializing in behavioral health and neuropsychological populations, college counseling centers, mental health centers, forensic sites, and placements specializing in the treatment of specific ethnic minority populations, women, gays/lesbians, and the disabled.

American University

Department of Psychology
Washington, DC 20016
phone#: (202) 885-1726
e-mail: cweissb@american.edu
Web address:
http://www.american.edu/cas/psych/clinicalprog.html

1	2	3	**4**	5	6	7

Clinically oriented   Equal emphasis   Research oriented

What percentage of your faculty subscribes to or practices in each of the following orientations?

Psychodynamic/Psychoanalytic	15%
Applied behavioral analysis/Radical behavioral	0%
Family systems/Systems	0%
Existential/Phenomenological/Humanistic	15%
Cognitive/Cognitive-behavioral	70%

What percentage of students applying for internship last year was accepted into APPIC-member internships? 100%

What courses are required for incoming students to have completed prior to enrolling?
None

Are there courses you recommend that are not mandatory?
Psychology major, including experimental psychology, statistics

GRE mean
Verbal 621   Quantitative 650 Advanced Psychology 704
Analytical Writing Data not available

GPA mean
Overall GPA 3.61 Psychology GPA 3.5

Number of applications/admission offers/incoming students in 2005
284 applied/13 admission offers/7 incoming

% of students receiving:
Tuition waiver only: 0%
Assistantship/fellowship only: 0%
Both tuition waiver & assistantship/fellowship: 57%

Approximate percentage of incoming students who entered with a B.A./B.S. only: 86% **Master's:** 14%

Approximate percentage of students who are Women: 86% **Ethnic Minority:** 14% **International:** No data

Average years to complete the doctoral program (including internship): 6.5 years

Personal interview
Required in person

Research areas	# Faculty	# Grants
addiction	2	2
anxiety disorders	1	0
child	1	0
coping	1	0
depression	1	0
eating disorders	1	0
treatment cost effectiveness	1	0

Clinical opportunities
cognitive-behavior therapy
externships
family therapy
neuropsychological testing
person-centered therapy
psychodynamic therapy
psychological testing

Antioch/New England Graduate School (Psy.D.)

Department of Clinical Psychology
40 Avon Street
Keene, NH 03431
phone#: (603) 357-3122
e-mail: rpeterson@antiochne.edu
Web address: http://www.antiochne.edu/cp/

1	2	**3**	4	5	6	7
Clinically oriented		Equal emphasis			Research oriented	

What percentage of your faculty subscribes to or practices in each of the following orientations?

Psychodynamic/Psychoanalytic	30%
Applied behavioral analysis/Radical behavioral	10%
Family systems/Systems	10%
Existential/Phenomenological/Humanistic	10%
Cognitive/Cognitive-behavioral	20%
Integrative	20%

What percentage of students applying for internship last year was accepted into APPIC-member internships? 7%

What courses are required for incoming students to have completed prior to enrolling?
Undergraduate or graduate degree in psychology is preferred, at a minimum at least 15 credits of relevant coursework is required.

Are there courses you recommend that are not mandatory?
No

GRE mean
Verbal 536   Quantitative 551

GPA mean
Overall GPA 3.0

Number of applications/admission offers/incoming students in 2003
118 applied/60 admission offers/30 incoming

% of students receiving:
Tuition waiver only: 0%
Assistantship/fellowship only: 18% (small stipends)
Both tuition waiver & assistantship/fellowship: 0%

Approximate percentage of incoming students who entered with a B.A./B.S. only: 64%   **Master's:** 36%

Approximate percentage of students who are Women: 82%   **Ethnic Minority:** 8%   **International:** 3%

Average years to complete the doctoral program (including internship): 7.2 years

Personal interview
Required in person

Research areas	# Faculty	# Grants
community services	2	2
children	2	0
health psychology	1	1
graduate training	2	0
group	1	0
multicultural psychology	1	0
outcome evaluation	2	0
women's issues	2	0

Clinical opportunities
assessment
battering/abuse
behavioral medicine
child clinical psychology
cognitive/behavioral therapy
conduct disorders
community services
counseling center
family therapy
forensic
gay and lesbian
group therapy
health psychology
neuropsychology/rehabilitation
personality disorders
psychodynamic
rural psychology
school based: substance abuse, supervision

Argosy University–Atlanta (Psy.D.)

Georgia School of Professional
980 Hammond Drive, Suite 100
Atlanta, GA 30328
phone#: (770) 671-1200 or (888) 671-4777
e-mail: jbinder@argosyu.edu
Web address: http://www.argosyu.edu/lcontent/
?location=1&parent=106&subpg=118

1	**2**	3	4	5	6	7
Clinically oriented		Equal emphasis			Research oriented	

What percentage of your faculty subscribes to or practices in each of the following orientations?

Psychodynamic/Psychoanalytic	33%
Applied behavioral analysis/Radical behavioral	0%
Family systems/Systems	25%
Existential/Phenomenological/Humanistic	8%
Cognitive/Cognitive-behavioral	33%

What percentage of students applying for internship last year was accepted into APPIC-member internships? 100%

What courses are required for incoming students to have completed prior to enrolling?
General psychology, statistics, tests & measures, abnormal, and personality

Are there courses you recommend that are not mandatory?
No

GRE mean
Verbal 500   Quantitative 500
Advanced Psychology N/A   Analytical Writing N/A

GPA mean
Overall GPA 3.25   Psychology GPA 3.25
Junior/Senior GPA 3.25

Number of applications/admission offers/incoming students in 2003
226 applied/89 admission offers/53 incoming

% of students receiving:
Tuition waiver only: 0%
Assistantship/fellowship only: 20%
Both tuition waiver & assistantship/fellowship: 0%

Approximate percentage of incoming students who entered with a B.A./B.S. only: 95%   **Master's:** 5%

**Approximate percentage of students who are
Women:** 77%   **Ethnic Minority:** 20%   **International:** 0%

Average years to complete the doctoral program (including internship): 5 years

Personal interview
Data not avaiilable

Research areas	# Faculty	# Grants
geropsychology	2	0
multicultural issues	3	0
neuropsychology	3	0
pediatric psychology	2	0
psychological assessment	4	0
short-term, dynamic therapy	1	0
teenage sexuality	2	0

Clinical opportunities
assessment
adult psychotherapy
child & adolescent psychotherapy
crisis intervention
educational assessments and consultation
forensic psychology
health psychology
inpatient and outpatient clinical services
neuropsychology
rehabilitation medicine
substance abuse rehabilitation

Argosy University–Chicago Campus (Psy.D.)
(Illinois School of Professional Psychology)

350 N. Orleans Street
Chicago, IL 60654
phone#: (312) 777-7600 or (800) 626-4123
Web address: http://www.argosyu.edu/lcontent/
?location=8&parent=131&subpg=112

1	**2**	3	4	5	6	7
Clinically oriented		Equal emphasis			Research oriented	

What percentage of your faculty subscribes to or practices in each of the following orientations?

Psychodynamic/Psychoanalytic	35%
Applied behavioral analysis/Radical behavioral	0%
Family systems/Systems	20%
Existential/Phenomenological/Humanistic	15%
Cognitive/Cognitive-behavioral	20%

What percentage of students applying for internship last year was accepted into APPIC-member internships? 95%

What courses are required for incoming students to have completed prior to enrolling?
Introductory psychology, abnormal psychology, statistics, tests and measures, personality

Are there courses you recommend that are not mandatory?
No

GRE mean
Data not available

GPA mean
Overall GPA 3.25   Psychology GPA 3.25
Junior/Senior GPA 3.25

Number of applications/admission offers/incoming students in 2005   Data not available

% of students receiving:
Tuition waiver only: 7% (partial)
Assistantship/fellowship only: 25% (partial)
Both tuition waiver & assistantship/fellowship: 0%

Approximate percentage of incoming students who entered with a B.A./B.S. only: 54%   **Master's:** 46%

**Approximate percentage of students who are
Women:** 80%   **Ethnic Minority:** 28%   **International:** 28%

Average years to complete the doctoral program (including internship): 5.7 years

131

Personal interview
Required in person
Preferred in person but telephone acceptable (international students only)

Research areas	# Faculty	# Grants
adolescence and delinquency	1	1
behavioral medicine	3	0
diverse students' needs	2	1
eating disorders	1	0
gay men adult development	2	0
mother–daughter cross-cultural patterns	1	0
personality disorders	1	0
sexual abuse	1	0
therapist development	2	0
therapy of severe mental illness	1	1

Clinical opportunities
behavioral medicine
child and adolescent psychology
chronic mental illness
cognitive-behavioral psychotherapy
community psychology
couples
eating disorders
EMDR
emergency crisis
ethnic-racial psychology
family psychology
forensic psychology
gay/lesbian/bisexual
gerontology
group therapy
health psychology
neuropsychology
person-centered and experiential psychotherapy
personality disorders
prevention
psychoanalytic psychotherapy
refugee populations/trauma and torture survivors
rehabilitation
religiously committed clients
school-based programs
sexual abuse
short-term psychotherapy
sports psychology
substance abuse
victim/abuse/battering

Argosy University–Chicago Northwest Campus (Psy.D.) (Illinois School of Professional Psychology)

Rolling Meadows, IL 60008
phone#: (847) 290-7400
e-mail: admissionscnw@argosyu.edu
Web address: http://www.argosyu.edu/

1	2	**3**	4	5	6	7

Clinically oriented   Equal emphasis   Research oriented

What percentage of your faculty subscribes to or practices in each of the following orientations?

Psychodynamic/Psychoanalytic	17%
Applied behavioral analysis/Radical behavioral	0%
Family systems/Systems	17%
Existential/Phenomenological/Humanistic	25%
Cognitive/Cognitive-behavioral	25%

What percentage of students applying for internship last year was accepted into APPIC-member internships? Data not available

What courses are required for incoming students to have completed prior to enrolling?
Introduction to psychology, abnormal psychology, tests and measurement (or intro to psychological assessment), personality theory, introductory statistics

Are there courses you recommend that are not mandatory?
—

GRE mean
N/A

GPA mean
Data not available

Number of applications/admission offers/incoming students in 2003
105 applied/54 admission offers/36 incoming

% of students receiving:
Tuition waiver only: 0%
Assistantship/fellowship only: 25%
Both tuition waiver & assistantship/fellowship: 0%

Approximate percentage of incoming students who entered with a B.A./B.S. only: 51%   **Master's:** 49%

Approximate percentage of students who are Women: 78%   **Ethnic Minority:** 14%
International: Data not available

Average years to complete the doctoral program (including internship): 5.2 years

Personal interview
Required in person

Research areas	# Faculty	# Grants
ADHD and child externalizing behaviors	1	0
cultural bias in psychological testing	2	0
effectiveness of process	2	1
experiential therapy	3	1
family therapy effectiveness	1	0
men's perception of psychotherapy	1	0
multicultural training	2	1
psychotherapy process and outcome	2	1
stigma in mental illness identity	1	1
substance abuse program evaluation	1	1
treatment of domestic violence	2	0

Clinical opportunities

Numerous sites available; more than 200 practicum sites in greater Chicago area. Specialization sites include:
child and pediatric psychology
college counseling center
community mental health
correctional psychology
family and marital counseling
forensics
health and medical psychology
inpatient psychiatric hospital, adult and adolescent
neuropsychological assessment
rehabilitation
severely mentally ill
substance abuse

Argosy University–Honolulu Campus (Psy.D.)

400 ASB Tower, 1001 Bishop Street
Honolulu, HI 96813
phone#: (808) 536-5555
e-mail: hawaii@argosyu.edu
Web address: http://www.argosyu.edu/lcontent/
?location=3&parent=216&subpg=217

1	**2**	3	4	5	6	7

Clinically oriented   Equal emphasis   Research oriented

What percentage of your faculty subscribes to or practices in each of the following orientations?

Psychodynamic/Psychoanalytic	10%
Applied behavioral analysis/Radical behavioral	0%
Family systems/Systems	30%
Existential/Phenomenological/Humanistic	20%
Cognitive/Cognitive-behavioral	40%

What percentage of students applying for internship last year was accepted into APPIC-member internships? 90%

What courses are required for incoming students to have completed prior to enrolling?

Introduction to general psychology, abnormal psychology, tests and measurements, personality theories, research methods or statistics

Are there courses you recommend that are not mandatory?

—

GRE mean

Data not available

GPA mean

Overall GPA 3.25

Number of applications/admission offers/incoming students in 2005

149 applied/79 admission offers/46 incoming

% of students receiving:

Tuition waiver only: 0%
Assistantship/fellowship only: 5%
Both tuition waiver & assistantship/fellowship: 0%

Approximate percentage of incoming students who entered with a B.A./B.S. only: 65%   Master's: 25%   Ph.D., J.D.: 10%

Approximate percentage of students who are Women: 77%   Ethnic Minority: 53%   International: 0%

Average years to complete the doctoral program (including internship): 5.4 years

Personal interview

Preferred in person but telephone acceptable

Research areas	# Faculty	# Grants
diversity education	5	0
gay/lesbian relationships	1	0
health psychology	3	0
neuropsychology	3	0
posttraumatic stress disorder	2	1

Clinical opportunities

adolescent
day treatment and hospice programs
community mental health centers
developmental evaluation clinics
outpatient treatment centers
parole agencies
psychiatric, medical, and veterans hospitals
public and private schools
state courts, prisons
substance abuse

Argosy University–Phoenix (Psy.D.)

Department of Psychology
2301 West Dunlap Avenue, Suite 211
Phoenix, AZ 85021
phone#: (602) 216-2600
e-mail: www.argosyu.edu
Web address: http://www.argosyu.edu/lcontent/?
location=11&parent=238&subpg=239

1	**2**	3	4	5	6	7

Clinically oriented   Equal emphasis   Research oriented

What percentage of your faculty subscribes to or practices in each of the following orientations?

Psychodynamic/Psychoanalytic	20%
Applied behavioral analysis/Radical behavioral	0%
Family systems/Systems	20%
Existential/Phenomenological/Humanistic	25%
Cognitive/Cognitive-behavioral	35%

What percentage of students applying for internship last year was accepted into APPIC-member internships? Data not available

What courses are required for incoming students to have completed prior to enrolling?

Foundation courses must be completed within 1 year of admission: introductory psychology, personality theory, abnormal psychology, test and measurement, psychological assessment, psychological measurement, statistics or research methods.

Are there courses you recommend that are not mandatory?
No

GRE mean
Data not available

GPA mean
Data not available

Number of applications/admission offers/incoming students in 2003
95 applied/67 admission offers/34 incoming

% of students receiving:
Tuition waiver only: 0%
Assistantship/fellowship only: 0%
Both tuition waiver & assistantship/fellowship: 0%

Approximate percentage of incoming students who entered with a B.A./B.S. only: 75% **Master's:** 25%

Approximate percentage of students who are Women: 80% **Ethnic Minority:** 16%
International: Data not available

Average years to complete the doctoral program (including internship): 5 years

Personal interview
Preferred in person but telephone acceptable

Research areas	# Faculty	# Grants
diversity	1	0
forensic psychology	2	0
learning disability/ADHD	1	0
neuropsychology	2	0
psychopharmacology	1	0
sexual trauma	2	0

Clinical opportunities
Not as a part of the school. We do offer a diverse array of practicum placement in specialty clinics, including but not limited to sexual offender treatment, substance abuse, pain management, neuropsychology, surgical centers, schools and specialty schools for the behaviorally or emotionally challenged, preschool age children, inpatient and outpatient psychotherapy, HIV/AIDS, and culturally diverse sites.

Argosy University–San Francisco Bay (Psy.D.)

Argosy University/San Francisco Bay Area
999A Canal Boulevard
Point Richmond, CA 94804
phone#: (510) 215-0277 or toll-free outside of the Bay Area, (866) 215-2777
e-mail: jstofan@argosyu.edu
Web address: http://www.argosyu.edu/lcontent/?location=5&parent=253&subpg=510
Program data unavailable

Argosy University–Tampa (Psy.D.)

Argosy University/Tampa
Parkside at Tampa Bay Park
4401 North Himes Avenue, Suite 150
Tampa, FL 33614
phone#: (813) 393-5290 or toll-free outside of the Tampa area, (800) 850-6488
e-mail: mgallagher@argosyu.edu
Web address: http://www.argosyu.edu/lcontent/?location=13&parent=338&subpg=339
Program data unavailable

Argosy University–Twin Cities Campus (Psy.D.)

Minnesota School of Professional Psychology
Graduate Admissions
Argosy University/Twin Cities
1515 Central Parkway
Eagan, MN 55121
phone#: (888) 844-2004
e-mail: tcadmissions@argosy.edu
Web address: http://www.argosyu.edu/lcontent/?location=7&parent=441&subpg=443

1	**2**	3	4	5	6	7
Clinically oriented		Equal emphasis			Research oriented	

What percentage of your faculty subscribes to or practices in each of the following orientations?

Psychodynamic/Psychoanalytic	25%
Applied behavioral analysis/Radical behavioral	0%
Family systems/Systems	25%
Existential/Phenomenological/Humanistic	25%
Cognitive/Cognitive-behavioral	25%

What percentage of students applying for internship last year was accepted into APPIC-member internships?
Data not available

What courses are required for incoming students to have completed prior to enrolling?
4 psychology courses and 1 statistics course

Are there courses you recommend that are not mandatory?
No

GRE mean
Verbal 536   Quantitative 656   Analytical 577

GPA mean
Data not available

Number of applications/admission offers/incoming students in 2003
141 applied/78 admission offers/38 incoming

% of students receiving:
Tuition waiver only: 0%
Assistantship/fellowship only: 35%
Both tuition waiver & assistantship/fellowship: 0%

Approximate percentage of incoming students who entered with a B.A./B.S. only: 70% **Master's:** 30%

Approximate percentage of students who are Women: 75% **Ethnic Minority:** 15%
International: Data not available

Average years to complete the doctoral program (including internship): 5 years

Personal interview
Required in person

Research areas	# Faculty	# Grants
psychometric properties of Rorschach	2	0
psychotherapy outcome research	1	0
reconciliation in psychotherapy	1	0

Clinical opportunities
—

Argosy University–Washington, DC Campus (Psy.D.)

1550 Wilson Boulevard, Suite 600
Washington, DC 22209
phone#: 703-526-5800
e-mail: dosullivan@argosyu.edu
Web address: http://www.argosyu.edu/lcontent/
?location=14&parent=197&subpg=198

1	2	3	4	5	6	7

Clinically oriented Equal emphasis Research oriented

What percentage of your faculty subscribes to or practices in each of the following orientations?

Psychodynamic/Psychoanalytic	57%
Applied behavioral analysis/Radical behavioral	0%
Family systems/Systems	21%
Existential/Phenomenological/Humanistic	36%
Cognitive/Cognitive-behavioral	64%

What percentage of students applying for internship last year was accepted into APPIC-member internships?
Data not available

What courses are required for incoming students to have completed prior to enrolling?
Intro to psychology, statistics or research methods, abnormal psychology, personality theories, psychological assessment

Are there courses you recommend that are not mandatory?
No

GRE mean
N/A

GPA mean
Data not available

Number of applications/admission offers/incoming students in 2003
265 applied/127 admission offers/75 incoming

% of students receiving:
Partial tuition waiver only: 0%
Assistantship/fellowship only: 11%
Both tuition waiver & assistantship/fellowship: 11%

Approximate percentage of incoming students who entered with a B.A./B.S. only: 51% **Master's:** 45%

Approximate percentage of students who are Women: 81.5% **Ethnic Minority:** 31%
International: Data not available

Average years to complete the doctoral program (including internship): 6 years

Personal interview
Preferred in person but telephone acceptable

Research areas	# Faculty	# Grants
cognitive attributions and appraisals	1	0
multicultural competence	1	0

Clinical opportunities
anxiety disorders/obsessive–compulsive disorders
child abuse
children's hospitals
forensic hospitals/prisons
gerontology
neuropsychology
posttraumatic stress disorder
sexual orientation
school mental health
substance abuse
university counseling center

University of Arizona

Department of Psychology
Psychology Building
Tucson, AZ 85721
phone#: (520) 621-1867
e-mail: varda@u.arizona.edu
Web address: http://psychology.arizona.edu/programs/
g_each/clinical.php

1	2	3	4	5	**6**	7

Clinically oriented Equal emphasis Research oriented

What percentage of your faculty subscribes to or practices in each of the following orientations?

Psychodynamic/Psychoanalytic	0%
Applied behavioral analysis/Radical behavioral	20%
Family systems/Systems	20%
Existential/Phenomenological/Humanistic	10%
Cognitive/Cognitive-behavioral	70%

What percentage of students applying for internship last year was accepted into APPIC-member internships?
Data not available

What courses are required for incoming students to have completed prior to enrolling?
B.A. or B.S. in psychology

Are there courses you recommend that are not mandatory?
No

GRE mean
Verbal 626   Quantitative 691
Advanced Psychology 701

GPA mean
Overall GPA 3.6

Number of applications/admission offers/incoming students in 2005
234 applied/9 admission offers/7 incoming

% of students receiving:
Tuition waiver only: 0%
Assistantship/fellowship only: 0%
Both tuition waiver & assistantship/fellowship: 100%

Approximate percentage of incoming students who entered with a B.A./B.S. only: 80%   **Master's:** 20%

Approximate percentage of students who are Women: 60%   **Ethnic Minority:** 22%
International: Data not available

Average years to complete the doctoral program (including internship): 6 years (median)

Personal interview
Preferred in person but telephone acceptable

Research areas	# Faculty	# Grants
clinical neuropsychology	2	2
depression	2	1
family systems	2	4
health psychology	6	6
mental health policy	2	1
sleep disorders	1	2
treatment outcome	4	4

Clinical opportunities
behavioral medicine
community psychology
couple and family therapy
depression
gerontology
neuropsychology/rehabilitation
sleep disorders

Arizona State University
Department of Psychology
Tempe, AZ 85287-1104
phone#: (480) 965-7606
e-mail: Manuel.Barrera@asu.edu
Web address: http://www.asu.edu/clas/psych/gprogram/clinical/

1	2	3	4	5	**6**	7
Clinically oriented		Equal emphasis			Research oriented	

What percentage of your faculty subscribes to or practices in each of the following orientations?

Psychodynamic/Psychoanalytic	0%
Applied behavioral analysis/Radical behavioral	5%
Family systems/Systems	30%
Existential/Phenomenological/Humanistic	0%
Cognitive/Cognitive-behavioral	65%

What percentage of students applying for internship last year was accepted into APPIC-member internships? 100%

What courses are required for incoming students to have completed prior to enrolling?
B.A. in psychology or equivalent

Are there courses you recommend that are not mandatory?
No

GRE mean
Verbal 633   Quantitative 713
Analytical Writing 5.5

GPA mean
Overall GPA 3.7

Number of applications/admission offers/incoming students in 2005
286 applied/14 admission offers/4 incoming

% of students receiving:
Tuition waiver only: 0%
Assistantship/fellowship only: 0%
Both tuition waiver & assistantship/fellowship: 100%

Approximate percentage of incoming students who entered with a B.A./B.S. only: 90%   **Master's:** 10%

Approximate percentage of students who are Women: 75%   **Ethnic Minority:** 27%   **International:** 8%

Average years to complete the doctoral program (including internship): 6.9 years

Personal interview
Preferred in person but telephone acceptable

Research areas	# Faculty	# Grants
adult psychopathology	3	3
aging/gerontology	3	3
behavioral medicine/health psychology	11	10
child clinical	5	5
community psychology	6	5
family interactions	4	4
gender roles	2	1
hispanic studies	5	4
minority mental health	5	4
personality assessment	1	1
prevention	6	5
psychoneuroimmunology	3	3
quantitative statistics	6	6
substance abuse	5	5

Clinical opportunities
behavioral analysis
behavioral medicine
child clinical psychology
child health psychology
family therapy

geropsychology
individual therapy
intellectual and academic assessment
interpersonal psychotherapy
marital/couples therapy
parenting groups
prevention programs

University of Arkansas

Department of Psychology
216 Memorial Hall
Fayetteville, AR 72701
phone#: (479) 575-4256
Web address:
http://www.uark.edu/depts/psyc/clinical.html

1	2	3	4	**5**	6	7

Clinically oriented   Equal emphasis   Research oriented

What percentage of your faculty subscribes to or practices in each of the following orientations?

Psychodynamic/Psychoanalytic   0%
Applied behavioral analysis/Radical behavioral   30%
Family systems/Systems   50%
Existential/Phenomenological/Humanistic   15%
Cognitive/Cognitive-behavioral   100%

What percentage of students applying for internship last year was accepted into APPIC-member internships? 100%

What courses are required for incoming students to have completed prior to enrolling?
Applicants who have not taken a course in history and systems will be expected to take these courses upon arrival.

Are there courses you recommend that are not mandatory?
18 semester hours in psychology including statistics, learning, and experimental psychology

GRE mean
Verbal 566   Quantitative 638
Analytical Writing 5.13

GPA mean
Overall GPA 3.67

Number of applications/admission offers/incoming students in 2005
123 applied/7 admission offers/5 incoming

% of students receiving:
Tuition waiver only: 0%
Assistantship/fellowship only: 0%
Both tuition waiver & assistantship/fellowship: 100%

Approximate percentage of incoming students who entered with a B.A./B.S. only: 50%   **Master's:** 50%

Approximate percentage of students who are Women: 65%   **Ethnic Minority:** 15%   **International:** 0%

Average years to complete the doctoral program (including internship): 6 years

Personal interview
Required in person

Research areas	# Faculty	# Grants
aggression & victimization	3	1
child and family interventions	2	0
cognitive vulnerability to anxiety and depression	2	0
emotion regulation and psychopathology	3	0
family, parent, systems intervention	1	0
science and psuedoscience in psychological practice	1	0

Clinical opportunities
ADHD clinic
community mental health
developmental pediatrics
primary health care setting

Auburn University

Department of Psychology
226 Thach
Auburn, AL 36849
phone#: (334) 844-6471
e-mail: BRYANGT@MAIL.AUBURN.EDU
Web address: http://www.cla.auburn.edu/psychology/gs/prospective/clinical/index.htm

1	2	**3**	4	5	6	7

Clinically oriented   Equal emphasis   Research oriented

What percentage of your faculty subscribes to or practices in each of the following orientations?

Psychodynamic/Psychoanalytic   10%
Applied behavioral analysis/Radical behavioral   30%
Family systems/Systems   10%
Existential/Phenomenological/Humanistic   0%
Cognitive/Cognitive-behavioral   50%

What percentage of students applying for internship last year was accepted into APPIC-member internships?
Data not available

What courses are required for incoming students to have completed prior to enrolling?
14 semester hours in theoretical or experimental psychology and quantitative methods

Are there courses you recommend that are not mandatory?
History of Psychology, second course in statistics

GRE mean
Verbal + Quantitative 1200

GPA mean
Overall GPA 3.7

Number of applications/admission offers/incoming students in 2003
109 applied/11 admission offers/9 incoming

% of students receiving:
Tuition waiver only: 0%
Assistantship/fellowship only: 0%
Both tuition waiver & assistantship/fellowship: 100%

Approximate percentage of incoming students who entered with a B.A./B.S. only: 78%   **Master's:** 22%

Approximate percentage of students who are Women: 70%   **Ethnic Minority:** 12%   **International:** Data not available

Average years to complete the doctoral program (including internship): 6.5 years

Personal interview
Required in person

Research areas	# Faculty	# Grants
anxiety disorders	2	1
child clinical/psychopathology	2	0
developmental disabilities	1	0
personality assessment	2	0
sexuality/deviation/dysfunction	1	1

Clinical opportunities
anxiety disorders
disorders in adolescence
hyperactivity
posttraumatic stress disorder
substance abuse

Azusa Pacific University (Psy.D.)
Department of Psychology
901 East Alosta Avenue
Azusa, CA 91702-7000
phone#: (626) 815-5008
e-mail: mstanton@apu.edu
Web address:
http://www.apu.edu/educabs/graduatepsychology/psyd/

1	2	**3**	4	5	6	7

Clinically oriented	Equal emphasis	Research oriented

What percentage of your faculty subscribes to or practices in each of the following orientations?
Psychodynamic/Psychoanalytic 42%
Applied behavioral analysis/Radical behavioral 0%
Family systems/Systems 58%
Existential/Phenomenological/Humanistic 25%
Cognitive/Cognitive-behavioral 33%

What percentage of students applying for internship last year was accepted into APPIC-member internships? 0%

What courses are required for incoming students to have completed prior to enrolling?
Master's level courses: child abuse (7 hours), family therapy, human sexuality/sex therapy, introduction to clinical practice, intro to psychological testing, psychopathology, psychotherapy and cultural diversity, theories of personality and psychotherapy.
Bachelor's level courses: Abnormal psychology, general/introduction to psychology, human growth and development, theories of personality, introduction to statistics

Are there courses you recommend that are not mandatory?
No

GRE mean
Verbal 504   Quantitative 554
Analytical Writing 3.0, 4.8

GPA mean
Overall GPA Master's 3.7   Bachelor's 3.47

Number of applications/admission offers/incoming students in 2005
82 applied/47 admission offers/28 incoming

% of students receiving:
Tuition waiver only: 0%
Assistantship/fellowship only: 2%
Both tuition waiver & assistantship/fellowship: 18%

Approximate percentage of incoming students who entered with a B.A./B.S. only: 78%   **Master's:** 22%

Approximate percentage of students who are Women: 70%   **Ethnic Minority:** 37%   **International:** 5%

Average years to complete the doctoral program (including internship): 5 years

Personal interview
Preferred in person but telephone acceptable

Research areas	# Faculty	# Grants
counseling skills	1	1
forensics	2	1
homelessness/HIV	1	0
moral development	2	1
religion/spirituality	3	1
Rorschach	1	0
school-based interventions	2	1

Clinical opportunities
behavior medicine
children and family
chronically mentally ill
community clinics
forensics
general population
geriatric
HIV/AIDS
inpatient: acute and chronic
school-based
substance abuse
university counseling

Baylor University (Psy.D.)

Department of Psychology
P.O. Box 97334
Waco, TX 76798-7334
phone#: (254) 710-2811
e-mail: M_Rudd@Baylor.edu
Web address: http://www.baylor.edu/
psychologyneuroscience/index.php?id=21323

1	**2**	3	4	5	6	7
Clinically oriented		Equal emphasis			Research oriented	

What percentage of your faculty subscribes to or practices in each of the following orientations?

Psychodynamic/Psychoanalytic	15%
Applied behavioral analysis/Radical behavioral	0%
Family systems/Systems	15%
Existential/Phenomenological/Humanistic	15%
Cognitive/Cognitive-behavioral	55%

What percentage of students applying for internship last year was accepted into APPIC-member internships?
Data not available

What courses are required for incoming students to have completed prior to enrolling?
None

Are there courses you recommend that are not mandatory?
Developmental psychology, psychopathology, statistics, biopsychology, personality, social

GRE mean
Verbal 630   Quantitative 631
Analytical Writing Data not available

GPA mean
Overall GPA 3.5   Psychology GPA 3.7
Junior/Senior GPA 3.7

Number of applications/admission offers/incoming students in 2003
150 applied/9 admission offers/8 incoming

% of students receiving:
Tuition waiver only: 0%
Assistantship/fellowship only: 0%
Both tuition waiver & assistantship/fellowship: 100%

Approximate percentage of incoming students who entered with a B.A./B.S. only: 78%   Master's: 22%

**Approximate percentage of students who are Women: 78%   Ethnic Minority: 11%
International:** Data not available

Average years to complete the doctoral program (including internship): 4 years

Personal interview
Required in person

Research areas	# Faculty	# Grants
behavioral medicine	1	0
child psychopathology	2	0
cognitive therapy	3	0
depression	3	0
group therapy	1	0
personality assessment	3	0

Clinical opportunities
alcohol and drug dependence
anxiety disorders
behavioral medicine
child psychotherapy
community psychology
crisis intervention
eating disorders
family therapy
gerontology
group dynamics
group therapy
health psychology
impulse control
mood disorders
neuropsychology
personality disorder
play therapy
rural psychology
schizophrenia/psychoses
school/educational
sexual offenders
suicide prevention
suicide risk assessment and treatment
victim/battering/abuse

Binghamton University/ State University of New York

Department of Psychology
Vestal Parkway East
Binghamton, NY 13902-6000
phone#: (607) 777-2334
e-mail: clinpsyc@binghamton.edu
Web address: http://psychology.binghamton.edu/
Clinical/index.html

1	2	3	4	**5**	6	7
Clinically oriented		Equal emphasis			Research oriented	

What percentage of your faculty subscribes to or practices in each of the following orientations?

Psychodynamic/Psychoanalytic	0%
Applied behavioral analysis/Radical behavioral	10%
Family systems/Systems	0%
Existential/Phenomenological/Humanistic	0%
Cognitive/Cognitive-behavioral	100%

What percentage of students applying for internship last year was accepted into APPIC-member internships? 100%

What courses are required for incoming students to have completed prior to enrolling?
Equivalent of a psychology major, with knowledge of experimental psychology and research methods

Are there courses you recommend that are not mandatory?
Physiological psychology

GRE mean
Verbal 623   Quantitative 655
Analytical Writing 5.0   Advanced Psychology 697

GPA mean
Overall GPA 3.7

Number of applications/admission offers/incoming students in 2003
223 applied/11 admission offers/8 incoming

% of students receiving:
Tuition waiver only: 0%
Assistantship/fellowship only: 0%
Both tuition waiver & assistantship/fellowship: 100%

Approximate percentage of students who are
Women: 74%   **Ethnic Minority:** 12%   **International:** 0%

Average years to complete the doctoral program (including internship): 6.25 years

Personal interview
Strongly preferred in person but telephone possible

Research areas	# Faculty	# Grants
adult psychopathology	8	2
anxiety disorders	2	1
assessment	4	0
behavioral medicine	1	1
child clinical	2	2
depression	1	1
developmental disabilities	1	2
hypnosis	1	1
learning disabilities	1	1
marital process and therapy	1	1
memory construction	2	0
neuropsychology	1	2
pain management	1	1
pediatric psychology	1	1
personality disorders	1	1
posttraumatic stress disorder/trauma	2	0
prevention	3	1
psychophysiology	2	0
social skills	1	0
substance abuse	1	1

Clinical opportunities
adolescent delinquency
adult psychopathology
anxiety disorders
autism spectrum disorders
behavioral medicine
conduct disorder
correctional facility
couples therapy
depression
disorders of childhood
family therapy
learning disabilities

neuropsychology
pain management
psychotherapy supervision
schizophrenia
school consultation
substance abuse

Biola University (Ph.D.)

Rosemead School of Psychology
13800 Biola Avenue
La Mirada, CA 90639
phone#: (562) 903-4752
e-mail: biola@admissions.edu
Web address:
http://www.rosemead.edu/programs/phd.cfm

1	2	3	**4**	5	6	7

Clinically oriented   Equal emphasis   Research oriented

What percentage of your faculty subscribes to or practices in each of the following orientations?

Psychodynamic/Psychoanalytic	39%
Applied behavioral analysis/Radical behavioral	0%
Family systems/Systems	17%
Existential/Phenomenological/Humanistic	10%
Cognitive/Cognitive-behavioral	34%

What percentage of students applying for internship last year was accepted into APPIC-member internships?
Data not available

What courses are required for incoming students to have completed prior to enrolling?
Introductory psychology, statistics, experimental psychology, abnormal psychology, personality, learning

Are there courses you recommend that are not mandatory?
Social psychology, history of psychology, physiological psychology, biology/zoology, developmental psychology

GRE mean
Verbal + Quantitative = 1310
Analytical Writing Data not available

GPA mean
Data not available

Number of applications/admission offers/incoming students in 2003
120 applied/9 admission offers/6 incoming

% of students receiving:
Tuition waiver only: 2%
Assistantship/fellowship only: 60%
Both tuition waiver & assistantship/fellowship: 0%

Approximate percentage of incoming students who entered with a B.A./B.S. only: 78%   **Master's:** 32%

Approximate percentage of students who are
Women: 78%   **Ethnic Minority:** 11%
International: Data not available

Average years to complete the doctoral program (including internship): 6 years

Personal interview
Required in person

Research areas	# Faculty	# Grants
cross-cultural adjustment	4	0
grief	1	0
neuropsychology	1	0
object relations	4	0
parenting behaviors	3	0
spirituality	4	2

Clinical opportunities
cultural and individual
diversity
family/child
individual
outpatient/inpatient
therapy and spirituality

Biola University (Psy.D.)

Rosemead School of Psychology
13800 Biola Avenue
La Mirada, CA 90639
phone#: (562) 903-4752
e-mail: biola@admissions.edu
Web address:
http://www.rosemead.edu/programs/psyd.cfm

1	**2**	3	4	5	6	7
Clinically oriented		Equal emphasis			Research oriented	

What percentage of your faculty subscribes to or practices in each of the following orientations?
Psychodynamic/Psychoanalytic	39%
Applied behavioral analysis/Radical behavioral	0%
Family systems/Systems	17%
Existential/Phenomenological/Humanistic	10%
Cognitive/Cognitive-behavioral	34%

What percentage of students applying for internship last year was accepted into APPIC-member internships?
Data not available

What courses are required for incoming students to have completed prior to enrolling?
Introductory psychology, statistics, experimental psychology, abnormal psychology, personality, learning

Are there courses you recommend that are not mandatory?
Social psychology, history of psychology, physiological psychology, biology/zoology, developmental psychology

GRE mean
Verbal + Quantitative = 1090
Analytical Writing Data not available

GPA mean
Data not available

Number of applications/admission offers/incoming students in 2003
120 applied/23 admission offers/19 incoming

% of students receiving:
Tuition waiver only: 5%
Assistantship/fellowship only: 60%
Both tuition waiver & assistantship/fellowship: 0%

Approximate percentage of incoming students who entered with a B.A./B.S. only: 58%   **Master's:** 42%

Approximate percentage of students who are Women: 60%   **Ethnic Minority:** 25%
International: Data not available

Average years to complete the doctoral program (including internship): 6 years

Personal interview
Required in person

Research areas	# Faculty	# Grants
cross-cultural adjustment	4	0
gender issues	2	1
grief	1	0
neuropsychology	1	1
object relations	4	0
parenting behaviors	3	0
spirituality	4	2

Clinical opportunities
cultural and individual
diversity
family/child
individual
outpatient/inpatient
therapy and spirituality

Boston University

Department of Psychology
64 Cummington Street
Boston, MA 02215
phone#: (617) 353-2587
e-mail: nclement@bu.edu
Web address: http://www.bu.edu/psych/graduate/clinical/

1	2	3	**4**	5	6	7
Clinically oriented		Equal emphasis			Research oriented	

What percentage of your faculty subscribes to or practices in each of the following orientations?
Psychodynamic/Psychoanalytic	5%
Applied behavioral analysis/Radical behavioral	0%
Family systems/Systems	17%
Existential/Phenomenological/Humanistic	0%
Cognitive/Cognitive-behavioral	70%
Neuropsychology	17%
Eclectic	10%

What percentage of students applying for internship last year was accepted into APPIC-member internships? 100%

What courses are required for incoming students to have completed prior to enrolling?
Introductory psychology, statistics, abnormal/clinical psychology, experimental

Are there courses you recommend that are not mandatory?
Broad liberal arts and science

GRE mean
Verbal + Quantitative 1300
Analytical Writing 4.5

GPA mean
Overall GPA 3.6

Number of applications/admission offers/incoming students in 2004
587 applied/15 admission offers/12 incoming

% of students receiving:
Tuition waiver only: 0%
Assistantship/fellowship only: 0%
Both tuition waiver & assistantship/fellowship: 92%

Approximate percentage of incoming students who entered with a B.A./B.S. only: 90% **Master's:** 10%

Approximate percentage of students who are
Women: 85% **Ethnic Minority:** 25% **International:** 10%

Average years to complete the doctoral program (including internship): 6.5 years

Personal interview
Required in person

Research areas	# Faculty	# Grants
affective disorders	2	2
anxiety disorders	7	5
behavioral genetics	1	1
community psychology	2	0
emotion	3	1
family	2	1
gender	1	0
gerontology	2	2
minority	2	0
neuropsychology	3	2
personality disorders	1	0
schizophrenia	1	1
substance abuse and addiction	1	1
victim/abuse	1	0
women's emotional health	1	0

Clinical opportunities
abuse/battering
adolescents
affective disorders
behavioral medicine
community psychology
couples therapy
dissociative disorders
eating disorders
family therapy
gerontology
neuropsychology
schizophrenia

Bowling Green State University

Department of Psychology
Bowling Green, OH 43403
phone#: (419) 372-2301
e-mail: pwatson@bgsu.edu
Web address: http://www.bgsu.edu/departments/
psych/Facultyprograms.html/ZAreaClinical.html

1	2	3	**4**	5	6	7
Clinically oriented		Equal emphasis			Research oriented	

What percentage of your faculty subscribes to or practices in each of the following orientations?

Psychodynamic/Psychoanalytic	20%
Applied behavioral analysis/Radical behavioral	0%
Family systems/Systems	30%
Existential/Phenomenological/Humanistic	20%
Cognitive/Cognitive-behavioral	65%

What percentage of students applying for internship last year was accepted into APPIC-member internships? 100%

What courses are required for incoming students to have completed prior to enrolling?
None

Are there courses you recommend that are not mandatory?
Science, math, statistics, introductory and advanced psychology courses, abnormal, abnormal, psychology lab courses

GRE mean
Verbal 562 Quantitative 665
Advanced Psychology 668
Analytical Writing Not used for admissions decisions

GPA mean
Overall GPA 3.73 Psychology GPA 3.79

Number of applications/admission offers/incoming students in 2005
159 applied/14 admission offers/9 incoming

% of students receiving:
Tuition waiver only: 0%
Assistantship/fellowship only: 0%
Both tuition waiver & assistantship/fellowship: 100%

Approximate percentage of students who are
Women: 84% **Ethnic Minority:** 17% **International:** 7%

Average years to complete the doctoral program (including internship): 6.3 years

Personal interview
Preferred in person but telephone acceptable

Research areas	# Faculty	# Grants
alcohol and substance abuse	1	0
child clinical psychology	2	1
child stress and adjustment	3	0
community psychology	1	1
family	2	0
health psychology	2	1
psychology of religion	1	1

Clinical opportunities
behavioral medicine
child clinical psychology
clinical health psychology
community mental health
community psychology
family
school-based assessment/intervention

Brigham Young University

Clinical Psychology Ph.D. Program
284 TLRB
Provo, UT 84602
phone#: (801) 422-4050
e-mail: clinical psychology@byu.edu
Web address: http://www.byu.edu/gradstudies/
index.php?action=programs.details&programid=100

1	2	**3**	4	5	6	7

Clinically oriented   Equal emphasis   Research oriented

What percentage of your faculty subscribes to or practices in each of the following orientations?

Psychodynamic/Psychoanalytic	20%
Applied behavioral analysis/Radical behavioral	20%
Family systems/Systems	10%
Existential/Phenomenological/Humanistic	50%
Cognitive/Cognitive-behavioral	70%

What percentage of students applying for internship last year was accepted into APPIC-member internships? 100%

What courses are required for incoming students to have completed prior to enrolling?
Introductory psychology, psychological statistics, research design, personality, abnormal psychology, learning or cognition, tests and measurements

Are there courses you recommend that are not mandatory?
Additional coursework in substantive areas of psychology are recommended.

GRE mean
Verbal 560   Quantitative 660
Analytical Writing Data not available

GPA mean
Overall GPA Data not available   Junior/Senior GPA 3.72

Number of applications/admission offers/incoming students in 2003
68 applied/15 admission offers/10 incoming

% of students receiving tuition waiver & assistantship/fellowship:
All 1st-year students receive assistantships and a waiver for part of their tuition. All 2nd-, 3rd-, and 4th-year students are funded in work settings, which are coordinated by the department and also receive a waiver for part of their tuition.

Approximate percentage of incoming students who entered with a B.A./B.S. only: 90%   **Master's:** 10%

Approximate percentage of students who are
Women: 41%   **Ethnic Minority:** 17%   **International:** 14%

Average years to complete the doctoral program (including internship): 5.5 years

Personal interview
Preferred in person but telephone acceptable

Research areas	# Faculty	# Grants
child/adolescent development	3	1
clinical assessment	2	0
cultural diversity/gender issues	3	1
depression and cognitive-behavioral therapy	1	1
eating disorders	1	1
group therapy, process and outcome	3	1
health psychology/behavioral medicine	2	1
individual psychotherapy, process and outcome	3	1
measurement	2	1
neuropsychology	2	4
posttraumatic stress disorder	1	1
psychopathology	2	0

Clinical opportunities
adolescent residential treatment facilities
community mental health centers
neuropsychology rehabilitation units
private general hospitals—behavioral medicine, ER, psychiatric units
private practices
residential facilities for eating disorders
school districts
state hospital
state prison
third world placements
university counseling centers—Utah and Hawaii

University of British Columbia

Department of Psychology
2316 West Mall
Vancouver, British Columbia V6T 1Z4, Canada
phone#: (604) 822-2755
e-mail: gradsec@psych.ubc.ca
Web address: http://www.psych.ubc.ca/graduate/
2005-06/g_clinical-sep05.pdf

1	2	3	4	5	**6**	7

Clinically oriented   Equal emphasis   Research oriented

What percentage of your faculty subscribes to or practices in each of the following orientations?

Psychodynamic/Psychoanalytic	10%
Applied behavioral analysis/Radical behavioral	0%
Family systems/Systems	10%
Existential/Phenomenological/Humanistic	0%
Cognitive/Cognitive-behavioral	80%

What percentage of students applying for internship last year was accepted into CCPPP-member internships? 100%

What courses are required for incoming students to have completed prior to enrolling?
None

Are there courses you recommend that are not mandatory?
Statistics, abnormal behavior, and a cross-section of other psychology courses

GRE mean
Verbal 610   Quantitative 704   Analytical 704

GPA mean
Overall GPA M = 86%

Number of applications/admission offers/incoming students in 2003
129 applied/7 admission offers/6 incoming

% of students receiving:
Tuition waiver only: 0%
Assistantship/fellowship only: 100%
Both tuition waiver & assistantship/fellowship: 0%

Approximate percentage of incoming students who entered with a B.A./B.S. only: 100%   **Master's:** 0%

Approximate percentage of students who are Women: 70%   **Ethnic Minority:** 10%
International: Data not available

Average years to complete the doctoral program (including internship): 7.2 years

Personal interview
Telephone required

Research areas	# Faculty	# Grants
anxiety disorders	3	5
attention-deficit disorder	1	2
behavioral medicine	3	7
health psychology	1	2
sexual dysfunction	1	1

Clinical opportunities
assessment
behavioral medicine
child and adult
couple therapy
forensic psychology
hospital settings

University at Buffalo/
State University of New York

Department of Psychology
Park Hall
Buffalo, NY 14260
phone#: (716) 645-3650, ext. #342
e-mail: robertsj@buffalo.edu
Web address: http://www.wings.buffalo.edu/psychology/doctoral/clinical.html

1	2	3	4	5	**6**	7

Clinically oriented   Equal emphasis   Research oriented

What percentage of your faculty subscribes to or practices in each of the following orientations?

Psychodynamic/Psychoanalytic	0%
Applied behavioral analysis/Radical behavioral	25%
Family systems/Systems	0%
Existential/Phenomenological/Humanistic	0%
Cognitive/Cognitive-behavioral	75%

What percentage of students applying for internship last year was accepted into APPIC-member internships? 100%

What courses are required for incoming students to have completed prior to enrolling?
Introductory psychology, research methods, statistics

Are there courses you recommend that are not mandatory?
Good science background, abnormal psychology, cognitive psychology, social psychology, developmental psychology

GRE mean
Verbal 640   Quantitative 680   Analytical Writing 5.0
Advanced Psychology 690

GPA mean
Data not available

Number of applications/admission offers/incoming students in 2005
165 applied/16 admission offers/7 incoming

% of students receiving:
Tuition waiver only: 0%
Assistantship/fellowship only: 0%
Both tuition waiver & assistantship/fellowship: 100%

Approximate percentage of incoming students who entered with a B.A./B.S. only: 72%   **Master's:** 28%

Approximate percentage of students who are Women: 68%   **Ethnic Minority:** 14%   **International:** 11%

Average years to complete the doctoral program (including internship): 6 years

Personal interview
Telephone required

Research areas	# Faculty	# Grants
addictions	2	2
anxiety disorders	3	2
attention-deficit disorder	3	8
behavioral medicine	1	1
childhood risk of psychopathology	3	1
depression	2	1
sexual dysfunction	1	0

Clinical opportunities
ADHD
anxiety disorders
child/adolescent externalizing disorders
depression
parent training
psychological services center

University of California–Berkeley

Department of Psychology
Berkeley, CA 94720
phone#: (510) 642-1382
e-mail: psychapp@socrates.berkeley.edu
Web address: http://psychology.berkeley.edu/
gradprograms/clinical/index.html

1	2	3	4	5	**6**	7

Clinically oriented　　Equal emphasis　　Research oriented

What percentage of your faculty subscribes to or practices in each of the following orientations?
Psychodynamic/Psychoanalytic　　　　　　　　0%
Applied behavioral analysis/Radical behavioral　0%
Family systems/Systems　　　　　　　　　　40%
Existential/Phenomenological/Humanistic　　　0%
Cognitive/Cognitive-behavioral　　　　　　　60%

What percentage of students applying for internship last year was accepted into APPIC-member internships? 100%

What courses are required for incoming students to have completed prior to enrolling?
None

Are there courses you recommend that are not mandatory?
Research design and methods, breadth in psychology

GRE mean
Verbal 688　Quantitative 737　Analytical 708
Advanced psychology 738　Analytical Writing 5.5

GPA mean
Overall GPA 3.73

Number of applications/admission offers/incoming students in 2005
298 applied/7 admission offers/6 incoming

% of students receiving:
Tuition waiver only: 0%
Assistantship/fellowship only: 0%
Both tuition waiver & assistantship/fellowship: 95%

Approximate percentage of incoming students who entered with a B.A./B.S. only: 80%　**Master's:** 20%

Approximate percentage of students who are Women: 76%　**Ethnic Minority:** 37%
International: Data not available

Average years to complete the doctoral program (including internship): 6.75 years

Personal interview
Preferred in person but telephone acceptable

Research areas	# Faculty	# Grants
ADHD externalizing behavior	1	2
classrooms, school, student achievement	1	0
emotion and aging	1	1
emotion and marriage	1	1
marriage and family	1	1
schizophrenia/depression	1	1

Clinical opportunities
—

University of California–Los Angeles

Department of Psychology
405 Hilgard Avenue
Los Angeles, CA 90095-1563
phone#: (310) 825-2617
e-mail: gradadm@psych.ucla.edu
Web address:
http://www.psych.ucla.edu/Grads/Areas/clinical.php

1	2	3	4	5	6	**7**

Clinically oriented　　Equal emphasis　　Research oriented

What percentage of your faculty subscribes to or practices in each of the following orientations?
Psychodynamic/Psychoanalytic　　　　　　　　0%
Applied behavioral analysis/Radical behavioral　0%
Family systems/Systems　　　　　　　　　　25%
Existential/Phenomenological/Humanistic　　　0%
Cognitive/Cognitive-behavioral　　　　　　　75%

What percentage of students applying for internship last year was accepted into APPIC-member internships?
Data not available

What courses are required for incoming students to have completed prior to enrolling?
Elementary statistics; two of the following: learning, physiological, or perception/information processing; two of the following: developmental, social, or personality/abnormal; one course in biology or zoology; two physical science courses (physics and/or chemistry) although a course in anthropology, philosophy, or sociology may be substituted for one of the physical science courses; at least one math course, preferably calculus or probability; advanced statistics

Are there courses you recommend that are not mandatory?
Research design and methods, psychology research labs, independent research courses; a broad background in the mathematical, biological and social sciences

GRE mean
Verbal 670　Quantitative 710
Analytical Writing 5.5　Advanced Psychology 725

GPA mean
Overall GPA 3.87

Number of applications/admission offers/incoming students in 2005
359 applied/19 admission offers/11 incoming

% of students receiving:
Tuition waiver only: 0%
Assistantship/fellowship only: 0%
Both tuition waiver & assistantship/fellowship: 80%–90%

Approximate percentage of incoming students who entered with a B.A./B.S. only: 99% **Master's:** 1%

Approximate percentage of students who are Women: 100% **Ethnic Minority:** 45% **International:** Data not available

Average years to complete the doctoral program (including internship): 6.2 years

Personal interview
Preferred in person but telephone acceptable

Research areas	# Faculty	# Grants
anxiety disorders and treatment	1	3
family issues	3	3
marital and couple relationships and treatments	2	2
medical issues	3	4
minority mental and physical health issues	3	3
mood disorders	1	1
schizophrenia	2	4
school mental health	1	1

Clinical opportunities
adoptions, families
child and adult affective disorders
child and adult anxiety disorders
community psychology, community mental health
couples/marital
developmental disabilities/autism
family/child
major mental illness, psychosis
minority populations
psychotherapy supervision
school mental health

Carlos Albizu University–Miami Campus (Psy.D.)

2173 NW 99th Avenue
Miami, FL 33172-2209
phone#: (305) 593-1223, ext. 129
e-mail: croca@albizu.edu
Web address:
http://mia.albizu.edu/web/academic_programs/psychology
/doctor_of_psychology_in_clinical_psychology.asp

1	2	3	4	5	6	7
Clinically oriented		Equal emphasis			Research oriented	

What percentage of your faculty subscribes to or practices in each of the following orientations?
Psychodynamic/Psychoanalytic 20%
Applied behavioral analysis/Radical behavioral 0%
Family systems/Systems 10%

Existential/Phenomenological/Humanistic 20%
Cognitive/Cognitive-behavioral 50%

What percentage of students applying for internship last year was accepted into APPIC-member internships?
Data not available

What courses are required for incoming students to have completed prior to enrolling?
Physiological psychology, research methodology, developmental psychology, abnormal psychology, statistics, theories of personality.

Are there courses you recommend that are not mandatory?
No.

GRE mean
Verbal 450 Quantitative 500 Analytical 570
Psychology Advanced Test 550
Analytical Writing Data not available

GPA mean
Data not available

Number of applications/admission offers/incoming students in 2003
44 applied/26 admission offers/26 incoming

% of students receiving:
Tuition waiver only: 0%
Assistantship/fellowship only: 5%
Both tuition waiver & assistantship/fellowship: 0%

Approximate percentage of incoming students who entered with a B.A./B.S. only: 40% **Master's:** 60%

Approximate percentage of students who are Women: 72% **Ethnic Minority:** 56% **International:** Data not available

Average years to complete the doctoral program (including internship): 4.9 years

Personal interview
Preferred in person but telephone acceptable

Research areas	# Faculty	# Grants
children and adolescents	3	0
depression	3	0
elderly	1	0
forensic psychology	1	0
multicultural issues	6	0
neuropsychology	2	0
positive psychology	1	0
psychotherapy	6	0

Clinical opportunities
In-house training clinic where students work with multiethnic populations of various ages, including children.

Carlos Albizu University–San Juan Campus (Ph.D.)

P.O. Box 9023711
San Juan, PR 00902-3711
phone#: (787) 725-6500, ext. 127
e-mail: escardalda@albizu.edu
Web address: http://sju.albizu.edu/student/
stuAcadConc.asp?cboConc=23

1	2	3	**4**	5	6	7
Clinically oriented		Equal emphasis			Research oriented	

What percentage of your faculty subscribes to or practices in each of the following orientations?

Psychodynamic/Psychoanalytic	10%
Applied behavioral analysis/Radical behavioral	10%
Family systems/Systems	10%
Existential/Phenomenological/Humanistic	10%
Cognitive/Cognitive-behavioral	10%

What percentage of students applying for internship last year was accepted into APPIC-member internships?
Data not available

What courses are required for incoming students to have completed prior to enrolling?
Experimental psychology and laboratory, physiological psychology and laboratory, abnormal psychology, introductory statistics, personality theories

Are there courses you recommend that are not mandatory?
—

GRE mean
Data not available

GPA mean
Data not available

Number of applications/admission offers/incoming students in 2005
23 applied/19 admission offers/19 incoming

% of students receiving:
Tuition waiver only: 0%
Assistantship/fellowship only: 9%
Both tuition waiver & assistantship/fellowship: 0%

Approximate percentage of incoming students who entered with a B.A./B.S. only: 100%   **Master's:** 0%

Approximate percentage of students who are Women: 79%   **Ethnic Minority:** 100%
International: Data not available

Average years to complete the doctoral program (including internship): 7 years

Personal interview
Required in person

Research areas	# Faculty	# Grants
attention-deficit disorder	1	1
elderly	1	1
high risk children/adolescents	3	1
impulsion-aggressive children	1	3
social skills	1	1

Clinical opportunities
COF Program
Domestic Violence Program
PAF Program
PAS Program

Carlos Albizu University–San Juan Campus (Psy.D.)

San Juan, PR 00902-3711
phone#: (787) 725-6500, ext. 52
e-mail: galtieri@prip.edu
Web address: http://sju.albizu.edu/student/
stuAcadConc.asp?cboConc=22

1	2	**3**	4	5	6	7
Clinically oriented		Equal emphasis			Research oriented	

What percentage of your faculty subscribes to or practices in each of the following orientations?

Psychodynamic/Psychoanalytic	10%
Applied behavioral analysis/Radical behavioral	10%
Family systems/Systems	30%
Existential/Phenomenological/Humanistic	10%
Cognitive/Cognitive-behavioral	40%

What percentage of students applying for internship last year was accepted into APPIC-member internships?
Data not available

What courses are required for incoming students to have completed prior to enrolling?
Experimental psychology and laboratory, physiological psychology and laboratory, abnormal psychology, introductory statistics, personality theories

Are there courses you recommend that are not mandatory?
—

GRE mean
Data not available

GPA mean
Data not available

Number of applications/admission offers/incoming students in 2005
103 applied/91 admission offers/81 incoming

% of students receiving:
Tuition waiver only: 0%
Assistantship/fellowship only: 0%
Both tuition waiver & assistantship/fellowship: 0%

Approximate percentage of incoming students who entered with a B.A./B.S. only: 90%   **Master's:** 10%

Approximate percentage of students who are Women: 83%   **Ethnic Minority:** 99%
International: Data not available

147

Average years to complete the doctoral program (including internship): 6.5 years

Personal interview
Required in person

Research areas	# Faculty	# Grants
health and well-being in elderly	2	0
sexual behavior	2	0
sport anxiety	2	0

Clinical opportunities
domestic violence
forensic psychology
program for sexual abuse victims
sex abuse therapy for children victims of abuse and their families
sexual disorders
sports psychology
victims of crime

Case Western Reserve University

Department of Psychology
Mather Memorial Building
11220 Bellflower Road
Cleveland, OH 44106
phone#: (216) 368-2686
e-mail: psychdept@cwru.edu
Web address:
http://www.case.edu/artsci/pscl/clinical.htm

1	2	3	**4**	5	6	7

Clinically oriented　　Equal emphasis　　Research oriented

What percentage of your faculty subscribes to or practices in each of the following orientations?

Psychodynamic/Psychoanalytic	50%
Applied behavioral analysis/Radical behavioral	0%
Family systems/Systems	25%
Existential/Phenomenological/Humanistic	0%
Cognitive/Cognitive-behavioral	50%

What percentage of students applying for internship last year was accepted into APPIC-member internships? Data not available

What courses are required for incoming students to have completed prior to enrolling?
Statistics, undergraduate psychology courses

Are there courses you recommend that are not mandatory?
Psychology major

GRE mean
Verbal + Quantitative 1200

GPA mean
Overall GPA 3.0

Number of applications/admission offers/incoming students in 2005
155 applied/9 admission offers/7 incoming

% of students receiving:
Tuition waiver only: 43%
Assistantship/fellowship only: 0%
Both tuition waiver & assistantship/fellowship: 57%

Approximate percentage of incoming students who entered with a B.A./B.S. only: 95%　**Master's:** 5%

Approximate percentage of students who are Women: 75%　**Ethnic Minority:** 16%
International: Data not available

Average years to complete the doctoral program (including internship): 6 years

Personal interview
Preferred in person but telephone acceptable

Research areas	# Faculty	# Grants
aging	2	1
behavioral medicine/ health psychology	1	0
chronic mental illness	1	0
developmental disabilities	1	1
learning disabilities	1	0
memory	2	0
parent–child interaction	2	0
personality disorders	1	0
self-psychology	1	0
temperament	1	1

Clinical opportunities
ADHD
affective disorders
aging and dementia
anxiety disorders
gerontology/Alzheimer's
juvenile bipolar disorder
obsessive–compulsive disorders
personality disorders
schizophrenia/psychosis

Catholic University of America

Department of Psychology
620 Michigan Avenue, NE
Washington, DC 20064
phone#: (202) 319-5729
e-mail: cua-psychology@cua.edu
Web address:
http://psychology.cua.edu/graduate/phdclprog.cfm

1	2	3	**4**	5	6	7

Clinically oriented　　Equal emphasis　　Research oriented

What percentage of your faculty subscribes to or practices in each of the following orientations?

Psychodynamic/Psychoanalytic	50%
Applied behavioral analysis/Radical behavioral	25%
Family systems/Systems	50%
Existential/Phenomenological/Humanistic	75%
Cognitive/Cognitive-behavioral	85%

What percentage of students applying for internship last year was accepted into APPIC-member internships? 100%

What courses are required for incoming students to have completed prior to enrolling?
Introductory psychology, statistics, research methods

Are there courses you recommend that are not mandatory?
Research experience in psychology; abnormal psychology; personality; developmental psychology; social psychology

GRE mean
Verbal 622   Quantitative 688
Advanced Psychology 667
Analytical Writing 5.31

GPA mean
Overall GPA 3.57

Number of applications/admission offers/incoming students in 2005
136 applied/15 admission offers/7 incoming

% of students receiving:
Tuition waiver only: 29%
Assistantship/fellowship only: 6%
Both tuition waiver & assistantship/fellowship: 65%

Approximate percentage of incoming students who entered with a B.A./B.S. only: 84%   **Master's:** 16%

Approximate percentage of students who are Women: 81%   **Ethnic Minority:** 19%   **International:** 5%

Average years to complete the doctoral program (including internship): 6.6 years

Personal interview
Required in person

Research areas	# Faculty	# Grants
adolescence	3	1
adult psychopathology	3	0
anxiety	1	0
anxiety disorders	2	0
assessment	2	0
attachment	2	0
child clinical	4	1
clinical training	1	0
cognition	3	0
community context	1	1
couples	1	1
developmental	4	1
developmental psychopathology	4	1
emotions	2	0
emotion regulation	1	0
family	2	1
interpersonal processes	2	0
language development	1	0
mood disorders	2	0
parent–child interactions	2	0
psychotherapy integration	2	0
psychotherapy outcome	3	0
psychotherapy practice	3	0
psychotherapy process	3	0
self-efficacy	1	0
social anxiety	2	0
sport psychology	1	0
stress and coping	3	1
suicide	2	0
violence	1	1

Clinical opportunities
adult psychotherapy
assessment batteries
child and adult assessment
couples therapy
family therapy
group therapy
minority mental health
neuropsychology

University of Central Florida Clinical Psychology (Ph.D.)

4000 Central Florida Blvd, Howard Phillips Hall, Room 302
Orlando, Florida, 32816-1390
phone#: (407) 823-4344
e-mail: psyinfo@mail.ucf.edu
Web address: http://www.cas.ucf.edu/psychology/ graduate_degrees_clinicalphd.php

1	2	3	4	5	6	7

Clinically oriented   Equal emphasis   Research oriented

What percentage of your faculty subscribes to or practices in each of the following orientations?
Data not available

What percentage of students applying for internship last year was accepted into APPIC-member internships?
Data not available

What courses are required for incoming students to have completed prior to enrolling?
If not coming from a psychology background, a minium of 15 semester hours of undergraduate psychology courses is required prior to matriculation.

Are there courses you recommend that are not mandatory?
Research experience is heavily weighted during admissions.

GRE mean
Quantitative 666   Verbal 566
Psychology Advanced Test N/A   Analytical Writing N/A

GPA mean
Overall GPA 3.63

Number of applications/admission offers/incoming students in 2005
120 applied/10 admission offers/6 incoming

REPORTS ON INDIVIDUAL CLINICAL PSYCHOLOGY PROGRAMS

% of students receiving:
Tuition waiver only: 0%
Assistantship/fellowship only: 0%
Both tuition waiver & assistantship/fellowship: 86%

Approximate percentage of incoming students who entered with a B.A./B.S. only: 100%   **Master's:** 0%

Approximate percentage of students who are Women: 81%   **Ethnic Minority:** 16%   **International:** 1%

Average years to complete the doctoral program (including internship): 5 years

Personal interview
Required in person

Research areas	# Faculty	# Grants
alcohol and substance abuse	1	
child/pediatric psychology	1	
developmental psychopathology	2	
eating behavior and body image	2	
multicultural	1	
personality testing	1	
prevention	1	
schizophrenia	1	

Clinical opportunities
children's learning
clinical neuroscience
eating, appearance, & health
family
substance use

Central Michigan University

Department of Psychology
Mt. Pleasant, MI 48859
phone#: (989) 774-6463
e-mail: Reid.Skeel@cmich.edu
Web address:
http://www.chsbs.cmich.edu/Clinical%5FPsychology/

1	2	3	**4**	5	6	7

Clinically oriented   Equal emphasis   Research oriented

What percentage of your faculty subscribes to or practices in each of the following orientations?
Psychodynamic/Psychoanalytic   10%
Applied behavioral analysis/Radical behavioral   10%
Family systems/Systems   25%
Existential/Phenomenological/Humanistic   10%
Cognitive/Cognitive-behavioral   70%

What percentage of students applying for internship last year was accepted into APPIC-member internships? 100%

What courses are required for incoming students to have completed prior to enrolling?
None

Are there courses you recommend that are not mandatory?
Statistics, experimental psychology, developmental

psychology, abnormal psychology, personality theory, measurement theory

GRE mean
Verbal 611   Quantitative 741
Analytical Writing 4.7

GPA mean
Overall GPA 3.53   Psychology GPA 3.68

Number of applications/admission offers/incoming students in 2005
101 applied/15 admission offers/7 incoming

% of students receiving:
Tuition waiver only: 0%
Assistantship/fellowship only: 0%
Both tuition waiver & assistantship/fellowship: 100%

Approximate percentage of incoming students who entered with a B.A./B.S. only: 100%   **Master's:** 0%

Approximate percentage of students who are Women: 57%   **Ethnic Minority:** 10%   **International:** 13%

Average years to complete the doctoral program (including internship): 6 years

Personal interview
Interview not required

Research areas	# Faculty	# Grants
anxiety disorders	1	1
assessment	1	0
children	1	2
diversity and sexual deviance	1	0
health psychology	1	1
neuropsychology	1	1
severe psychopathology	1	1
violence and agression	1	0

Clinical opportunities
adult clinical
behavior therapy
child clinical
cognitive-behavioral therapy
forensic psychology
neuropsychology/rehabilitation
parent–child interaction therapy
psychodynamic therapy
psychological assessment
school-based interventions

Chicago School of Professional Psychology (Psy.D.)

47 West Polk
Chicago, IL 60605
phone#: (312) 786-9443
e-mail: admissions@csopp.edu
Web address: http://www.csopp.edu/abouttheschool/
default.asp?pagename=clinicalpsyd

1	**2**	3	4	5	6	7

Clinically oriented   Equal emphasis   Research oriented

What percentage of your faculty subscribes to or practices in each of the following orientations?

Psychodynamic/Psychoanalytic	30%
Applied behavioral analysis/Radical behavioral	10%
Family systems/Systems	20%
Existential/Phenomenological/Humanistic	15%
Cognitive/Cognitive-behavioral	25%

What percentage of students applying for internship last year was accepted into APPIC-member internships?
Data not available

What courses are required for incoming students to have completed prior to enrolling?
18 hours in psychology, including statistics, theories of personality, abnormal psychology

Are there courses you recommend that are not mandatory?
No

GRE mean
Verbal + Quantitative 1015
Analytical Writing Data not available

GPA mean
Overall GPA 3.35

Number of applications/admission offers/incoming students in 2005
353 applied/217 admission offers/83 incoming

% of students receiving:
Tuition waiver only: 9%
Assistantship/fellowship only: 21%
Both tuition waiver & assistantship/fellowship: 28%

Approximate percentage of incoming students who entered with a B.A./B.S. only: 61%   **Master's:** 39%

Approximate percentage of students who are Women: 69%   **Ethnic Minority:** 20%
International: Data not available

Average years to complete the doctoral program (including internship): 5.8 years

Personal interview
Preferred in person but telephone acceptable

Research areas	# Faculty	# Grants
behavioral intervention	1	0
diversity and cultural competence training	5	1
forensic psychology	3	0
Latino early education	2	1
multigenerational health	2	0
pediatric obesity	2	0
trauma	2	0

Clinical opportunities
child and adolescent
college counseling center
community mental health
community psychology
correctional/forensic settings
creative and expressive arts
cross-cultural/international

early education/head start/infants
forensic
health
inner city and rural populations
inpatient/outpatient/partial hospitalization
mental health administration
multicultural
organizational
private and group practice
school based intervention
sexual orientation and gender identity
teaching
veterans

University of Cincinnati
Department of Psychology
429 Dyer Hall
Cincinnati, OH 45221-0376
phone#: (513) 556-5580
e-mail: Paula.Shear@uc.edu
Web address:
http://asweb.artsci.uc.edu/psychology/grad/clinical.cfm

1	2	3	4	5	**6**	7
Clinically oriented		Equal emphasis			Research oriented	

What percentage of your faculty subscribes to or practices in each of the following orientations?

Psychodynamic/Psychoanalytic	20%
Applied behavioral analysis/Radical behavioral	10%
Family systems/Systems	5%
Existential/Phenomenological/Humanistic	10%
Cognitive/Cognitive-behavioral	55%

What percentage of students applying for internship last year was accepted into APPIC-member internships? 100%

What courses are required for incoming students to have completed prior to enrolling?
Preference given to applicants with coursework in psychology

Are there courses you recommend that are not mandatory?
Abnormal psychology, statistics and research methods

GRE mean
Verbal 547   Quantitative 629
Analytical Writing 5.4
Advanced Psychology (optional) 637

GPA mean
Overall GPA 3.6

Number of applications/admission offers/incoming students in 2005
236 applied/16 admission offers/10 incoming

% of students receiving:
Tuition waiver only: 0%
Assistantship/fellowship only: 0%
Both tuition waiver & assistantship/fellowship: 100%

Approximate percentage of incoming students who entered with a B.A./B.S. only: 90%   **Master's:** 10%

Approximate percentage of students who are Women: 75%   **Ethnic Minority:** 25%
International: Data not available

Average years to complete the doctoral program (including internship): 6 years

Personal interview
Preferred in person but telephone acceptable

Research areas	# Faculty	# Grants
addictive behaviors	5	2
adolescence	2	1
adult development	1	1
child clinical	3	2
domestic abuse	2	1
health psychology	5	2
homelessness	2	1
neuropsychology	5	2
serious mental illness	3	2

Clinical opportunities
addictive behaviors
child clinical psychology
clinical neuropsychology
community mental health
developmental disorders
health psychology
serious mental illness
university counseling center

City University of New York at City College

Department of Psychology
138th Street and Covenant Avenue
New York, NY 10031
phone#: (212) 650-5672/5674
e-mail: sbtuber@hotmail.com
Web address:
http://web.gc.cuny.edu/Psychology/clinical/index.html

1	2	**3**	4	5	6	7

Clinically oriented   Equal emphasis   Research oriented

What percentage of your faculty subscribes to or practices in each of the following orientations?

Psychodynamic/Psychoanalytic	60%
Applied behavioral analysis/Radical behavioral	0%
Family systems/Systems	30%
Existential/Phenomenological/Humanistic	10%
Cognitive/Cognitive-behavioral	20%

What percentage of students applying for internship last year was accepted into APPIC-member internships? 100%

What courses are required for incoming students to have completed prior to enrolling?
Experimental, statistics

Are there courses you recommend that are not mandatory?
Abnormal, developmental

GRE mean
Verbal 650   Quantitative 600 Analytic 600
Advanced Psychology 600
Analytical Writing Data not available

GPA mean
Overall GPA 3.7   Psychology GPA 3.8
Junior/Senior GPA 3.8

Number of applications/admission offers/incoming students in 2005
275 applied/14 admission offers/12 incoming

% of students receiving:
Tuition waiver only: 10%
Assistantship/fellowship only: 20%
Both tuition waiver & assistantship/fellowship: 35%

Approximate percentage of incoming students who entered with a B.A./B.S. only: 80%   **Master's:** 20%

Approximate percentage of students who are Women: 65%   **Ethnic Minority:** 40%   **International:** 20%

Average years to complete the doctoral program (including internship): 6.5 years

Personal interview
Preferred in person but telephone acceptable (if student is out of country)

Research areas	# Faculty	# Grants
African American adolescents	1	0
attachment	3	1
object relations	4	1
social policies in mental health	1	0
racism	1	0
psychotherapy outcome	3	0

Clinical opportunities
adult clinic
child clinic
family clinic

Clark University

Frances L. Hiatt School of Psychology
950 Main Street
Worcester, MA 01610
phone#: (508) 793-7269
e-mail: maddis@clarku.edu
Web address: http://www.clarku.edu/departments/
psychology/grad/clinical.shtml

1	2	3	4	**5**	6	7

Clinically oriented   Equal emphasis   Research oriented

What percentage of your faculty subscribes to or practices in each of the following orientations?

Psychodynamic/Psychoanalytic	40%
Applied behavioral analysis/Radical behavioral	40%
Family systems/Systems	40%
Existential/Phenomenological/Humanistic	0%
Cognitive/Cognitive-behavioral	60%

What percentage of students applying for internship last year was accepted into APPIC-member internships?
Data not available

What courses are required for incoming students to have completed prior to enrolling?
Statistics, research design, abnormal psychology

Are there courses you recommend that are not mandatory?
Psychology major, substantial research experience

GRE mean
Verbal 640   Quantitative 680
Advanced Psychology 680

GPA mean
Overall GPA 3.5

Number of applications/admission offers/incoming students in 2005
135 applied/9 admission offers/4 incoming

% of students receiving:
Tuition waiver only: 0%
Assistantship/fellowship only: 0%
Both tuition waiver & assistantship/fellowship: 100%

Approximate percentage of incoming students who entered with a B.A./B.S. only: 75%   **Master's:** 25%

Approximate percentage of students who are Women: 75%   **Ethnic Minority:** 25%
International: Data not available

Average years to complete the doctoral program (including internship): 7 years

Personal interview
Required in person

Research areas	# Faculty	# Grants
adult psychopathology	2	1
affective disorders	1	1
assessment/diagnosis/classification	1	0
child abuse and children at-risk	1	1
child clinical/child psychopathology	2	1
family research/therapy	3	2
gender roles/sex differences	1	0
motivation	1	1
parent–child interaction	3	1
personality disorders	1	0
prevention	3	0
psychotherapy process and outcome	1	0
social learning	1	0

Clinical opportunities
child therapy/assessment
couples/family therapy
preventive interventions
school-based interventions

University of Colorado
Department of Psychology
UCB 345
Muenzinger 244, Campus Box 345
Boulder, CO 80309-0345
phone#: (303) 492-8805
Web address: http://psych.colorado.edu/~clinical/

1	2	3	4	5	**6**	7
Clinically oriented		Equal emphasis			Research oriented	

What percentage of your faculty subscribes to or practices in each of the following orientations?

Psychodynamic/Psychoanalytic	10%
Applied behavioral analysis/Radical behavioral	10%
Family systems/Systems	10%
Existential/Phenomenological/Humanistic	0%
Cognitive/Cognitive-behavioral	90%

What percentage of students applying for internship last year was accepted into APPIC-member internships? 100%

What courses are required for incoming students to have completed prior to enrolling?
Psychology or the equivalent (30 semester hours in psychology)

Are there courses you recommend that are not mandatory?
Psychological assessment, psychopathology, psychotherapy, research methods, statistics, developmental psychology, social psychology/personality, biological psychology

GRE mean
Verbal 664   Quantitative 726
Psychology Subject 726
Analytical Writing 5.125

GPA mean
Overall GPA 3.2

Number of applications/admission offers/incoming students in 2004
135 applied/8 admission offers/5 incoming

% of students receiving:
Tuition waiver only: 0%
Assistantship/fellowship only: 0%
Both tuition waiver & assistantship/fellowship: 100%

Approximate percentage of incoming students who entered with a B.A./B.S. only: 66%   **Master's:** 33%

Approximate percentage of students who are Women: 80%   **Ethnic Minority:** 20%   **International:** 7%

Average years to complete the doctoral program (including internship): 5.5 years

Personal interview
Required in person

Research areas	# Faculty	# Grants
adult psychopathology	4	2
affective disorders	3	2
assessment/diagnosis/classification	2	2
child clinical	3	2

developmental	2	2
eating disorders	1	0
family research	1	1
genetics	1	1
marriage/couples	1	0
personality disorders	1	0
prevention	3	1
psychotherapy outcome/process	4	2
substance abuse	1	1
violence/abuse	1	0

Clinical opportunities
assessment
behavior therapy
cognitive therapy
family therapy
group therapy
interpersonal treatment
marital therapy
psychodynamic psychotherapy
substance abuse

Columbia University–Teachers College

Clinical Psychology Program
525 West 120th Street
New York, NY 10027
phone#: (212) 678-3267
fax#: (212) 678-4048
e-mail: tcinfo@www.tc.columbia.edu
Web address: http://www.tc.columbia.edu/academic/
ccp/clinical/degree.asp?id=Degree+Description%3A+
Doctor+of+Philosophy

1	2	3	**4**	5	6	7

Clinically oriented   Equal emphasis   Research oriented

What percentage of your faculty subscribes to or practices in each of the following orientations?

Psychodynamic/Psychoanalytic	60%
Applied behavioral analysis/Radical behavioral	0%
Family systems/Systems	0%
Existential/Phenomenological/Humanistic	0%
Cognitive/Cognitive-behavioral	40%

What percentage of students applying for internship last year was accepted into APPIC-member internships? 100%

What courses are required for incoming students to have completed prior to enrolling?
Statistics and 9 credits from among: experimental psychology, personality, history and systems, developmental psychology, or social psychology

Are there courses you recommend that are not mandatory?
Abnormal psychology

GRE mean
Verbal 610   Quantitative 630
Advanced Psychology 720
Analytical Writing Data not available

GPA mean
Overall GPA 3.7

Number of applications/admission offers/incoming students in 2003
303 applied/15 admission offers/10 incoming

% of students receiving:
Tuition waiver only: 87.5% (partial)
Assistantship/fellowship only: 0%
Both tuition waiver & assistantship/fellowship: 10%

Approximate percentage of incoming students who entered with a B.A./B.S. only: 25%   **Master's:** 75%

Approximate percentage of students who are Women: 70%   **Ethnic Minority:** 12.5%   **International:** 20%

Average years to complete the doctoral program (including internship): 7 years

Personal interview
Required in person

Research areas	# Faculty	# Grants
altruism	1	0
child abuse	1	1
geriatrics	1	1
psychotherapy research	3	2
risk and resilience	2	2
spirituality	1	1
trauma, stress and coping	2	2

Clinical opportunities
child therapy
psychodynamic/psychoanalytic therapy

Concordia University

Department of Psychology, PY 119-2
7141 Sherbrooke Street West
Montreal, Quebec H4B 1R6 Canada
phone#: (514) 848-2424 ext. 2205
e-mail: black@vax2.concordia.ca
Web address: http://psychology.concordia.ca/Grads/
admissionsPhD.html

1	2	3	4	**5**	6	7

Clinically oriented   Equal emphasis   Research oriented

What percentage of your faculty subscribes to or practices in each of the following orientations?

Psychodynamic/Psychoanalytic	15%
Applied behavioral analysis/Radical behavioral	0%
Family systems/Systems	25%
Existential/Phenomenological/Humanistic	0%
Cognitive/Cognitive-behavioral	60%

What percentage of students applying for internship last year was accepted into APPIC-member internships? Data not available

What courses are required for incoming students to have completed prior to enrolling?
Honors (B.A./B.Sc.) in psychology

Are there courses you recommend that are not mandatory?
No

GRE mean
Verbal 575   Quantitative 555
Advanced Psychology 710
Note: GRE's are recommended, but optional

GPA mean
Overall GPA 3.5
Note: Based on Concordia's scale of 4.3

Number of applications/admission offers/incoming students in 2003
128 applied/14 admission offers/9 incoming

% of students receiving:
Tuition waiver only: 0%
Assistantship/fellowship only: 78%
Both tuition waiver & assistantship/fellowship: 22%

Approximate percentage of incoming students who entered with a B.A./B.S. only: 89%   **Master's:** 11%

Approximate percentage of students who are Women: 89%   **Ethnic Minority:** 22%   **International:** Data not available

Personal interview
Preferred in person but telephone acceptable

Research areas	# Faculty	# Grants
anxiety	2	3
behavioral medicine	1	1
developmental/infancy	8	10
developmental psychopathology	3	5
gender roles	2	1
health psychology	1	0
major mental disorder/psychopathology	2	1
neuropsychology	2	5
neuroscience/psychobiology	9	12
perception/cognition	4	5
social competence	1	1

Clinical opportunities
adult
child/adolescent
cognitive/cognitive-behavioral
couples
family
psychodynamic

University of Connecticut
Department of Psychology
U-1020, Babbidge Road
Storrs, CT 06269-1020
phone#: (860) 486-3528 (Admissions information)
e-mail: psychadm@uconnvm.uconn.edu
Web address: http://web.uconn.edu/psychology/

1	2	3	4	**5**	6	7
Clinically oriented		Equal emphasis			Research oriented	

What percentage of your faculty subscribes to or practices in each of the following orientations?

Psychodynamic/Psychoanalytic	8%
Applied behavioral analysis/Radical behavioral	17%
Family systems/Systems	33%
Existential/Phenomenological/Humanistic	0%
Cognitive-behavioral	90%

What percentage of students applying for internship last year was accepted into APPIC-member internships? 100%

What courses are required for incoming students to have completed prior to enrolling?
None

Are there courses you recommend that are not mandatory?
abnormal psychology, research methods

GRE mean
Verbal 601   Quantitative 657   Analytical 605
Analytical Writing 4.9   Advanced Psychology 669

GPA mean
Overall GPA 3.50

Number of applications/admission offers/incoming students in 2005
302 applied/11 admission offers/10 incoming

% of students receiving:
Tuition waiver only: 0%
Assistantship/fellowship only: 0%
Both tuition waiver & assistantship/fellowship: 100%

Approximate percentage of incoming students who entered with a B.A./B.S. only: 60%   **Master's:** 40%

Approximate percentage of students who are Women: 75%   **Ethnic Minority:** 22%   **International:** 6%

Average years to complete the doctoral program (including internship): 5.65 years

Personal interview
Preferred in person but telephone acceptable

Research areas	# Faculty	# Grants
adult psychopathology	5	1
aging	1	0
anxiety disorders	1	0
autism	2	3
child psychopathology	6	2
developmental psychopathology	3	1
domestic violence	2	0
health psychology	3	2
multicultural psychology	2	1
neuropsychological assessment	3	1
trauma	3	0

Clinical opportunities
autistic children
childhood psychopathology
chronic mental health
corporate stress management
health psychology
multicultural psychology
neuroimaging
neuropsychological assessment

155

traumatic brain injury
traumatic stress disorders

Dalhousie University

Department of Psychology
Halifax, Nova Scotia B3H 4J1 Canada
phone #: (902) 494-1580
e-mail: beatrice@dal.ca
Web address:
http://psychology.dal.ca/PsychWeb/grad.html

1	2	3	4	**5**	6	7

Clinically oriented   Equal emphasis   Research oriented

What percentage of your faculty subscribes to or practices in each of the following orientations?

Psychodynamic/Psychoanalytic	10%
Applied behavioral analysis/Radical behavioral	10%
Family systems/Systems	10%
Existential/Phenomenological/Humanistic	0%
Cognitive/Cognitive-behavioral	100%

What percentage of students applying for internship last year was accepted into APPIC-member internships? 100%

What courses are required for incoming students to have completed prior to enrolling?
An honors degree in psychology

Are there courses you recommend that are not mandatory?
—

GRE mean
Verbal 680   Quantitative 670

GPA mean
Overall GPA 4.3

Number of applications/admission offers/incoming students in 2005
100 applied/11 admission offers/7 incoming

% of students receiving:
Tuition waiver only: 0%
Assistantship/fellowship only: 100%
Both tuition waiver & assistantship/fellowship: 0%

Approximate percentage of incoming students who entered with a B.A./B.S. only: 72%   **Master's:** 28%

Approximate percentage of students who are Women: 84%   **Ethnic Minority:** Not reported
International: 7%

Average years to complete the doctoral program (including internship): 6.5 years

Personal interview
Interview not required

Research areas	# Faculty	# Grants
addictions	1	10
adolescent mental health	1	1

anxiety	2	6
depression	2	5
disruptive behavior	2	3
forensic psychology	1	3
neuropsychology	1	3
pain in children	2	9
peer relationships	2	4
psychometrics	1	1
sleep in children	1	1

Clinical opportunities
Extensive range of practicum opportunities available from core faculty and in local agencies/hospitals.

University of Delaware

Department of Psychology
Newark, DE 19716
phone#: (302) 831-2271
e-mail: rkobak@udel.edu
Web address:
http://w3.psych.udel.edu/graduate/clinical/index.asp

1	2	3	4	5	**6**	7

Clinically oriented   Equal emphasis   Research oriented

What percentage of your faculty subscribes to or practices in each of the following orientations?

Psychodynamic/Psychoanalytic	12.5%
Applied behavioral analysis/Radical behavioral	12.5%
Family systems/Systems	12.5%
Existential/Phenomenological/Humanistic	12.5%
Cognitive/Cognitive-behavioral	75%

What percentage of students applying for internship last year was accepted into APPIC-member internships?
Data not available

What courses are required for incoming students to have completed prior to enrolling?
None

Are there courses you recommend that are not mandatory?
Statistics, biopsychology, abnormal psychology, history and systems, cognitive, developmental

GRE mean
Verbal 660   Quantitative 710
Analytical Writing Data not available

GPA mean
Overall GPA 3.6

Number of applications/admission offers/incoming students in 2005
145 applied/8 admission offers/7 incoming

% of students receiving:
Tuition waiver only: 0%
Assistantship/fellowship only: 0%
Both tuition waiver & assistantship/fellowship: 100%

Approximate percentage of incoming students who entered with a B.A./B.S. only: 90% **Master's:** 10%

Approximate percentage of students who are Women: 75% **Ethnic Minority:** 10% **International:** Data not available

Average years to complete the doctoral program (including internship): 5 years

Personal interview
Required in person

Research areas	# Faculty	# Grants
anxiety, stress, and coping	2	1
attachment theory	2	2
child clinical	4	5
developmental risk for pathology	4	4
emotions	4	1
foster care	1	2
personality	2	1
psychophysiology	3	1
psychotherapy	1	1

Clinical opportunities
anxiety disorders
child assessment
conduct disorder
developmental disabilities/autism
family therapy
neuropsychology/rehabilitation
pediatric
sexual assault/abuse

University of Denver (Ph.D.)

Department of Psychology
University Park
Denver, CO 80210
phone#: (303) 871-3803
e-mail: phoughta@nova.psy.du.edu
Web address: http://www.du.edu/psychology/research/child_clinical.htm

1	2	3	4	5	**6**	7

Clinically oriented   Equal emphasis   Research oriented

What percentage of your faculty subscribes to or practices in each of the following orientations?

Psychodynamic/Psychoanalytic	16%
Applied behavioral analysis/Radical behavioral	0%
Family systems/Systems	67%
Existential/Phenomenological/Humanistic	0%
Cognitive/Cognitive-behavioral	67%

What percentage of students applying for internship last year was accepted into APPIC-member internships? 100%

What courses are required for incoming students to have completed prior to enrolling?
None

Are there courses you recommend that are not mandatory?
Statistics

GRE mean
Verbal + Quantitative 1325
Analytical Writing Data not available

GPA mean
Overall GPA 3.7

Number of applications/admission offers in 2005
183 applied/13 admission offers

% of students receiving:
Tuition waiver only: 0%
Assistantship/fellowship only: 0%
Both tuition waiver & assistantship/fellowship: 100%

Approximate percentage of incoming students who entered with a B.A./B.S. only: 90% **Master's:** 10%

Approximate percentage of students who are Women: 75% **Ethnic Minority:** 33% **International:** 7%

Average years to complete the doctoral program (including internship): 6.5 years

Personal interview
Preferred in person but telephone acceptable

Research areas	# Faculty	# Grants
adolescent psychopathology	3	1
behavioral genetics	1	1
child psychopathology	1	2
close relationships	2	2
community	1	1
developmental disabilities	1	2
family	3	1
marital	1	1
multicultural	3	0
neuropsychology	1	1
poverty	1	0
prevention	1	1
psychotherapy	1	1
sexual abuse	1	0
trauma	3	1

Clinical opportunities
developmental disorders
family
inpatient adolescents
marital/couples
minority/cross-cultural
neuropsychology
pediatrics

University of Denver (Psy.D.)

Graduate School of Professional Psychology
2450 South Vine Street
Denver, CO 80208-0208
phone#: (303) 871-3873
e-mail: gsppinfo@du.edu
Web address: http://www.du.edu/gspp

	1	**2**	3	4	5	6	7	
Clinically oriented			Equal emphasis			Research oriented		

What percentage of your faculty subscribes to or practices in each of the following orientations?

Psychodynamic/Psychoanalytic	40%
Applied behavioral analysis/Radical behavioral	20%
Family systems/Systems	20%
Existential/Phenomenological/Humanistic	10%
Cognitive/Cognitive-behavioral	10%

What percentage of students applying for internship last year was accepted into APPIC-member internships? 90%

What courses are required for incoming students to have completed prior to enrolling?
Statistics, learning theory, personality theory, experimental psychology, child psychology, abnormal psychology, history of psychology (or at least 90th percentile [660] on the Psychology Subject Test of the GREs)

Are there courses you recommend that are not mandatory?
Physiological psychology

GRE mean
Verbal 550   Quantitative 550   Analytical 4.5

GPA mean
Overall GPA 3.5

Number of applications/admission offers/incoming students in 2004
350 applied/60 admission offers/39 incoming

% of students receiving:
Tuition waiver only: 2%
Assistantship/fellowship only: 35%
Both tuition waiver & assistantship/fellowship: 5%

Approximate percentage of incoming students who entered with a B.A./B.S. only: 60%   **Master's:** 39%

**Approximate percentage of students who are
Women:** 76%   **Ethnic Minority:** 11%   **International:** 5%

Average years to complete the doctoral program (including internship): 4 years

Personal interview
Required in person

Research areas	# Faculty	# Grants
behavioral medicine/therapy	1	0
cognitive issues	1	0
couples and family therapy	2	0
forensic issues	2	0
multicultural issues	1	0

Clinical opportunities
assessment
behavioral medicine
cognitive therapy
group therapy
hypnosis
international disaster psychology
psychodynamic/psychoanalytic therapy
psychotherapy supervision

DePaul University

Department of Psychology
2219 North Kenmore
Chicago, IL 60614
phone#: (773) 325-7787
e-mail: gradpsych@depaul.edu
Web address: http://condor.depaul.edu/%7Epsych/clwebsite/clinical_program.html

	1	2	3	**4**	5	6	7	
Clinically oriented			Equal emphasis			Research oriented		

What percentage of your faculty subscribes to or practices in each of the following orientations?

Psychodynamic/Psychoanalytic	0%
Applied behavioral analysis/Radical behavioral	22%
Family systems/Systems	55%
Existential/Phenomenological/Humanistic	0%
Cognitive/Cognitive-behavioral	33%

What percentage of students applying for internship last year was accepted into APPIC-member internships? 100%

What courses are required for incoming students to have completed prior to enrolling?
24 semester hours in psychology, 3 semester hours of statistics, and 3 semester hours in experimental psychology

Are there courses you recommend that are not mandatory?
Science, computer, and math courses

GRE mean
Verbal 589   Quantitative 655
Analytical Writing Data not available

GPA mean
Overall GPA 3.57

Number of applications/admission offers/incoming students in 2004
211 applied/9 admission offers/7 incoming

% of students receiving:
Tuition waiver only: 0%
Assistantship/fellowship only: 0%
Both tuition waiver & assistantship/fellowship: 100%

Approximate percentage of incoming students who entered with a B.A./B.S. only: 71%   **Master's:** 29%

**Approximate percentage of students who are
Women:** 57%   **Ethnic Minority:** 43%   **International:** 7%

Average years to complete the doctoral program (including internship): 8 years

Personal interview
Preferred in person but telephone acceptable

Research areas	# Faculty	# Grants
adolescent depression	2	2
child abuse and neglect	1	1
chronic fatigue syndrome	1	3
disability	2	2
HIV/AIDS adolescent prevention	1	3
minority mental health	3	1
parent–child interaction	1	1
program evaluation	3	1
smoking cessation	1	1
social support	1	1
teenage pregnancy	2	1
violence prevention		

Clinical opportunities
assessment
child and adolescent
community psychology
family therapy
group therapy
minority/diversity

University of Detroit–Mercy
Department of Psychology
4001 W. McNichols Road
Detroit, MI 48221-3038
phone#: (313) 578-0570
e-mail: mccownja@udmercy.edu
Web address:
http://liberalarts.udmercy.edu/psychology/pycphd.html

1	2	**3**	4	5	6	7

Clinically oriented   Equal emphasis   Research oriented

What percentage of your faculty subscribes to or practices in each of the following orientations?

Psychodynamic/Psychoanalytic	75%
Applied behavioral analysis/Radical behavioral	10%
Family systems/Systems	10%
Existential/Phenomenological/Humanistic	10%
Cognitive/Cognitive-behavioral	25%

What percentage of students applying for internship last year was accepted into APPIC-member internships?
Data not available

What courses are required for incoming students to have completed prior to enrolling?
Statistics, experimental, research methods, personality, abnormal psychology, research course

Are there courses you recommend that are not mandatory?
Physiological psychology

GRE mean
Verbal 530   Quantitative 600
Analytical Writing Data not available

GPA mean
Overall GPA 3.3

Number of applications/admission offers/incoming students in 2005
65 applied/20 admission offers/10 incoming

% of students receiving:
Tuition waiver only: 0%
Assistantship/fellowship only: 0%
Both tuition waiver & assistantship/fellowship: 100%
(all students in first 2 years of program)

Approximate percentage of incoming students who entered with a B.A./B.S. only: 56%   **Master's:** 44%

**Approximate percentage of students who are
Women:** 80%   **Ethnic Minority:** 25%
International: Data not available

Average years to complete the doctoral program (including internship): 6 years

Personal interview
Required in person

Research areas	# Faculty	# Grants
alcohol abuse	1	1
critical incident response	2	0
helping behavior	1	0
identity development	2	0
intellectual assessment using human figure drawings	1	0
marital and family relationships	2	0
perception and eye movement	1	1
posttraumatic stress disorder	2	0
psychiatric diagnosis, ethnicity, and clinical judgment	1	0
psychotherapy process and outcome	4	0
self-esteem/body image	2	0
spirituality	3	0

Clinical opportunities
Practicums and internships are completed at one of over 30 agencies in the metropolitan area. Students are also encouraged to apply nationally for internship if their circumstances permit.

Drexel University
Department of Psychology
Main Campus Office
3141 Chestnut Street
Philadelphia, PA 19104
phone#: (215) 895-1895
Web address: http://www.drexel.edu/coas/psychology/programs/graduate/phdprog.asp

1	2	3	**4**	5	6	7

Clinically oriented   Equal emphasis   Research oriented

What percentage of your faculty subscribes to or practices in each of the following orientations?

Psychodynamic/Psychoanalytic	0%
Applied behavioral analysis/Radical behavioral	0%

159

Family systems/Systems	10%	
Existential/Phenomenological/Humanistic	0%	
Cognitive/Cognitive-behavioral	90%	

What percentage of students applying for internship last year was accepted into APPIC-member internships?
Data not available

What courses are required for incoming students to have completed prior to enrolling?
None

Are there courses you recommend that are not mandatory?
Foundation courses in psychology

GRE mean
Verbal 537   Quantitative 605   Analytical 616
Advanced Psychology 650
Analytical Writing Data not available

GPA mean
Overall GPA 3.5

Number of applications/admission offers/incoming students in 2005
275 applied/13 admission offers/10 incoming

% of students receiving:
Tuition waiver only: 0%
Assistantship/fellowship only: 0%
Both tuition waiver & assistantship/fellowship: 100%
(1st-year class)
**All students in subsequent yeas currently receive at least a tuition waiver, and approximately 50% receive additional support)

Approximate percentage of incoming students who entered with a B.A./B.S. only: 80%   **Master's:** 20%

Approximate percentage of students who are Women: 86%   **Ethnic Minority:** 14%
International: Data not available

Average years to complete the doctoral program (including internship): 5.8 years

Personal interview
Preferred in person but telephone acceptable

Research areas	# Faculty	# Grants
child abuse/neglect	1	0
childhood illness/family coping	1	1
childhood loss	2	2
chronic illness and coping (adult)	1	0
conscious/unconscious processes	1	0
divorce	1	1
family systems	4	1
family violence	2	2
health psychology (AIDS, polio, head injury)	2	0
homeless families	1	0
inner-city children	4	2
low birthweight children	1	0
neuropsychology	6	0
peer relations/social skills in children	2	2
personality disorders	2	0
psychotherapy research	5	0
schizophrenia	1	0
social competence in children	2	0
substance abuse	2	2
television violence	1	1

Clinical opportunities
adult
child and family

Duke University
Department of Psychology
Durham, NC 27708
phone#: (919) 660-5716
e-mail: lkc@duke.edu
Web address:
http://www.psych-shs.duke.edu/grad/clinical/index.php

1	2	3	4	5	**6**	7
Clinically oriented		Equal emphasis			Research oriented	

What percentage of your faculty subscribes to or practices in each of the following orientations?

Psychodynamic/Psychoanalytic	20%
Applied behavioral analysis/Radical behavioral	0%
Family systems/Systems	15%
Existential/Phenomenological/Humanistic	0%
Cognitive/Cognitive-behavioral	65%

What percentage of students applying for internship last year was accepted into APPIC-member internships?
Data not available

What courses are required for incoming students to have completed prior to enrolling?
None

Are there courses you recommend that are not mandatory?
Broad background, statistics, personality theory

GRE mean
Verbal 580   Quantitative 660
Analytical Writing Data not available

GPA mean
Overall GPA 3.6

Number of applications/admission offers/incoming students in 2005
303 applied/11 admission offers/6 incoming

% of students receiving:
Tuition waiver only: 0%
Assistantship/fellowship only: 0%
Both tuition waiver & assistantship/fellowship: 100%

Approximate percentage of incoming students who entered with a B.A./B.S. only: 100%   **Master's:** 0%

Approximate percentage of students who are Women: 75%   **Ethnic Minority:** 23%
International: Data not available

Average years to complete the doctoral program (including internship): 5.5 years

Personal interview
Required in person

Research areas	# Faculty	# Grants
affective disorders	3	2
behavioral medicine	4	6
conduct disorders	2	3
eating disorders	1	0
developmental psychopathology	5	5
neuropsychology	1	0
posttraumatic stress disorder	2	0
school/educational	5	2
sexual abuse	2	0
social cognition	2	2
social skills	3	2
stress and coping	6	6

Clinical opportunities
adolescents
affective disorders
behavioral cardiology
behavioral medicine
behavior disorders of children
child abuse
cognitive/dialectical behavior therapy
eating disorders
neuropsychology
pediatric psychology
posttraumatic stress disorder
public sector impairment treatment
school/educational
substance abuse

Emory University

Department of Psychology
Kilgo Circle
Atlanta, GA 30322
phone#: (404) 727-7456
e-mail:TLEGGE@EMORY.EDU
Web address:
http://www.psychology.emory.edu/clinical/index.html

1	2	3	4	5	**6**	7

Clinically oriented   Equal emphasis   Research oriented

What percentage of your faculty subscribes to or practices in each of the following orientations?

Psychodynamic/Psychoanalytic	10%
Applied behavioral analysis/Radical behavioral	10%
Family systems/Systems	30%
Existential/Phenomenological/Humanistic	0%
Cognitive/Cognitive-behavioral	40%

What percentage of students applying for internship last year was accepted into APPIC-member internships? 83%

What courses are required for incoming students to have completed prior to enrolling?
No

Are there courses you recommend that are not mandatory?
Statistics, methodology, psychopathology, personality

GRE mean
Verbal 570   Quantitative 650   Analytical 680
Analytical Writing 5.5

GPA mean
Overall GPA 3.5

Number of applications/admission offers/incoming students in 2005
225 applied/8 admission offers/6 incoming

% of students receiving:
Tuition waiver only: 0%
Assistantship/fellowship only: 0%
Both tuition waiver & assistantship/fellowship: 100%

Approximate percentage of incoming students who entered with a B.A./B.S. only: 80%   **Master's:** 20%

Approximate percentage of students who are Women: 85%   **Ethnic Minority:** 10%   **International:** 5%

Average years to complete the doctoral program (including internship): 5 years

Personal interview
Required in person

Research areas	# Faculty	# Grants
adolescent psychopathology	2	1
attention-deficit disorder	1	1
behavior control	1	0
behavioral genetics	2	1
eating disorders	1	0
infant development	1	2
neuropsychology	1	0
personality and personality disorders	3	2
schizophrenia	2	1

Clinical opportunities
assessment
behavioral medicine
behavior therapy
cognitive therapy
interpersonal therapy
neuropsychology
psychodynamic therapy

Fairleigh Dickinson University

Department of Psychology
Teaneck–Hackensack Campus
1000 River Road
Teaneck, NJ 07666
phone#: (201) 692-2315
e-mail: massoth@alpha.fdu.edu
Web address:
http://alpha.fdu.edu/ucoll/psychology/psyphd.html

1	2	3	**4**	5	6	7

Clinically oriented   Equal emphasis   Research oriented

What percentage of your faculty subscribes to or practices in each of the following orientations?

Psychodynamic/Psychoanalytic	60%
Applied behavioral analysis/Radical behavioral	10%
Family systems/Systems	15%
Existential/Phenomenological/Humanistic	20%
Cognitive/Cognitive-behavioral	60%

What percentage of students applying for internship last year was accepted into APPIC-member internships? 100%

What courses are required for incoming students to have completed prior to enrolling?
18 credits in psychology including statistics, introductory developmental, experimental, social

Are there courses you recommend that are not mandatory?
Psychopathology, physiological, assessment

GRE mean
Verbal 582 Quantitative 640 Analytical 680
Advanced Psychology 666
Analytical Writing 5.0

GPA mean
Overall GPA 3.5

Number of applications/admission offers/incoming students in 2005
210 applied/33 admission offers/16 incoming

% of students receiving:
Tuition waiver only: 0%
Assistantship/fellowship only: 100% (can be taken as tuition remission)
Both tuition waiver & assistantship/fellowship: 0%

Approximate percentage of incoming students who entered with a B.A./B.S. only: 60%   **Master's:** 40%

Approximate percentage of students who are Women: 66%   **Ethnic Minority:** 20%   **International:** 4%

Average years to complete the doctoral program (including internship): 5.5 years

Personal interview
Required in person

Research areas	# Faculty	# Grants
assessment	6	2
behavioral medicine	3	1
child clinical	4	2
community psychology	3	0
depression	1	0
eating disorders	1	0
ethical issues	2	0
forensic	2	0
minority issues	2	0
relationship	4	0
sexual abuse	3	0
statistics	2	0
stress—disasters	2	1
women's studies	4	0

Clinical opportunities
anxiety disorders
assessment
behavioral medicine
community psychology
family therapy
gerontology
minority populations
neuropsychology
substance abuse

Fielding Graduate Institute

School of Psychology
2112 Santa Barbara Street
Santa Barbara, CA 93105
phone#: (800) 340-1099
e-mail: admissions@fielding.edu
Web address: http://www.fielding.edu/psy/index.htm

1	2	3	4	**5**	6	7
Clinically oriented		Equal emphasis			Research oriented	

What percentage of your faculty subscribes to or practices in each of the following orientations?

Psychodynamic/Psychoanalytic	20%
Applied behavioral analysis/Radical behavioral	0%
Family systems/Systems	13%
Existential/Phenomenological/Humanistic	30%
Cognitive/Cognitive-behavioral	37%

What percentage of students applying for internship last year was accepted into APPIC-member internships? 40%

What courses are required for incoming students to have completed prior to enrolling?
A bachelor's degree is the minimum. Strong psychological background recommended.

Are there courses you recommend that are not mandatory?
This is a networked distributed learning organization only appropriate for adult students with professional experience.

GRE mean
Not used

GPA mean
Data not available

Number of applications/admission offers/incoming students in 2004
378 applied/97 admission offers/77 incoming

% of students receiving:
Tuition waiver only: 0%
Assistantship/fellowship only: 0%
Both tuition waiver & assistantship/fellowship: 0%

Approximate percentage of incoming students who entered with a B.A./B.S. only: 16%   **Master's:** 84%

Approximate percentage of students who are Women: 72%   **Ethnic Minority:** 19%   **International:** 4%

Average years to complete the doctoral program (including internship): 7–8 years

Personal interview
Required in person

Research areas
health psychology
neuropsychology
prevention
violence

Clinical opportunities
Cognitive-behavioral, psychoanalytic/psychodynamic, and
TA-Gestalt training tracks

University of Florida

Department of Clinical and Health Psychology
Box 100165 University of Florida Health Science Center
Gainesville, FL 32610
phone#: (352) 273-6455
e-mail: vcarter@hp.ufl.edu
Web address: http://www.phhp.ufl.edu/chp/
prospectivestudents/doctoral_program/index.html

1	2	3	**4**	5	6	7
Clinically oriented		Equal emphasis			Research oriented	

What percentage of your faculty subscribes to or practices in each of the following orientations?

Psychodynamic/Psychoanalytic	20%
Applied behavioral analysis/Radical behavioral	10%
Family systems/Systems	60%
Existential/Phenomenological/Humanistic	20%
Cognitive/Cognitive-behavioral	80%

What percentage of students applying for internship last year was accepted into APPIC-member internships?
Data not available

What courses are required for incoming students to have completed prior to enrolling?
Statistics

Are there courses you recommend that are not mandatory?
Undergraduate courses in experimental psychology, developmental psychology, social psychology, personality, physiological, perception, statistics

GRE mean
Data not available

GPA mean
Data not available

Number of applications/admission offers/incoming students in 2003
322 applied/23 admission offers/16 incoming

% of students receiving:
Tuition waiver only: 0%
Assistantship/fellowship only: 0%
Both tuition waiver & assistantship/fellowship: 95% all students; 100% incoming

Approximate percentage of incoming students who entered with a B.A./B.S. only: 80% **Master's:** 20%

Approximate percentage of students who are
Women: 78% **Ethnic Minority:** 20%
International: Data not available

Average years to complete the doctoral program (including internship): 5.5 years

Personal interview
Preferred in person but telephone acceptable

Research areas	# Faculty	# Grants
anxiety disorders and emotions	2	3
child clinical psychology	3	3
clinical/medical psychology	3	3
functional neuroimaging		
neuropsychology	4	4
obesity treatment	1	1
pain	2	3
pediatric psychology	3	4
rural health	1	2
telehealth	1	1

Clinical opportunities
anxiety
child clinical psychology
fear
forensic psychology
inpatient consultation/liaison
medical psychology
neuropsychology
pain and stress
parent training'
pediatric consultation
rural behavioral health
weight loss

Florida Institute of Technology (Psy.D.)

School of Psychology
150 West University Boulevard
Melbourne, FL 32901
phone#: (407) 674-8105
e-mail: rkrishna@fit.edu
Web address:
http://www.fit.edu/AcadRes/psych/clinical/index.htm

1	2	**3**	4	5	6	7
Clinically oriented		Equal emphasis			Research oriented	

What percentage of your faculty subscribes to or practices in each of the following orientations?

Psychodynamic/Psychoanalytic	10%
Applied behavioral analysis/Radical behavioral	10%
Family systems/Systems	20%
Existential/Phenomenological/Humanistic	20%
Cognitive/Cognitive-behavioral	40%

What percentage of students applying for internship last year was accepted into APPIC-member internships? 21%

What courses are required for incoming students to have completed prior to enrolling?
Statistics, learning, personality, physiological psychology, abnormal psychology, social psychology

Are there courses you recommend that are not mandatory?
Data not available

GRE mean
Verbal + Quantitative 1048
Analytical Writing 4.5

GPA mean
Overall GPA 3.54

Number of applications/admission offers/incoming students in 2005
91 applied/54 admission offers/20 incoming

% of students receiving:
Tuition waiver only: 0%
Assistantship/fellowship only: 0%
Both tuition waiver & assistantship/fellowship: 56%

Approximate percentage of incoming students who entered with a B.A./B.S. only: 65%   **Master's:** 35%

Approximate percentage of students who are Women: 95%   **Ethnic Minority:** 10%   **International:** 4%

Average years to complete the doctoral program (including internship): 5 years

Personal interview
Preferred in person but telephone acceptable

Research areas	# Faculty	# Grants
aging	2	0
eating disorders	1	0
family psychology	2	0
health psychology	3	2
neuropsychology	2	1
personality assessment	3	0
sexual abuse	1	1
supervision	1	0
Vietnam veterans	1	0
(posttraumatic stress syndrome)		

Clinical opportunities
behavioral medicine/health psychology
eating disorders
family and marital therapy
forensic settings
neuropsychology
sexual abuse (offenders and victims)
Vietnam veterans (posttraumatic stress syndrome)

Florida State University

Department of Psychology
Tallahassee, FL 32306-1051
phone#: (850) 644-2499
e-mail: dilworth@psy.fsu.edu
Web address: http://www.psy.fsu.edu

1	2	3	4	5	6	**7**

Clinically oriented   Equal emphasis   Research oriented

What percentage of your faculty subscribes to or practices in each of the following orientations?

Psychodynamic/Psychoanalytic	0%
Applied behavioral analysis/Radical behavioral	0%
Family systems/Systems	0%
Existential/Phenomenological/Humanistic	15%
Cognitive/Cognitive-behavioral	100%

What percentage of students applying for internship last year was accepted into APPIC-member internships? 100%

What courses are required for incoming students to have completed prior to enrolling?
Undergraduate degree

Are there courses you recommend that are not mandatory?
No

GRE mean
Verbal 653   Quantitative 723
Analytical Writing 4.9

GPA mean
Junior/Senior GPA 3.9

Number of applications/admission offers/incoming students in 2005
259 applied/14 admission offers/6 incoming

% of students receiving:
Tuition waiver only: 0%
Assistantship/fellowship only: 0%
Both tuition waiver & assistantship/fellowship: 100%

Approximate percentage of incoming students who entered with a B.A./B.S. only: 80%   **Master's:** 20%

Approximate percentage of students who are Women: 81%   **Ethnic Minority:** 23%   **International:** 2%

Average years to complete the doctoral program (including internship): 7 years

Personal interview
Preferred in person but telephone acceptable

Research areas	# Faculty	# Grants
addictive behavior, especially alcohol abuse	2	1
conduct disorder and anti-social behavior	1	1
depression, bulimia nervosa, and anxiety	3	3
developmental psychopathology	3	3
early intervention and its effects on cognitive, behavioral, and social development	2	1
epidemiological psychology	1	1
prediction of criminal behavior	1	0
problematic social interactions of children	1	1
suicide	1	0

Clinical opportunities

adolescent delinquency
anxiety disorders
behavioral health
child academic, behavioral and emotional problems
juvenile felony offenders
migrant workers
state psychiatric hospital

Fordham University

Department of Psychology
Fordham Road and Southern Boulevard
Bronx, NY 10458
phone#: (718) 817-3782
fax#: (718) 817-3785
e-mail: cboyle@fordham.edu
Web address: http://www.fordham.edu/psychology/
updated/Clinical/clinical%20home%20page.html

1	2	3	**4**	5	6	7
Clinically oriented		Equal emphasis			Research oriented	

What percentage of your faculty subscribes to or practices in each of the following orientations?

Psychodynamic/Psychoanalytic	20%
Applied behavioral analysis/Radical behavioral	10%
Family systems/Systems	20%
Existential/Phenomenological/Humanistic	10%
Cognitive/Cognitive-behavioral	40%

What percentage of students applying for internship last year was accepted into APPIC-member internships?
Data not available

What courses are required for incoming students to have completed prior to enrolling?
Statistics, experimental psychology, introductory psychology

Are there courses you recommend that are not mandatory?
No

GRE mean
Data not available

GPA mean
Data not available

Number of applications/admission offers/incoming students in 2005
290 applied/25 admission offers/13 incoming

% of students receiving:
Tuition waiver only: 15%
Assistantship/fellowship only: 0%
Both tuition waiver & assistantship/fellowship: 50%

Approximate percentage of incoming students who entered with a B.A./B.S. only: 80% **Master's:** 20%

**Approximate percentage of students who are
Women:** 66% **Ethnic Minority:** 20%
International: Data not available

Average years to complete the doctoral program (including internship): 7.1 years

Personal interview
No preference given

Research areas	# Faculty	# Grants
adolescent development	1	0
assessment	3	0
attachment relationships in couples	1	0
clinical child psychology	1	0
family systems	1	0
health psychology/behavioral medicine	1	0
MMPI	1	0
neuropsychology	1	0
parent–child relationships	2	0
personality disorders	1	0
prevention	1	0
social support	1	0
stress and coping	2	0
substance abuse	1	0

Clinical opportunities

Clinical externships available at numerous inpatient and outpatient specialty clinics in the New York metropolitan area. Appropriate training sites can be found in any area.

Forest Institute of Professional Psychology (Psy.D.)

2885 West Battlefield Road
Springfield, MO 65807
phone#: (417) 823-3477 or
(800) 424-7793
e-mail: praleigh@forest.edu (Director of Admissions); DCarpenter@forest.edu (Graduate Training Director)
Web address: http://www.forest.edu/academics/courses/psyd/index.html

1	2	3	4	5	6	7
Clinically oriented		Equal emphasis			Research oriented	

What percentage of your faculty subscribes to or practices in each of the following orientations?

Psychodynamic/Psychoanalytic	40%
Applied behavioral analysis/Radical behavioral	10%
Family systems/Systems	20%
Existential/Phenomenological/Humanistic	10%
Cognitive/Cognitive-behavioral	20%

What percentage of students applying for internship last year was accepted into APPIC-member internships? 90%

What courses are required for incoming students to have completed prior to enrolling?
Psy.D.: 18 hours of psychology
M.A.: 12 hours of psychology

Are there courses you recommend that are not mandatory?
General psychology, history and systems, abnormal psychology, theories of personality, statistics, biological sciences

GRE mean
Verbal 550   Quantitative 490
Analytical Writing Data not available

GPA mean
Data not available

Number of applications/admission offers/incoming students in 2003
102 applied/81 admission offers/65 incoming

% of students receiving:
Tuition waiver only: 6%
Assistantship/fellowship only: 0%
Both tuition waiver & assistantship/fellowship: 0%

Approximate percentage of incoming students who entered with a B.A./B.S. only: 54%   **Master's:** 46%

Approximate percentage of students who are Women: 81%   **Ethnic Minority:** 10%
International: Data not available

Average years to complete the doctoral program (including internship): 4–5 years

Personal interview
Required in person

Research areas	# Faculty	# Grants
autoimmune disorders and psychological indices	2	1
depression	2	1
electro-stimulation and stress	2	1
pain management	2	1

Clinical opportunities
biofeedback
child therapy
corrections/forensics
integrated healthcare
marriage and family therapy
multicultural center
neuropsychology (adult and child/adolescent)
pain management
psychopharmacology
underserved populations

Fuller Theological Seminary (Ph.D. & Psy.D.)

(Part of Fuller Theological Seminary)
180 North Oakland Avenue
Pasadena, CA 91101
phone#: (626) 584-5500
e-mail: tkelly@fuller.edu
Web address:
http://www.fuller.edu/admiss/degrees/phdpsy.asp and
http://www.fuller.edu/admiss/degrees/psyd.asp

1	2	3	**4**	5	6	7

Clinically oriented   Equal emphasis   Research oriented

What percentage of your faculty subscribes to or practices in each of the following orientations?
Psychodynamic/Psychoanalytic	20%
Applied behavioral analysis/Radical behavioral	0%
Family systems/Systems	30%
Existential/Phenomenological/Humanistic	10%
Cognitive/Cognitive-behavioral	40%

What percentage of students applying for internship last year was accepted into APPIC-member internships?
Data not available

What courses are required for incoming students to have completed prior to enrolling?
6 courses in psychology and a B.A. from an accredited school

Are there courses you recommend that are not mandatory?
Courses in the areas of abnormal, developmental, experimental, physiological, social psychology, statistics, tests and measures, learning, motivation, and personality

GRE mean
Verbal + Quantitative 1190

GPA mean
Psychology GPA 3.85

Number of applications/admission offers/incoming students in 2003
151 applied/63 (+9 deferrals) admission offers/48 incoming

% of students receiving:
Tuition waiver only: 0%
Assistantship/fellowship only: 70%
Both tuition waiver & assistantship/fellowship: 0%

Approximate percentage of incoming students who entered with a B.A./B.S. only: 76%   **Master's:** 24%

Approximate percentage of students who are Women: 62%   **Ethnic Minority:** 30%
International: Data not available

Average years to complete the doctoral program (including internship): 6 years

Personal interview
Preferred in person but telephone acceptable

Research areas	# Faculty	# Grants
biopsychosocial	3	2
child clinical	3	1
cognition	1	0
cross-cultural psychology	2	0
depression	1	0
developmental	3	1
family	2	1
group processes	1	0
health psychology/behavioral medicine	3	0
marriages	4	0
neuropsychology	1	0
posttraumatic stress disorders	2	0
relaxation/biofeedback	1	0
religion	7	0
stress and coping	1	0
substance abuse	1	0

Clinical opportunities
assessment
child/adolescent therapy
chronic mental illness
family therapy
forensic population
gerontology
group therapy
inpatient adult population
interpersonal psychotherapy
marital/couples therapy
neuropsychology/rehabilitation
supervision
victim/battering

Gallaudet University

Department of Psychology
8th and Florida Avenue, NE
Washington, DC 20002-3695
phone#: (202) 651-5540
e-mail: Patrick.Brice@Gallaudet.edu
Web address: http://www.gallaudet.edu/x718.xml

1	2	**3**	4	5	6	7

Clinically oriented   Equal emphasis   Research oriented

What percentage of your faculty subscribes to or practices in each of the following orientations?

Psychodynamic/Psychoanalytic   60%
Applied behavioral analysis/Radical behavioral   20%
Family systems/Systems   0%
Existential/Phenomenological/Humanistic   20%
Cognitive/Cognitive-behavioral   40%

What percentage of students applying for internship last year was accepted into APPIC-member internships?
Data not available

What courses are required for incoming students to have completed prior to enrolling?
Major or minor in undergraduate psychology including statistics and experimental psychology

Are there courses you recommend that are not mandatory?
Social psychology, personality, learning, cognition, perception

GRE mean
Verbal 485 Quantitative 512
Advanced Psychology is not required
Analytical Writing Data not available

GPA mean
Overall GPA 3.3 Psychology GPA 3.5

Number of applications/admission offers/incoming students in 2005
20 applied/7 admission offers/7 incoming

% of students receiving:
Tuition waiver only: 20%

Assistantship/fellowship only: 70%
Both tuition waiver & assistantship/fellowship: 5%

Approximate percentage of incoming students who entered with a B.A./B.S. only: 88% **Master's:** 12%

**Approximate percentage of students who are
Women:** 88% **Ethnic Minority:** 12%
International: Data not available
Deaf or Hard of Hearing: 33% **Hearing:** 67%

Average years to complete the doctoral program (including internship): 6.25 years

Personal interview
Preferred in person but telephone acceptable

Research areas	# Faculty	# Grants
adult development issues for deaf lesbians and gay men	1	0
assessment of attachment in deaf persons	2	1
assessment of attention in deaf children	1	1
assessment of depression in deaf clients	1	0
cognitive processing and memory in deaf persons	1	0
ethics in mental health and deafness	1	0
neuropsychological assessment of deaf clients	1	0
parental involvement with education of ethnic minority deaf children	1	1

Clinical opportunities
Assessment and therapy with deaf and hard-of-hearing clients through our multidisciplinary mental health clinic. More than 60 externship programs available in Washington, D.C. metropolitan area.

George Fox University (Psy.D.)

Graduate Department of Clinical Psychology
School of Behavioral and Health Sciences
414 North Meridian Street
Newburg, OR 97132-2697
phone#: (503) 554-2263
e-mail: amcconaughey@georgefox.edu
Web address: http://psyd.georgefox.edu

1	2	3	**4**	5	6	7

Clinically oriented   Equal emphasis   Research oriented

What percentage of your faculty subscribes to or practices in each of the following orientations?

Psychodynamic/Psychoanalytic   10%
Applied behavioral analysis/Radical behavioral   10%
Family systems/Systems   10%
Existential/Phenomenological/Humanistic   10%
Cognitive/Cognitive-behavioral   50%

What percentage of students applying for internship last year was accepted into APPIC-member internships? 100%

What courses are required for incoming students to have completed prior to enrolling?
18 semester hours or the equivalent (no specific courses required)

Are there courses you recommend that are not mandatory?
Personality, developmental, statistics, social, experimental, abnormal psychobiology

GRE mean
Verbal + Quantitative 1180
Analytical Writing Data not used

GPA mean
Overall GPA 3.69

Number of applications/admission offers/incoming students in 2004
60 applied/28 admission offers/22 incoming

% of students receiving:
Tuition waiver only: 15%
Assistantship/fellowship only: 25%
Both tuition waiver & assistantship/fellowship: 5%

Approximate percentage of incoming students who entered with a B.A./B.S. only: 75%   **Master's:** 25%

Approximate percentage of students who are Women: 55%   **Ethnic Minority:** 9%   **International:** 2%

Average years to complete the doctoral program (including internship): 5.2 years

Personal interview
Preferred in person but telephone acceptable

Research areas	# Faculty	# Grants
adjudicated youth/adults	1	0
child and geriatric memory	1	0
clinical supervision	1	0
coping skills in high-risk junior high students	1	1
marriage relationships	1	1
memory assessment	1	1
mission school consultation	1	0
pain management	1	1
shame	1	0
spirituality and mental health	1	1
Stroop effect	1	1
values and psychologist training	1	0

Clinical opportunities
addictions
adolescent residential
assessment
child psychopathology
community mental health
corrections
emergency room consultation
geriatics
health psychology
inpatient hospital consultation
Native American
out-patient hospital consultation/treatment
pain managment
public school
rural psychology
spirituality in psychotherapeutic intervention

George Mason University

Department of Psychology
4400 University Drive
Fairfax, VA 22030-4444
phone#: (703) 993-1342
e-mail: dwiggin3@gmu.edu
Web address:
http://mason.gmu.edu/%7Ejshort/clinical.html

1	2	3	**4**	5	6	7
Clinically oriented		Equal emphasis			Research oriented	

What percentage of your faculty subscribes to or practices in each of the following orientations?

Psychodynamic/Psychoanalytic	20%
Applied behavioral analysis/Radical behavioral	10%
Family systems/Systems	0%
Existential/Phenomenological/Humanistic	40%
Cognitive/Cognitive-behavioral	80%

What percentage of students applying for internship last year was accepted into APPIC-member internships? 90%

What courses are required for incoming students to have completed prior to enrolling?
Statistics, abnormal psychology, any laboratory science course

Are there courses you recommend that are not mandatory?
Tests and measurements/psychometrics, personality

GRE mean
Verbal 631   Quantitative 694
Analytical Writing N/A

GPA mean
Overall GPA 3.45

Number of applications/admission offers/incoming students in 2005
178 applied/11 admission offers/9 incoming

% of students receiving:
Tuition waiver only: 0%
Assistantship/fellowship only: 0%
Both tuition waiver & assistantship/fellowship: 100%

Approximate percentage of incoming students who entered with a B.A./B.S. only: 89%   **Master's:** 11%

Approximate percentage of students who are Women: 78%   **Ethnic Minority:** 12%   **International:** 5%

Average years to complete the doctoral program (including internship): 6 years

Personal interview
Required in person

Research areas	# Faculty	# Grants
cognition and affect	4	0
domestic violence	1	0
forensics	1	1
gay and lesbian issues	1	0
personality—shame and guilt	1	1
positive human functioning	3	0
psychotherapy/counseling process	1	0
self-efficacy	1	0
social anxiety	1	0
stress and coping	2	0

Clinical opportunities
child/adult assessment
cognitive-behavioral psychotherapy
community consultation/education
group/marriage psychotherapy
individual adult psychotherapy
neuropsychological assessment

George Washington University (Ph.D.)

Department of Psychology
2125 G Street, NW
Washington, DC 20052
phone#: (202) 994-6544
e-mail: roilp@gwu.edu
Web address: http://www.gwu.edu/~clinpsyc

1	2	3	4	**5**	6	7
Clinically oriented		Equal emphasis			Research oriented	

What percentage of your faculty subscribes to or practices in each of the following orientations?

Psychodynamic/Psychoanalytic	10%
Applied behavioral analysis/Radical behavioral	10%
Family systems/Systems	20%
Existential/Phenomenological/Humanistic	10%
Cognitive/Cognitive-behavioral	50%

What percentage of students applying for internship last year was accepted into APPIC-member internships? 100%

What courses are required for incoming students to have completed prior to enrolling?
At least a minor in psychology, statistics, research methods (or experimental course), basic psychology theory courses (from neuropsychology, physiological psychology, abnormal psychology, social psychology, learning, developmental psychology)

Are there courses you recommend that are not mandatory?
History and systems (if not taken must then take without credit)

GRE mean
Verbal 600   Quantitative 670
Analytical Writing Data not available

GPA mean
Overall GPA 3.5

Number of applications/admission offers/incoming students in 2005
270 applied/8 admission offers/5 incoming

% of students receiving:
Tuition waiver only: 0%
Assistantship/fellowship only: 0%
Both tuition waiver & assistantship/fellowship: 100%

Approximate percentage of incoming students who entered with a B.A./B.S. only: 100%   **Master's:** 0%

Approximate percentage of students who are
Women: 80%   **Ethnic Minority:** 40%   **International:** 0%

Average years to complete the doctoral program (including internship): 6.5 years

Personal interview
Preferred in person but telephone acceptable

Research areas	# Faculty	# Grants
adolescence	3	3
AIDS	1	2
anxiety disorders	1	0
behavioral medicine	1	0
child	2	1
community	2	1
depression	1	1
family	1	1
health	1	0
minority mental health	4	3
relaxation/biofeedback	1	0
stress	2	0

Clinical opportunities
adolescent problems
AIDS
adolescent delinquency
affective disorders/depression
anxiety disorders
assessment
behavioral medicine
child assessment and therapy
conduct disorder
developmental disabilities/autism
dissociative disorder
eating disorders
family therapy
forensic psychology
group therapy
health
hyperactivity
impulse control/aggression
marital/couples therapy
minority/cross-cultural
neuropsychology/rehabilitation
obsessive–compulsive disorder
personality disorders
psychodynamic/psychoanalytic therapy
schizophrenia/psychoses
substance abuse
victim/battering abuse

George Washington University (Psy.D.)

Center for Professional Psychology
2300 M Street, NW, Suite 910
Washington, DC 20037
phone#: (202) 496-6260
e-mail: psyd@gwu.edu
Web address: http://www.gwu.edu/~psyd/index.htm

1	2	**3**	4	5	6	7

Clinically oriented   Equal emphasis   Research oriented

What percentage of your faculty subscribes to or practices in each of the following orientations?

Psychodynamic/Psychoanalytic	90%
Applied behavioral analysis/Radical behavioral	0%
Family systems/Systems	0%
Existential/Phenomenological/Humanistic	0%
Cognitive/Cognitive-behavioral	10%

What percentage of students applying for internship last year was accepted into APPIC-member internships?
Data not available

What courses are required for incoming students to have completed prior to enrolling?
B.A./B.S.

Are there courses you recommend that are not mandatory?
Psychodynamic/psychoanalytic theory, personality, development, psychodynamic/psychoanalytic therapy, cognitive development and a course in statistics

GRE mean
Verbal 569   Quantitative 634   Analytical 641
Analytical Writing Data not available

GPA mean
Overall GPA 3.4

Number of applications/admission offers/incoming students in 2005
400 applied/70 admission offers/30 incoming

% of students receiving:
Tuition waiver only: 33%
Assistantship/fellowship only: 0%
Both tuition waiver & assistantship/fellowship: 0%

Approximate percentage of incoming students who entered with a B.A./B.S. only: 63%   **Master's:** 17%

Approximate percentage of students who are Women: 76%   **Ethnic Minority:** 28%
International: Data not available

Average years to complete the doctoral program (including internship): 4.3 years

Personal interview
Required in person

Research areas	# Faculty	# Grants
adult psychopathology	4	0
child clinical	2	1
child development	2	2
community intervention	3	1
group process	3	0
infant and early childhood research	1	1
intellectual assessment	3	0
personality assessment	3	0

Clinical opportunities
assessment
clinical intervention with children
clinical outcome studies
developmental disorders
family therapy
learning disorders
psychotherapy
schizophrenia

University of Georgia

Department of Psychology
Athens, GA 30602
phone#: (706) 542-1787
e-mail: gradadm@arches.uga.edu
Web address: http://www.uga.edu/psychology/graduate/clinical/index.html

1	2	3	**4**	5	6	7

Clinically oriented   Equal emphasis   Research oriented

What percentage of your faculty subscribes to or practices in each of the following orientations?

Psychodynamic/Psychoanalytic	0%
Applied behavioral analysis/Radical behavioral	0%
Family systems/Systems	10%
Existential/Phenomenological/Humanistic	0%
Cognitive/Cognitive-behavioral	100%

What percentage of students applying for internship last year was accepted into APPIC-member internships? 100%

What courses are required for incoming students to have completed prior to enrolling?
None

Are there courses you recommend that are not mandatory?
Abnormal psychology, statistics

GRE mean
Data not available

GPA mean
Overall GPA 3.5

Number of applications/admission offers/incoming students in 2005
206 applied/11 admission offers/6 incoming

% of students receiving:
Tuition waiver only: 0%
Assistantship/fellowship only: 0%
Both tuition waiver & assistantship/fellowship: 100%

Approximate percentage of incoming students who entered with a B.A./B.S. only: 83%   **Master's:** 17%

Approximate percentage of students who are
Women: 82%   **Ethnic Minority:** 23%   **International:** 8%

Average years to complete the doctoral program
(including internship): 5 years

Personal interview
Preferred in person but telephone acceptable

Research areas	# Faculty	# Grants
AIDS	1	0
adolescence	1	1
adult psychopathology	4	1
affective disorder/depression	1	0
aggression	1	1
aging/gerontology	1	2
alcohol use and stress	1	1
anxiety disorders	1	0
applied behavioral analysis	1	0
battering	2	0
behavioral medicine	2	2
behavioral pharmacology	1	0
cardiovascular function	1	1
child clinical/child psychopathology	3	1
depression	2	0
developmental psychopathology	1	1
emotions	1	1
family/therapy/systems	1	1
interpersonal processes	1	1
marriage/couples	2	1
minority mental health	1	0
neuropsychology	1	2
pain management/control	1	0
parent–child interaction	2	1
pediatric psychology	1	1
prevention	3	2
psychology of women	1	0
schizophrenia/psychoses	1	0
stress and coping	2	1
substance abuse	1	0
violence/abuse/victim–offender	2	1
women's issues in therapy	1	0

Clinical opportunities
affective disorders/depression
anxiety disorders
assessment
behavior therapy
behavioral medicine
developmental disorders/autism
dissociative disorders
eating disorders
family therapy
hyperactivity
impulse control/aggression
marital/couples
minority/cross-cultural
neuropsychology
pediatric psychology
personality disorders
psychotherapy supervision
sex therapy
stress management
substance abuse
victim/battering/abuse

Georgia State University

Department of Psychology
University Plaza
P.O. Box 5010
Atlanta, GA 30303
phone#: (404) 651-2284
Web address:
http://www2.gsu.edu/~wwwpsy/ClinProg.htm

1	2	3	**4**	5	6	7
Clinically oriented		Equal emphasis			Research oriented	

What percentage of your faculty subscribes to or practices in each of the following orientations?

Psychodynamic/Psychoanalytic/Interpersonal	10%
Applied behavioral analysis/Radical behavioral	0%
Family systems/Systems	20%
Existential/Phenomenological/Humanistic	0%
Cognitive/Cognitive-behavioral	40%
Clinical Neuropsychology	30%

What percentage of students applying for internship last year was accepted into APPIC-member internships?
Data not available

What courses are required for incoming students to have completed prior to enrolling?
Research methods, psychological statistics, and two additional Junior/Senior-level psychology courses

Are there courses you recommend that are not mandatory?
Abnormal psychology

GRE mean
Verbal 640 (Median)   Quantitative 660 (Median)

GPA mean
Overall GPA 3.5

Number of applications/admission offers/incoming students in 2005
386 applied/15 admission offers/11 incoming

% of students receiving:
Tuition waiver only: 0%
Assistantship/fellowship only: 0%
Both tuition waiver & assistantship/fellowship: 100%

Approximate percentage of incoming students who entered with a B.A./B.S. only: 90%   **Master's:** 10%

Approximate percentage of students who are
Women: 80%   **Ethnic Minority:** 40%   **International:** 11%

Average years to complete the doctoral program
(including internship): 6 years

Personal interview
Preferred in person but telephone acceptable

Research areas	# Faculty	# Grants
acquired brain injuries	3	0
cognitive therapy	1	1
depression	1	0
couples therapy	2	0
crime and delinquency	2	1

171

eating disorders	1	1
early brain injury and visiospatial and attention skills	1	0
emotion and executive functioning	3	0
developmental neuropsychology	3	1
family traumatology	2	2
families and developmental disabilities	1	4
functional neuroimaging	3	1
HIV and families	1	1
HIV prevention	1	3
gender issues	1	1
multicultural issues	3	0
male parenting	1	1
parentification	1	0
reading/dyslexia	1	4
treatment of anxiety disorders	1	1

Clinical opportunities

adjustment problems of childhood, adolescence, and adulthood
anxiety disorders
behavioral assessment
chronic health conditions
clinical-community psychology
clinical neuropsychology and treatment
depressive disorders
developmental disabilities
eating disorders and body image
health psychology
HIV/AIDS prevention and therapy
individual, couples, family, and group therapy
neuropsychological assessment
personality assessment
personality disorders
psychopathology of childhood
psychosocial rehabilitation
psychotherapy supervision
violence prevention

University of Hartford (Psy.D.)

Graduate Institute of Professional Psychology
103 Woodland Street, 4th Floor
Hartford, CT 06105
phone#: (860) 520-1147/51
e-mail: owahl@uhavax.hartford.edu
Web address: http://www.hartford.edu/gipp

1	**2**	3	4	5	6	7

Clinically oriented   Equal emphasis   Research oriented

What percentage of your faculty subscribes to or practices in each of the following orientations?

Psychodynamic/Psychoanalytic	32%
Applied behavioral analysis/Radical behavioral	16%
Family systems/Systems	16%
Existential/Phenomenological/Humanistic	16%
Cognitive/Cognitive-behavioral	16%

What percentage of students applying for internship last year was accepted into APPIC-member internships?
Data not available

What courses are required for incoming students to have completed prior to enrolling?
None

Are there courses you recommend that are not mandatory?
Psychology major, abnormal, social, research methods/experimental, personality theory, developmental, statistics

GRE mean
Data not available

GPA mean
Data not available

Number of applications/admission offers/incoming students in 2003
170 applied/62 admission offers/28 incoming

% of students receiving:
Tuition waiver only: 0%
Assistantship/fellowship only: 64%
Both tuition waiver & assistantship/fellowship: 0%

Approximate percentage of incoming students who entered with a B.A./B.S. only: 71%   **Master's:** 29%

Approximate percentage of students who are Women: 74%   **Ethnic Minority:** 21%
International: Data not available

Average years to complete the doctoral program (including internship): 5.5 years

Personal interview
Required in person (unless international students)

Research areas	# Faculty	# Grants
adolescent	1	0
aesthetics of therapy	1	1
community treatment	1	0
group therapy (therapist orientation)	1	0
mentoring women students	2	0
mother–daughter relationships	1	0
therapist–client match	1	0
therapy termination	1	0

Clinical opportunities
acute psychiatry/mental health
anxiety disorders
chronically mentally ill
mentally retarded adults
obsessive–compulsive disorder
70 other sites, including community mental health centers, hospital-based psychology departments, and residential schools

University of Hawaii at Manoa

Department of Psychology
2430 Campus Road
Honolulu, HI 96822
phone#: (808) 956-7644
e-mail: (Charles Mueller, Director) cmueller@hawaii.edu
(Vicky Keogh, Secretary) ckeough@hawaii.edu
Web address: http://www.psychology.hawaii.edu/
forms_manuals/clinical.pdf

1	2	3	4	5	**6**	7

Clinically oriented	Equal emphasis	Research oriented

What percentage of your faculty subscribes to or practices in each of the following orientations?

Psychodynamic/Psychoanalytic	0%
Behavioral	50%
Family systems/Systems	15%
Existential/Phenomenological/Humanistic	0%
Cognitive/Cognitive-behavioral	85%

What percentage of students applying for internship last year was accepted into APPIC-member internships? 80%

What courses are required for incoming students to have completed prior to enrolling?
Psychology major or approximately 5–10 selected psychology courses

Are there courses you recommend that are not mandatory?
No

GRE mean
Verbal 640   Quantitative 700
Advanced Psychology No longer required
Analytical Writing 5.0

GPA mean
Overall GPA 3.58

Number of applications/admission offers/incoming students in 2004
135 applied/11 admission offers/9 incoming

% of students receiving:
Tuition waiver only: 0%
Assistantship/fellowship only: 0%
Both tuition waiver & assistantship/fellowship: 100%

Approximate percentage of incoming students who entered with a B.A./B.S. only: 67%   **Master's:** 33%

Approximate percentage of students who are Women: 85%   **Ethnic Minority:** 41%   **International:** 12.3%

Average years to complete the doctoral program (including internship): 7 years

Personal interview
Telephone required

Research areas	# Faculty	# Grants
anxiety	1	1
assessment	7	2
behavioral medicine	1	0
childhood clinical	3	4
cross-cultural	2	1
data-based case management	2	0
depression	2	0
eating disorders	2	0
ethnic minority	2	2
health care compliance	2	0
mental health systems	5	6
neurocognitive assessment	1	0
schizophrenia	5	1
substance use prevention	1	3
treatment outcome	4	4

Clinical opportunities
assessment
behavioral medicine
case and system consultation
child clinical
cross-cultural
developmental disabilities
dual diagnoses
eating disorders
neuropsychology
rehabilitation psychology
severely mentally ill
substance use prevention

University of Houston

Department of Psychology
126 Heyne Building
Houston, TX 77204-5022
phone#: (713) 743-8600
e-mail: jvincent@uh.edu
Web address: http://www.Psychology.uh.edu/
GraduatePrograms/Clinical/

1	2	3	**4**	5	6	7

Clinically oriented	Equal emphasis	Research oriented

What percentage of your faculty subscribes to or practices in each of the following orientations?

Psychodynamic/Psychoanalytic	6%
Applied behavioral analysis/Radical behavioral	5%
Family systems/Systems	20%
Existential/Phenomenological/Humanistic	0%
Cognitive/Cognitive-behavioral	100%

What percentage of students applying for internship last year was accepted into APPIC-member internships? 88%

What courses are required for incoming students to have completed prior to enrolling?
None

Are there courses you recommend that are not mandatory?
Statistics, introductory psychology, history and systems, physiological psychology, abnormal psychology, experimental, social psychology, developmental psychology, methods

GRE mean
Verbal 600   Quantitative 720   Analytical 750
Analytical Writing 5.0

GPA mean
Overall GPA 3.7

Number of applications/admission offers/incoming students in 2005
203 applied/30 admission offers/12 incoming

% of students receiving:
Tuition waiver only: 0%
Assistantship/fellowship only: 10%
Both tuition waiver & assistantship/fellowship: 100%

Approximate percentage of incoming students who entered with a B.A./B.S. only: 91.7%   **Master's:** 8.3%

Approximate percentage of students who are Women: 67%   **Ethnic Minority:** 16.7%   **International:** 3%

Average years to complete the doctoral program (including internship): Data not available

Personal interview
Preferred in person but telephone acceptable

Research areas	# Faculty	# Grants
adult psychopathology	6	3
affective disorder/depression	3	1
anxiety disorder	3	1
child clinical	3	2
chronic mental illness	3	1
cross-cultural	3	2
family research/therapy	3	2
forensic psychology	2	1
marriage/couples	2	1
neuropsychology	3	3
parent–child interaction	2	1
schizophrenia/psychoses	2	1
social skills	4	2

Clinical opportunities
adolescent suicide
Alzheimer's/dementia
anxiety disorders
child custody evaluation
child depression/anxiety
child victimization
clinical assessment
cognitive therapy
conduct disorder
couples therapy
domestic violence
family therapy
forensic psychology
health psychology
interpersonal psychotherapy
learning disabilities
multicultural
post traumatic stress disorder
rehabilitation
neuropsychology
schizophrenia/psychoses
traumatic brain injury
stroke

Howard University
Department of Psychology
520 Bryant Street, NW
Washington, DC 20059
phone#: (202) 806-6805
e-mail: olewis-jack@howard.edu
Web address: http://www.founders.howard.edu/
psychology-dept/Clinical%20Program%2020050412.html

1	2	3	**4**	5	6	7
Clinically oriented		Equal emphasis			Research oriented	

What percentage of your faculty subscribes to or practices in each of the following orientations?

Psychodynamic/Psychoanalytic	30%
Applied behavioral analysis/Radical behavioral	0%
Family systems/Systems	20%
Existential/Phenomenological/Humanistic	20%
Cognitive/Cognitive-behavioral	30%

What percentage of students applying for internship last year was accepted into APPIC-member internships?
Data not available

What courses are required for incoming students to have completed prior to enrolling?
Psychology major, including the following: introductory psychology, statistics, abnormal psychology, experimental psychology, developmental psychology

Are there courses you recommend that are not mandatory?
Yes, Psychological Testing or Statistics 11

GRE mean
Note: Required but not used for admission
Verbal 450   Quantitative 450
Analytical Writing Data not available

GPA mean
Data not available

Number of applications/admission offers/incoming students in 2003
175 applied/9 admission offers/8 incoming

% of students receiving:
Tuition waiver only: 0%
Assistantship/fellowship only: 12%
Both tuition waiver & assistantship/fellowship: 10%

Approximate percentage of incoming students who entered with a B.A./B.S. only: 50%   **Master's:** 50%

Approximate percentage of students who are Women: 80%   **Ethnic Minority:** 95%
International: Data not available

Average years to complete the doctoral program (including internship): 6 years

Personal interview
Preferred in person but telephone acceptable

Research areas	# Faculty	# Grants
adolescent development	3	2
behavioral medicine	3	3

clinical training	6	0
family therapy	2	0
minority mental health	4	4
neuropsychology	2	2
psychophysiology	1	0
suicide prevention	1	0

Clinical opportunities
anxiety disorders
behavioral medicine
child violence prevention
community psychology
crisis intervention
diagnosis and treatment of substance use disorders
family
minority
neuropsychology
psychoneuroimmunology
schizophrenia
victim/battering

Idaho State University

Psychology Department
Box 8112
Idaho State University
Pocatello ID 83209
phone#: (208) 282-2462
e-mail: robemark@isu.edu
Web address: http://www.isu.edu/departments/psych/
clinicalprogram.shtml

1	2	3	**4**	5	6	7

Clinically oriented   Equal emphasis   Research oriented

What percentage of your faculty subscribes to or practices in each of the following orientations?

Psychodynamic/Psychoanalytic	10%
Applied behavioral analysis/Radical behavioral	10%
Family systems/Systems	100%
Existential/Phenomenological/Humanistic	60%
Cognitive/Cognitive-behavioral	100%

What percentage of students applying for internship last year was accepted into APPIC-member internships? 71%

What courses are required for incoming students to have completed prior to enrolling?
Psychology major or its equivalent. The stronger the major, the better, i.e., methodology courses plus undergraduate courses in the major areas: history and systems, developmental, cognitive/learning, social, physiological, and personality. The methodology courses are mandatory.

Are there courses you recommend that are not mandatory?
—

GRE mean
Verbal 552   Quantitative 642
Analytical Writing 5.3
Advanced Psychology 624

GPA mean
Overall GPA 3.80

Number of applications/admission offers/incoming students in 2005
76 applied/10 admission offers/5 incoming

% of students receiving:
Tuition waiver only: 0%
Assistantship/fellowship only: 35%
Both tuition waiver & assistantship/fellowship: 61%

Approximate percentage of incoming students who entered with a B.A./B.S. only: 100%   **Master's:** 0%

Approximate percentage of students who are Women: 83%   **Ethnic Minority:** 9%   **International:** 20%

Average years to complete the doctoral program (including internship): 6.2 years

Personal interview
Preferred in person but telephone acceptable

Research areas	# Faculty	# Grants
addictions	2	0
behavioral pharmocology	1	2
developmental psychopathology	1	1
mood and decision making	1	0
parent–child interaction therapy	1	0
sexual assault	1	1
trauma	2	1
working memory	1	0

Clinical opportunities
cognitive-behavioral marital therapy
cognitive behavioral treatments for anxiety & trauma
family systems therapy
parent–child interaction therapy
relapse prevention group therapy (addictions)

University of Illinois at Chicago

Department of Psychology
1007 West Harrison
Chicago, IL 60680
phone#: (312) 996-1469
e-mail: robinm@uic.edu
Web address: http://www3.psch.uic.edu/
clinicalprog.asp?sm=clinical_program

1	2	3	4	5	**6**	7

Clinically oriented   Equal emphasis   Research oriented

What percentage of your faculty subscribes to or practices in each of the following orientations?

Psychodynamic/Psychoanalytic	0%
Applied behavioral analysis/Radical behavioral	5%
Family systems/Systems	15%
Existential/Phenomenological/Humanistic	0%
Cognitive/Cognitive-behavioral	80%
Community psychology	40%

What percentage of students applying for internship last year was accepted into APPIC-member internships? 100%

What courses are required for incoming students to have completed prior to enrolling?
None

Are there courses you recommend that are not mandatory?
Statistics, science courses, independent research (for psychology majors), other research experience

GRE mean
Verbal 625 Quantitative 743
Advanced Psychology 725
Analytical Writing 5.6

GPA mean
Psychology GPA (not available) Junior/Senior GPA 3.66 (M)

Number of applications/admission offers/incoming students in 2004
181 applied/7 admission offers/3 incoming

% of students receiving:
Tuition waiver only: 0%
Assistantship/fellowship only: 0%
Both tuition waiver & assistantship/fellowship: 100%

Approximate percentage of incoming students who entered with a B.A./B.S. only: 80% **Master's:** 20%

Approximate percentage of students who are Women: 83% **Ethnic Minority:** 18% **International:** 17%

Average years to complete the doctoral program (including internship): 7 years

Personal interview
Preferred in person but telephone acceptable

Research areas	# Faculty	# Grants
AIDS	1	1
alcohol relapse, models of relapse	1	0
anxiety	1	0
cognitive deficits in schizophrenia	1	4
community psychology	2	1
depression	1	0
eating disorders and obesity	1	0
health behavior change	4	1
neurobehavioral and genetic aspects of autism	1	4
tobacco use, etiology, prevention and cessation	3	5

Clinical opportunities
adjustment reactions
anxiety and depression
health-related behaviors
HIV prevention
preventive intervention with youth
smoking cessation
weight reduction

University of Illinois at Urbana–Champaign

Department of Psychology
Psychology Building
603 East Daniel Street
Champaign, IL 61820
phone#: (217) 333-2169
e-mail: gradstdy@s.psych.uiuc.edu
Web address: http://www.psych.uiuc.edu/divisions/clinicalcommunity.php

1	2	3	4	5	**6**	7

Clinically oriented   Equal emphasis   Research oriented

What percentage of your faculty subscribes to or practices in each of the following orientations?

Psychodynamic/Psychoanalytic	18%
Applied behavioral analysis/Radical behavioral	18%
Family systems/Systems	27%
Existential/Phenomenological/Humanistic	27%
Cognitive/Cognitive-behavioral	63%

What percentage of students applying for internship last year was accepted into APPIC-member internships? 80%

What courses are required for incoming students to have completed prior to enrolling?
None

Are there courses you recommend that are not mandatory?
Psychology major, undergraduate statistics

GRE mean
Verbal 555 Quantitative 695 Subject 720
Analytical Writing 5.1

GPA mean
Overall GPA 3.84

Number of applications/admission offers/incoming students in 2005
126 applied/19 admission offers/11 incoming

% of students receiving:
Tuition waiver only: 0%
Assistantship/fellowship only: 0%
Both tuition waiver & assistantship/fellowship: 100%

Approximate percentage of incoming students who entered with a B.A./B.S. only: 100% **Master's:** 0%

Approximate percentage of students who are Women: 78% **Ethnic Minority:** 45% **International:** 6%

Average years to complete the doctoral program (including internship): 7.5 years

Personal interview
Telephone required

Research areas	# Faculty	# Grants
behavior genetics	1	0
children, law, and mental health policy	3	1
clinical neuropsychology	2	1
clinical psychophysiology	2	1

community psychology	4	1
emotion and psychopathology	5	3
marital/family/child	3	1
minority mental health	3	0
minority populations/mentoring	2	0
mutual-help organizations	1	0
psychotherapy/systems	1	0
schizophrenia	2	0
women's issues	3	2

Clinical opportunities
anxiety
child assessment
child protective services
community & economic development
community psychology
custody evaluations
feminist and women's issues
forensic evaluations
group therapy
individual adult psychotherapy
inpatient assessment/psychosis
juvenile justice services
marital and family/therapy
mutual-help organizations
neighborhood organization
neuropsychological assessment
school consultation
school and educational settings and policy
voluntary organizations

Illinois Institute of Technology

Department of Psychology
IIT Center, LS252
Chicago, IL 60616
phone#: (312) 562-3503, 567-3500
e-mail: myoung@charlie.cns.iit.edu or youngm@iit.edu
Web address: http://www.iit.edu/colleges/psych/current/
progs/clinical/clinical.html

1	2	**3**	4	5	6	7
Clinically oriented		Equal emphasis			Research oriented	

What percentage of your faculty subscribes to or practices in each of the following orientations?

Psychodynamic/Psychoanalytic	0%
Applied behavioral analysis/Radical behavioral	0%
Family systems/Systems	10%
Existential/Phenomenological/Humanistic	0%
Cognitive/Cognitive-behavioral	90%

What percentage of students applying for internship last year was accepted into APPIC-member internships? 92%

What courses are required for incoming students to have completed prior to enrolling?
18 credits in psychology including experimental and statistics

Are there courses you recommend that are not mandatory?
No

GRE mean
Verbal 540   Quantitative 620
Analytical Writing Data not available

GPA mean
Overall GPA 3.6

Number of applications/admission offers/incoming students in 2003
90 applied/25 admission offers/13 incoming

% of students receiving:
Tuition waiver only: 7%
Assistantship/fellowship only: 70%
Both tuition waiver & assistantship/fellowship: 0%

Approximate percentage of incoming students who entered with a B.A./B.S. only: 80%   **Master's:** 20%

Approximate percentage of students who are Women: 80%   **Ethnic Minority:** 17%   **International:** 6%

Average years to complete the doctoral program (including internship): 5.5 years

Personal interview
Preferred in person but telephone acceptable

Research areas	# Faculty	# Grants
ADHD	1	0
affective disorders	1	1
child behavior	2	1
family	1	0
health	1	1
marital	1	1
pediatric	2	1
severe mental illness	2	1
social support	1	0
sports psychology	1	0
rehabilitation	2	1

Clinical opportunities
affective disorders
child
family
health/behavioral medicine
marital/couples
minority/cross-cultural
neuropsychology
pain
severe mental illness

Immaculata College (Psy.D.)

Department of Graduate Psychology
Immaculata, PA 19345-0500
phone#: (610) 647-4400, ext. 3503
e-mail: jyalof@immaculata.edu
Web address: http://www.immaculata.edu/Academics/
Departments/Graduate%20Psychology/
Psy.D.%20in%20Clinical%20Psychology.htm

1	**2**	3	4	5	6	7
Clinically oriented		Equal emphasis			Research oriented	

What percentage of your faculty subscribes to or practices in each of the following orientations?

Psychodynamic/Psychoanalytic	75%
Applied behavioral analysis/Radical behavioral	0%
Family systems/Systems	0%
Existential/Phenomenological/Humanistic	25%
Cognitive/Cognitive-behavioral	0%

What percentage of students applying for internship last year was accepted into APPIC-member internships?
Data not available

What courses are required for incoming students to have completed prior to enrolling?
Need M.A. in clinical or allied field, preferably

Are there courses you recommend that are not mandatory?
—

GRE mean
Verbal 600   Quantitative 600

GPA mean
Overall GPA 3.5

Number of applications/admission offers/incoming students in 2003
67 applied/31 admission offers/23 incoming

% of students receiving:
Tuition waiver only: 0%
Assistantship/fellowship only: 0%
Both tuition waiver & assistantship/fellowship: 0%

Approximate percentage of incoming students who entered with a B.A./B.S. only: 26%   **Master's:** 74%

Approximate percentage of students who are Women: 77%   **Ethnic Minority:** 9%
International: Data not available

Average years to complete the doctoral program (including internship): 6 years

Personal interview
No preference given

Research areas	# Faculty	# Grants
child, adolescent	2	0
development	3	0
existential-humanistic	2	0
gender	3	0
psychotherapy process	1	0
parenting	2	0
resilience and hopefulness	2	0
Rorschach	2	0
school psychology	2	0
sexism	2	0

Clinical opportunities
—

Indiana State University (Psy.D.)

Department of Psychology
Root Hall
Terre Haute, IN 47809
phone#: (812) 237-4314
e-mail: lizo@indstate.edu
Web address:
http://www.indstate.edu/psych/doctoral_prog.htm

1	2	3	**4**	5	6	7
Clinically oriented		Equal emphasis			Research oriented	

What percentage of your faculty subscribes to or practices in each of the following orientations?

Psychodynamic/Psychoanalytic	15%
Applied behavioral analysis/Radical behavioral	0%
Family systems/Systems	15%
Existential/Phenomenological/Humanistic	5%
Cognitive/Cognitive-behavioral	70%

What percentage of students applying for internship last year was accepted into APPIC-member internships? 100%

What courses are required for incoming students to have completed prior to enrolling?
Introductory psychology, abnormal psychology, personality, experimental psychology, statistics, learning or cognition (24 credits in undergraduate psychology)

Are there courses you recommend that are not mandatory?
Physiological psychology

GRE mean
Data not available   Analytical Writing 5.0

GPA mean
Data not available

Number of applications/admission offers/incoming students in 2004
140 applied/8 admission offers/8 incoming

% of students receiving:
Tuition waiver only: 0%
Assistantship/fellowship only: 0%
Both tuition waiver & assistantship/fellowship: 100%

Approximate percentage of incoming students who entered with a B.A./B.S. only: 80%   **Master's:** 20%

Approximate percentage of students who are Women: 70%   **Ethnic Minority:** 20%   **International:** 5%

Average years to complete the doctoral program (including internship): 5.5 years

Personal interview
Preferred in person but telephone acceptable

Research areas	# Faculty	# Grants
adult psychopathology	2	0
affective disorders/depression	2	0
anxiety disorders	0	0
assessment	2	0
behavioral medicine	3	1
child clinical psychopathology	1	0

clinical judgment	1	0
eating disorders	2	1
friendship/relationships/intimacy	1	0
gender roles	3	0
organizational/industrial	1	1
personality disorders	1	0
professional training	1	0
stress and coping	2	0
substance abuse	1	1
women's studies	2	0

Clinical opportunities
ADHD assessment/treatment
behavioral medicine
forensic psychology
rural psychology

Indiana University

Department of Psychology
Bloomington, IN 47405
phone#: (812) 855-2311
e-mail: shiricha@indiana.edu
Web address: http://www.indiana.edu/%7Eclinpsy/

1	2	3	4	5	6	**7**

Clinically oriented   Equal emphasis   Research oriented

What percentage of your faculty subscribes to or practices in each of the following orientations?
Psychodynamic/Psychoanalytic 0%
Applied behavioral analysis/Radical behavioral 0%
Family systems/Systems 100%
Existential/Phenomenological/Humanistic 0%
Cognitive/Cognitive-behavioral 100%
Note: Our faculty doesn't really have particular "orientations" apart from an "empirical science" commitment.

What percentage of students applying for internship last year was accepted into APPIC-member internships?
Data not available

What courses are required for incoming students to have completed prior to enrolling?
Psychology major

Are there courses you recommend that are not mandatory?
Basic sciences, math

GRE mean
Data not available

GPA mean
Data not available

Number of applications/admission offers/incoming students in 2003
73 applied/6 admission offers/3 incoming

% of students receiving:
Tuition waiver only: 0%
Assistantship/fellowship only: 0%
Both tuition waiver & assistantship/fellowship: 100%

Approximate percentage of incoming students who entered with a B.A./B.S. only: 100%   **Master's:** 0%

Approximate percentage of students who are Women: 75%   **Ethnic Minority:** 32%
International: Data not available

Average years to complete the doctoral program (including internship): 6.2 years

Personal interview
Preferred in person but telephone acceptable

Research areas	# Faculty	# Grants
alcoholism/psychophysiology	1	1
behavioral genetics	4	2
child health interventions	1	1
childhood/temperament/family	3	3
health psychology	5	4
marital violence	1	1
mathematical models of causality	2	1
obsessive–compulsive disorder	2	0
schizophrenia	2	2
social information processing and social interaction	3	1

Clinical opportunities
anxiety disorders
assessment of health-related family adjustment problems
child and family therapy
depression
marital violence/marital therapy
neuropsychology
obsessive–compulsive disorder
schizophrenia
school/Head Start consultation
sexual dysfunction
smoking cessation

Indiana University of Pennsylvania (Psy.D.)

Department of Psychology
201 Uhler Hall
Indiana, PA 15705
phone#: (412) 357-4519
e-mail: goodwin@iup.edu
Web address: http://www.iup.edu/psychology/PsyD/

1	2	**3**	4	5	6	7

Clinically oriented   Equal emphasis   Research oriented

What percentage of your faculty subscribes to or practices in each of the following orientations?
Psychodynamic/Psychoanalytic 0%
Applied behavioral analysis/Radical behavioral 35%
Family systems/Systems 22%
Existential/Phenomenological/Humanistic 5%
Cognitive/Cognitive-behavioral 38%

What percentage of students applying for internship last year was accepted into APPIC-member internships? 100%

What courses are required for incoming students to have completed prior to enrolling?

Introductory psychology, personality, statistics or methods, abnormal psychology, learning, social psychology

Are there courses you recommend that are not mandatory?

6 credits in other areas of psychology

GRE mean

Verbal 500   Quantitative 500
Advanced Psychology 500

GPA mean

Overall GPA 3.0   Psychology GPA 3.0
Junior/Senior GPA 3.0

Number of applications/admission offers/incoming students in 2005

122 applied/25 admission offers/11 incoming

% of students receiving:

Tuition waiver only: 0%
Assistantship/fellowship only: 0%
Both tuition waiver & assistantship/fellowship: 100%

Approximate percentage of incoming students who entered with a B.A./B.S. only: 72%   **Master's:** 18%

Approximate percentage of students who are Women: 78%   **Ethnic Minority:** 9%   **International:** 9%

Average years to complete the doctoral program (including internship): 5 years

Personal interview

Required in person

Research areas	# Faculty	# Grants
abortion	1	0
aging	1	0
behavioral medicine	1	0
clinical judgment	1	0
cross-cultural	2	0
death and dying	1	0
ethical issues	1	0
family therapy	3	0
gender roles	1	0
minority mental health	1	0
parent–child	1	0
prevention	1	0
professional issues	1	0
psychopathology	1	0
psychopharmacology	1	0
women's studies	3	0

Clinical opportunities

assessment
behavioral medicine
family therapy
intake interviews
stress and habit disorders

Indiana University–Purdue University Indianapolis

Clinical Rehabilitation Ph.D. Program
402 North Blackford Street, LD124
Indianapolis, IN 46202-3275
phone#: (317) 274-6945
e-mail: gradpsy@IUPUI.edu
Web address: http://www.psynt.iupui.edu/

1	2	3	4	5	**6**	7

Clinically oriented   Equal emphasis   Research oriented

What percentage of your faculty subscribes to or practices in each of the following orientations?

Psychodynamic/Psychoanalytic	0%
Applied behavioral analysis/Radical behavioral	0%
Family systems/Systems	5%
Existential/Phenomenological/Humanistic	0%
Cognitive/Cognitive-behavioral	90%

What percentage of students applying for internship last year was accepted into APPIC-member internships? 60%

What courses are required for incoming students to have completed prior to enrolling?

Tests and measurements, statistics, physiology, abnormal psychology

Are there courses you recommend that are not mandatory?

No

GRE mean

Verbal 515   Quantitative 635
Analytical Writing 5.28

GPA mean

Overall GPA 3.2

Number of applications/admission offers/incoming students in 2004

30 applied/7 admission offers/3 incoming

% of students receiving:

Tuition waiver only: 100%
Assistantship/fellowship only: 100%
Both tuition waiver & assistantship/fellowship: 100%

Approximate percentage of incoming students who entered with a B.A./B.S. only: 100%   **Master's:** 0%

Approximate percentage of students who are Women: 78%   **Ethnic Minority:** 17%   **International:** 9%

Average years to complete the doctoral program (including internship): 7 years

Personal interview

Required in person

Research areas	# Faculty	# Grants
health psychology	3	1
neuropsychology	2	2–3
psychobiology	3	5–6
severe mental illness	2	3–4

Clinical opportunities
adaptive educational services (students with disabilities)
adult behavioral medicine (community cancer care)
crisis intervention unit (Wishard)
hospice
neuropsychological assessment
neurorehabilitation intervention
pediatric behavioral medicine
severe mental illness
women's prison—female offenders with psychiatric
   and medical problems

University of Indianapolis (Psy.D.)

School of Psychological Sciences
1400 East Hanna Avenue
Good Hall Room 109
Indianapolis, IN 46227-3697
phone#: (317) 788-3353
e-mail: ddowning@uindy.edu or rholigrocki@uindy.edu
Web address: http://psych.uindy.edu/psyd/index.php

1	2	**3**	4	5	6	7
Clinically oriented		Equal emphasis			Research oriented	

What percentage of your faculty subscribes to or practices in each of the following orientations?

Psychodynamic/Psychoanalytic	25%
Applied behavioral analysis/Radical behavioral	12.5%
Family systems/Systems	12.5%
Existential/Phenomenological/Humanistic	12.5%
Cognitive/Cognitive-behavioral	37.5%

What percentage of students applying for internship last year was accepted into APPIC-member internships? 8%

What courses are required for incoming students to have completed prior to enrolling?
18 credit hours of psychology

Are there courses you recommend that are not mandatory?
Abnormal psychology, child/development, statistics, personality

GRE mean
Verbal 511.6   Quantitative 591.5
Advanced Psychology 624.4
Analytical Writing 4.8

GPA mean
Overall GPA 3.69

Number of applications/admission offers/incoming students in 2005
145 applied/50 admission offers/25 incoming

% of students receiving:
Tuition waiver only: 8%
Assistantship/fellowship only: 16%
Both tuition waiver & assistantship/fellowship: 0%

Approximate percentage of incoming students who entered with a B.A./B.S. only: 88%   **Master's:** 12%

Approximate percentage of students who are
Women: 88%   **Ethnic Minority:** 4%   **International:** 0%

Average years to complete the doctoral program (including internship): 5 years

Personal interview
Preferred in person but telephone acceptable

Research areas	# Faculty	# Grants
adult sibling relationships	1	1
child/family treatment outcome	1	0
intimate relationships	1	0
memory	1	0
multicultural mental health	2	1
parent–child relationships	1	1
posttraumatic stress disorders	1	0

Clinical opportunities
assessment
behavioral medicine
child/adolescent
forensics/prison populations
neuropsychological assessment
pain management
VA medical centers/hospitals

University of Iowa

Department of Psychology
E-11 Seashore Hall
Iowa City, IA 52242-1407
phone#: (319) 335-2406
e-mail: mike-ohara@uiowa.edu
Web address:
http://www.psychology.uiowa.edu/training3.html

1	2	3	4	5	**6**	7
Clinically oriented		Equal emphasis			Research oriented	

What percentage of your faculty subscribes to or practices in each of the following orientations?

Psychodynamic/Psychoanalytic	0%
Applied behavioral analysis/Radical behavioral	0%
Family systems/Systems	0%
Existential/Phenomenological/Humanistic	0%
Cognitive/Cognitive-behavioral	100%

What percentage of students applying for internship last year was accepted into APPIC-member internships? 100%

What courses are required for incoming students to have completed prior to enrolling?
None

Are there courses you recommend that are not mandatory?
Undergraduate psychology major, statistics, abnormal psychology, laboratory research, strong science background

GRE mean
Verbal 650   Quantitative 700
Analytical Writing 5.2

GPA mean
Overall GPA 3.7   Psychology GPA 3.7
Junior/Senior GPA 3.7

Number of applications/admission offers/incoming students in 2005
132 applied/13 admission offers/12 incoming

% of students receiving:
Tuition waiver only: 0%
Assistantship/fellowship only: 58%
Both tuition waiver & assistantship/fellowship: 42%

Approximate percentage of incoming students who entered with a B.A./B.S. only: 92%   **Master's:** 8%

Approximate percentage of students who are Women: 82%   **Ethnic Minority:** 13%   **International:** 5%

Average years to complete the doctoral program (including internship): 7 years

Personal interview
Preferred in person but telephone acceptable

Research areas	# Faculty	# Grants
assessment	1	0
child abuse	2	2
deafness	1	0
depression	2	2
eating disorders	1	1
health psychology/behavioral medicine	3	3
marital therapy	1	0
personality disorders	1	1
psychophysiology	1	0
substance abuse	1	0

Clinical opportunities
abuse
adult psychiatry
child psychiatry/pediatrics
cognitive-behavioral therapy
deafness
depression
eating disorders
health psychology/behavioral medicine
infancy/postpartum
neuropsychology

Jackson State University

Department of Psychology
Clinical Psychology Ph.D. Program
P.O. Box 17550
Jackson, MS 39216-0350
phone#: (601) 979-5990
e-mail: cassisi@att.net
Web address:
http://www.jsums.edu/%7Epsycdept/grad/index.htm

1	2	3	4	**5**	6	7

Clinically oriented   Equal emphasis   Research oriented

What percentage of your faculty subscribes to or practices in each of the following orientations?
Psychodynamic/Psychoanalytic   10%
Applied behavioral analysis/Radical behavioral   0%
Family systems/Systems   0%
Existential/Phenomenological/Humanistic   0%
Cognitive/Cognitive-behavioral   90%

What percentage of students applying for internship last year was accepted into APPIC-member internships?
Data not available

What courses are required for incoming students to have completed prior to enrolling?
24 hours of previous coursework in psychology is required

Are there courses you recommend that are not mandatory?
Experimental, learning, statistics, physiological, abnormal

GRE mean
Verbal 490   Quantitative 460
Analytical Writing 4.0

GPA mean
Data not available

Number of applications/admission offers/incoming students in 2003
42 applied/9 admission offers/8 incoming

% of students receiving:
Tuition waiver only: 5%
Assistantship/fellowship only: 80%
Both tuition waiver & assistantship/fellowship: 5%

Approximate percentage of incoming students who entered with a B.A./B.S. only: 60%   **Master's:** 30%

Approximate percentage of students who are Women: 75%   **Ethnic Minority:** 60%
International: Data not available

Average years to complete the doctoral program (including internship): 7 years

Personal interview
Preferred in person but telephone acceptable

Research areas	# Faculty	# Grants
alcohol/substance abuse	2	0
childhood obesity	1	0
chronic pain/headache	3	1
depression	1	0
health care disparities	3	0
HIV/AIDS	3	3
posttraumatic stress disorder	1	0
psychological assessment	6	0
stigma	2	0

Clinical opportunities
behavioral medicine
campus counseling center
forensic
inpatient pediatric
inpatient psychiatric
neuropsychiatric rehab
outpatient pediatric
outpatient psychiatric

University of Kansas

Clinical Child Psychology Program
2010 Dole Human Development Center
University of Kansas
100 Sunnyside Avenue
Lawrence, KS 66045
phone#: (785) 864-4226
e-mail: clchild@ku.edu
Web address:
http://www.psych.ku.edu/clinical_home.html

1	2	3	**4**	5	6	7

Clinically oriented   Equal emphasis   Research oriented

What percentage of your faculty subscribes to or practices in each of the following orientations?

Psychodynamic/Psychoanalytic	5%
Applied behavioral analysis/Radical behavioral	5%
Family systems/Systems	25%
Existential/Phenomenological/Humanistic	5%
Cognitive/Cognitive-behavioral	60%

What percentage of students applying for internship last year was accepted into APPIC-member internships? 100%

What courses are required for incoming students to have completed prior to enrolling?

Major in psychology or a minimum of 15–18 hours including: research methods, statistics, developmental/child psychology, developmental psychopathology (abnormal child psychology) or Advanced Psychology GRE

Are there courses you recommend that are not mandatory?

None

GRE mean

Verbal 700   Quantitative 614
Analytical Writing Data not available

GPA mean

Overall GPA 3.86

Number of applications/admission offers/incoming students in 2005

126 applied/3 admission offers/3 incoming

% of students receiving:

Tuition waiver only: 0%
Assistantship/fellowship only: 25%
Both tuition waiver & assistantship/fellowship: 75%

Approximate percentage of incoming students who entered with a B.A./B.S. only: 75%   **Master's:** 25%

Approximate percentage of students who are Women: 58%   **Ethnic Minority:** 33%   **International:** 0%

Average years to complete the doctoral program (including internship): 6.5 years

Personal interview

Preferred in person but telephone acceptable

Research areas	# Faculty	# Grants
children with chronic illness (adherence/adjustment/functioning)	2	1
disasters and children	2	1
domestic violence	1	0
ethnicity/cultural issues	3	0
health promotion	2	1
school-based services for serious emotional disorders	2	1
stress & coping	2	1
violence and children (bullying)	2	1

Clinical opportunities

community mental health center
early in-home intervention
intensive services for serious emotional disorders
pediatric psychology

Kent State University

Department of Psychology
Kent, OH 44242
phone#: (330) 672-2166
e-mail: gradpsyc@kent.edu
Web address: http://dept.kent.edu/psychology/
gradprograms/clinical.htm

1	2	3	4	**5**	6	7

Clinically oriented   Equal emphasis   Research oriented

What percentage of your faculty subscribes to or practices in each of the following orientations?

Psychodynamic/Psychoanalytic	25%
Applied behavioral analysis/Radical behavioral	15%
Family systems/Systems	10%
Existential/Phenomenological/Humanistic	0%
Cognitive/Cognitive-behavioral	50%

What percentage of students applying for internship last year was accepted into APPIC-member internships? 92%

What courses are required for incoming students to have completed prior to enrolling?

None

Are there courses you recommend that are not mandatory?

Prefer 15–20 hours in psychology, including 1–2 statistics courses and at least 1 psychology class, which has a lab associated with it

GRE mean

Verbal 613   Quantitative 702
Analytical Writing Not used

GPA mean

Overall GPA 3.66

Number of applications/admission offers/incoming students in 2005

221 applied/19 admission offers/12 incoming

% of students receiving:

Tuition waiver only: 0%
Assistantship/fellowship only: 0%
Both tuition waiver & assistantship/fellowship: 100%

Approximate percentage of incoming students who entered with a B.A./B.S. only: 89%   **Master's:** 11%

Approximate percentage of students who are Women: 67%   **Ethnic Minority:** 12%   **International:** 10%

Average years to complete the doctoral program (including internship): 6 years

Personal interview
Preferred in person but telephone acceptable

Research areas	# Faculty	# Grants
AIDS	2	1
aggression	1	1
anxiety and depression	2	0
eating disorders	1	0
family research	2	2
gerontology	1	0
MMPI	2	2
schizophrenia	1	1
stress and coping	4	2

Clinical opportunities
child/family therapy
eating disorders
forensic assessments
health psychology
marital therapy
neuropsychology
objective personality assessment
schizophrenia

University of Kentucky

Department of Psychology
Kastle Hall
Lexington, KY 40506-0044
phone#: (859) 257-8662
e-mail: dlyna1@uky.edu
Web address: http://www.uky.edu/AS/Psychology/graduate/clinical.html

1	2	3	4	**5**	6	7

Clinically oriented   Equal emphasis   Research oriented

What percentage of your faculty subscribes to or practices in each of the following orientations?

Psychodynamic/Psychoanalytic	10%
Applied behavioral analysis/Radical behavioral	10%
Family systems/Systems	10%
Existential/Phenomenological/Humanistic	10%
Cognitive/Cognitive-behavioral	100%

What percentage of students applying for internship last year was accepted into APPIC-member internships? 100%

What courses are required for incoming students to have completed prior to enrolling?
Experimental methodology, statistics

Are there courses you recommend that are not mandatory?
Abnormal psychology, tests & measures, personality

GRE mean
Verbal 588   Quantitative 651
Analytical Writing Data not available

GPA mean
Overall GPA 3.59

Number of applications/admission offers/incoming students in 2005
177 applied/9 admission offers/9 incoming

% of students receiving:
Tuition waiver only: 0%
Assistantship/fellowship only: 0%
Both tuition waiver & assistantship/fellowship: 100%
First 4 years in program, in-state tuition is not always waived.

Approximate percentage of incoming students who entered with a B.A./B.S. only: 78%   **Master's:** 22%

Approximate percentage of students who are Women: 55%   **Ethnic Minority:** 22%   **International:** 5%

Average years to complete the doctoral program (including internship): 6.3 years

Personal interview
Preferred in person but telephone acceptable

Research areas	# Faculty	# Grants
adolescent development	2	1
adult psychopathology	4	3
assessment/diagnosis/classification	3	0
behavioral medicine	2	1
child clinical	3	1
developmental psychopathology	2	1
eating disorders	1	1
neuropsychology	2	1
pain	1	1
personality assessment	3	0
personality disorders	2	0
psychoneuroimmunology	1	1
psychophysiology	2	1
substance abuse	4	2
violence/agression	2	2

Clinical opportunities
assessment
behavioral medicine
child
chronic mental illness
cognitive-behavioral therapies
community mental health
dialectical behavior therapy
neuropsychology
orofacial pain

University of La Verne (Psy.D.)

Program in Clinical-Community Psychology
1950 Third Street
La Verne, CA 91750
phone#: (909) 593-3511 ext. 4413
email: BPerlmutter@ulv.edu
Web address: http://www.ulv.edu/psyd/

1	2	**3**	4	5	6	7

Clinically oriented	Equal emphasis	Research oriented

What percentage of your faculty subscribes to or practices in each of the following orientations?

Psychodynamic/Psychoanalytic	50%
Applied behavioral analysis/Radical behavioral	0%
Family systems/Systems	50%
Existential/Phenomenological/Humanistic	50%
Cognitive/Cognitive-behavioral	50%

What percentage of students applying for internship last year was accepted into APPIC-member internships?
Data not available

What courses are required for incoming students to have completed prior to enrolling?
Courses must include introductory psychology, statistics, experimental psychology or research methods, physiological psychology, and abnormal psychology. In addition, one course from among the following is required: history & systems, social psychology, theories of personality, human development, and clinical or community psychology.

Are there courses you recommend that are not mandatory?
No

GRE mean
Data not available

GPA mean
Overall GPA 3.51

Number of applications/admission offers/incoming students in 2005
84 applied/39 admission offers/18 incoming

% of students receiving:
(Partial) tuition waiver only: 0%
Assistantship/fellowship only: 33%
Both tuition waiver & assistantship/fellowship: 0%

Approximate percentage of incoming students who entered with a B.A./B.S. only: 83% **Master's:** 17%

Approximate percentage of students who are Women: 70% **Ethnic Minority:** 35% **International:** 10%

Average years to complete the doctoral program (including internship): 5 years

Personal interview
Data not available

Research areas	# Faculty	# Grants
multiculturalism	7	2
clinical forensics	2	0
community psychology	12	0
psychotherapy services	3	0
gender issues & sexuality	2	0
values and moral development	2	0

Clinical opportunities
children and adolescents
clinical forensics
college counseling center
families
HIV/AIDS
substance abuse
Multiple other specialty clinics are available to our students through clinical practica.

Loma Linda University (Ph.D.)

Department of Psychology
Loma Linda, CA 92350
phone#: (909) 558-8577 (Central Office)
e-mail: lortiz@univ.llu.edu
Web address: http://www.llu.edu/llu/grad/psychology

1	2	3	4	**5**	6	7

Clinically oriented	Equal emphasis	Research oriented

What percentage of your faculty subscribes to or practices in each of the following orientations?

Psychodynamic/Psychoanalytic	36%
Applied behavioral analysis/Radical behavioral	0%
Family systems/Systems	0%
Existential/Phenomenological/Humanistic	28%
Cognitive/Cognitive-behavioral	36%

What percentage of students applying for internship last year was accepted into APPIC-member internships?
Data not available

What courses are required for incoming students to have completed prior to enrolling?
History and systems, learning, personality, statistics, social psychology, developmental psychology, psychobiology

Are there courses you recommend that are not mandatory?
Computer literacy, math, research methods, sociology, biology

GRE mean
Data not available

GPA mean
Data not available

Number of applications/admission offers/incoming students in 2005
28 applied/12 admission offers/8 incoming

% of students receiving:
Tuition waiver only: 17%
Assistantship/fellowship only: 4%
Both tuition waiver & assistantship/fellowship: 0%

Approximate percentage of incoming students who entered with a B.A./B.S. only: 60%   **Master's:** 40%

Approximate percentage of students who are Women: 78%   **Ethnic Minority:** 46%
International: Data not available

Average years to complete the doctoral program (including internship): 6 years

Personal interview
Preferred in person but telephone acceptable

Research areas	# Faculty	# Grants
adult health psychology	4	2
anxiety disorders	1	0
childhood sexual abuse	2	0
conflict resolution	1	0
ethical decision making	1	0
neurodegenerative diseases	1	0
pediatric health psychology	1	2
posttraumatic stress disorder	2	0
psychobiology	2	0
psychology and religion	2	0
psychotherapy process outcomes	1	0
statistical methods	2	0

Clinical opportunities
adult behavioral medicine
community outpatient mental health
pediatric behavioral medicine

Loma Linda University (Psy.D.)

Department of Psychology
Loma Linda, CA 92350
phone#: (909) 558-8577 (central office)
e-mail: lortiz@psych.llu.edu
Web address: http://www.llu.edu/llu/grad/psychology

1	2	**3**	4	5	6	7

Clinically oriented   Equal emphasis   Research oriented

What percentage of your faculty subscribes to or practices in each of the following orientations?
Psychodynamic/Psychoanalytic   36%
Applied behavioral analysis/Radical behavioral   0%
Family systems/Systems   0%
Existential/Phenomenological/Humanistic   28%
Cognitive/Cognitive-behavioral   36%

What percentage of students applying for internship last year was accepted into APPIC-member internships?
Data not available

What courses are required for incoming students to have completed prior to enrolling?
History and systems, learning, personality, statistics, social psychology, developmental psychology, psychobiology

Are there courses you recommend that are not mandatory?
Computer literacy, math, sociology, biology

GRE mean
Data not available

GPA mean
Data not available

Number of applications/admission offers/incoming students in 2003
27 applied/16 admission offers/13 incoming

% of students receiving:
Tuition waiver only: 13%
Assistantship/fellowship only: 0%
Both tuition waiver & assistantship/fellowship: 0%

Approximate percentage of incoming students who entered with a B.A./B.S. only: 69%   **Master's:** 31%

Approximate percentage of students who are Women: 62%   **Ethnic Minority:** 23%
International: Data not available

Average years to complete the doctoral program (including internship): 5 years

Personal interview
Preferred in person but telephone acceptable

Research areas	# Faculty	# Grants
anxiety disorders	1	0
childhood sexual abuse	2	0
conflict resolution	1	0
ethical decision making	1	0
health psychology	4	2
neurodegenerative diseases	1	0
pediatric health psychology	1	2
posttraumatic stress disorder	2	0
psychobiology	2	0
psychology and religion	2	0
psychotherapy process outcome	1	0
statistics methods	2	0

Clinical opportunities
adult behavioral medicine
community outpatient
pediatric behavioral medicine

Long Island University

Department of Psychology
University Plaza
Brooklyn, NY 11201
phone#: (718) 488-1164
e-mail: nicholas.papouchis@liu.edu
Web address: http://www.brooklyn.liu.edu/psych/phdprogram/index.html

1	2	3	**4**	5	6	7

Clinically oriented   Equal emphasis   Research oriented

What percentage of your faculty subscribes to or practices in each of the following orientations?

Psychodynamic/Psychoanalytic	70%
Applied behavioral analysis/Radical behavioral	5%
Family systems/Systems	20%
Existential/Phenomenological/Humanistic	30%
Cognitive/Cognitive-behavioral	30%

What percentage of students applying for internship last year was accepted into APPIC-member internships?
Data not available

What courses are required for incoming students to have completed prior to enrolling?
Experimental, statistics, abnormal, developmental, personality

Are there courses you recommend that are not mandatory?
Social, history and systems, physiological psychology, learning

GRE mean
Verbal 630   Quantitative 625   Analytical 635
Advanced Psychology 625   Analytical Writing 5.25

GPA mean
Overall GPA 3.59   Psychology GPA 3.65

Number of applications/admission offers/incoming students in 2005
187 applied/30 admission offers/15 incoming

% of students receiving:
Tuition waiver only: 0%
Both tuition waiver & assistantship/fellowship: 20%
Half tuition waiver & assistantship: 80%

Approximate percentage of incoming students who entered with a B.A./B.S. only: 66%   **Master's:** 34%

Approximate percentage of students who are Women: 75%   **Ethnic Minority:** 20%   **International:** 5%

Average years to complete the doctoral program (including internship): 6.2 years

Personal interview
Required in person

Research areas	# Faculty	# Grants
aging and mental health	1	1
cultural/cross-cultural	4	0
developmental issues	4	1
developmental psychopathology	2	0
forensic issues	3	0
health psychology	1	1
neuropsychology	1	0
projective techniques	1	0
psychotherapy process	3	1
sociodevelopment	1	1
socioemotional development	1	0
trauma	1	1

Clinical opportunities
behavioral clinics
child clinics and child hospital settings
college counseling
community mental health
family therapy
forensic units
homeless shelters
hospital inpatient/outpatient
neuropsychology
substance abuse

Long Island University–C.W. Post Campus (Psy.D.)

Department of Psychology
College of Liberal Arts and Sciences
Brookville, NY 11548
phone#: (516) 299-2090
e-mail: doctoral.psychology@cwpost.liu.edu
Web address:
http://www.cwpost.liu.edu/cwis/cwp/clas/psych/doctoral

1	**2**	3	4	5	6	7

Clinically oriented   Equal emphasis   Research oriented

What percentage of your faculty subscribes to or practices in each of the following orientations?

Psychodynamic/Psychoanalytic	50%
Applied behavioral analysis/Radical behavioral	12%
Family systems/Systems	0%
Existential/Phenomenological/Humanistic	0%
Cognitive/Cognitive-behavioral	38%

What percentage of students applying for internship last year was accepted into APPIC-member internships? Data not available

What courses are required for incoming students to have completed prior to enrolling?
18 credits of undergraduate psychology

Are there courses you recommend that are not mandatory?
Yes

GRE mean
Verbal 550   Quantitative 598
Advanced psychology 608
Analytical Writing Data not available

GPA mean
Data not available

Number of applications/admission offers/incoming students in 2003
204 applied/30 admission offers/12 incoming

% of students receiving:
Tuition waiver only: 25%
Assistantship/fellowship only: 40%
Both tuition waiver & assistantship/fellowship: 0%

Approximate percentage of incoming students who entered with a B.A./B.S. only: 75%   **Master's:** 25%

Approximate percentage of students who are Women: 67%   **Ethnic Minority:** 20%
International: Data not available

Average years to complete the doctoral program (including internship): 5.5 years

Personal interview
Required in person

Research areas	# Faculty	# Grants
anger management	1	0
attachment	1	1
developmental disabilities	1	0
marital violence	2	0
parent training	1	0
professional discipline	1	0
schizophrenia	1	0

Clinical opportunities
adult difficulties as follows:
  behavior modification for habit control
  behavior patterns
  depression
  domestic violence
  eating disorders and compulsive
  marital and relationship therapy
  phobias and anxiety disorders
child and family difficulties as follows:
  academic and school-related problems
  aggressive behavior/anger management
  developmental difficulties (treatment)
  family conflicts/family therapy
  family violence
  hyperactivity/low attention span
  parent/child conflicts
  socialization difficulties
group therapy as follows:
  anger management for children and adults
  assertiveness training
  parent training
  social skills for children
  stress management
individual psychotherapy
psychological assessment as follows:
  achievement and intelligence testing
  emotional and behavioral assessment
  neuropsychological assessment
  personality assessment
short-term and psychodynamic therapy

Louisiana State University

Department of Psychology
Audobon Hall, Room 236
Baton Rouge, LA 70803
phone#: (225) 578-8745
fax#: (225) 578-4125
e-mail: psrose@lsu.edu
Web address:
http://www.lsu.edu/psychology/graduate/Clinical.html

1	2	3	4	5	**6**	7
Clinically oriented		Equal emphasis			Research oriented	

What percentage of your faculty subscribes to or practices in each of the following orientations?

Psychodynamic/Psychoanalytic	0%
Applied behavioral analysis/Radical behavioral	100%
Family systems/Systems	0%
Existential/Phenomenological/Humanistic	0%
Cognitive/Cognitive-behavioral	50%

What percentage of students applying for internship last year was accepted into APPIC-member internships? Data not available

What courses are required for incoming students to have completed prior to enrolling?
None

Are there courses you recommend that are not mandatory?
Intro psych, stats, experimental, physiological psych, psychology of learning

GRE mean
Data not available

GPA mean
Data not available

Number of applications/admission offers/incoming students in 2003
350 applied/12 admission offers/12 incoming

% of students receiving:
Tuition waiver only: 0%
Assistantship/fellowship only: 0%
Both tuition waiver & assistantship/fellowship: 100%

Approximate percentage of incoming students who entered with a B.A./B.S. only: 50%   **Master's:** 50%

Approximate percentage of students who are Women: 75%   **Ethnic Minority:** 10%
International: Data not available

Average years to complete the doctoral program (including internship): 5 years

Personal interview
No preference given

Research areas	# Faculty	# Grants
anxiety disorders	1	1
autism	1	1
depression	1	1
eating disorders	1	1
mental retardation	1	1
neuropsychology	1	0
parent skills training	1	0
psychophysiology	1	0
social skills	2	1
stress and coping	1	0

Clinical opportunities
anxiety disorders
autism
behavioral medicine
deafness disorder
eating disorders
family
mental retardation

neuropsychology
obsessive–compulsive
schizophrenia
school/educational

University of Louisville

Department of Psychological and Brain Sciences
Louisville, KY 40292
phone#: (502) 852-6775
e-mail: rich.lewine_@louisville.edu
Web address:
http://www.louisville.edu/a-s/psychology/clinical/

1	2	3	4	**5**	6	7
Clinically oriented		Equal emphasis		Research oriented		

What percentage of your faculty subscribes to or practices in each of the following orientations?

Psychodynamic/Psychoanalytic	0%
Interpersonal-ego relations	10%
Applied behavioral analysis/Radical behavioral	0%
Family systems/Systems	0%
Existential/Phenomenological/Humanistic	0%
Cognitive/Cognitive-behavioral	80%
Eclectic	10%

What percentage of students applying for internship last year was accepted into APPIC-member internships? 84%

What courses are required for incoming students to have completed prior to enrolling?
None

Are there courses you recommend that are not mandatory?
History, abnormal, personality, social, statistics, physiological, learning

GRE mean
Verbal 568   Quantitative 621
Analytical Writing Data not available

GPA mean
Junior/Senior GPA 3.6

Number of applications/admission offers/incoming students in 2003
137 applied/9 admission offers/7 incoming

% of students receiving:
Tuition waiver only: 0%
Assistantship/fellowship only: 0%
Both tuition waiver & assistantship/fellowship: 100%

Approximate percentage of incoming students who entered with a B.A./B.S. only: 80%   **Master's:** 20%

Approximate percentage of students who are Women: 62%   **Ethnic Minority:** 12%   **International:** 2%

Average years to complete the doctoral program (including internship): 6 years

Personal interview
Preferred in person but telephone acceptable

Research areas	# Faculty	# Grants
anxiety disorders	3	1
behavioral medicine	2	1
chronic mental illness	1	0
forensic psychology	1	0
gerontology/aging	2	0
stress and coping	2	0
substance abuse	1	0

Clinical opportunities
affective disorders
anxiety disorders
behavioral primary care
child clinical psychology
developmental disabilities
forensic psychology
gerontology/aging
health psychology
interpersonal psychotherapy
psychosis

Loyola College in Maryland (Psy.D.)

Department of Psychology
Baltimore, MD 21210-2699
phone#: (410) 617-2696
e-mail: jlating@loyola.edu
Web address:
http://graduate.loyola.edu/graduate/academics/psy/

1	2	**3**	4	5	6	7
Clinically oriented		Equal emphasis		Research oriented		

What percentage of your faculty subscribes to or practices in each of the following orientations?

Psychodynamic/Psychoanalytic	15%
Applied behavioral analysis/Radical behavioral	10%
Family systems/Systems	5%
Existential/Phenomenological/Humanistic	10%
Cognitive/Cognitive-behavioral	65%

What percentage of students applying for internship last year was accepted into APPIC-member internships? 92%

What courses are required for incoming students to have completed prior to enrolling?
Introductory psychology, social psychology, statistics or research methods, abnormal psychology, personality theory, tests and measurements, learning theory or cognitive psychology

Are there courses you recommend that are not mandatory?
No

GRE mean
Verbal 588   Quantitative 637   Analytical 659

GPA mean
Overall GPA 3.56

Number of applications/admission offers/incoming students in 2005
248 applied/25 admission offers/17 incoming

% of students receiving:
Tuition waiver only: 0%
Assistantship/fellowship only: 40%
Both tuition waiver & assistantship/fellowship: 0%

Approximate percentage of incoming students who entered with a B.A./B.S. only: 65% Master's: 35%

Approximate percentage of students who are Women: 94% Ethnic Minority: 12% International: 0%

Average years to complete the doctoral program (including internship): 5.5 years

Personal interview
Required in person

Research areas	# Faculty	# Grants
child psychopathology	5	0
domestic violence	1	0
ethics and legal issues	2	0
gambling	1	0
gerontology	2	0
health psychology	3	0
homophobia	1	0
multicultural	3	0
neuropsychology	2	0
nonverbal communication	1	0
posttraumatic stress disorder	4	0
psychotherapy outcomes	1	0
sexuality	2	0
spirituality	2	0
social psychology	1	0
trichotillomania	1	0
women's issues	2	0

Clinical opportunities
adult inpatient
behavioral medicine
child and family
eating disorders
juvenile forensics
outpatient private practice
prison settings
stress and anxiety
The Loyola Clinics: multidisciplinary assessment centers
  (child and adult)

Loyola University Chicago

Graduate Enrollment Services
820 North Michigan Avenue
Chicago, IL 60611
phone#: (312) 915-8900
e-mail: gradinfo@luc.edu
Web address:
http://www.luc.edu/depts/psychology/overview.htm

1	2	3	4	**5**	6	7

Clinically oriented   Equal emphasis   Research oriented

What percentage of your faculty subscribes to or practices in each of the following orientations?

Psychodynamic/Psychoanalytic	22%
Applied behavioral analysis/Radical behavioral	0%
Family systems/Systems	22%
Existential/Phenomenological/Humanistic	0%
Cognitive/Cognitive-behavioral	55%

What percentage of students applying for internship last year was accepted into APPIC-member internships? 88%

What courses are required for incoming students to have completed prior to enrolling?
Research methods/experimental and statistics plus any 6 other psychology courses (24 hours, total)

Are there courses you recommend that are not mandatory?
No

GRE mean
Verbal 590   Quantitative 669
Analytical Writing 5.17

GPA mean
Overall GPA 3.5

Number of applications/admission offers/incoming students in 2005
256 applied/13 admission offers/7 incoming

% of students receiving:
Tuition waiver only: 0%
Assistantship/fellowship only: 0%
Both tuition waiver & assistantship/fellowship: 100%

Approximate percentage of incoming students who entered with a B.A./B.S. only: 90% Master's: 10%

Approximate percentage of students who are Women: 76% Ethnic Minority: 37% International: 7%

Average years to complete the doctoral program (including internship): 6 years

Personal interview
Preferred in person but telephone acceptable

Research areas	# Faculty	# Grants
AIDS	2	1
adolescence	3	4
adult psychopathology	2	0
affective disorders	1	0
African American men	1	0
clinical-child/psychopathology	5	4
community psychology	3	0
death/bereavement	1	0
developmental psychopathology	4	3
disabilities	1	2
ethical issues	1	0
extracurricular activities	1	0
minority mental health	3	3
personality	2	0
prevention	3	2
psychotherapy	4	1
sexuality/dysfunctions	1	0
utilization of health services	1	0

Clinical opportunities
assessment (child and adult)
eating disorders
family psychology
health psychology
HIV/AIDS
neuropsychological assessment (child and adult)
personality disorders
psychotherapy (child and adult)
substance abuse
victims of abuse

University of Maine

Department of Psychology
5742 Little Hall
Orono, ME 04469-5742
phone#: (207) 581-2038
e-mail: Douglas.nangle@umit.maine.edu
Web address: http://www.hutchinsoncenter.umaine.edu/
psychology/clinical.html

1	2	3	4	**5**	6	7

Clinically oriented　　Equal emphasis　　Research oriented

What percentage of your faculty subscribes to or practices in each of the following orientations?
Psychodynamic/Psychoanalytic　　0%
Applied behavioral analysis/Radical behavioral　　20%
Family systems/Systems　　0%
Existential/Phenomenological/Humanistic　　0%
Cognitive/Cognitive-behavioral　　80%

What percentage of students applying for internship last year was accepted into APPIC-member internships? 100%

What courses are required for incoming students to have completed prior to enrolling?
At least three to four advanced undergraduate psychology courses; background in natural sciences and mathematics

Are there courses you recommend that are not mandatory?
Learning, developmental, cognition

GRE mean
Verbal 560　Quantitative 650
Advanced Psychology 603
Analytical Writing Data not available

GPA mean
Overall GPA 3.60

Number of applications/admission offers/incoming students in 2005
98 applied/10 admission offers/5 incoming

% of students receiving:
Tuition waiver only: 0%
Assistantship/fellowship only: 0%
Both tuition waiver & assistantship/fellowship: 100% for the 1st-year students, 100% of the 2nd- to 4th-year students

Approximate percentage of incoming students who entered with a B.A./B.S. only: 80%　**Master's:** 20%

Approximate percentage of students who are
Women: 70%　**Ethnic Minority:** 5%　**International:** 0%

Average years to complete the doctoral program (including internship): 6 years

Personal interview
Preferred in person but telephone acceptable

Research areas	# Faculty	# Grants
anxiety disorders	2	0
behavioral medicine	1	0
children's regulation of affect	1	0
depression	1	0
forensic psychology	3	0
psychotherapy outcome	3	0
social development	1	0
women's health	1	0

Clinical opportunities
ADHD clinic
anxiety disorders clinic
behavioral-developmental pediatrics
body dysmorphic disorder clinic
community mental health
crisis services—outpatient
Head Start
juvenile offenders
residential program for children at risk

University of Manitoba

Psychology Graduate Office P514
Duff Roblin Building
Winnipeg, Manitoba R3T 2N2, Canada
phone#: (204) 474-6377
fax #: (204) 474-7917
e-mail: inglislf@ms.umanitoba.ca
Web address: http://www.umanitoba.ca/faculties/arts/
psychology/grad/programs/clinical.php

1	2	3	**4**	5	6	7

Clinically oriented　　Equal emphasis　　Research oriented

What percentage of your faculty subscribes to or practices in each of the following orientations?
Psychodynamic/Psychoanalytic　　10%
Applied behavioral analysis/Radical behavioral　　20%
Clinical neuropsychology　　14%
Family systems/Systems　　20%
Existential/Phenomenological/Humanistic　　10%
Cognitive/Cognitive-behavioral　　30%

What percentage of students applying for internship last year was accepted into APPIC-member internships? 80%

What courses are required for incoming students to have completed prior to enrolling?
Eight half (3 credit hour) courses in psychology, which include introductory psychology, research methods, and a second course in either research methods, statistics, or computer science

Are there courses you recommend that are not mandatory?

Psychological measurement and assessment; psychological tests or design and analysis for psychological experiments; physiological psychology or sensory processes

GRE mean

Verbal 557 Quantitative 625
Subject score for one of the following: psychology, biology, zoology 695
Analytical Writing Not required

GPA mean

Data not available

Number of applications/admission offers/incoming students in 2005

72 applied/7 admission offers/5 incoming

% of students receiving:

Tuition waiver only: 0%
Assistantship/fellowship only: 25%
Both tuition waiver & assistantship/fellowship: 0%

Approximate percentage of incoming students who entered with a B.A./B.S. only: 25%   B.A. Honors: 50% Master's: 25%

Approximate percentage of students who are

Women: 67%   Ethnic Minority: 10%   International: 1%

Average years to complete the doctoral program (including internship): 7 years

Personal interview

Interview not required

Research areas	# Faculty	# Grants
anxiety disorders	4	0
applied behavioral analysis	3	2
childhood psychopathology	1	0
chronic illness	1	1
chronic pain	1	0
clinical supervision	1	0
community psychology	1	0
compliance issues	2	0
developmental disabilities	3	0
eating disorders	2	0
health psychology	2	1
hypnosis	1	0
neuropsychology	2	1
offender/abuse	2	0
psychoneuroimmunology	1	0
psychopathology	1	0
psychotherapy outcome	3	0
schizophrenia	1	0
sports psychology	1	1
trauma effects	3	0
victim/abuse	3	0

Clinical opportunities

anxiety disorders
behavioral medicine
child/play therapy
clinical supervision
cognitive behavioral
community psychology
couples
eating disorders
developmental disabilities
family
health psychology
neuropsychology
obsessive–compulsive disorders
sports psychology
victim/battering/abuse

Marquette University

Psychology Department
P.O. Box 1881
Milwaukee, WI 53201-1881
phone#: (414) 288-7218
e-mail: Stephen.Saunders@mu.edu
Web address:
http://www.marquette.edu/psyc/doctoralprogram.html

1	2	3	**4**	5	6	7
Clinically oriented		Equal emphasis			Research oriented	

What percentage of your faculty subscribes to or practices in each of the following orientations?

Psychodynamic/Psychoanalytic	15%
Applied behavioral analysis/Radical behavioral	10%
Family systems/Systems	40%
Existential/Phenomenological/Humanistic	15%
Cognitive/Cognitive-behavioral	80%

What percentage of students applying for internship last year was accepted into APPIC-member internships? 80%

What courses are required for incoming students to have completed prior to enrolling?

Research methods, statistics, developmental, abnormal, personality, social, cognition, neuroscience

Are there courses you recommend that are not mandatory?

History and systems

GRE mean

Verbal 600   Quantitative 600   Analytical Writing N/A

GPA mean

Overall GPA 3.5

Number of applications/admission offers/incoming students in 2005

111 applied/11 admission offers/4 incoming

% of students receiving:

Tuition waiver only: 10%
Assistantship/fellowship only: 0%
Both tuition waiver & assistantship/fellowship: 90%

Approximate percentage of incoming students who entered with a B.A./B.S. only: 100%   Master's: 0%

Approximate percentage of students who are

Women: 70%   Ethnic Minority: 20%   International: 5%

Average years to complete the doctoral program (including internship): 6.5 years

Personal interview

Preferred in person but telephone acceptable

Research areas	# Faculty	# Grants
adult development	1	0
ADHD	1	0
alcohol treatment	1	1
Alzheimer's disease	1	0
chaos theory	1	1
child development	3	1
child–parent relationships	3	1
depression	1	0
family conflict	2	1
friendships	1	0
help-seeking	1	1
memory problems	1	2
mental imagery	1	0
neuropsychology	2	0
pediatric psychology	1	0
psychosocial aspects of medical illness	1	0
psychotherapy research	3	0

Clinical opportunities

adult neuropsychology
adult psychotherapy
child neuropsychology
child psychotherapy
family therapy
geriatric clinic
pain clinic
pediatric neuropsychology

University of Maryland

Department of Psychology
Biology–Psychology Building
College Park, MD 20742-4411
phone#: (301) 405-5866
e-mail: bpadgett@psyc.umd.edu
Web address:
http://www.bsos.umd.edu/psyc/clinicalpsyc/index.htm

1	2	3	4	5	**6**	7

Clinically oriented   Equal emphasis   Research oriented

What percentage of your faculty subscribes to or practices in each of the following orientations?

Psychodynamic/Psychoanalytic	0%
Applied behavioral analysis/Radical behavioral	0%
Family systems/Systems	0%
Existential/Phenomenological/Humanistic	10%
Cognitive/Cognitive-behavioral	90%

What percentage of students applying for internship last year was accepted into APPIC-member internships?

Data not available

What courses are required for incoming students to have completed prior to enrolling?

B.A. or B.S. in psychology or related areas

Are there courses you recommend that are not mandatory? Statistics, laboratory courses in psychology

GRE mean

Verbal 584   Quantitative 650
Analytical Writing Data not available

GPA mean

Overall GPA 3.62

Number of applications/admission offers/incoming students in 2003

296 applied/12 admission offers/7 incoming

% of students receiving:

Tuition waiver only: 0%
Assistantship/fellowship only: 0%
Both tuition waiver & assistantship/fellowship: 100%

Approximate percentage of incoming students who entered with a B.A./B.S. only: 90%   **Master's:** 10%

Approximate percentage of students who are Women: 78%   **Ethnic Minority:** 40%
International: Data not available

Average years to complete the doctoral program (including internship): 7.96 years

Personal interview

Required in person

Research areas	# Faculty	# Grants
addictive behaviors	2	2
anxiety disorder	2	2
behavioral undercontrol	2	1
personality and physiology	1	0
psychotherapy outcome	3	2
serious mental illnesses	2	2

Clinical opportunities

Multiple opportunities in in-house training clinic, extern, and intern levels in inpatient, outpatient, and specialized settings

University of Maryland, Baltimore County

Department of Psychology
1000 Hilltop Circle
Baltimore, MD 21250
phone#: (410) 455-2567
e-mail: psycdept@umbc.edu
Web address:
http://www.umbc.edu/psyc/grad/hspclindata.html

1	2	3	4	**5**	6	7

Clinically oriented   Equal emphasis   Research oriented

What percentage of your faculty subscribes to or practices in each of the following orientations?

Psychodynamic/Psychoanalytic	20%
Applied behavioral analysis/Radical behavioral	10%
Family systems/Systems	40%
Existential/Phenomenological/Humanistic	0%
Cognitive/Cognitive-behavioral	80%

What percentage of students applying for internship last year was accepted into APPIC-member internships? 100%

What courses are required for incoming students to have completed prior to enrolling?
Introductory psychology, statistics, abnormal psychology

Are there courses you recommend that are not mandatory?
Personality, physiological, developmental, experimental psychology

GRE mean
Verbal 610   Quantitative 689
Advanced Psychology 691
Analytical Writing 5.38

GPA mean
Overall GPA 3.68

Number of applications/admission offers/incoming students in 2005
112 applied/20 admission offers/10 incoming

% of students receiving:
Tuition waiver only: 0%
Assistantship/fellowship only: 0%
Both tuition waiver & assistantship/fellowship: 100%

Approximate percentage of incoming students who entered with a B.A./B.S. only: 90%   **Master's:** 10%

Approximate percentage of students who are Women: 80%   **Ethnic Minority:** 20%   **International:** 0%

Average years to complete the doctoral program (including internship): 7 years

Personal interview
Preferred in person but telephone acceptable

Research areas	# Faculty	# Grants
addictive disorders	2	2
behavioral medicine	4	3
cardiovascular/cerebrovascular disease	1	1
community psychology	4	2
delinquency	1	1
domestic violence	1	1
family therapy	1	1
interpersonal processes	1	0
psychology of religion	1	0
psychoneuroimmunology	1	0
suicide	1	0

Clinical opportunities
addictive disorders
applied behavior
analysis
domestic abuse
emergency mental
health services
family therapy
forensic psychology
medical liaison
neuropsychology
pediatric psychology
prevention
rehabilitation psychology
school-based mental health services
severe and chronic mental illness

University of Massachusetts at Amherst
Department of Psychology
Tobin Hall
Amherst, MA 01003
phone#: (413) 545-0662
e-mail: wisocki@psych.umass.edu
Web address:
http://www.umass.edu/psychology/div4/main/

1	2	3	**4**	5	6	7
Clinically oriented			Equal emphasis			Research oriented

What percentage of your faculty subscribes to or practices in each of the following orientations?

Psychodynamic/Psychoanalytic	15%
Applied behavioral analysis/Radical behavioral	0%
Family systems/Systems	5%
Existential/Phenomenological/Humanistic	0%
Cognitive/Cognitive-behavioral	35%
Integrative	45%

What percentage of students applying for internship last year was accepted into APPIC-member internships? 86%

What courses are required for incoming students to have completed prior to enrolling?
An undergraduate background in psychology which, at a minimum, consists of: introduction to psychology, statistics, methods, and 3 advanced subjects in psychology

Are there courses you recommend that are not mandatory?
No

GRE mean
Verbal 600   Quantitative 600

GPA mean
Overall GPA 3.5

Number of applications/admission offers/incoming students in 2005
202 applied/13 admission offers/7 incoming

% of students receiving:
Tuition waiver only: 0%
Assistantship/fellowship only: 0%
Both tuition waiver & assistantship/fellowship: 100%

Approximate percentage of incoming students who entered with a B.A./B.S. only: 66%   **Master's:** 33%

Approximate percentage of students who are Women: 100%   **Ethnic Minority:** 29% (incoming class)
International: 29%

Average years to complete the doctoral program (including internship): 6 years

Personal interview
Preferred in person but telephone acceptable

Research areas	# Faculty	# Grants
adjustment issues	1	0
aging/gerontology	2	0
developmental psychopathology	1	1
family relationships	2	2

psychotherapy process	1	1
psychotherapist's development	1	1
stress and coping	1	0

Clinical opportunities
child and adolescent therapy
cognitive-behavior therapy
cultural diversity experience
geropsychology
psychoanalytic therapy
psychotherapy supervision

University of Massachusetts at Boston

Department of Psychology
Boston, MA 02125-3393
phone#: (617) 287-6340
e-mail: clinical.Psych@umb.edu
Web address: http://www.umb.edu/academics/graduate/
clinical_psychology/index.html

1	2	3	**4**	5	6	7

Clinically oriented   Equal emphasis   Research oriented

What percentage of your faculty subscribes to or practices in each of the following orientations?
Psychodynamic/Psychoanalytic	50%
Applied behavioral analysis/Radical behavioral	0%
Family systems/Systems	30%
Existential/Phenomenological/Humanistic	0%
Cognitive/Cognitive-behavioral	50%

What percentage of students applying for internship last year was accepted into APPIC-member internships?
Data not available

What courses are required for incoming students to have completed prior to enrolling?
Statistics; 6 courses total in psychology

Are there courses you recommend that are not mandatory?
Development, abnormal, personality, research methods

GRE mean
Verbal 613   Quantitative 704
Advanced Psychology 696
Analytical Writing Data not available

GPA mean
Overall GPA 3.5   Psychology GPA 3.8
Junior/Senior GPA 3.7

Number of applications/admission offers/incoming students in 2003
339 applied/14 admission offers/8 incoming

% of students receiving:
Tuition waiver only: 0%
Assistantship/fellowship only: 0%
Both tuition waiver & assistantship/fellowship: 100%

Approximate percentage of incoming students who entered with a B.A./B.S. only: 87.5%   Master's: 12.5%

Approximate percentage of students who are
Women: 77%   **Ethnic Minority:** 42%
International: Data not available

Average years to complete the doctoral program (including internship): 6.5 years

Personal interview
Required in person

Research areas	# Faculty	# Grants
cross-cultural	3	0
family	3	2
media and psychology	1	0
severe psychopathology	2	1
social stereotypes	1	0
trauma	4	1

Clinical opportunities
—

Massachusetts School of Professional Psychology (Psy.D.)

221 Rivermoor Street
Boston, MA 02132
phone#: (617) 327-6777
toll free (888) 664-MSPP
e-mail: admissions@mspp.edu
Web address: http://www.mspp.edu/
index.asp?action=15&what=100017

1	2	**3**	4	5	6	7

Clinically oriented   Equal emphasis   Research oriented

What percentage of your faculty subscribes to or practices in each of the following orientations?
Psychodynamic/Psychoanalytic	50%
Applied behavioral analysis/Radical behavioral	0%
Family systems/Systems	19%
Existential/Phenomenological/Humanistic	12%
Cognitive/Cognitive-behavioral	19%

What percentage of students applying for internship last year was accepted into APPIC-member internships? 100%

What courses are required for incoming students to have completed prior to enrolling?
Introduction to psychology, abnormal, developmental/child, personality theory

Are there courses you recommend that are not mandatory?
All psychology related

GRE mean
Verbal 540   Quantitative 603
Analytical Writing 4.5

GPA mean
Overall GPA 3.0

Number of applications/admission offers/incoming students in 2005
335 applied/92 admission offers/55 incoming

% of students receiving:
Tuition waiver only: 0%
Assistantship/fellowship only: 45%
Both tuition waiver & assistantship/fellowship: 0%

Approximate percentage of incoming students who entered with a B.A./B.S. only: 60%   **Master's:** 40%

Approximate percentage of students who are Women: 75%   **Ethnic Minority:** 12%   **International:** 12%

Average years to complete the doctoral program (including internship): 4.5 years

Personal interview
Required in person

Research areas	# Faculty	# Grants
—		

Clinical opportunities
We have 160 sites per year in diverse areas. If your area is not covered, we will find a site. Optional specialty tracks in health and forensic psychology are available.

McGill University

Department of Psychology
1205 Avenue Docteur Penfield
Montreal, Quebec H3A 1B1, Canada
phone#: (514) 398-6124
e-mail: gradapp@psych.mcgill.ca
Web address:
http://www.psych.mcgill.ca/grad/clnprg.htm

1	2	3	4	5	**6**	7
Clinically oriented		Equal emphasis			Research oriented	

What percentage of your faculty subscribes to or practices in each of the following orientations?
Psychodynamic/Psychoanalytic   20%
Applied behavioral analysis/Radical behavioral   0%
Family systems/Systems   0%
Existential/Phenomenological/Humanistic   0%
Cognitive/Cognitive-behavioral   80%

What percentage of students applying for internship last year was accepted into APPIC-member internships? 100%

What courses are required for incoming students to have completed prior to enrolling?
Courses in the biological, cognitive and social bases of behavior as well as statistics.

Are there courses you recommend that are not mandatory?
No

GRE mean
Verbal and Quantitative 660; Do not require GREs for non-native speakers of English
Analytical Writing Data not available

GPA mean
Overall GPA 3.7

Number of applications/admission offers/incoming students in 2004/2005
180 applied/5 admission offers/4 incoming

% of students receiving:
Tuition waiver only: 0%
Assistantship/fellowship only: 100%
Both tuition waiver & assistantship/fellowship: 0%

Approximate percentage of incoming students who entered with a B.A./B.S. only: 95%   **Master's:** 5%

Approximate percentage of students who are Women: 66%   **Ethnic Minority:** 10%   **International:** 20%

Average years to complete the doctoral program (including internship): 6 years

Personal interview
Telephone required

Research areas	# Faculty	# Grants
aggression	1	1
aging (including Alzheimer's)	2	1
assessment/diagnosis	2	0
attention-deficit disorder	1	1
behavior therapy	1	0
behavioral genetics	1	1
behavioral medicine	2	2
child	1	1
child psychopathology	1	1
cognitive information processing	1	0
depression	2	2
developmental	1	1
eating disorders	1	1
emotion	1	1
family	2	1
gender	1	1
health psychology	2	2
interpersonal relations	2	2
memory	2	1
neuropsychology	1	1
olfaction	1	1
personality	1	1
personality assessment	2	0
psychopathology	2	2
psychopharmacology	2	1
psychophysiology	2	1
psychotherapy process and outcome	1	1
sexual dysfunction	1	1
stress	1	1
substance abuse	1	1

Clinical opportunities
The McGill University Psychology Internship Consortium is closely associated with our graduate program in clinical psychology. The Consortium consists of departments of psychology in 3 university teaching hospitals, a children's hospital, and a psychiatric hospital.

University of Memphis

Department of Psychology
Memphis, TN 38152
phone#: (901) 678-3015
e-mail: j.johnson@mail.psyc.memphis.edu
Web address: http://www.psyc.memphis.edu/programs/
grad/clinical/clinicalhome.html

1	2	3	4	5	**6**	7
Clinically oriented		Equal emphasis			Research oriented	

What percentage of your faculty subscribes to or practices in each of the following orientations?

Psychodynamic/Psychoanalytic	0%
Applied behavioral analysis/Radical behavioral	0%
Family systems/Systems	20%
Existential/Phenomenological/Humanistic	10%
Cognitive/Cognitive-behavioral	70%

What percentage of students applying for internship last year was accepted into APPIC-member internships? 100%

What courses are required for incoming students to have completed prior to enrolling?
12–18 psychology credits preferred; statistics and experimental psychology are required

Are there courses you recommend that are not mandatory?
No

GRE mean
Verbal 580   Quantitative 670
Analytical Writing 5.0

GPA mean
Overall GPA 3.5

Number of applications/admission offers/incoming students in 2005
129 applied/12 admission offers/9 incoming

% of students receiving:
Tuition waiver only: 0%
Assistantship/fellowship only: 0%
Both tuition waiver & assistantship/fellowship: 100%

Approximate percentage of incoming students who entered with a B.A./B.S. only: 65%   **Master's:** 35%

Approximate percentage of students who are Women: 65%   **Ethnic Minority:** 15%   **International:** 0%

Average years to complete the doctoral program (including internship): 5.6 years

Personal interview
Interview not required

Research areas	# Faculty	# Grants
addictions	2	3
behavioral medicine	4	7
child clinical	2	1
psychopathology and psychotherapy	3	0

Clinical opportunities
addiction
affective disorders
anxiety disorders
behavioral medicine
cancer and emotional adjustment
developmental disabilities/autism
eating disorders
family therapy
gambling
inpatient psychology
minority/cross-cultural
school/educational
sleep disorders

University of Miami

Department of Psychology
P.O. Box 249229
Coral Gables, FL 33124
phone#: (305) 284-5720
e-mail: INQUIRE@miami.edu
Web address: http://www.psy.miami.edu/

1	2	3	4	5	**6**	7
Clinically oriented		Equal emphasis			Research oriented	

What percentage of your faculty subscribes to or practices in each of the following orientations?

Psychodynamic/Psychoanalytic	10%
Applied behavioral analysis/Radical behavioral	0%
Family systems/Systems	30%
Existential/Phenomenological/Humanistic	10%
Cognitive/Cognitive-behavioral	80%

What percentage of students applying for internship last year was accepted into APPIC-member internships? 95%

What courses are required for incoming students to have completed prior to enrolling?
Statistics, experimental psychology

Are there courses you recommend that are not mandatory?
Strong science background, especially biology, and mathematics

GRE mean
Verbal 640   Quantitative 730
Analytical Writing Data not available

GPA mean
Overall GPA 3.5

Number of applications/admission offers/incoming students in 2005
288 applied/16 admission offers/11 incoming

% of students receiving:
Tuition waiver only: 0%
Assistantship/fellowship only: 0%
Both tuition waiver & assistantship/fellowship: 100%

Approximate percentage of incoming students who entered with a B.A./B.S. only: 90%   **Master's:** 10%

Approximate percentage of students who are Women: 70%   **Ethnic Minority:** 30%   **International:** 1%

Average years to complete the doctoral program (including internship): 5.5 years

Personal interview
Required in person

Research areas	# Faculty	# Grants
AIDS	6	2
adult psychopathology	6	2
affective disorders	3	1
cancer	4	1
cardiovascular disease	4	2
child clinical psychology	6	2
child psychopathology	5	2
diabetes	3	2
family therapy	2	1
health psychology	14	2
hypertension	3	1
pediatric psychology	3	2
psychoneuroimmunology	6	2
stress and coping	9	2
trauma	4	2

Clinical opportunities
abuse
AIDS
behavioral medicine
conduct disorder
developmental disabilities/autism
diabetes
eating disorders
family therapy
group therapy
long-term care
marital therapy
minority/cross-cultural
neuropsychology
pediatrics
substance abuse

Miami University
Department of Psychology
Oxford, OH 45056
phone#: (513) 529-2400
e-mail: KNUDSORM@muohio.edu
Web address: http://www.units.muohio.edu/psychology/clinical/index.html

1	2	3	**4**	5	6	7
Clinically oriented		Equal emphasis			Research oriented	

What percentage of your faculty subscribes to or practices in each of the following orientations?
Psychodynamic/Psychoanalytic   17%
Applied behavioral analysis/Radical behavioral   0%
Family systems/Systems   25%

Existential/Phenomenological/Humanistic   25%
Cognitive/Cognitive-behavioral   17%
Developmental/Developmental Psychopathology   17%

What percentage of students applying for internship last year was accepted into APPIC-member internships? 100%

What courses are required for incoming students to have completed prior to enrolling?
1 course in statistics

Are there courses you recommend that are not mandatory?
No

GRE mean
Verbal 600   Quantitative 660   Analytical 670
Analytical Writing 5.5/6

GPA mean
Overall GPA 3.6

Number of applications/admission offers/incoming students in 2005
114 applied/20 admission offers/9 incoming

% of students receiving:
Tuition waiver only: 0%
Assistantship/fellowship only: 0%
Both tuition waiver & assistantship/fellowship: 100%

Approximate percentage of incoming students who entered with a B.A./B.S. only: 66%   **Master's:** 34%

Approximate percentage of students who are Women: 70%   **Ethnic Minority:** 7%
International: Data not available

Average years to complete the doctoral program (including internship): 6 years

Personal interview
Preferred in person but telephone acceptable

Research areas	# Faculty	# Grants
action research	2	1
anxiety disorders	3	0
bullying youth	3	1
child psychopathology	2	0
consultation/school improvement	2	1
dreams	1	0
early childhood mental health	1	0
eating disorders	1	0
family research	1	0
fetal alcohol spectrum disorders	1	0
immigration/acculturation	2	0
interparental conflict & violence	1	0
narrative methodologies	2	0
parent–child boundary dissolution	1	1
personality disorders	1	0
program development/program evaluation	2	1
psychotherapy process	3	0
school-based mental health	1	1
school–family community partnership	2	1
training/technical assistance	2	1
trauma recovery	2	0

Clinical opportunities
assessment
community mental health
conduct disorder
developmental disabilities
family therapy
hyperactivity
inpatient mental health
marital/couples therapy
personality disorders
rural mental health
school-based mental health

University of Michigan

Department of Psychology
530 Church Street
Ann Arbor, MI 48109-1109
phone#: (734) 764-6332
e-mail: psych2sect@umich.edu
Web address:
http://www.lsa.umich.edu/psych/areas/clinical/

	1	2	3	4	**5**	6	7

Clinically oriented   Equal emphasis   Research oriented

What percentage of your faculty subscribes to or practices in each of the following orientations?

Psychodynamic/Psychoanalytic	33%
Applied behavioral analysis/Radical behavioral	0%
Family systems/Systems	33%
Existential/Phenomenological/Humanistic	0%
Cognitive/Cognitive-behavioral	33%

What percentage of students applying for internship last year was accepted into APPIC-member internships? 100%

What courses are required for incoming students to have completed prior to enrolling?
None

Are there courses you recommend that are not mandatory?
Basic course work in psychology

GRE mean
Verbal 700 Quantitative 705
Analytical Writing Data not available

GPA mean
Overall GPA 3.75 Psychology GPA 3.9

Number of applications/admission offers/incoming students in 2005
321 applied/7 admission offers/7 incoming
(1 deferred from last year)

% of students receiving:
Tuition waiver only: 0%
Assistantship/fellowship only: 0%
Both tuition waiver & assistantship/fellowship: 100%

Approximate percentage of incoming students who entered with a B.A./B.S. only: 90% **Master's:** 10%

Approximate percentage of students who are
Women: 100% **Ethnic Minority:** 50%
International: Data not available

Average years to complete the doctoral program (including internship): 5 years

Personal interview
Preferred in person but telephone acceptable

Research areas	# Faculty	# Grants
child abuse/neglect	1	0
childhood illness/family coping	1	1
childhood loss	2	2
chronic illness and coping (adult)	1	0
conscious/unconscious processes	1	0
divorce	1	1
family systems	4	1
family violence	2	2
health psychology (AIDS, polio, head injury)	2	0
homeless families	1	0
inner city children	4	2
low birthweight children	1	0
neuropsychology	6	0
peer relations/social skills in children	2	2
personality disorders	2	0
psychotherapy research	5	0
schizophrenia	1	0
social competence in children	2	0
substance abuse	2	2
television violence	1	1

Clinical opportunities
adult
child and family

Michigan State University

Department of Psychology
East Lansing, MI 48824
phone#: (517) 432-9953
e-mail: mcvay@msu.edu
Web address:
http://psychology.msu.edu/academic/clinical/index.htm

	1	2	3	4	**5**	6	7

Clinically oriented   Equal emphasis   Research oriented

What percentage of your faculty subscribes to or practices in each of the following orientations?

Psychodynamic/Psychoanalytic	40%
Applied behavioral analysis/Radical behavioral	0%
Family systems/Systems	40%
Existential/Phenomenological/Humanistic	0%
Cognitive/Cognitive-behavioral	40%
Feminist	10%

What percentage of students applying for internship last year was accepted into APPIC-member internships? 100%

What courses are required for incoming students to have completed prior to enrolling?
12 hours of psychology courses at the bachelor's level

Are there courses you recommend that are not mandatory?
Quantitative methods, research design, advanced competence with the use of computer programs (SPSS, SYSTAT, etc.)

GRE mean
Verbal 553 Quantitative 631
Advanced Psychology 629
Analytical Writing 5.0

GPA mean
Overall GPA 3.55

Number of applications/admission offers/incoming students in 2005
197 applied/15 admission offers/5 incoming

% of incoming students receiving:
Tuition waiver only: 0%
Assistantship/fellowship only: 0%
Both tuition waiver & assistantship/fellowship: 100%

Approximate percentage of incoming students who entered with a B.A./B.S. only: 100%   Master's: 0%

Approximate percentage of students who are Women: 93%   Ethnic Minority: 40%   International: 9%

Average years to complete the doctoral program (including internship): 6.7 years

Personal interview
Preferred in person but telephone acceptable

Research areas	# Faculty	# Grants
ADHD	1	3
aging/gerontology	1	0
antisocial behavior	1	1
eating disorders	1	2
family research/systems	4	1
family violence	4	1
intimate partner violence	2	1
neuropsychology of alcholism	1	1
neuroscience of anxiety	1	2
racial harassment/gendered bullying	1	2

Clinical opportunities
assessment (child, adult, aging, ADHD, clinical neuropsychology)
couples therapy
depression and anxiety
eating disorders
family therapy
gerontology/aging
intimate partner violence
loss and trauma group therapy
minority/cross-cultural
play therapy

University of Minnesota
Department of Psychology
N218 Elliot Hall, 75 East River Road
Minneapolis, MN 55455
phone#: (612) 625-2546
e-mail: cspr@umn.edu
Web address:
http://www.psych.umn.edu/areas/clinical/index.htm

1	2	3	4	5	**6**	7

Clinically oriented   Equal emphasis   Research oriented

What percentage of your faculty subscribes to or practices in each of the following orientations?

Psychodynamic/Psychoanalytic	17%
Applied behavioral analysis/Radical behavioral	17%
Family systems/Systems	0%
Existential/Phenomenological/Humanistic	0%
Cognitive/Cognitive-behavioral	83%

What percentage of students applying for internship last year was accepted into APPIC-member internships?
Data not available

What courses are required for incoming students to have completed prior to enrolling?
Statistics, abnormal psychology

Are there courses you recommend that are not mandatory?
No

GRE mean
Verbal 632 Quantitative 683
Analytical Writing Data not available

GPA mean
Overall GPA 3.75

Number of applications/admission offers/incoming students in 2005
213 applied/12 admission offers/8 incoming

% of students receiving:
Tuition waiver only: 0%
Assistantship/fellowship only: 0%
Both tuition waiver & assistantship/fellowship: 100%

Approximate percentage of incoming students who entered with a B.A./B.S. only: 86%   Master's: 14%

**Approximate percentage of students who are Women: 79%   Ethnic Minority: 21%
International: Data not available**

Average years to complete the doctoral program (including internship): 6 years

Personal interview
Interview not required

Research areas	# Faculty	# Grants
affective disorders	3	1
anxiety disorders	3	1
behavioral genetics	4	4
cross-cultural psychology	1	0
developmental psychopathology	5	5

eating disorders	2	1
personality assessment	6	3
personality disorders	5	1
psychophysiology/neuroimaging	4	3
responses to extreme stress	2	0
schizophrenia	3	0

Clinical opportunities
ADHD
affective disorders
antisocial personality disorders
anxiety disorders
behavior therapy
childhood disorders and therapy
cognitive therapy
community psychology
conduct disorder
crisis intervention
eating disorders
family therapy
forensic psychology
gerontology/aging
long-term psychodynamic psychotherapy
neuropsychology
obsessive–compulsive disorder
panic disorder
psychopathic personality
psychotic disorders
schizophrenia
substance abuse

University of Mississippi

Department of Psychology
University, MS 38677
phone#: (662) 915-7383
e-mail: pygross@olemiss.edu
Web address: http://www.olemiss.edu/depts/psychology/
Clinical/index.html

1	2	3	4	**5**	6	7
Clinically oriented		Equal emphasis			Research oriented	

What percentage of your faculty subscribes to or practices in each of the following orientations?

Psychodynamic/Psychoanalytic	0%
Applied behavioral analysis/Radical behavioral	29%
Family systems/Systems	14%
Existential/Phenomenological/Humanistic	14%
Cognitive/Cognitive-behavioral	71%

(some faculty not easily categorized, e.g. applied behavioral/behavioral)

What percentage of students applying for internship last year was accepted into APPIC-member internships? 100%

What courses are required for incoming students to have completed prior to enrolling?
Introductory psychology, statistics, lab course

Are there courses you recommend that are not mandatory?
Physiological psychology, abnormal psychology, developmental psychology, and some grounding in biology/physiology/chemistry

GRE mean
Verbal 554   Quantitative 674
Verbal + Quantitative 1228
Advanced Psychology 635
Analytical Writing N/A

GPA mean
Overall GPA 3.72   Psychology GPA 3.5
Junior/Senior GPA 3.5

Number of applications/admission offers/incoming students in 2005
115 applied/15 admission offers/7 incoming

% of students receiving:
Tuition waiver only: 0%
Assistantship/fellowship only: 0%
Both tuition waiver & assistantship/fellowship: 100%

Approximate percentage of incoming students who entered with a B.A./B.S. only: 86%   **Master's:** 14%

Approximate percentage of students who are
Women: 84%   **Ethnic Minority:** 20%   **International:** 0%

Average years to complete the doctoral program (including internship): 6 years

Personal interview
Preferred in person but telephone acceptable

Research areas	# Faculty	# Grants
behavior problems in children	3	0
community psychology	2	0
compliance	1	0
computer-based research	1	1
emotion	2	1
posttraumatic stress disorder	1	0
psychological assessment	2	0
race relations	1	0
rape	2	0
rural mental health	2	0
smoking cessation/addiction/ substance abuse	1	1
social skills/competence	2	0

Clinical opportunities
child/adolescent
children's social skills
chronic mental illness
clinical assessment
community mental health
consultation
eating disorders
family/marital therapy
health psychology
mental retardation
posttramatic stress disorder
sexual aggression
smoking cessation
substance abuse/alcohol abuse

University of Missouri–Columbia

Department of Psychology
210 McAlester Hall
Columbia, MO 65211
phone#: (573) 882-6860
e-mail: BellDolanD@Missouri.edu
Web address:
http://psychology.missouri.edu/programs/clinical.htm

1	2	3	4	5	**6**	7
Clinically oriented		Equal emphasis			Research oriented	

What percentage of your faculty subscribes to or practices in each of the following orientations?

Psychodynamic/Psychoanalytic	10%
Applied behavioral analysis/Radical behavioral	0%
Family systems/Systems	10%
Existential/Phenomenological/Humanistic	0%
Cognitive/Cognitive-behavioral	80%

What percentage of students applying for internship last year was accepted into APPIC-member internships? 100%

What courses are required for incoming students to have completed prior to enrolling?
None

Are there courses you recommend that are not mandatory?
Other sciences, statistics/mathematics

GRE mean
Verbal + Quantitative = 1257
Analytical Writing Data not available

GPA mean
Overall GPA 3.67   Psychology GPA 3.78
Junior/Senior GPA 3.82

Number of applications/admission offers/incoming students in 2005
87 applied/9 admission offers/3 incoming

% of students receiving:
Tuition waiver only: 0%
Assistantship/fellowship only: 0%
Both tuition waiver & assistantship/fellowship: 100%

Approximate percentage of incoming students who entered with a B.A./B.S. only: 90%   **Master's:** 10%

Approximate percentage of students who are Women: 70%   **Ethnic Minority:** 17%
International: Data not available

Average years to complete the doctoral program (including internship): 5.4 years

Personal interview
Preferred in person but telephone acceptable

Research areas	# Faculty	# Grants
addictions	4	15
anxiety disorders	1	1
bipolar disorder	1	1
eating disorders	1	1
multisystemic therapy	1	1
schizophrenia	1	0
sexual dysfunction	1	0

Clinical opportunities
adult and child, outpatient and inpatient
health psychology
medical center
rehabilitation psychology
research protocol assessment and prevention
state hospital
VA hospital

University of Missouri-Kansas City

Department of Psychology
4825 Troost, Room 215
Kansas City, MO 64110
phone#: (816) 235-1318
e-mail: psychology@umkc.edu
Web address: http://cas.umkc.edu/psyc/grad/clinical.htm
Program data unavailable

University of Missouri–St. Louis

Department of Psychology
One University Blvd.
St. Louis, MO 63121
phone#: (314) 516-5391
Web address: http://www.umsl.edu/divisions/
artscience/psychology/clinical/index.html

1	2	3	**4**	5	6	7
Clinically oriented		Equal emphasis			Research oriented	

What percentage of your faculty subscribes to or practices in each of the following orientations?

Psychodynamic/Psychoanalytic	25%
Applied behavioral analysis/Radical behavioral	0%
Family systems/Systems	0%
Existential/Phenomenological/Humanistic	35%
Cognitive/Cognitive-behavioral	40%

What percentage of students applying for internship last year was accepted into APPIC-member internships? 100%

What courses are required for incoming students to have completed prior to enrolling?
A total of 24 undergraduate credits: introductory psychology, psychological statistics, research methods in psychology

Are there courses you recommend that are not mandatory?
Personality, social psychology, learning and motivation, history and systems, physiological psychology, developmental

GRE mean
Verbal 648   Quantitative 688
Advanced Psychology 738
Analytical Writing 5.2

GPA mean
Overall GPA 3.76   Psychology GPA 3.78

Number of applications/admission offers/incoming students in 2005
106 applied/9 admission offers/6 incoming

% of students receiving:
Tuition waiver only: 0%
Assistantship/fellowship only: 0%
Both tuition waiver & assistantship/fellowship: 100% in first 2 years

Approximate percentage of incoming students who entered with a B.A./B.S. only: 83%   **Master's:** 17%

Approximate percentage of students who are Women: 75%   **Ethnic Minority:** 16%   **International:** 9.4%

Average years to complete the doctoral program (including internship): 6.2 years

Personal interview
Preferred in person but telephone acceptable

Research areas	# Faculty	# Grants
behavioral health	1	1
bereavement	1	1
caretakers of the elderly	1	1
child and health	1	0
children's play	1	0
psychology of women	1	0
trauma studies	1	1

Clinical opportunities
adult
behavioral health
children and families
feminist therapy
interventions for caregivers of the elderly
psychotherapy with older populations
treatment of rape victims

University of Montana
Department of Psychology
Missoula, MT 59812
phone#: (406) 243-4521
e-mail: PSYCGRAD@SELWAY.UMT.EDU
Web address: http://psychweb.psy.umt.edu/www/default.asp?file=graduate_clinical_about

1	2	3	**4**	5	6	7

Clinically oriented   Equal emphasis   Research oriented

What percentage of your faculty subscribes to or practices in each of the following orientations?
Psychodynamic/Psychoanalytic   25%
Applied behavioral analysis/Radical behavioral   12%
Family systems/Systems   25%
Existential/Phenomenological/Humanistic   12%
Cognitive/Cognitive-behavioral   50%

What percentage of students applying for internship last year was accepted into APPIC-member internships? 100%

What courses are required for incoming students to have completed prior to enrolling?
None

Are there courses you recommend that are not mandatory?
Research methods, statistics, abnormal psychology, Personality, physiological psychology

GRE mean
Verbal 525   Quantitative 550
Advanced Psychology Not Required
Analytical Writing Data not available

GPA mean
Overall GPA 3.42

Number of applications/admission offers/incoming students in 2003
136 applied/9 admission offers/7 incoming

% of students receiving:
Tuition waiver only: 0%
Assistantship/fellowship only: 0%
Both tuition waiver & assistantship/fellowship: 71%

Approximate percentage of incoming students who entered with a B.A./B.S. only: 85%   **Master's:** 15%

Approximate percentage of students who are Women: 85%   **Ethnic Minority:** 28%   **International:** 3%

Average years to complete the doctoral program (including internship): 6 years

Personal interview
Preferred in person but telephone acceptable

Research areas	# Faculty	# Grants
assessment	1	0
attention-deficit disorder	1	0
behavioral medicine/health psychology	3	1
child psychopathology	1	1
closed-head injury	1	0
cross-cultural (Native American)	1	0
depression	1	0
emotion regulation	1	1
gender issues	2	1
malingering	1	1
neuropsychology	1	0
nonlinear dynamic systems	1	0
psychotherapy process and outcome	2	1
schizophrenia	1	0
sexuality	1	0
substance abuse	1	1

Clinical opportunities
adolescent and child
anxiety disorders
assessment
attachment disorder
borderline personality disorder
community health
couples/family
depression

domestic violence
functional analytic therapy
motivational interviewing
neuropsychology
pain management
prison populations
rural psychology
schizophrenia/psychoses
substance abuse
trauma

University of Nebraska–Lincoln

Department of Psychology
209 Burnett Hall
Lincoln, NE 68588-0311
phone#: (402) 472-3229
e-mail: rbarnes1@unl.edu
Web address: http://psycweb.unl.edu/psypage/
dynamic.asp?dir=grad&page=clinical.htm

1	2	3	**4**	5	6	7

Clinically oriented   Equal emphasis   Research oriented

What percentage of your faculty subscribes to or practices in each of the following orientations?

Psychodynamic/Psychoanalytic	0%
Applied behavioral analysis/Radical behavioral	10%
Family systems/Systems	25%
Existential/Phenomenological/Humanistic	10%
Cognitive/Cognitive-behavioral	85%

What percentage of students applying for internship last year was accepted into APPIC-member internships? 100%

What courses are required for incoming students to have completed prior to enrolling?
Psychology major preferred

Are there courses you recommend that are not mandatory?
Methodology and quantitative courses

GRE mean
Verbal 590   Quantitative 660
Analytical Writing Data not available

GPA mean
Overall GPA 3.58

Number of applications/admission offers/incoming students in 2005
136 applied/13 admission offers/7 incoming

% of students receiving:
Tuition waiver only: 0%
Assistantship/fellowship only: 0%
Both tuition waiver & assistantship/fellowship: 100%

Approximate percentage of incoming students who entered with a B.A./B.S. only: 87%   **Master's:** 23%

Approximate percentage of students who are
Women: 65%   **Ethnic Minority:** 20%   **International:** 5%

Average years to complete the doctoral program (including internship): 6.5 years

Personal interview
Preferred in person but telephone acceptable

Research areas	# Faculty	# Grants
anxiety disorders	2	2
child abuse/family violence	2	2
child/adolescence	2	1
chronically mentally ill	1	1
forensic	2	2
neuropsychology	1	0
psychopathology	3	2

Clinical opportunities
alcoholism
anxiety disorders
child abuse/family violence
chronically mentally ill
forensic
minority issues

University of Nevada–Reno

Department of Psychology
MSS 298
Reno, NV 89557
Web address:
http://www.unr.edu/psych/clinical/index.html

1	2	3	4	**5**	6	7

Clinically oriented   Equal emphasis   Research oriented

What percentage of your faculty subscribes to or practices in each of the following orientations?

Psychodynamic/Psychoanalytic	0%
Applied behavioral analysis/Radical behavioral	40%
Family systems/Systems	15%
Existential/Phenomenological/Humanistic	0%
Cognitive/Cognitive-behavioral	45%

What percentage of students applying for internship last year was accepted into APPIC-member internships? 100%

What courses are required for incoming students to have completed prior to enrolling?
Abnormal psychology, statistics

Are there courses you recommend that are not mandatory?
Behavioral principles (e.g., behavior analysis, learning), research methodology

GRE mean
Verbal 640   Quantitative 661
Advanced Psychology 700
Analytical Writing Not required

GPA mean
Overall GPA 3.7   Psychology GPA 3.85

Number of applications/admission offers/incoming students in 2005
93 applied/7 admission offers/6 incoming

% of students receiving:
Tuition waiver only: 0%
Assistantship/fellowship only: 0%
Both tuition waiver & assistantship/fellowship: 100%

Approximate percentage of incoming students who entered with a B.A./B.S. only: 67%   **Master's:** 33%

Approximate percentage of students who are Women: 70%   **Ethnic Minority:** 10%   **International:** 2%

Average years to complete the doctoral program (including internship): 7.5 years

Personal interview
Preferred in person but telephone acceptable

Research areas	# Faculty	# Grants
aging	1	2
anxiety disorders	2	0
behavior analysis	3	0
behavioral assessment	3	0
behavioral health	2	0
couples	2	0
drug and alcohol abuse	2	1
gerontology	1	2
health care administration	1	1
incest survivors	2	0
minority mental health	1	0
mood disorders	1	0
prevention	4	2
sexual offenders	1	1
social skills	3	0
suicide	1	0
treatment development	3	1
verbal behavior	4	0

Clinical opportunities
AIDS
anxiety disorders
behavioral health care
couples
depression
drug and alcohol abuse
gerontology
health care administration
incest survivors
personality disorders
posttraumatic stress disorder

University of New Mexico

Department of Psychology
MSCO3 2220
Albuquerque, NM 87131-0001
phone#: (505) 277-4121
e-mail: dougher@unm.edu (director) or
advising@unm.edu (graduate office) or
trishara@unm.edu (coordinator)
Web address: http://psych.unm.edu/grad_clinical.htm

1	2	3	4	**5**	6	7
Clinically oriented		Equal emphasis			Research oriented	

What percentage of your faculty subscribes to or practices in each of the following orientations?

Psychodynamic/Psychoanalytic	0%
Clinical behavior analysis/Applied behavioral analysis/Radical behavioral	20%
Family systems/Systems	38%
Existential/Phenomenological/Humanistic	25%
Cognitive/Cognitive-behavioral	50%

What percentage of students applying for internship last year was accepted into APPIC-member internships? 100%

What courses are required for incoming students to have completed prior to enrolling?
Statistics, research methods, psychology major or equivalent course work

Are there courses you recommend that are not mandatory?
Basic science courses, laboratory courses, supervised research

GRE mean
Verbal 620   Quantitative 709   Analytical 716
Advanced Psychology 685
Analytical Writing Data not available

GPA mean
Overall GPA 3.72

Number of applications/admission offers/incoming students in 2005
175 applied/16 admission offers/8 incoming

% of students receiving:
Tuition waiver only: 0%
Assistantship/fellowship only: 0%
Both tuition waiver & assistantship/fellowship: 100%

Approximate percentage of incoming students who entered with a B.A./B.S. only: 100%   **Master's:** 0%

Approximate percentage of students who are Women: 80%   **Ethnic Minority:** 20%   **International:** 2%

Average years to complete the doctoral program (including internship): 7 years

Personal interview
Preferred in person but telephone acceptable

Research areas	# Faculty	# Grants
eating disorders	1	1
family interactions	2	3
minority/cultural issues	3	1
health psychology	3	0
human learning/language	1	0
neuropsychology	2	4
pediatric psychology	1	0
sexual victimization		
substance abuse	6	8

Clinical opportunities
behavioral medicine
forensic settings/domestic violence
inpatient/oupatient psychotherapy
multicultural
neuroimaging
neuropsychological assessment
pediatrics

personality assessment
school setting (children, adolescents, families,
adults, couples)
substance abuse

New School University

(formerly listed as New School for Social Research)
Graduate Faculty, Department of Psychology
65 Fifth Avenue, A/L 330
New York, NY 10003
phone#: (212) 229-5756
e-mail: gfadmit@newschool.edu
Web address: http://www.newschool.edu/gf/psy/
degree-programs.htm#ClinicalPhD

1	2	3	**4**	5	6	7
Clinically oriented		Equal emphasis			Research oriented	

What percentage of your faculty subscribes to or practices in each of the following orientations?

Psychodynamic/Psychoanalytic — 90%
Applied behavioral analysis/Radical behavioral — 0%
Family systems/Systems — 0%
Existential/Phenomenological/Humanistic — 0%
Cognitive/Cognitive-behavioral — 10%

What percentage of students applying for internship last year was accepted into APPIC-member internships?
Data not available

What courses are required for incoming students to have completed prior to enrolling?
The clinical Ph.D. program requires 1 course in each of the following: personality, social, developmental; psychopathology I and II; 1 course in assessment of individual differences; 1 course in statistics; 1 research methods course.

Are there courses you recommend that are not mandatory?
Undergraduate major in psychology recommended, But not mandatory

GRE mean
Verbal 525 Quantitative 590 Analytical 610
Advanced Psychology 595
Analytical Writing Data not available

GPA mean
GPA 3.63

Number of applications/admission offers/incoming students in 2005
40 applied/17 admission offers/17 incoming
Note: Only applications from New School University master's students in psychology are considered for enrollment.

% of students receiving:
Tuition waiver only: 6% (33% partial tuition waiver)
Assistantship/fellowship only: 6%
Both tuition waiver & assistantship/fellowship: 2%

Approximate percentage of incoming students who entered with a B.A./B.S. only: 0% **Master's:** 100%

Approximate percentage of students who are Women: 80% **Ethnic Minority:** 17% **International:** 9%

Average years to complete the doctoral program (including internship): 7 years

Personal interview
Required in person

Research areas	# Faculty	# Grants
assessment/diagnosis	2	1
child clinical	1	1
developmental	1	0
emotions	1	0
memory	2	1
moral development	1	0
narrative methodologies	2	0
personality assessment	1	0
prevention	2	1
psychoanalysis	2	0
psychopathology	2	0
psychotherapy process and outcome	3	1

Clinical opportunities
Our 1st-year students gain clinical experience at the New School–Beth Israel Center for clinical training and research, where they conduct intake interviews with psychiatric outpatients, and lead therapeutic groups in 1 of 3 different inpatient units.

University of North Carolina at Chapel Hill

Department of Psychology
Davie Hall 013A
Chapel Hill, NC 27514
phone#: (919) 962-5082
fax#: (919) 962-2537
Web address: http://www.unc.edu/depts/clinpsy/

1	2	3	4	**5**	6	7
Clinically oriented		Equal emphasis			Research oriented	

What percentage of your faculty subscribes to or practices in each of the following orientations?

Psychodynamic/Psychoanalytic — 20%
Applied behavioral analysis/Radical behavioral — 0%
Family systems/Systems — 20%
Existential/Phenomenological/Humanistic — 20%
Cognitive/Cognitive-behavioral — 40%

What percentage of students applying for internship last year was accepted into APPIC-member internships? 100%

What courses are required for incoming students to have completed prior to enrolling?
A psychology major or its equivalent (8 or more courses). These courses must include training in statistics.

Are there courses you recommend that are not mandatory?
No

GRE mean
Verbal + Quantitative 1350

GPA mean
Psychology GPA 3.5 Junior/Senior GPA 3.5

Number of applications/admission offers/incoming students in 2003
344 applied/9 admission offers/7 incoming

% of students receiving:
Tuition waiver only: 0%
Assistantship/fellowship only: 4%
Both tuition waiver & assistantship/fellowship: 95%

Approximate percentage of incoming students who entered with a B.A./B.S. only: 85% **Master's:** 15%
Approximate percentage of students who are
Women: 71% **Ethnic Minority:** 28%
International: Data not available

Average years to complete the doctoral program (including internship): 6 years

Personal interview
Preferred in person but telephone acceptable

Research areas	# Faculty	# Grants
adolescent drug use	1	1
assessment	1	0
behavioral medicine	1	2
children's peer relationships	2	2
family systems/therapy	1	2
marriage/couples	1	1
neuropsychology of aging	2	1
rural–migrant families	1	1
schizophrenia	1	1
self-esteem/minority	1	0

Clinical opportunities
assessment
behavioral medicine
cognitive-behavioral
developmental disabilities
family therapy
marital therapy
pediatric
psychodynamic
victim/battering/abuse

University of North Carolina at Greensboro

Department of Psychology
296 Eberhart Building
Greensboro, NC 27402-6170
phone#: (336) 256-0006
e-mail: ada@uncg.edu
Web address:
http://www.uncg.edu/psy/areas_clinical.htm

1	2	3	**4**	5	6	7

Clinically oriented	Equal emphasis	Research oriented

What percentage of your faculty subscribes to or practices in each of the following orientations?

Psychodynamic/Psychoanalytic	0%
Applied behavioral analysis/Radical behavioral	12%
Family systems/Systems	62%
Existential/Phenomenological/Humanistic	0%
Cognitive/Cognitive-behavioral	100%

What percentage of students applying for internship last year was accepted into APPIC-member internships? 86%

What courses are required for incoming students to have completed prior to enrolling?
Equivalent of undergraduate major in psychology which typically includes introductory psychology, statistics, and 4 other courses in psychology

Are there courses you recommend that are not mandatory?
Courses in psychology as a natural science (e.g., physiological psychology), abnormal psychology, statistics, learning/cognitive psychology

GRE mean
Verbal 580 Quantitative 681
Advanced Psychology 640
Analytical Writing Data not available

GPA mean
Overall GPA 3.8

Number of applications/admission offers/incoming students in 2005
237 applied/7 admission offers/7 incoming

% of students receiving:
Tuition waiver only: 0%
Assistantship/fellowship only: 43%
Both tuition waiver & assistantship/fellowship: 57%

Approximate percentage of incoming students who entered with a B.A./B.S. only: 72% **Master's:** 28%

Approximate percentage of students who are
Women: 86% **Ethnic Minority:** 28%
International: Data not available

Average years to complete the doctoral program (including internship): 6 years

Personal interview
Required in person

Research areas	# Faculty	# Grants
ADHD	1	2
adolescents' externalizing disorder	1	0
behavioral analysis	1	0
behavioral assessment	1	0
children's internalizing disorder	1	0
children's social relationships	2	2
depression	1	0
personality disorders	1	0
schizophrenia	1	1

Clinical opportunities
family practice setting in local hospital
university-based community clinic
university counseling center

University of North Dakota

Department of Psychology
Box 8380
Grand Forks, ND 58202
phone#: (701) 777-3451
e-mail: alan_king@UND.nodak.edu
Web address:
http://ndwild.psych.und.nodak.edu/dept/clinical.html

1	2	3	4	**5**	6	7

Clinically oriented	Equal emphasis	Research oriented

What percentage of your faculty subscribes to or practices in each of the following orientations?

Psychodynamic/Psychoanalytic	5%
Applied behavioral analysis/Radical behavioral	15%
Family systems/Systems	0%
Existential/Phenomenological/Humanistic	5%
Cognitive/Cognitive-behavioral	75%

What percentage of students applying for internship last year was accepted into APPIC-member internships? 100%

What courses are required for incoming students to have completed prior to enrolling?
Psychology courses (at least 18 hours) in general developmental, abnormal psychology, statistics, experimental or research methods. One semester of college algebra and a year of biological science.

Are there courses you recommend that are not mandatory?
A background in social and natural sciences

GRE mean
Verbal + Quantitative 1085
Analytical Writing Data not available

GPA mean
Overall GPA 3.65

Number of applications/admission offers/incoming students in 2005
76 applied/17 admission offers/9 incoming

% of students receiving:
Tuition waiver only: 0%
Assistantship/fellowship only: 0%
Both tuition waiver & assistantship/fellowship: 100%

Approximate percentage of incoming students who entered with a B.A./B.S. only: 66%   **Master's:** 33%

Approximate percentage of students who are Women: 67%   **Ethnic Minority:** 33%   **International:** <1%

Average years to complete the doctoral program (including internship): 6.1 years

Personal interview
Preferred in person but telephone acceptable

Research areas	# Faculty	# Grants
adult psychopathology	6	0
anxiety disorders	1	0
applied behavioral analysis	2	0
behavioral medicine	2	0
community psychology	2	0
cross-cultural psychology	2	1
friendship/relationships	2	0
gender roles	2	0
minority mental health	2	0
pain management/control	1	0
personality assessment	2	0
personality disorders	3	0
psychophysiology	1	0
relaxation/biofeedback	3	0
rural psychology	2	2
stress and coping	6	0
substance abuse	1	0
women's studies	2	0

Clinical opportunities
affective disorders
anxiety disorders
assessment
behavioral medicine
community psychology
interpersonal psychotherapy
marital/couples therapy
minority/cross-cultural
obsessive–compulsive disorder
personality disorders
rural psychology
substance abuse
victim/battering abuse

University of North Texas

Clinical Psychology Program
Department of Psychology
Box 13587
Denton, TX 76203
phone#: (940) 565-2652
e-mail: AMYG@UNT.EDU
Web address: http://www.psyc.unt.edu/grad.shtml

1	2	3	**4**	5	6	7

Clinically oriented	Equal emphasis	Research oriented

What percentage of your faculty subscribes to or practices in each of the following orientations?

Psychodynamic/Psychoanalytic	25%
Applied behavioral analysis/Radical behavioral	0%
Family systems/Systems	25%
Existential/Phenomenological/Humanistic	37%
Cognitive/Cognitive-behavioral	37%

What percentage of students applying for internship last year was accepted into APPIC-member internships? 88%

What courses are required for incoming students to have completed prior to enrolling?
Statistics, experimental, learning, and history and systems

Are there courses you recommend that are not mandatory?
Physiological psychology, social psychology, abnormal psychology, personality, tests and measurements

GRE mean
Verbal 531   Quantitative 648

GPA mean
Data not available

Number of applications/admission offers/incoming students in 2005
144 applied/13 admission offers/8 incoming

% of students receiving:
Tuition waiver only: 0%
Assistantship/fellowship only: 35%
Both tuition waiver & assistantship/fellowship: 25%

Approximate percentage of incoming students who entered with a B.A./B.S. only: 100%   **Master's:** 0%

Approximate percentage of students who are Women: 75%   **Ethnic Minority:** 15%   **International:** 5%

Average years to complete the doctoral program (including internship): 6 years (mode)

Personal interview
Required in person

Research areas	# Faculty	# Grants
abuse	2	0
AIDS	1	0
affect management	1	0
aging	1	1
children	1	1
disaster intervention	2	0
forensics	2	1
malingering	2	2
neuropsychology	1	0
posttraumatic stress disorder	2	1
schizophrenia	2	1
stress	2	1

Clinical opportunities
attention-deficit disorder
children
depression
forensic psychology
neuropsychology
posttraumatic stress disorder

Northern Illinois University

Department of Psychology
DeKalb, IL 60115
phone#: (815) 753-0772
e-mail: MLOVEJOY@NIU.EDU
Web address: http://www.niu.edu/psyc/grad_clinical/clinical_index.shtml

1	2	3	**4**	5	6	7

Clinically oriented   Equal emphasis   Research oriented

What percentage of your faculty subscribes to or practices in each of the following orientations?

Psychodynamic/Psychoanalytic	17%
Applied behavioral analysis/Radical behavioral	56%
Family systems/Systems	34%
Existential/Phenomenological/Humanistic	17%
Cognitive/Cognitive-behavioral	100%

What percentage of students applying for internship last year was accepted into APPIC-member internships? 100%

What courses are required for incoming students to have completed prior to enrolling?
None

Are there courses you recommend that are not mandatory?
Statistics, research methods, laboratory course, history

GRE mean
Verbal 561   Quantitative 649
Analytical Writing 5.3

GPA mean
Overall GPA 3.65

Number of applications/admission offers/incoming students in 2005
153 applied/14 admission offers/8 incoming

% of students receiving:
Tuition waiver only: 0%
Assistantship/fellowship only: 0%
Both tuition waiver & assistantship/fellowship: 100%

Approximate percentage of incoming students who entered with a B.A./B.S. only: 75%   **Master's:** 25%

Approximate percentage of students who are Women: 75%   **Ethnic Minority:** 25%   **International:** 4%

Average years to complete the doctoral program (including internship): 6.5 years

Personal interview
Preferred in person but telephone acceptable

Research areas	# Faculty	# Grants
adolescents	3	0
adult psychopathology	6	1
anxiety disorders	3	0
child sexual abuse	3	2
developmental psychopathology	5	1
physical abuse	2	2
prevention	3	2
psychometrics	4	1
sexual aggression	3	3
suicide	1	0

Clinical opportunities
ADHD clinic
anxiety disorders
assessment
child psychotherapy
developmental disabilities
family therapy
forensic evaluations

individual psychotherapy
parent training
personality and cognitive assessment
victim/battering/abuse

Northwestern University

Department of Psychology
102 Swift Hall, 2029 Sheridan Road
Evanston, IL 60208-2710
phone#: (847) 491-5190
e-mail: mineka@northwestern.edu
Web address: http://www.wcas.northwestern.edu/psych/
programs/clinical.html

1	2	3	4	5	6	**7**

Clinically oriented	Equal emphasis	Research oriented

What percentage of your faculty subscribes to or practices in each of the following orientations?

Psychodynamic/Psychoanalytic	10%
Applied behavioral analysis/Radical behavioral	0%
Family systems/Systems	10%
Existential/Phenomenological/Humanistic	0%
Cognitive/Cognitive-behavioral	80%

What percentage of students applying for internship last year was accepted into APPIC-member internships?
Data not available

What courses are required for incoming students to have completed prior to enrolling?
None

Are there courses you recommend that are not mandatory?
Psychology major, undergraduate statistics

GRE mean
Verbal 680 Quantitative 750 Analytical 750
Advanced Psychology 750
Analytical Writing Data not available

GPA mean
Overall GPA 3.83 Junior/Senior GPA 3.88

Number of applications/admission offers/incoming students in 2005
89 applied/5 admission offers/1 incoming

% of students receiving:
Tuition waiver only: 0%
Assistantship/fellowship only: 0%
Both tuition waiver & assistantship/fellowship: 100%

Approximate percentage of incoming students who entered with a B.A./B.S. only: 90% **Master's:** 10%

Approximate percentage of students who are Women: 50% **Ethnic Minority:** 10%
International: Data not available

Average years to complete the doctoral program (including internship): 6 years

Personal interview
Telephone required

Research areas

	# Faculty	# Grants
anxiety	2	1
behavioral genetics	1	0
cognitive functioning	1	1
depression	2	0
personality	2	1
psychotherapy	1	0

Clinical opportunities
anxiety disorders
behavioral medicine
couples
crisis intervention
depression
family
neuropsychology
psychosis

Northwestern University, Feinberg School of Medicine

Department of Psychiatry and Behavioral Sciences
Division of Psychology
Abbott Hall, Suite 1205
710 North Lakeshore Drive
Chicago, IL 60611
phone#: (312) 908-8262
e-mail: j-johnson6@northwestern.edu or
clinpsych@northwestern.edu
Web address:
http://www.clinpsych.northwestern.edu/doc_prog.htm

1	2	3	**4**	5	6	7

Clinically oriented	Equal emphasis	Research oriented

What percentage of your faculty subscribes to or practices in each of the following orientations?

Psychodynamic/Psychoanalytic	50%
Applied behavioral analysis/Radical behavioral	0%
Family systems/Systems	0%
Existential/Phenomenological/Humanistic	10%
Cognitive/Cognitive-behavioral	40%

What percentage of students applying for internship last year was accepted into APPIC-member internships? 83%

What courses are required for incoming students to have completed prior to enrolling?
Statistics, research designs, experimental, abnormal

Are there courses you recommend that are not mandatory?
Advanced statistics

GRE mean
Verbal 620 Quantitative 640
Advanced Psychology 650
Analytical Writing Data not available

GPA mean
Data not available

Number of applications/admission offers/incoming students in 2005
150 applied/7 admission offers/6 incoming

% of students receiving:
Half tuition waiver only: 50%
Assistantship/fellowship only: 0%
Half tuition & research assistantship: 25%
Both tuition waiver & assistantship/fellowship: 25%

Approximate percentage of incoming students who entered with a B.A./B.S. only: 80% **Master's:** 20%

**Approximate percentage of students who are
Women:** 70% **Ethnic Minority:** 15% **International:** 10%

Average years to complete the doctoral program (including internship): 6 years

Personal interview
Required in person

Research areas	# Faculty	# Grants
adolescent depression	2	1
child mental health	3	1
mental health services and policy	2	3
neuropsychology	3	1
personality	1	0
psycho-legal studies (youth in criminal justice system)	2	1

Clinical opportunities
adult, adolescent, and child outpatient clinics
chronic mental illness
neuropsychology (adult and pediatric)
student mental health

Nova Southeastern University (Ph.D.)

Dean, Center for Psychological Studies
3301 College Avenue
Fort Lauderdale, FL 33314
phone#: (954) 262-5700
e-mail: cpsinfo@nova.edu
Web address: http://www.cps.nova.edu

1	2	3	4	5	**6**	7

Clinically oriented　　Equal emphasis　　Research oriented

What percentage of your faculty subscribes to or practices in each of the following orientations?
Psychodynamic/Psychoanalytic　22%
Applied behavioral analysis/Radical behavioral　3%
Family systems/Systems　9%
Existential/Phenomenological/Humanistic　3%
Cognitive/Cognitive-behavioral　63%

What percentage of students applying for internship last year was accepted into APPIC-member internships?
Data not available

What courses are required for incoming students to have completed prior to enrolling?
18 credits in psychology and 3 credits in statistics

Are there courses you recommend that are not mandatory?
Calculus, intermediate statistics, experimental psychology, and hard rather than soft courses in psychology, biology, and philosophy

GRE mean
Verbal 550　Quantitative 596
Advanced Psychology 624
Analytical Writing Data not available

GPA mean
Data not available

Number of applications/admission offers/incoming students in 2003
225 applied/35 admission offers/19 incoming

% of students receiving:
Tuition waiver only: 0%
Assistantship/fellowship only: 24%
Both tuition waiver & assistantship/fellowship: 24%

Approximate percentage of incoming students who entered with a B.A./B.S. only: 79% **Master's:** 21%

**Approximate percentage of students who are
Women:** 71% **Ethnic Minority:** 41%
International: Data not available

Average years to complete the doctoral program (including internship): 5.6 years

Personal interview
Required in person

Research areas	# Faculty	# Grants
ADHD	3	0
alcohol/substance abuse	3	5
anxiety disorders	1	0
behavior therapy	8	0
biofeedback	2	0
child/adolescent depression	2	0
child/adolescent psychotherapy	5	0
child neuropsychology	4	0
community mental health	4	0
cross-cultural counseling	2	0
domestic/interpersonal violence	2	0
forensic psychology	3	2
gerontology	2	0
health psychology	7	2
long-term mental illness	2	0
MMPI-2	1	0
neuropsychology	5	2
posttraumatic stress disorder	4	0
psychoanalysis	2	0
psychology of men	1	0
survivors of sexual abuse/assault	2	0
trauma and victimization	7	0

Clinical opportunities
anxiety disorders
behavioral modification
biofeedback

child/adolescent assessment and treatment
child/adolescent depression
community support services
crisis assessment and intervention
day treatment
depression
dual diagnosis
family and multifamily therapy
forensic evaluation and testimony
geriatric
group therapy
interpersonal violence
medication management
multilingual services
neuropsychological assessment and evaluation
pain management
parenting skills training
psychodynamic psychotherapy
psychological consultation
psychological testing
serious emotional disturbance
skills treatment and enhancement program (STEP)
stress management
student counseling
substance abuse

Nova Southeastern University (Psy.D.)

Dean, Center for Psychological Studies
3301 College Avenue
Fort Lauderdale, FL 33314
phone#: (954) 262-5700
e-mail: cpsinfo@cps.acast.nova.edu
Web address: www.cps.nova.edu

1	2	**3**	4	5	6	7
Clinically oriented		Equal emphasis			Research oriented	

What percentage of your faculty subscribes to or practices in each of the following orientations?

Psychodynamic/Psychoanalytic	22%
Applied behavioral analysis/Radical behavioral	3%
Family systems/Systems	9%
Existential/Phenomenological/Humanistic	3%
Cognitive/Cognitive-behavioral	63%

What percentage of students applying for internship last year was accepted into APPIC-member internships?
Data not available

What courses are required for incoming students to have completed prior to enrolling?
18 credits in psychology and 3 credits in statistics

Are there courses you recommend that are not mandatory?
Experimental psychology; hard rather than soft courses in psychology, biology, and philosophy

GRE mean
Verbal 494 Quantitative 544 Analytical 574
Advanced Psychology 578

Analytical Writing Data not available

GPA mean
Overall GPA 3.43

Number of applications/admission offers/incoming students in 2003
263 applied/129 admission offers/80 incoming

% of students receiving:
Tuition waiver only: 0%
Assistantship/fellowship only: 24%
Both tuition waiver & assistantship/fellowship: 24%

Approximate percentage of incoming students who entered with a B.A./B.S. only: 91% **Master's:** 9%

Approximate percentage of students who are Women: 81% **Ethnic Minority:** 24%
International: Data not available

Average years to complete the doctoral program (including internship): 5 years

Personal interview
Required in person

Research areas	# Faculty	# Grants
ADHD	3	0
alcohol/substance abuse	3	5
anxiety disorders	1	0
behavior therapy	8	0
biofeedback	2	0
child/adolescent depression	2	0
child/adolescent psychotherapy	5	0
child neuropsychology	4	0
community mental health	4	0
cross-cultural counseling	2	0
domestic/interpersonal violence	2	0
forensic psychology	3	2
gerontology	2	0
health psychology	7	2
long-term mental illness	2	0
MMPI-2	1	0
neuropsychology	5	2
posttraumatic stress disorder	4	0
psychoanalysis	2	0
psychology of men	1	0
survivors of sexual abuse/assault	2	0
trauma and victimization	7	0

Clinical opportunities
anxiety disorders
behavioral modification
biofeedback
child/adolescent assessment and treatment
child/adolescent traumatic stress and depression
community support services
crisis assessment and intervention
day treatment
depression
dual diagnosis and day treatment
family and multifamily treatment
forensic evaluation and testimony
geriatric residential treatment
group therapy
interpersonal violence

medication management
multilingual services
neuropsychological assessment and evaluation
pain management
parenting skills and training
psychodynamic psychotherapy
psychological consultation
psychological testing
serious emotional disturbance
skills treatment and enhancement program (STEP)
stress management
student counseling
substance abuse

Ohio State University

Department of Psychology
238 Townshend Hall
1885 Neil Avenue Mall
Columbus, OH 43210
phone#: (614) 292-4112
e-mail: sexton.3@osu.edu
Web address:
http://www2.psy.ohio-state.edu/programs/clinical/

1	2	3	4	5	**6**	7
Clinically oriented		Equal emphasis			Research oriented	

What percentage of your faculty subscribes to or practices in each of the following orientations?

Psychodynamic/Psychoanalytic	14%
Applied behavioral analysis/Radical behavioral	0%
Family systems/Systems	0%
Existential/Phenomenological/Humanistic	0%
Cognitive/Cognitive-behavioral	86%

What percentage of students applying for internship last year was accepted into APPIC-member internships? 94%

What courses are required for incoming students to have completed prior to enrolling?
Experimental psychology, abnormal psychology, statistics, personality

Are there courses you recommend that are not mandatory?
No

GRE mean
Verbal 647   Quantitative 646
Analytical Writing 5.5

GPA mean
Psychology GPA 3.8

Number of applications/admission offers/incoming students in 2005
187 applied/16 admission offers/7 incoming

% of students receiving:
Tuition waiver only: 0%
Assistantship/fellowship only: 0%
Both tuition waiver & assistantship/fellowship: 100%

Approximate percentage of incoming students who entered with a B.A./B.S. only: 100%   **Master's:** 0%

**Approximate percentage of students who are
Women:** 87%   **Ethnic Minority:** 22%   **International:** 7%

Average years to complete the doctoral program (including internship): 6 years

Personal interview
Preferred in person but telephone acceptable

Research areas	# Faculty	# Grants
anxiety disorders	2	1
cardiovascular health	3	4
child psychopathology	3	4
childhood mood disorders	2	4
depression	3	1
oncology	1	2
pediatric neuropsychology	3	3
personality	1	0
psychoneuroimmunology	2	5
psychosocial aspects of pediatric oncology	2	3

Clinical opportunities
anxiety disorder
child and adolescent psychopathology
childhood mood disorders
crisis intervention
depressive disorders
eating disorders
family
gerontology
health psychology
neuropsychology
oncology
psycho-education evaluations
sex therapy

Ohio University

Department of Psychology
Athens, OH 45701-2979
phone#: (740) 593-1707
Web address: http://www.psych.ohiou.edu/academics/grad_studies/clinical.html

1	2	3	**4**	5	6	7
Clinically oriented		Equal emphasis			Research oriented	

What percentage of your faculty subscribes to or practices in each of the following orientations?

Psychodynamic/Psychoanalytic	20%
Applied behavioral analysis/Radical behavioral	0%
Family systems/Systems	30%
Existential/Phenomenological/Humanistic	0%
Cognitive/Cognitive-behavioral	50%

What percentage of students applying for internship last year was accepted into APPIC-member internships?
Data not available

What courses are required for incoming students to have completed prior to enrolling?
27 quarter hours of undergraduate psychology, introductory psychology, experimental psychology, statistics

Are there courses you recommend that are not mandatory?
Computer science, abnormal psychology, personality

GRE mean
Verbal 552   Quantitative 638   Psychology 643

GPA mean
Data not available

Number of applications/admission offers/incoming students in 2005
173 applied/17 admission offers/10 incoming

% of students receiving:
Tuition waiver only: 0%
Assistantship/fellowship only: 0
Both tuition waiver & assistantship/fellowship: 100%

Approximate percentage of incoming students who entered with a B.A./B.S. only: 80%   **Master's:** 20%

Approximate percentage of students who are Women: 70%   **Ethnic Minority:** 5%
International: Data not available

Average years to complete the doctoral program (including internship): 6 years

Personal interview
Preferred in person but telephone acceptable

Research areas	# Faculty	# Grants
adult psychopathology	2	0
family and child	3	0
health psychology	4	3
psychotherapy	2	2
sexual assault	1	2

Clinical opportunities
adult inpatient and outpatient
child and family
neuropsychological assessment
pain management and cardiac rehabilitation
substance abuse

Oklahoma State University
Department of Psychology
215 North Murray Hall
Stillwater, OK 74078
phone#: (405) 744-6983
e-mail: FRANKLC@OKSTATE.EDU
Web address:
http://psychology.okstate.edu/grad/index.html#clinical

1	2	3	4	**5**	6	7

Clinically oriented   Equal emphasis   Research oriented

What percentage of your faculty subscribes to or practices in each of the following orientations?

Psychodynamic/Psychoanalytic	0%
Applied behavioral analysis/Radical behavioral	12.5%
Family systems/Systems	12.5%
Existential/Phenomenological/Humanistic	0%
Cognitive/Cognitive-behavioral	75%

What percentage of students applying for internship last year was accepted into APPIC-member internships? 100%

What courses are required for incoming students to have completed prior to enrolling?
Introductory psychology, statistics, experimental psychology

Are there courses you recommend that are not mandatory?
Abnormal psychology, history and systems

GRE mean
Verbal 600   Quantitative 550
Advanced Psychology 550
Analytical Writing Data not available

GPA mean
Overall GPA 3.2

Number of applications/admission offers/incoming students in 2003
96 applied/11 admission offers/9 incoming

% of students receiving:
Tuition waiver only: 0%
Assistantship/fellowship only: 0%
Both tuition waiver & assistantship/fellowship: 100%

Approximate percentage of incoming students who entered with a B.A./B.S. only: 100%   **Master's:** 0%

Approximate percentage of students who are Women: 66%   **Ethnic Minority:** 34%
International: Data not available

Average years to complete the doctoral program (including internship): 6.4 years

Personal interview
No preference given

Research areas	# Faculty	# Grants
anxiety disorders	1	0
health psychology	2	0
pediatric psychology	2	0
sexual abuse	1	0
substance abuse	1	0

Clinical opportunities
anxiety disorder
behavioral medicine
family therapy
marital therapy

University of Oregon

Department of Psychology
Eugene, OR 97403
phone#: (541) 346-5060
e-mail: gradsec@psych.uoregon.edu
Web address:
http://psychweb.uoregon.edu/gradprog/gpmain.htm

	1	2	3	4	**5**	6	7

Clinically oriented   Equal emphasis   Research oriented

What percentage of your faculty subscribes to or practices in each of the following orientations?

Psychodynamic/Psychoanalytic	0%
Applied behavioral analysis/Radical behavioral	20%
Family systems/Systems	20%
Existential/Phenomenological/Humanistic	0%
Cognitive/Cognitive-behavioral	55%

What percentage of students applying for internship last year was accepted into APPIC-member internships?
Data not available

What courses are required for incoming students to have completed prior to enrolling?
Good background in psychology

Are there courses you recommend that are not mandatory?
Research, statistics or math background

GRE mean
All GRE scores should be in the high 600 or 700 range or higher
Analytical Writing 5.23

GPA mean
Data not available

Number of applications/admission offers/incoming students in 2005
200 applied/8 admission offers/6 incoming

% of students receiving:
Tuition waiver only: 0%
Assistantship/fellowship only: 0%
Both tuition waiver & assistantship/fellowship: 100%

Approximate percentage of incoming students who entered with a B.A./B.S. only: 71.5% **Master's:** 28.5%

Approximate percentage of students who are Women: 85.7% **Ethnic Minority:** 71.5% **International:** 17%

Average years to complete the doctoral program (including internship): 5 years

Personal interview
Preferred in person but telephone acceptable *under special circumstances*

Research areas	# Faculty	# Grants
affective disorders	3	2
anxiety disorders	2	2
developmental psychopathology	2	1
life stress	1	0
neuropsychology	2	2

Clinical opportunities
anxiety disorders
behavioral genetics
child, family, and adult assessment
cognitive therapy
depression
marital
neuropsychology

University of Ottawa

School of Psychology
Lamoureux Hall
145 Jean-Jacques Lussier
Ottawa, Ontario K1N 6N5, Canada
phone#: (613) 562-5801
Web address: http://www.grad.uottawa.ca/programs/doctorates/psychology/program_objective.html

	1	2	3	**4**	5	6	7

Clinically oriented   Equal emphasis   Research oriented

What percentage of your faculty subscribes to or practices in each of the following orientations?

Psychodynamic/Psychoanalytic	5%
Applied behavioral analysis/Radical behavioral	0%
Family systems/Systems	15%
Existential/Phenomenological/Humanistic	18%
Cognitive/Cognitive-behavioral	62%

What percentage of students applying for internship last year was accepted into APPIC-member internships?
Data not available

What courses are required for incoming students to have completed prior to enrolling?
Canadian Honors B.A. degree or its equivalent (60 credits in psychology, plus research experience similar to the honors thesis)

Are there courses you recommend that are not mandatory?
History and systems

GRE mean
GRE is not required for admission

GPA mean
Overall GPA 8 on a scale of 10

Number of applications/admission offers/incoming students in 2003
119 applied/15 admission offers/13 incoming

% of students receiving:
Tuition waiver only: 0%
Assistantship/fellowship only: 94%
Both tuition waiver & assistantship/fellowship: 66%

Approximate percentage of incoming students who entered with a B.A./B.S. only: 92% **Master's:** 8%

Approximate percentage of students who are
Women: 87%   **Ethnic Minority:** Data not available
International: Data not available

Average years to complete the doctoral program
(including internship): 6.4 years

Personal interview
Interview not required

Research areas	# Faculty	# Grants
adult psychopathology	2	3
behavior problems in children	3	1
family functioning	1	1
forensic psychology	1	0
health psychology	3	5
marital therapy	1	0
psychotherapy and counselling	4	0
social development of children	2	2

Clinical opportunities
anxiety
community psychology
couples therapy
depression
external rotations to
community agencies
family therapy
play therapy
posttraumatic stress disorders

Pacific Graduate School of Psychology

Department of Clinical Psychology
935 East Meadow
Palo Alto, CA 94303
phone#: (650) 843-3419
e-mail: admissions@pgsp.edu
Web address: http://www.pgsp.edu/

1	2	3	**4**	5	6	7

Clinically oriented   Equal emphasis   Research oriented

What percentage of your faculty subscribes to or practices in each of the following orientations?

Psychodynamic/Psychoanalytic	40%
Applied behavioral analysis/Radical behavioral	0%
Family systems/Systems	20%
Existential/Phenomenological/Humanistic	0%
Cognitive/Cognitive-behavioral	40%

What percentage of students applying for internship last year was accepted into APPIC-member internships? 80%

What courses are required for incoming students to have completed prior to enrolling?
None

Are there courses you recommend that are not mandatory?
Statistics, personality or abnormal, developmental psychology, physiological psychology. Also solid academic background.

GRE mean
Verbal + Quantitative 1145
Analytical Writing 4.5

GPA mean
Undergraduate GPA 3.31

Number of applications/admission offers/incoming students in 2005
136 applied/120 admission offers/44 incoming

% of students receiving:
Tuition waiver only: 0%
Assistantship/fellowship only: 35%
Both tuition waiver & assistantship/fellowship: 0%

Approximate percentage of incoming students who entered with a B.A./B.S. only: 75%   **Master's:** 25%

Approximate percentage of students who are
Women: 78%   **Ethnic Minority:** 33%   **International:** 7%

Average years to complete the doctoral program
(including internship): 6.5 years

Personal interview
Interview not required

Research areas	# Faculty	# Grants
adult psychopathology	7	2
assessment	5	1
child and adolescent development	4	0
culture	4	0
health psychology	2	1
neuropsychology	2	1
substance abuse	2	1

Clinical opportunities
AIDS
assessment
child psychology
family
health psychology
minority
neuropsychology

Pacific University (Psy.D.)

Department of Clinical Psychology
School of Professional Psychology
2004 Pacific Avenue
Forest Grove, OR 97116
phone#: (503) 352-2240
e-mail: admissions@pacificu.edu (Admissions)
Web address:
http://www.pacificu.edu/spp/clinical/index.cfm

1	2	3	**4**	5	6	7

Clinically oriented   Equal emphasis   Research oriented

What percentage of your faculty subscribes to or practices in each of the following orientations?

Psychodynamic/Psychoanalytic	18%
Applied behavioral analysis	0%

Family systems/Systems	6%
Existential/Phenomenological/Humanistic	11%
Cognitive/Cognitive-behavioral	65%

What percentage of students applying for internship last year was accepted into APPIC-member internships?
Data not available

What courses are required for incoming students to have completed prior to enrolling?
A strong undergraduate background in psychology

Are there courses you recommend that are not mandatory?
Yes, 4 of the 7 following courses: introduction to psychology, personality theory, abnormal psychology, experimental psychology, physiological psychology, social psychology, behavioral statistics.

GRE mean
Verbal 540   Quantitative 556
Advanced Psychology 614
Analytical Writing 4.8

GPA mean
Junior/Senior GPA 3.47

Number of applications/admission offers/incoming students in 2005
189 applied/87 admission offers/49 incoming

% of students receiving:
Tuition waiver only: 16%
Assistantship/fellowship only: 20%
Both tuition waiver & assistantship/fellowship: 4%

Approximate percentage of incoming students who entered with a B.A./B.S. only: 86%   **Master's:** 14%

Approximate percentage of students who are Women: 71%   **Ethnic Minority:** 14%
International: Data not available

Average years to complete the doctoral program (including internship): 5.5 years

Personal interview
Required in person

Research areas	# Faculty	# Grants
anxiety disorders	2	0
behavioral health	1	0
behavior therapy	7	0
child psychopathology	4	6
dynamic psychotherapy	2	0
forensic psychology	2	0
gestalt therapy	1	0
integrative approaches	2	0
neuropsychology	1	1
organizational behavior	4	0
posttraumatic stress disorders	1	0
psychology of women	2	0
psychotherapy with minorities	4	0
single case research	1	0
training, supervision and consultation	3	2

Clinical opportunities
The school maintains a large psychological service center in downtown Portland plus 38 community sites.

University of Pennsylvania
Department of Psychology
3815 Walnut Street
Philadelphia, PA 19104
phone#: (215) 898-5663
e-mail: re@psych.upenn.edu
Web address:
http://www.psych.upenn.edu/grad/clinprog.htm

1	2	3	4	5	6	**7**
Clinically oriented		Equal emphasis			Research oriented	

What percentage of your faculty subscribes to or practices in each of the following orientations?

Psychodynamic/Psychoanalytic	5%
Applied behavioral analysis/Radical behavioral	10%
Family systems/Systems	0%
Existential/Phenomenological/Humanistic	10%
Cognitive/Cognitive-behavioral	85%

What percentage of students applying for internship last year was accepted into APPIC-member internships? 100%

What courses are required for incoming students to have completed prior to enrolling?
None

Are there courses you recommend that are not mandatory?
Statistics

GRE mean
Verbal 688   Quantitative 756
Advanced Psychology 800
Analytical Writing Data not available

GPA mean
Overall GPA 3.76

Number of applications/admission offers/incoming students in 2005
263 applied/10 admission offers/4 incoming

% of students receiving:
Tuition waiver only: 0%
Assistantship/fellowship only: 0%
Both tuition waiver & assistantship/fellowship: 100%

Approximate percentage of incoming students who entered with a B.A./B.S. only: 80%   **Master's:** 20%

Approximate percentage of students who are Women: 50%   **Ethnic Minority:** 5%   **International:** 15%

Average years to complete the doctoral program (including internship): 6 years

Personal interview
Required in person

Research areas	# Faculty	# Grants
anxiety disorders	2	5
depression	3	4
family/community	1	0
psychodynamic treatment	2	2
psychopharmacology	3	3
substance abuse	1	1

Clinical opportunities
assessment and diagnostic interviewing
behavioral health
behavioral therapy
cognitive-behavioral therapy
neuropsychology
psychodynamic therapy

Pennsylvania State University

Department of Psychology
417 Bruce V. Moore Building
University Park, PA 16802
phone#: (814) 863-1751
e-mail: kac8@psu.edu
Web address: http://psych.la.psu.edu/Clinical/index.html

1	2	3	**4**	5	6	7
Clinically oriented		Equal emphasis			Research oriented	

What percentage of your faculty subscribes to or practices in each of the following orientations?
Psychodynamic/Psychoanalytic	20%
Applied behavioral analysis/Radical behavioral	0%
Family systems/Systems	20%
Existential/Phenomenological/Humanistic	10%
Cognitive/Cognitive-behavioral	50%

What percentage of students applying for internship last year was accepted into APPIC-member internships?
Data not available

What courses are required for incoming students to have completed prior to enrolling?
No course requirements. Broad psychology background preferred.

Are there courses you recommend that are not mandatory?
Statistics and methodology

GRE mean
Verbal 670   Quantitative 680
Analytical Writing Data not available

GPA mean
Overall GPA 3.88

Number of applications/admission offers/incoming students in 2003
265 applied/16 admission offers/12 incoming

% of students receiving:
Tuition waiver only: 0%
Assistantship/fellowship only: 0%
Both tuition waiver & assistantship/fellowship: 100%

Approximate percentage of incoming students who entered with a B.A./B.S. only: 100%   Master's: 0%

Approximate percentage of students who are
Women: 72%   Ethnic Minority: 21%
International: Data not available

Average years to complete the doctoral program (including internship): 7.6 years

Personal interview
Preferred in person but telephone acceptable

Research areas	# Faculty	# Grants
adult psychopathology	5	1
affective disorders	2	0
anxiety disorders	7	3
behavioral medicine	2	0
child clinical/child psychopathology	3	2
cognition/information processing	2	0
cross-cultural psychology	1	1
developmental/childhood and adolescence	2	1
developmental disabilities	3	1
emotions	5	1
family research/therapy	2	1
hypnosis	1	0
neuropsychology	2	1
parent–child interactions	3	2
personality assessment	3	1
personality development	1	0
personality disorders	2	0
psychoanalysis/psychodynamics	2	0
psychophysiology	2	0
psychotherapy process and outcome	4	3
relaxation/biofeedback	2	1
rural psychology	1	1
violence/abuse	2	0

Clinical opportunities
Since we serve as a mental health center for this area, we offer a broad range of clinical experiences involving a variety of psychopathologies. The only significant area in which we do not offer experience in our clinic is with drug and alcohol dependence.

Pepperdine University (Psy.D.)

Department of Psychology
Graduate School of Education and Psychology
400 Corporate Pointe
Culver City, CA 90230
phone#: (310) 568-5600
e-mail: cheryl.saunders@pepperdine.edu
Web address: http://gsep.pepperdine.edu/academics/psychology/psycd-clinicalpsyc/

1	**2**	3	4	5	6	7
Clinically oriented		Equal emphasis			Research oriented	

What percentage of your faculty subscribes to or practices in each of the following orientations?
Psychodynamic/Psychoanalytic	30%
Applied behavioral analysis/Radical behavioral	5%
Family systems/Systems	20%
Existential/Phenomenological/Humanistic	15%
Cognitive/Cognitive-behavioral	30%

What percentage of students applying for internship last year was accepted into APPIC-member internships? Data not available

What courses are required for incoming students to have completed prior to enrolling?
Applicants for doctoral study should possess a master's degree in psychology or a closely related field that reflects a master's-level foundation of knowledge in the following domains: biological aspects of behavior; cognitive and affective aspects of behavior; social aspects of behavior; psychological measurement; research methodology; and techniques of data analysis.

Are there courses you recommend that are not mandatory?
No

GRE mean
Verbal 600   Quantitative 600
Advanced Psychology 600
Analytical Writing Data not available

GPA mean
Overall GPA 3.31   Master's GPA 3.87

Number of applications/admission offers/incoming students in 2003
95 applied/44 admission offers/26 incoming

% of students receiving:
Partial scholarship: 68%
Assistantship/fellowship only: 12%
Both tuition waiver & assistantship/fellowship: 0%

Approximate percentage of incoming students who entered with a B.A./B.S. only: 0%   **Master's:** 100%

Approximate percentage of students who are Women: 78%   **Ethnic Minority:** 27%
International: Data not available

Average years to complete the doctoral program (including internship): 5.4 years

Personal interview
Preferred in person but telephone acceptable

Research areas	# Faculty	# Grants
ADHD	1	2
posttraumatic stress disorder	1	2
program evaluation	1	1
psychotherapy process and outcome	6	1
psychiatric diagnosis	1	1

Clinical opportunities
ADHD
adolescence
AIDS
aging
assessment
behavior therapy
behavioral medicine (oncology)
child clinical
cognitive behavioral therapy
chronically mentally ill
existential-humanistic psychotherapy
forensic
group
inpatient
marital/family/systemic psychotherapy
neuropsychology
posttraumatic stress disorder
psychodynamic psychotherapy
rehabilitation
religious
schizophrenia
substance abuse

University of Pittsburgh

Department of Psychology
Psychology Graduate Office
Sennott Square, 3rd Floor
210 South Bouquet Street
Pittsburgh, PA 15260
phone#: (412) 624-4502
e-mail: psygrad@pitt.edu
Web address: http://www.psychology.pitt.edu/graduate/clinical/index.php

1	2	3	4	5	**6**	7

Clinically oriented	Equal emphasis	Research oriented

What percentage of your faculty subscribes to or practices in each of the following orientations?

Psychodynamic/Psychoanalytic	0%
Applied behavioral analysis/Radical behavioral	0%
Family systems/Systems	30%
Existential/Phenomenological/Humanistic	0%
Cognitive/Cognitive-behavioral	70%

What percentage of students applying for internship last year was accepted into APPIC-member internships? 100%

What courses are required for incoming students to have completed prior to enrolling?
None

Are there courses you recommend that are not mandatory?
Basic psychology courses, including research methods and statistics; background in biology, math, and computer science

GRE mean
Verbal 621   Quantitative 723
Advanced Psychology 706
Analytical Writing Data not available

GPA mean
Overall GPA 3.7

Number of applications/admission offers/incoming students in 2005
238 applied/16 admission offers/8 incoming

% of students receiving:
Tuition waiver only: 0%
Assistantship/fellowship only: 0%
Both tuition waiver & assistantship/fellowship: 100%

Approximate percentage of incoming students who entered with a B.A./B.S. only: 90% **Master's:** 10%

Approximate percentage of students who are Women: 80% **Ethnic Minority:** 12% **International:** 8%

Average years to complete the doctoral program (including internship): 7 years

Personal interview
Preferred in person but telephone acceptable

Research areas	# Faculty	# Grants
adult psychopathology	10	17
affective/mood disorders/depression	5	7
at-risk adolescents	7	10
attention-deficit disorder	2	2
autism	2	3
behavioral genetics	3	4
behavioral medicine/health psychology	14	30
cancer/behavioral oncology	3	3
cardiovascular behavioral medicine	3	11
child/family/developmental/ psychopathology	12	18
chronic disease	3	4
clinical cognitive neuroscience	3	5
disaster/trauma	1	1
emotion	3	4
obesity/eating disorders	1	3
posttraumatic stress disorder	1	1
prevention	2	2
psychoneuroimmunology	3	5
psychopharmacology	3	4
psychophysiology	5	7
schizophrenia	1	1
social cognition	4	6
statistics	2	2
stress and coping	3	5
substance abuse/addictions	9	15

Clinical opportunities
adolescent treatment
affective disorders/depression
anxiety disorders
assessment (preschool, school age, and adult)
attention-deficit disorder
autism
behavioral medicine
child treatment
cognitive-behavioral therapy
conduct disorder
eating disorders
emergency room assessment
family therapy
gay/lesbian
inpatient
neuropsychological assessment
obsessive-compulsive
pain management
parent training
pediatric
personality disorders
posttraumatic stress disorder
schizophrenia
smoking cessation
substance abuse
suicide prevention
victim/violence/sexual abuse
weight management

Ponce School of Medicine
Ponce School of Medicine
Admissions Office
Clinical Psychology Doctorate Program
P. O. Box 7004
Ponce PR   00732
phone#: (787) 840-2575
e-mail: admissions@psm.edu
Web address: http://www.psm.edu/Academic%20
Affair%20&%20Programs/programs/PsyD/index.html
Program data not available

Purdue University
Department of Psychological Sciences
703 Third Street
West Lafayette, IN 47907-2081
phone#: (765) 494-6977
e-mail: (secretary) dlbatta@psych.purdue.edu
(director) rollock@psych.purdue.edu
Web address:
http://www2.psych.purdue.edu/Clinical/index.html

1	2	3	4	**5**	6	7
Clinically oriented		Equal emphasis			Research oriented	

What percentage of your faculty subscribes to or practices in each of the following orientations?

Psychodynamic/Psychoanalytic	10%
Applied behavioral analysis/Radical behavioral	20%
Family systems/Systems	10%
Existential/Phenomenological/Humanistic	0%
Cognitive/Cognitive-behavioral	60%

What percentage of students applying for internship last year was accepted into APPIC-member internships?
Data not available

What courses are required for incoming students to have completed prior to enrolling?
Background in psychology, especially methodology and statistics

Are there courses you recommend that are not mandatory?
Science, mathematics, statistics and research experience with a university researcher

GRE mean
Data not available

GPA mean
Data not available

Number of applications/admission offers/incoming students in 2003
167 applied/10 admission offers/7 incoming

% of students receiving:
Tuition waiver only: 0%
Assistantship/fellowship only: 0%
Both tuition waiver & assistantship/fellowship: 100%

Approximate percentage of incoming students who entered with a B.A./B.S. only: 100%   Master's: 0%

Approximate percentage of students who are Women: 57%   Ethnic Minority: 29%
International: Data not available

Average years to complete the doctoral program (including internship): 6.9 years

Personal interview
Preferred in person but telephone acceptable

Research areas	# Faculty	# Grants
adolescence	1	0
affective disorders	1	0
anxiety disorders	1	0
disruptive behavior disorders/ ADHD	1	3
disruptive behavior disorders/ conduct disorders and prevention	1	1
disruptive behavior disorders/ developmental disabilities	1	0
ethnicity/culture	4	0
family processes	2	1
personality and psychopathology	1	0

Clinical opportunities
ADHD (child)
anxiety (adult and child)
depression (adult)
developmental disorders
family and adolescence
Headstart consultations
oppositional defiant disorders, and other disruptive behavior and conduct problems (child)
personality disorders (adult)

Purdue University Philadelphia College of Osteopathic Medicine

Philadelphia College of Osteopathic Medicine
Office of Admissions
4170 City Avenue
Philadelphia, PA 19131
phone#: (800) 999-6998
e-mail: gradadmissions@pcom.edu
Web address:
http://www.pcom.edu/Academic_Programs/
aca_psych/PsyD_in_Clinical_Psychology/
psyd_in_clinical_psychology.html
Program data not available

Queen's University

Department of Psychology
Kingston, Ontario K7L 3N6, Canada
phone#: (613) 533-6004
e-mail: Leachj@psyc.queensu.ca
Web address:
http://psyc.queensu.ca/gradbeta1/clinicalprogram.html

1	2	3	4	5	**6**	7
Clinically oriented		Equal emphasis			Research oriented	

What percentage of your faculty subscribes to or practices in each of the following orientations?

Psychodynamic/Psychoanalytic	1%
Applied behavioral analysis/Radical behavioral	2%
Family systems/Systems	1%
Existential/Phenomenological/Humanistic	0%
Cognitive/Cognitive-behavioral	98%

What percentage of students applying for internship last year was accepted into APPIC-member internships? 100%

What courses are required for incoming students to have completed prior to enrolling?
Undergraduate thesis required; history and systems; biological, cognitive-affective; social; (2) abnormal psychology

Are there courses you recommend that are not mandatory?
No

GRE mean
Verbal 600   Quantitative 600
Advanced Psychology 600
Analytical Writing 5.5

GPA mean
Psychology GPA 3.8

Number of applications/admission offers/incoming students in 2005
106 applied/8 admission offers/5 incoming

% of students receiving:
Tuition waiver only: 0%
Assistantship/fellowship only: 100%
Both tuition waiver & assistantship/fellowship: 0%

Approximate percentage of incoming students who entered with a B.A./B.S. (Honors) only: 90%   Master's: 10%

Approximate percentage of students who are Women: 82%   Ethnic Minority: 0%   International: 0%

Average years to complete the doctoral program (including internship): 6 years

Personal interview
Interview not required

Research areas	# Faculty	# Grants
—		

Clinical opportunities
child and family
children and adolescents

developmental disabilities
education
forensic
geriatric
inpatient and outpatient facilities
neuropsychology
rehabilitation
young offenders

Regent University

Doctoral Program in Clinical Psychology
CRB 154
1000 Regent University Drive
Virginia Beach, VA 23464
phone#: (800) 373-5504 ext. 4498
e-mail: psycoun@regent.edu
Web address: http://www.regent.edu/psyd

1	2	**3**	4	5	6	7

Clinically oriented　　Equal emphasis　　Research oriented

What percentage of your faculty subscribes to or practices in each of the following orientations?
Psychodynamic/Psychoanalytic　　　　　　　　30%
Applied behavioral analysis/Radical behavioral　20%
Family systems/Systems　　　　　　　　　　40%
Existential/Phenomenological/Humanistic　　　30%
Cognitive/Cognitive-behavioral　　　　　　　60%

What percentage of students applying for internship last year was accepted into APPIC-member internships? 92%

What courses are required for incoming students to have completed prior to enrolling?
18 hours of psychology (undergrad)

Are there courses you recommend that are not mandatory?
Statistics, research methods, personality theories, human growth and development, abnormal psychology, social psychology, physiological psychology

GRE mean
Verbal and Quantitative Data not available
Analytical Writing 3.5

GPA mean
Data not available

Number of applications/admission offers/incoming students in 2005
71 applied/37 admission offers/27 incoming

% of students receiving:
Tuition waiver only: 100% (at least partial support)
Assistantship/fellowship only: 13%
Both tuition waiver & assistantship/fellowship: 13%

Approximate percentage of incoming students who entered with a B.A./B.S. (Honors) only: 79%　**Master's:** 21%

Approximate percentage of students who are Women: 68%　**Ethnic Minority:** 18%　**International:** 4%

Average years to complete the doctoral program (including internship): 5 years

Personal interview
Required in person

Research areas	# Faculty	# Grants
ADHD	1	0
consultation to religious and community organizations by clinicians	4	3
diversity issues in the military	1	0
personality, religion, and adjustment	1	1
marital functioning and spirituality	2	1
sexual and religious identity	1	3
traumatic brain injury	1	1

Clinical opportunities
behavioral medicine
child mental health settings
Christian counseling centers
forensic settings
military mental health and VA
neuropsychology
psychiatric hospitals

University of Rhode Island

Department of Psychology
Chafee Center
Kingston, RI 02881
phone#: (401) 874-2193
e-mail: alberman@uri.edu
Web address:
http://www.uri.edu/artsci/psy/clinical/index.html

1	2	3	**4**	5	6	7

Clinically oriented　　Equal emphasis　　Research oriented

What percentage of your faculty subscribes to or practices in each of the following orientations?
Psychodynamic/Psychoanalytic　　　　　　　　10%
Applied behavioral analysis/Radical behavioral　0%
Family systems/Systems　　　　　　　　　　40%
Existential/Phenomenological/Humanistic　　　30%
Cognitive/Cognitive-behavioral　　　　　　　50%
Feminist　　　　　　　　　　　　　　　　10%

What percentage of students applying for internship last year was accepted into APPIC-member internships? 100%

What courses are required for incoming students to have completed prior to enrolling?
Sufficient background in undergraduate psychology courses

Are there courses you recommend that are not mandatory?
Psychological tests and measurements

GRE mean
Verbal 583　Quantitative 600
Analytical Writing Data not available

GPA mean
Undergraduate GPA 3.64

Number of applications/admission offers/incoming students in 2005
183 applied/9 admission offers/8 incoming

% of students receiving:
Tuition waiver only: 5%
Assistantship/fellowship only: 7%
Both tuition waiver & assistantship/fellowship: 83%

Approximate percentage of incoming students who entered with a B.A./B.S. only: 50% **Master's:** 50%

Approximate percentage of students who are Women: 74% **Ethnic Minority:** 37% **International:** 10%

Average years to complete the doctoral program (including internship): 6.8 years

Personal interview
Required in person

Research areas	# Faculty	# Grants
behavioral medicine/health psychology	3	10
child clinical	1	0
clinical judgment	1	0
community psychology	1	4
family research	1	0
multicultural issues	1	0

Clinical opportunities
child therapy
community psychology
family therapy
health psychology
individual psychotherapy
marriage and couples therapy
sex therapy

University of Rochester

Department of Psychology
Meliora Hall
Rochester, NY 14627-0266
phone#: (585) 275-8704
e-mail: gilbert@psych.rochester.edu
Web address:
http://www.psych.rochester.edu/graduate/clinical/

1	2	3	4	**5**	6	7
Clinically oriented		Equal emphasis			Research oriented	

What percentage of your faculty subscribes to or practices in each of the following orientations?

Psychodynamic/Psychoanalytic	25%
Applied behavioral analysis/Radical behavioral	25%
Family systems/Systems	0%
Existential/Phenomenological/Humanistic	10%
Cognitive/Cognitive-behavioral	50%

What percentage of students applying for internship last year was accepted into APPIC-member internships? 100%

What courses are required for incoming students to have completed prior to enrolling?
Equivalent of psychology major

Are there courses you recommend that are not mandatory?
No

GRE mean
Verbal 608   Quantitative 680
Analytical Writing 5.4

GPA mean
Overall GPA 3.5

Number of applications/admission offers/incoming students in 2005
115 applied/4 admission offers/4 incoming

% of students receiving:
Tuition waiver only: 0%
Assistantship/fellowship only: 0%
Both tuition waiver & assistantship/fellowship: 100%

Approximate percentage of students who are Women: 75% **Ethnic Minority:** 16% **International:** 6%

Average years to complete the doctoral program (including internship): 5–6 years

Personal interview
Required in person

Research areas	# Faculty	# Grants
attention-deficit disorder	1	1
autism	2	2
child abuse	1	4
cognition	3	2
marriage	1	0
motivation	3	2

Clinical opportunities
attention-deficit disorder
autism
child mistreatment/abuse
psychodynamic therapy
smoking prevention

Rosalind Franklin University of Medicine and Science

Department of Psychology
3333 Green Bay Road
North Chicago, IL 60064
phone#: (847) 578-3305
e-mail: CHINNI.CHILAMKURTI@FINCHCMS.EDU
http://www.rosalindfranklin.edu/sgpds/psychology/

1	2	3	**4**	5	6	7
Clinically oriented		Equal emphasis			Research oriented	

What percentage of your faculty subscribes to or practices in each of the following orientations?

Psychodynamic/Psychoanalytic	5%
Applied behavioral analysis/Radical behavioral	5%
Family systems/Systems	15%
Existential/Phenomenological/Humanistic	5%
Cognitive/Cognitive-behavioral	70%

What percentage of students applying for internship last year was accepted into APPIC-member internships? 100%

What courses are required for incoming students to have completed prior to enrolling?
Statistics and biological/physiological psychology

Are there courses you recommend that are not mandatory?
abnormal psychology, developmental psychology, social psychology

GRE mean
Verbal 539   Quantitative 634
Advanced Psychology 685
Analytical Writing 4.5

GPA mean
Overall GPA 3.54

Number of applications/admission offers/incoming students in 2003
81 applied/14 admission offers/8 incoming

% of students receiving:
Tuition waiver only: 0%
Assistantship/fellowship only: 0%
Both tuition waiver & assistantship/fellowship: 100%

Approximate percentage of incoming students who entered with a B.A./B.S. only: 85%   **Master's:** 15%

Approximate percentage of students who are Women: 75%   **Ethnic Minority:** 15%   **International:** 4%

Average years to complete the doctoral program (including internship): 7 years

Personal interview
Preferred in person but telephone acceptable

Research areas	# Faculty	# Grants
aging	1	1
anxiety disorders	1	1
cancer	1	0
diabetes	1	0
epilepsy/neuropsychology	1	2
pain	1	1
psychopathy	1	0
risk behaviors in adolescents	1	0
schizophrenia	1	0
sports concussion	1	0

Clinical opportunities
anxiety disorders
behavioral medicine
neuropsychiatric
neuropsychological

Rutgers University (Ph.D.)

Department of Psychology
Graduate School of Arts and Sciences
New Brunswick, NJ 08903
Web address: http://psych.rutgers.edu/
program_areas/clin/clin.html

1	2	3	4	**5**	6	7
Clinically oriented		Equal emphasis			Research oriented	

What percentage of your faculty subscribes to or practices in each of the following orientations?

Psychodynamic/Psychoanalytic	6.7%
Applied behavioral analysis/Radical behavioral	13.3%
Family systems/Systems	0%
Existential/Phenomenological/Humanistic	0%
Cognitive/Cognitive-behavioral	80%

What percentage of students applying for internship last year was accepted into APPIC-member internships? 100%

What courses are required for incoming students to have completed prior to enrolling?
A major in psychology or equivalent courses

Are there courses you recommend that are not mandatory?
No

GRE mean
Verbal 670   Quantitative 700
Advanced Psychology 750
Analytical Writing Data not available

GPA mean
Overall GPA 3.77

Number of applications/admission offers/incoming students in 2005
354 applied/9 admission offers/7 incoming

% of students receiving:
Tuition waiver only: 0%
Assistantship/fellowship only: 0%
Both tuition waiver & assistantship/fellowship: 100%

Approximate percentage of incoming students who entered with a B.A./B.S. only: 100%   **Master's:** 0%

Approximate percentage of students who are Women: 85%   **Ethnic Minority:** 20%   **International:** 10%

Average years to complete the doctoral program (including internship): 6 years

Personal interview
Preferred in person but telephone acceptable

Research areas	# Faculty	# Grants
applied behavioral analysis	2	0
autism	1	1
behavioral medicine	5	6
depression	1	0
developmental psychopathology	1	1
eating disorders	1	1
ethical issues	1	0
marriage/couples	2	1

philosophical issues	2	0
prevention	2	1
program design and evaluation	1	1
psychopathology	1	1
psychotherapy process and outcome	5	4
somatization disorders	1	1
substance abuse	3	5

Clinical opportunities
adolescent delinquency
affective disorders
alcohol use disorders
anxiety disorders
assessment
behavioral medicine
community psychology
conduct disorder
depression
developmental disabilities
eating disorders
family therapy
minority
obsessive–compulsive disorder
personality disorders
sex therapy
somatization disorders
substance abuse

Rutgers University (Psy.D.)
Graduate School of Applied and Professional
Psychology
152 Frelinghuysen Road
Piscataway, NJ 08854-8085
phone#: (732) 445-2004
e-mail: clinpsyd@rcu.rutgers.edu
Web address:
http://gsappweb.rutgers.edu/gsappweb/clincal.htm

1	2	**3**	4	5	6	7
Clinically oriented		Equal emphasis			Research oriented	

What percentage of your faculty subscribes to or practices in each of the following orientations?

Psychodynamic/Psychoanalytic	35%
Applied behavioral analysis/Radical behavioral	10%
Family systems/Systems	20%
Existential/Phenomenological/Humanistic	10%
Cognitive/Cognitive-behavioral	25%

What percentage of students applying for internship last year was accepted into APPIC-member internships? 100%

What courses are required for incoming students to have completed prior to enrolling?
Introductory psychology, statistics, abnormal psychology, And the biological bases of psychology

Are there courses you recommend that are not mandatory?
Students also should have taken 1 and preferably 2 courses in 1 of the following: cognitive psychology, psychology of perception, conditioning and learning, developmental psychology, psychology of personality and social psychology. We prefer that 1 of the above have a laboratory component.

GRE mean
Data not available

GPA mean
Overall GPA 3.5

Number of applications/admission offers/incoming students in 2005
386 applied/24 admission offers/16 incoming

% of students receiving:
Tuition waiver only: 0%
Scholarships: 60%
Both tuition waiver & assistantship/fellowship: 40%

Approximate percentage of incoming students who entered with a B.A./B.S. only: 87.5% **Master's:** 12.5%

Approximate percentage of students who are Women: 75% **Ethnic Minority:** 37.5%
International: Data not available

Average years to complete the doctoral program (including internship): 4.5 years

Personal interview
Preferred in person but telephone acceptable

Research areas	# Faculty	# Grants
adolescence	4	1
adoption	1	1
anxiety depressive disorders	3	1
applied and behavioral analysis	1	1
autism	1	1
community	2	1
developmental disabilities	3	2
diagnosis and classification	2	0
dissociative disorders	1	0
eating disorders	1	1
empirically supported treatment research	2	1
ethical issues	1	0
family/marriage/couples	4	2
feminist theory and psychology	1	0
mental health policy	2	1
mind/body/health	1	0
multicultural issues	2	0
organizational psychology	2	0
personality disorders	2	0
philosophy and psychology	5	1
program design and evaluation	1	0
psychiatric disabilities	1	1
psychoanalytic theory	7	1
psychology and the arts	1	0
psychophysiological disorders	1	0
psychotherapy process and outcome	3	0
severe mental illness	2	1
social learning theory	1	1
substance abuse	4	4

Clinical opportunities
AIDS
adolescent delinquency

affective disorders
anxiety disorders
assessment
behavioral medicine
community psychology
conduct disorder
developmental disabilities
dissociative disorder
eating disorders
family therapy
forensic psychology
gerontology
group therapy
hyperactivity
hypnosis
impulse control
infancy/postpartum
interpersonal psychotherapy
marital/couples therapy
minority
neuropsychology
obsessive–compulsive disorder
organizational psychology
personality disorders
psychodynamic/psychoanalytic therapy
rational-emotive psychotherapy
schizophrenia
school psychology
sex therapy
substance abuse
victim/abuse

St. John's University

Department of Psychology
8000 Utopia Parkway
Jamaica, NY 11439
phone#: (718) 990-6369
e-mail: nevidj@stjohns.edu
Web address: http://www.stjohns.edu/academics/
graduate/liberalarts/departments/psychology/
programs/phd_cp

1	2	3	**4**	5	6	7
Clinically oriented		Equal emphasis			Research oriented	

What percentage of your faculty subscribes to or practices in each of the following orientations?

Psychodynamic/Psychoanalytic	30%
Applied behavioral analysis/Radical behavioral	0%
Family systems/Systems	10%
Existential/Phenomenological/Humanistic	0%
Cognitive/Cognitive-behavioral	60%

What percentage of students applying for internship last year was accepted into APPIC-member internships? 100%

What courses are required for incoming students to have completed prior to enrolling?
Introductory psychology, statistics, experimental laboratory

Are there courses you recommend that are not mandatory?
No

GRE mean
Verbal 623   Quantitative 693
Advanced Psychology 683
Analytical Writing 5.36

GPA mean
Overall GPA 3.67   Psychology GPA 3.78

Number of applications/admission offers/incoming students in 2005
253 applied/25 admission offers/12 incoming

% of incoming students receiving:
Tuition waiver only: 8%
Assistantship/fellowship only: 0%
Both tuition waiver & assistantship/fellowship: 92% (some partial support)

Approximate percentage of incoming students who entered with a B.A./B.S. only: 92%   **Master's:** 8%

**Approximate percentage of students who are
Women:** 83%   **Ethnic Minority:** 17%   **International:** 0%

Average years to complete the doctoral program (including internship): 7 years

Personal interview
Preferred in person but telephone acceptable

Research areas	# Faculty	# Grants
anxiety disorders	2	0
autism	1	1
bilingualism	2	0
bullying behavior/victimization	1	0
child abuse	1	2
gender issues	2	0
health psychology	2	1
minority mental health	5	1
moral development	3	0
physiological psychology	1	1
psychotherapy research	1	1
schizophrenia	1	0
smoking cessation	1	0
stress management	1	1

Clinical opportunities
clinical child psychology
cognitive-behavioral therapy
family therapy
group therapy
neuropsychological assessment
psychodynamic/psychoanalytic therapy
Opportunities in the greater New York City area include leading medical centers, municipal hospitals, outpatient clinics, and research institutes.

St. Louis University

Department of Psychology
221 North Grand Boulevard
St. Louis, MO 63103
phone#: (314) 977-2278
Web address: http://www.slu.edu/graduate/degrees/
degree_index.php?id=105

1	2	3	**4**	5	6	7
Clinically oriented		Equal emphasis			Research oriented	

What percentage of your faculty subscribes to or practices in each of the following orientations?

Psychodynamic/Psychoanalytic	15%
Applied behavioral analysis/Radical behavioral	0%
Family systems/Systems	25%
Existential/Phenomenological/Humanistic	15%
Cognitive/Cognitive-behavioral	70%

What percentage of students applying for internship last year was accepted into APPIC-member internships? 100%

What courses are required for incoming students to have completed prior to enrolling?
Introductory psychology, statistics, abnormal psychology, and 6 upper division psychology courses

Are there courses you recommend that are not mandatory?
Personality, learning, social psychology, physiological psychology, developmental psychology, tests and measurement

GRE mean
Verbal 535   Quantitative 615
Analytical Writing 4.0

GPA mean
Overall GPA 3.6

Number of applications/admission offers/incoming students in 2005
125 applied/12 admission offers/8 incoming

% of students receiving:
Tuition waiver only: 0%
Assistantship/fellowship only: 0%
Tuition waiver & assistantship/fellowship: 100% for first year

Approximate percentage of incoming students who entered with a B.A./B.S. only: 85%   **Master's:** 15%

Approximate percentage of students who are Women: 70%   **Ethnic Minority:** 20%   **International:** 10%

Average years to complete the doctoral program (including internship): 6 years

Personal interview
Preferred in person but telephone acceptable

Research areas	# Faculty	# Grants
abuse/violence	2	1
adjustment	2	0
assessment	3	0
child/adolescent	2	0
community	1	0
depression	2	0
ethical issues	3	0
family	3	0
personality disorders	2	0
professional issues	3	0
stress and coping	2	0

Clinical opportunities
anxiety
assessment
clinical neuropsychology
ethnic diversity
family therapy
hyperactivity
learning disabilities
marital
parent skills training
personality disorders
psychodynamic therapy
victims of abuse and assault

San Diego State University/ University of California–San Diego

College of Sciences/School of Medicine
San Diego, CA 92182
phone#: (619) 594-2246
e-mail: akienle@psychology.sdsu.edu
Web address: http://www.psychology.sdsu.edu/doctoral/

1	2	3	4	5	**6**	7
Clinically oriented		Equal emphasis			Research oriented	

What percentage of your faculty subscribes to or practices in each of the following orientations?

Psychodynamic/Psychoanalytic	5%
Applied behavioral analysis/Radical behavioral	30%
Family systems/Systems	10%
Existential/Phenomenological/Humanistic	5%
Cognitive/Cognitive-behavioral	50%

What percentage of students applying for internship last year was accepted into APPIC-member internships? Data not available

What courses are required for incoming students to have completed prior to enrolling?
Psychology major or 18 semester hours in psychology including: personality, abnormal, social, statistics, testing, experimental with lab, physiological.

Are there courses you recommend that are not mandatory?
Advanced courses in perception and learning, biology, mathematics, linguistics, computer science, medical physics.

GRE mean
Verbal 637   Quantitative 671
Advanced Psychology 3.73
Analytical Writing Data not available

GPA mean
Overall GPA 3.67   Psychology GPA 3.80

Number of applications/admission offers/incoming students in 2003
306 applied/19 admission offers/11 incoming

% of students receiving:
Tuition waiver only: 0%
Assistantship/fellowship only: 0%
Tuition waiver & assistantship/fellowship: 100%

Approximate percentage of incoming students who entered with a B.A./B.S. only: 73% **Master's:** 27%

Approximate percentage of students who are Women: 78% **Ethnic Minority:** 22%
International: Data not available

Average years to complete the doctoral program (including internship): 6 years

Personal interview
Preferred in person but telephone acceptable

Research areas	# Faculty	# Grants
AIDS	7	1
aging	8	1
Alzheimer's/dementia	6	0
anxiety	4	1
applied behavioral analysis	4	0
autism	2	0
behavioral medicine		
bereavement	2	0
biofeedback	1	0
cancer disparities	4	0
cancer prevention	2	2
cardiovascular disease	4	1
child, marriage, and family	5	0
childhood brain damage	2	0
chronic disease	4	1
cognition and memory	13	0
cognitive psychology/therapy	2	0
community psychology	1	0
cross-cultural psychology	10	0
decision making	1	0
depression	3	2
developmental neuropsychology	7	0
developmental psychopathology	3	0
ethnicity and health	2	0
exercise	2	1
gender and health	2	0
gender issues	2	0
information processing	4	0
interpersonal psychology	1	0
neuropsychological testing	2	1
nutrition	3	0
pain	2	0
PNI	3	0
posttraumatic stress disorder	1	0
problem solving	1	0
psychological testing	4	0
psychology of humor	1	0
psychopathology	3	0
psychopharmacology	6	2
psychophysiology	5	0
psychotherapy process and outcome	4	0
schizophrenia/psychosis	7	2
sexuality	1	0
sleep	4	0
smoking	7	1
social skills training	1	0
social support	2	0
statistics	4	0
stress and coping	13	0
substance abuse	12	5
women's health	3	0

Clinical opportunities
anxiety disorders
behavioral medicine
child and family therapy
cognitive therapy
neuropsychology
school psychology

University of Saskatchewan
Department of Psychology
Doctoral Program in Clinical Psychology
Saskatoon, Saskatchewan S7N 5A5, Canada
e-mail: psychology@usask.ca
Web address: http://www.usask.ca/psychology/
programs/clinprog/welcome/index.html

1	2	3	**4**	5	6	7
Clinically oriented		Equal emphasis			Research oriented	

What percentage of your faculty subscribes to or practices in each of the following orientations?

Psychodynamic/Psychoanalytic	12.5%
Applied behavioral analysis/Radical behavioral	12.5%
Family systems/Systems	12.5%
Existential/Phenomenological/Humanistic	25%
Cognitive/Cognitive-behavioral	50%

What percentage of students applying for internship last year was accepted into APPIC-member internships? 80%

What courses are required for incoming students to have completed prior to enrolling?
An honors B.A. or B.Sc. degree in psychology or its equivalent, including statistics, research methods, and an honors thesis

Are there courses you recommend that are not mandatory?
Basic area courses, for example, biological, cognitive, and social bases of behavior

GRE mean
Mean percentiles for class admitted 2005:
Verbal 66   Quantitative 52   Advanced Psychology 71
Analytical Writing 79

GPA mean
Overall GPA 84%

Number of applications/admission offers/incoming students in 2005
76 applied/9 admission offers/6 incoming

% of students receiving:
Tuition waiver only: 0%
Assistantship/fellowship only: 100%
Tuition waiver & assistantship/fellowship: 0%

Approximate percentage of incoming students who entered with a B.A./B.S. only: 100% Master's: 0%

Approximate percentage of students who are Women: 66% Ethnic Minority: 33% International: 0%

Average years to complete the doctoral program (including internship): 6.9 years

Personal interview
Preferred in person but telephone acceptable

Research areas	# Faculty	# Grants
bereavement	1	0
child trauma and violence	1	1
forensic/psychopathy	3	2
health psychology	3	3
metaphor/narrative	1	1
neuropsychology	1	1
psychotherapy process	2	1

Clinical opportunities
adult psychotherapy
child clinical psychology
behavioral medicine
developmental disabilities
inpatient forensic
neuropsychology
young offenders

Simon Fraser University

Department of Psychology
Burnaby, British Columbia V5A 1S6, Canada
phone#: (604) 291-3354
e-mail: kumpula@sfu.ca
Web address: http://www.psyc.sfu.ca/grad/
index.php?topic=clin_overview

1	2	3	**4**	5	6	7

Clinically oriented   Equal emphasis   Research oriented

What percentage of your faculty subscribes to or practices in each of the following orientations?

Psychodynamic/Psychoanalytic	25%
Applied behavioral analysis/Radical behavioral	0%
Family systems/Systems	35%
Existential/Phenomenological/Humanistic	0%
Cognitive/Cognitive-behavioral	40%

What percentage of students applying for internship last year was accepted into APPIC-member internships? Data not available

What courses are required for incoming students to have completed prior to enrolling?
96 semester hours in experimental areas and statistics

Are there courses you recommend that are not mandatory?
Psychology honors program; advanced undergraduate courses across all substantive areas of psychology

GRE mean
Verbal 588   Quantitative 725
Advanced Psychology 748
Analytical Writing Data not available

GPA mean
Overall GPA 3.73   Psychology GPA 3.73

Number of applications/admission offers/incoming students in 2005
124 applied/13 admission offers/6 incoming

% of students receiving:
Tuition waiver only: 0%
Assistantship/fellowship only: 100%
Both tuition waiver & assistantship/fellowship: 0%

Approximate percentage of incoming students who entered with a B.A./B.S. only: 95% Master's: 5%

Approximate percentage of students who are Women: 70% Ethnic Minority: 30% International: Data not available

Average years to complete the doctoral program (including internship): 7 years

Personal interview
Preferred in person but telephone acceptable

Research areas	# Faculty	# Grants
behavioral medicine	1	0
child clinical	3	3
child psychopathology	3	3
cognition	6	4
depression	2	1
developmental	6	6
family	3	3
forensic	4	4
gender	2	1
neuropsychology	4	2
psychopathology	8	8
sex offenders	2	2
stress and coping	1	0
violence and abuse	5	5

University of South Carolina

Department of Psychology
Columbia, SC 29208
phone#: (803) 777-4137
e-mail: doris@gwm.sc.edu
Web address:
http://www.cas.sc.edu/psyc/grad_psyccc/ccprog.html

1	2	3	**4**	5	6	7

Clinically oriented   Equal emphasis   Research oriented

What percentage of your faculty subscribes to or practices in each of the following orientations?

Psychodynamic/Psychoanalytic	30%
Applied behavioral analysis/Radical behavioral	20%
Family systems/Systems	10%
Existential/Phenomenological/Humanistic	0%
Cognitive/Cognitive-behavioral	40%

What percentage of students applying for internship last year was accepted into APPIC-member internships?
Data not available

What courses are required for incoming students to have completed prior to enrolling?
18 hours in psychology, including statistics

Are there courses you recommend that are not mandatory?
Research methods, learning, biopsychology, abnormal, social, developmental, personality

GRE mean
Verbal 667   Quantitative 691
Advanced Psychology 710
Analytical Writing Data not available

GPA mean
Overall GPA 3.68   Psychology GPA 3.82
Junior/Senior GPA 3.85

Number of applications/admission offers/incoming students in 2005
147 applied/15 admission offers/7 incoming

% of students receiving:
Tuition waiver only: 0%
Assistantship/fellowship only: 0%
Both tuition waiver & assistantship/fellowship: 100%

Approximate percentage of incoming students who entered with a B.A./B.S. only: 80%   Master's: 20%

**Approximate percentage of students who are Women: 65%   Ethnic Minority: 25%
International: Data not available**

Average years to complete the doctoral program (including internship): 6 years

Personal interview
Preferred in person but telephone acceptable

Research areas	# Faculty	# Grants
citizen participation	1	0
community coalition development	1	1
conduct disorders	1	1
marital relationships	4	0
neuropschology	2	1
prevention (racism/cross-cultural intolerance and other prevention topics)	5	3
self-perception in minority youth	1	1
violence/rape/battering	2	1

Clinical opportunities
community psychology
family therapy
neuropsychology

University of South Dakota

Department of Psychology
Vermillion, SD 57069
phone#: (605) 677-5353
e-mail: byutrzen@usd.edu
Web address: http://www.usd.edu/psyc/ctp

1	2	3	**4**	5	6	7

Clinically oriented   Equal emphasis   Research oriented

What percentage of your faculty subscribes to or practices in each of the following orientations?

Psychodynamic/Psychoanalytic	30%
Applied behavioral analysis/Radical behavioral	0%
Family systems/Systems	30%
Existential/Phenomenological/Humanistic	10%
Cognitive/Cognitive-behavioral	100%

What percentage of students applying for internship last year was accepted into APPIC-member internships?
Data not available

What courses are required for incoming students to have completed prior to enrolling?
18 semester hours in psychology within a distribution among standard coursework in general and experimental psychology

Are there courses you recommend that are not mandatory?
Research design, statistics, history/systems, learning/memory, abnormal psychology, physiological

GRE mean
Verbal 573   Quantitative 611
Advanced Psychology 606
Analytical Writing Data not available

GPA mean
Data not available

Number of applications/admission offers/incoming students in 2005
55 applied/14 admission offers/9 incoming

% of students receiving:
Tuition waiver only: 0%
Assistantship/fellowship only: 100% (all students on assistantships also receive tuition reduction to 1/3 of in-state tuition costs)
Both tuition waiver & assistantship/fellowship: 0%

Approximate percentage of incoming students who entered with a B.A./B.S. only: 78%   Master's: 22%

**Approximate percentage of students who are Women: 62%   Ethnic Minority: 23%
International: Data not available**

Average years to complete the doctoral program (including internship): 6 years

Personal interview
Interview not required *but preferred*

Research areas	# Faculty	# Grants
child clinical	3	0
cross-cultural	10	2

depression	2	0
disaster mental health	5	2
ethics	1	0
family violence	2	0
health psychology	2	0
psychosis/serious mental illness	2	0
rural community psychology	4	0
substance abuse	1	1

Clinical opportunities

crisis intervention
disaster mental health
minority/cross-cultural (specific emphasis in American Indian mental health)
rural/community psychology
severe mental illness

University of South Florida

Department of Psychology
4202 Fowler Avenue, PCP 4118G
Tampa, FL 33620
phone#: (813) 974-2492
e-mail: phares@luna.cas.usf.edu
Web address: http://www.cas.usf.edu/psychology/
gra_cli_stud_index.htm

1	2	3	4	5	**6**	7

Clinically oriented   Equal emphasis   Research oriented

What percentage of your faculty subscribes to or practices in each of the following orientations?

Psychodynamic/Psychoanalytic	0%
Applied behavioral analysis/Radical behavioral	9%
Family systems/Systems	9%
Existential/Phenomenological/Humanistic	9%
Cognitive/Cognitive-behavioral	73%

What percentage of students applying for internship last year was accepted into APPIC-member internships? 100%

What courses are required for incoming students to have completed prior to enrolling?
None

Are there courses you recommend that are not mandatory?
Research design, statistics

GRE mean
Verbal 567   Quantitative 667
Analytical Writing 4.8

GPA mean
Junior/Senior GPA 3.70

Number of applications/admission offers/incoming students in 2005
253 applied/13 admission offers/9 incoming

% of students receiving:
Tuition waiver only: 0%
Assistantship/fellowship only: 10%
Both tuition waiver & assistantship/fellowship: 90%

Approximate percentage of incoming students who entered with a B.A./B.S. only: 67%   **Master's:** 33%

Approximate percentage of students who are Women: 85%   **Ethnic Minority:** 23%   **International:** 14%

Average years to complete the doctoral program (including internship): 8 years

Personal interview
Preferred in person but telephone acceptable

Research areas	# Faculty	# Grants
child/adolescent	4	2
depression	1	0
eating disorders	2	1
emotions	2	0
family dysfunction	1	0
health psychology	5	5
neuropsychology	1	0
personality assessment	1	0
psychosocial oncology	2	5
substance abuse/addictions	2	5
suicidality	1	1

Clinical opportunities

ADHD
adult and child clinical assessment
adult neuropsychology
anxiety—child and adult
child and adolescent disorders
depression/anxiety
eating disorders
family dysfunction
health psychology
intellectual assessment
learning disorders assessment
oppositional defiant disorder
psychosocial oncology
selective mutism
substance abuse
survivors of torture
weight management

University of Southern California

Department of Psychology
University Park, SGM 501
Los Angeles, CA 90089-1061
phone#: (213) 740-2296
Web address: http://www.usc.edu/dept/LAS/
psychology/clinical.html

1	2	3	4	5	**6**	7

Clinically oriented   Equal emphasis   Research oriented

What percentage of your faculty subscribes to or practices in each of the following orientations?

Psychodynamic/Psychoanalytic	0%
Applied behavioral analysis/Radical behavioral	20%
Family systems/Systems	20%
Existential/Phenomenological/Humanistic	0%
Cognitive/Cognitive-behavioral	80%

What percentage of students applying for internship last year was accepted into APPIC-member internships? 100%

What courses are required for incoming students to have completed prior to enrolling?
None are required

Are there courses you recommend that are not mandatory?
Introductory psychology, elementary statistics, research methods or experimental psychology, and courses in biology, physical and social sciences mathematics

GRE mean
Verbal 645   Quantitative 671
Analytical Writing Data not available

GPA mean
Overall GPA 3.58

Number of applications/admission offers/incoming students in 2005
283 applied/12 admission offers/6 incoming

% of students receiving:
Tuition waiver only: 0%
Assistantship/fellowship only: 0%
Both tuition waiver & assistantship/fellowship: 100%

Approximate percentage of incoming students who entered with a B.A./B.S. only: 66%   **Master's:** 26%

Approximate percentage of students who are Women: 77%   **Ethnic Minority:** 34%
International: Data not available

Average years to complete the doctoral program (including internship): 5.5 years

Personal interview
Preferred in person but telephone acceptable

Research areas	# Faculty	# Grants
adolescent substance abuse	3	1
alcohol use/abuse	2	2
behavioral medicine	3	5
child psychopathology	4	0
childhood victimization	3	2
clinical neuroscience/experimental	6	3
cognitive behavioral therapy/ assessment	2	0
gerontology	3	3
marital and family research/abuse	6	2

Clinical opportunities
community
gerontology
individual adult
marital/family
minority mental health

Southern Illinois University

Department of Psychology
Life Science Building II, Room 281
Carbondale, IL 62901
phone#: (618) 453-3564 (graduate program secretary)
e-mail: DOLLNGR@SIU.EDU
Web address: http://www.psychology.siu.edu/clinical.htm

1	2	3	**4**	5	6	7

Clinically oriented   Equal emphasis   Research oriented

What percentage of your faculty subscribes to or practices in each of the following orientations?
Psychodynamic/Psychoanalytic   0%
Applied behavioral analysis/Radical behavioral   0%
Family systems   10%
Existential/Phenomenological/Humanistic   0%
Cognitive/Cognitive-behavioral   90%

What percentage of students applying for internship last year was accepted into APPIC-member internships? 90%

What courses are required for incoming students to have completed prior to enrolling?
None

Are there courses you recommend that are not mandatory?
History and systems, tests and measurements, abnormal psychology, personality, learning, developmental, physiological, statistics, social psychology

GRE mean
Data not available

GPA mean
Data not available

Number of applications/admission offers/incoming students in 2005
100 applied/10 admission offers/7 incoming

% of students receiving:
Tuition waiver only: 0%
Assistantship/fellowship only: 0%
Both tuition waiver & assistantship/fellowship: 100%

Approximate percentage of incoming students who entered with a B.A./B.S. only: 85%   **Master's:** 15% (average over multiple years)

Approximate percentage of students who are Women: 70%   **Ethnic Minority:** 20%   **International:** 15%

Average years to complete the doctoral program (including internship): 7.5 years

Personal interview
No preference given
Note: Short-listed applicants are invited to an open house in February.

Research areas	# Faculty	# Grants
abortion issues	1	0
abuse	1	0
AIDS attitudes	1	0
adolescent issues	2	0

anxiety disorders	3	0
assessment	8	0
behavioral genetics	1	0
behavioral medicine	2	0
child clinical	3	0
child sexual abuse	1	0
clinical judgment	1	0
community psychology	1	0
delinquency	1	1
depression	2	0
family systems	1	0
gender roles	1	0
learning disabilities	2	0
marital	1	0
pediatric psychology	1	0
personality (five-factor model)	3	0
personality assessment	4	0
psychology of religion	1	0
relationships	2	0
sleep (child)	1	0
smoking	1	1
stress, coping, and social support	1	0

Clinical opportunities
family therapy
forensic psychology
juvenile corrections
neuropsychology/rehabilitation
severe psychopathology
sexual abuse
substance abuse

University of Southern Mississippi

Department of Psychology
Box 5025 Southern Station
Hattiesburg, MS 39406-5025
phone#: (601) 266-4588
e-mail: mitchell.berman@usm.edu
Web address: http://www.usm.edu/psy/
clinical/home.htm

1	2	3	4	**5**	6	7
Clinically oriented		Equal emphasis			Research oriented	

What percentage of your faculty subscribes to or practices in each of the following orientations?

Psychodynamic/Psychoanalytic	12%
Applied behavioral analysis/Radical behavioral	13%
Family systems/Systems	0%
Existential/Phenomenological/Humanistic	0%
Cognitive/Cognitive-behavioral	75%

What percentage of students applying for internship last year was accepted into APPIC-member internships? 100%

What courses are required for incoming students to have completed prior to enrolling?
None

Are there courses you recommend that are not mandatory?
Experimental, statistics, history and systems

GRE mean
Verbal 516 Quantitative 658
Analytical Writing Data not available

GPA mean
Overall GPA 3.78

Number of applications/admission offers/incoming students in 2005
65 applied/8 admission offers/8 incoming

% of students receiving:
Tuition waiver only: 0%
Assistantship/fellowship only: 0%
Both tuition waiver & assistantship/fellowship: 100%

Approximate percentage of incoming students who entered with a B.A./B.S. only: 75% **Master's:** 25%

Approximate percentage of students who are Women: 60% **Ethnic Minority:** 20% **International:** 8%

Average years to complete the doctoral program (including internship): 5.3 years

Personal interview
Required in person

Research areas	**# Faculty**	**# Grants**
adult clinical psychology	5	1
child clinical psychology	3	0

Clinical opportunities
adult clinical psychology
child clinical psychology

Spalding University (Psy.D.)

School of Professional Psychology
851 South Fourth Street
Louisville, KY 40203
phone#: (502) 585-7127
e-mail: esimpson@spalding.edu
Web address:
http://www.spalding.edu/frame.asp?pg=db2.asp?id=419

1	**2**	3	4	5	6	7
Clinically oriented		Equal emphasis			Research oriented	

What percentage of your faculty subscribes to or practices in each of the following orientations?

Psychodynamic/Psychoanalytic	10%
Applied behavioral analysis/Radical behavioral	0%
Family systems/Systems	30%
Existential/Phenomenological/Humanistic	20%
Cognitive/Cognitive-behavioral	50%

What percentage of students applying for internship last year was accepted into APPIC-member internships? 10%

What courses are required for incoming students to have completed prior to enrolling?
18 hours of undergraduate work.

Are there courses you recommend that are not mandatory?
Undergraduate research, physiological psychology

GRE mean
Verbal 550 Quantitative 590
Analytical 630

GPA mean
Overall GPA 3.5

Number of applications/admission offers/incoming students in 2005
98 applied/69 admission offers/39 incoming

% of students receiving:
Tuition waiver only: 0%
Assistantship/fellowship only: 17%
Both tuition waiver & assistantship/fellowship: 0%

Approximate percentage of incoming students who entered with a B.A./B.S. only: 67% **Master's:** 33%

Approximate percentage of students who are Women: 74% **Ethnic Minority:** 9% **International:** 7%

Average years to complete the doctoral program (including internship): 6 years

Personal interview
Preferred in person but telephone acceptable

Research areas	# Faculty	# Grants
child development	1	0
clinical supervision	2	0
health psychology	2	1
program evaluation	1	0
sports psychology	2	0

Clinical opportunities
family/systems psychology
health psychology

Stony Brook University/ State University of New York

Department of Psychology
Stony Brook, NY 11794-2500
phone#: (516) 632-7830
e-mail: K.D.OLeary@sunysb.edu
Web address: http://www.psychology.sunysb.edu/
psychology/index.php?graduate/areasofstudy/clinical

1	2	3	4	5	**6**	7
Clinically oriented		Equal emphasis			Research oriented	

What percentage of your faculty subscribes to or practices in each of the following orientations?

Psychodynamic/Psychoanalytic	0%
Applied behavioral analysis/Radical behavioral	13%
Family systems/Systems	0%
Existential/Phenomenological/Humanistic	0%
Cognitive/Cognitive-behavioral	87%

What percentage of students applying for internship last year was accepted into APPIC-member internships?
Data not available

What courses are required for incoming students to have completed prior to enrolling?
None

Are there courses you recommend that are not mandatory?
Statistics, introductory psychology, experimental with lab, abnormal psychology, research methods

GRE mean
Verbal 628 Quantitative 704
Analytical Writing Data not available

GPA mean
Overall GPA 3.86

Number of applications/admission offers/incoming students in 2003
287 applied/13 admission offers/8 incoming

% of students receiving:
Tuition waiver only: 0%
Assistantship/fellowship only: 0%
Both tuition waiver & assistantship/fellowship: 100%

Approximate percentage of incoming students who entered with a B.A./B.S. only: 100% **Master's:** 12.5%

Approximate percentage of students who are Women: 70% **Ethnic Minority:** 10%
International: Data not available

Average years to complete the doctoral program (including internship): 6 years

Personal interview
Preferred in person but telephone acceptable

Research areas	# Faculty	# Grants
affective disorders	1	1
attachment/close relationships/ psychopathology	1	1
developmental disabilities	1	1
marriage/spousal abuse	3	6
parent–child interactions	1	2
problem solving	1	0
psychotherapy process and outcome	1	0
reading difficulties	1	1

Clinical opportunities
psychological center, marital clinic, university hospital, student counseling center, various community agencies

Suffolk University

Department of Psychology
41 Temple St., 6th Floor
Boston, MA 02114-4280
phone#: (617) 573-8293
e-mail: phd@suffolk.edu
Web address: http://www.cas.suffolk.edu/psychology/

	1	2	3	**4**	5	6	7	
Clinically oriented		Equal emphasis			Research oriented			

What percentage of your faculty subscribes to or practices in each of the following orientations?

Psychodynamic/Psychoanalytic	29%
Applied behavioral analysis/Radical behavioral	0%
Family systems/Systems	53%
Existential/Phenomenological/Humanistic	41%
Cognitive/Cognitive-behavioral	65%

What percentage of students applying for internship last year was accepted into APPIC-member internships? 92%

What courses are required for incoming students to have completed prior to enrolling?
5 courses in psychology including statistics, research methods

Are there courses you recommend that are not mandatory?
—

GRE mean
Verbal 576   Quantitative 653   Analytical N/A
Advanced Psychology 673
Analytical Writing 5

GPA mean
Overall GPA 3.74

Number of applications/admission offers/incoming students in 2005
261 applied/32 admission offers/14 incoming

% of students receiving:
Tuition waiver only: 0%
Assistantship/fellowship only: 100%
Both tuition waiver & assistantship/fellowship: 0%

Approximate percentage of incoming students who entered with a B.A./B.S. only: 60%   **Master's:** 40% (include Ph.D.s)

Approximate percentage of students who are Women: 60%   **Ethnic Minority:** 20%   **International:** 7%

Average years to complete the doctoral program (including internship): 6.9 years

Personal interview
Required; may occur in person or by telephone

Research areas   # Faculty   # Grants
14 full-time faculty; 3 half-time
8 faculty are recipients of grants or contracts
See Web site for specific research areas.
General areas include:
cultural diversity
development

family
developmental psychopathology
neuropsychology
psychological assessment
treatment process & outcome

Clinical opportunities
adult inpatient and outpatient
child and adolescent inpatient and outpatient
college/university counseling center
forensic
neuropsychological assessment

Syracuse University

Department of Psychology
430 Huntington Hall
Syracuse, NY 13244-2340
phone#: (315) 443-2760
e-mail: kemaster@syr.edu
Web address: http://www.psychweb@syr.edu/graduate/programs/clininfo.htm

	1	2	3	4	**5**	6	7	
Clinically oriented		Equal emphasis			Research oriented			

What percentage of your faculty subscribes to or practices in each of the following orientations?

Psychodynamic/Psychoanalytic	0%
Applied behavioral analysis/Radical behavioral	0%
Family systems/Systems	11%
Existential/Phenomenological/Humanistic	0%
Cognitive/Cognitive-behavioral	89%

What percentage of students applying for internship last year was accepted into APPIC-member internships? 100%

What courses are required for incoming students to have completed prior to enrolling?
15 credits of psychology courses, statistics, laboratory course

Are there courses you recommend that are not mandatory?
Numerous laboratory courses, research experience, science courses

GRE mean
Data not available

GPA mean
Overall GPA 3.6   Psychology GPA 3.6

Number of applications/admission offers/incoming students in 2005
110 applied/13 admission offers/6 incoming

% of students receiving:
Tuition waiver only: 0%
Assistantship/fellowship only: 0%
Both tuition waiver & assistantship/fellowship: 100%

Approximate percentage of incoming students who entered with a B.A./B.S. only: 80%   **Master's:** 20%

Approximate percentage of students who are
Women: 75%   **Ethnic Minority:** 10%   **International:** 25%

**Average years to complete the doctoral program
(including internship):** 6 years

Personal interview
Preferred in person but telephone acceptable

Research areas	# Faculty	# Grants
family	1	1
psychophysiology	2	1
sexual health, AIDS prevention	2	2
substance abuse	2	4

Clinical opportunities
addictions
anxiety disorders
behavioral medicine
community psychology
couples
crisis intervention
family
neuropsychology
school/educational

Temple University

Department of Psychology
Broad and Montgomery Streets
Philadelphia, PA 19122
phone#: (215) 204-1561
Web address:
http://www.temple.edu/psychology/Clinical/index.html

1	2	3	4	5	**6**	7

Clinically oriented   Equal emphasis   Research oriented

**What percentage of your faculty subscribes to or practices
in each of the following orientations?**

Psychodynamic/Psychoanalytic	27%
Applied behavioral analysis/Radical behavioral	18%
Family systems/Systems	36%
Existential/Phenomenological/Humanistic	27%
Cognitive/Cognitive-behavioral	73%

**What percentage of students applying for internship last
year was accepted into APPIC-member internships?** 100%

**What courses are required for incoming students to have
completed prior to enrolling?**
Applicants to the doctoral program must hold a B.A. or B.S.
degree and have completed at least 4 minimally 3-credit
courses in psychology, including 1 laboratory course. In
addition, a natural sciences lab course and a statistics course
required.

**Are there courses you recommend that are not
mandatory?**
No

GRE mean
Verbal + Quantitative 1300

GPA mean
GPA 3.64

**Number of applications/admission offers/incoming
students in 2005**
244 applied/26 admission offers/11 incoming

% of students receiving:
Tuition waiver only: 0%
Assistantship/fellowship only: 0%
Both tuition waiver & assistantship/fellowship: 100%

**Approximate percentage of incoming students who
entered with a B.A./B.S. only:** 80%   **Master's:** 20%

**Approximate percentage of students who are
Women:** 73%   **Ethnic Minority:** 18%
International: Data not available

**Average years to complete the doctoral program
(including internship):** 6 years

Personal interview
Required in person

Research areas	# Faculty	# Grants
adult anxiety disorders	1	2
child/adolescent anxiety disorders	1	3
conduct disorder	1	0
depression and bipolar	1	2
early learning/Head Start	1	1
emotions and psychotherapy	1	1
juvenile delinquency/juvenile justice	1	6
neuropsychology	1	0
psychophysiology of emotions	1	1
trauma/rape victims	2	0

Clinical opportunities
anxiety disorders in children
adult social phobia
Many specialty clinics in a large urban area

University of Tennessee

Department of Psychology
Austin Peay Psychology Building
Knoxville, TN 37996-0900
phone#: (865) 974-3328
e-mail: cjogle@utk.edu
Web address:
http://psychology.utk.edu/gradstudy/clinproc.html

1	2	3	**4**	5	6	7

Clinically oriented   Equal emphasis   Research oriented

**What percentage of your faculty subscribes to or practices
in each of the following orientations?**

Psychodynamic/Psychoanalytic	50%
Applied behavioral analysis/Radical behavioral	30%
Family systems/Systems	30%
Existential/Phenomenological/Humanistic	0%
Cognitive/Cognitive-behavioral	30%

What percentage of students applying for internship last year was accepted into APPIC-member internships? 100%

What courses are required for incoming students to have completed prior to enrolling?
None

Are there courses you recommend that are not mandatory?
No

GRE mean
Verbal 583   Quantitative 667
Advanced Psychology 599

GPA mean
Overall GPA 3.45

Number of applications/admission offers/incoming students in 2005
85 applied/10 admission offers/9 incoming

% of students receiving:
Tuition waiver only: 0%
Assistantship/fellowship only: 11% [Fulbright]
Both tuition waiver & assistantship/fellowship: 89%

Approximate percentage of incoming students who entered with a B.A./B.S. only: 67%   **Master's:** 33%

Approximate percentage of students who are Women: 78%   **Ethnic Minority:** 0%
International: Data not available

Average years to complete the doctoral program (including internship): 5.5 years

Personal interview
Preferred in person but telephone acceptable

Research areas	# Faculty	# Grants
adult psychopathology	4	1
developmental psychopathology	4	2
health psychology	1	1

Clinical opportunities
conduct disordered children
dysfunctional families
long-term psychotherapy
personality disorders
sexual deviation

Texas A&M University
Department of Psychology
College Station, TX 77843-4235
phone#: (979) 845-2581
e-mail: d-snyder@tamu.edu
Web address: http://psychology.tamu.edu/AOS.php?ID=1

1	2	3	4	**5**	6	7

Clinically oriented   Equal emphasis   Research oriented

What percentage of your faculty subscribes to or practices in each of the following orientations?
Psychodynamic/Psychoanalytic — 20%
Applied behavioral analysis/Radical behavioral — 0%
Family systems/Systems — 15%
Existential/Phenomenological/Humanistic — 15%
Cognitive/Cognitive-behavioral — 50%

What percentage of students applying for internship last year was accepted into APPIC-member internships? 100%

What courses are required for incoming students to have completed prior to enrolling?
Introductory statistics, abnormal psychology, and at least 3 other psychology courses including a course in a core basic experimental area

Are there courses you recommend that are not mandatory?
Advanced research-based seminars

GRE mean
Verbal 600   Quantitative 650
Analytical Writing Not required

GPA mean
Overall GPA 3.5

Number of applications/admission offers/incoming students in 2005
150 applied/8 admission offers/7 incoming

% of students receiving:
Tuition waiver only: 0%
Assistantship/fellowship only: 0%
Both tuition waiver & assistantship/fellowship: 100%

Approximate percentage of incoming students who entered with a B.A./B.S. only: 70%   **Master's:** 30%

Approximate percentage of students who are Women: 60%   **Ethnic Minority:** 30%   **International:** 10%

Average years to complete the doctoral program (including internship): 5 years

Personal interview
Preferred in person but telephone acceptable

Research areas	# Faculty	# Grants
addictive disorders	1	1
aging	2	1
anxiety disorders	3	1
assessment	3	0
child behavior disorders	4	3
health psychology	2	1
marital/family studies	5	3
psychopathology	2	1
psychotherapy	7	2

Clinical opportunities
community
family
forensic
neuropsychology
rural psychology
substance abuse

237

University of Texas at Austin

Department of Psychology
1 University Station A8000
Austin, TX 78712
phone#: (512) 471-3393
e-mail: gradoffice@psy.utexas.edu
Web address:
http://www.psy.utexas.edu/psy/clinical/index.html

1	2	3	4	5	**6**	7

Clinically oriented   Equal emphasis   Research oriented

What percentage of your faculty subscribes to or practices in each of the following orientations?

Psychodynamic/Psychoanalytic	0%
Applied behavioral analysis/Radical behavioral	0%
Family systems/Systems	0%
Existential/Phenomenological/Humanistic	25%
Cognitive/Cognitive-behavioral	75%

What percentage of students applying for internship last year was accepted into APPIC-member internships? 100%

What courses are required for incoming students to have completed prior to enrolling?
None

Are there courses you recommend that are not mandatory?
Abnormal psychology, biopsychology, research methods, statistics

GRE mean
Verbal + Quantitative 1344
Analytical Writing Data not available

GPA mean
Psychology GPA 3.75

Number of applications/admission offers/incoming students in 2005
263 applied/8 admission offers/5 incoming

% of students receiving:
Tuition waiver only: 0%
Assistantship/fellowship only: 0%
Both tuition waiver & assistantship/fellowship: 100%

Approximate percentage of incoming students who entered with a B.A./B.S. only: 80% **Master's:** 20%

Approximate percentage of students who are Women: 60% **Ethnic Minority:** 40% **International:** 9%

Average years to complete the doctoral program (including internship): 6.6 years

Personal interview
Telephone required

Research areas	# Faculty	# Grants
addictions	1	1
ADHD	1	1
anxiety	1	0
cross-cultural	1	0
depression	1	1
developmental disabilities	1	1
epidemiology	1	0
health psychology	1	1
neurological disorders (animal models)	1	1
neuropsychology	1	0
sexual dysfunction	1	1
stress and coping	1	1

Clinical opportunities
anxiety disorders
behavioral medicine
child/family
community
crisis intervention
depression
marital
neuropsychology
obsessive–compulsive disorder
personality disorders
schizophrenia
sleep psychology
student counseling center
survivors of torture

University of Texas Southwestern

Medical Center at Dallas
Graduate Program in Clinical Psychology
5323 Harry Hines Boulevard
Dallas, Texas 75390-9044
phone#: (214) 648-5277
e-mail: Alyce.Cadena@utsouthwestern.edu
Web address: http://www8.utsouthwestern.edu/utsw/
home/education/psychology/index.html

1	2	3	**4**	5	6	7

Clinically oriented   Equal emphasis   Research oriented

What percentage of your faculty subscribes to or practices in each of the following orientations?

Psychodynamic/Psychoanalytic	30%
Applied behavioral analysis/Radical behavioral	10%
Family systems/Systems	20%
Existential/Phenomenological/Humanistic	5%
Cognitive/Cognitive-behavioral	35%

What percentage of students applying for internship last year was accepted into APPIC-member internships?
Data not available

What courses are required for incoming students to have completed prior to enrolling?
Introduction to psychology, learning, statistics; a bachelor's degree or its equivalent

Are there courses you recommend that are not mandatory?
Developmental, physiological, experimental

GRE mean
Verbal + Quantitative 1200
Analytical Writing Data not available

GPA mean
Overall GPA 3.5

Number of applications/admission offers/incoming students in 2005
155 applied/16 admission offers/10 incoming

% of students receiving:
Tuition waiver only: 0%
Assistantship/fellowship: 100% (in 3rd semester of 1st year through end of 4th year)
Both tuition waiver & assistantship/fellowship: 0%

Approximate percentage of incoming students who entered with a B.A./B.S. only: 60%   Master's: 40%

Approximate percentage of students who are
Women: 70%   **Ethnic Minority:** 20%
International: Data not available

Average years to complete the doctoral program (including internship): 4.5 years

Personal interview
Required in person

Research areas	# Faculty	# Grants
Alzheimer's	1	1
child depression	2	1
community mental health	1	0
cultural issues in psychology	2	0
depression	3	3
developmental psychology	1	1
health psychology	3	3
health services research	1	1
learning disabilities	1	0
neurobiological aspects of psychological disorders	2	2
neuropsychological profiles associated with medical disease	2	2
pain management	1	1
pediatric psychology	1	0
rehabilitation psychology	1	1
sleep disorders	1	1

Clinical opportunities
affective disorders
behavioral psychology
clinical child
community mental health
deafness
developmental disabilities
family therapy
forensic psychology
health/medical psychology
inpatient psychiatry
neuropsychology
outpatient psychotherapy
personality disorders
primary care clinic consultation
psychiatric emergency care
rehabilitation psychology
sleep disorders
vocational assessment/counseling

Texas Tech University
Department of Psychology
P.O. Box 42501
Lubbock, TX 79409
phone#: (806) 742-3711
fax#: (806) 742-0818
e-mail: kay.hill@ttu.edu (for admission information)
lee.cohen@ttu.edu (for other information)
Web address: http://www.depts.ttu.edu/psy/
psy.php?page=graduate/clinical/clinical

1	2	3	**4**	5	6	7
Clinically oriented		Equal emphasis			Research oriented	

What percentage of your faculty subscribes to or practices in each of the following orientations?
Psychodynamic/Psychoanalytic	14%
Applied behavioral analysis/Radical behavioral	14%
Family systems/Systems	57%
Existential/Phenomenological/Humanistic	14%
Constructivist	14%
Cognitive–Interpersonal	14%
Cognitive/Cognitive-behavioral	100%

What percentage of students applying for internship last year was accepted into APPIC-member internships? 100%

What courses are required for incoming students to have completed prior to enrolling?
18 semester hours of psychology

Are there courses you recommend that are not mandatory?
Statistics, abnormal psychology, developmental psychology, physiological psychology, and a research course such as experimental design or independent research with a faculty member

GRE mean
Verbal 500   Quantitative 636
Analytical Writing 5.2

GPA mean
Overall GPA 3.57

Number of applications/admission offers/incoming students in 2005
82 applied/13 admission offers/8 incoming

% of students receiving:
Tuition waiver only: 0%
Assistantship/fellowship only: 0%
Both tuition waiver & assistantship/fellowship: 100% (of incoming students)

Approximate percentage of incoming students who entered with a B.A./B.S. only: 88%   Master's: 12%

Approximate percentage of students who are
Women: 66%   **Ethnic Minority:** 24%   **International:** 0%

Average years to complete the doctoral program (including internship): 6 years

Personal interview
In-person interviews strongly encouraged but telephone interviews acceptable

Research areas	# Faculty	# Grants
addictions	1	1
behavioral assessment	1	0
behavioral medicine	1	1
behavioral parent training	1	0
child depression and anxiety	1	0
child maltreatment and abuse	1	0
cognitive-behavioral therapies	3	0
community interventions	1	0
eating disorders	1	0
ethics/regulatory issues	1	0
ethnic minority/cultural issues	1	2
health psychology	2	0
high-risk patients/suicide	1	0
high-risk youth	1	0
informant discrepancies/rater biases in child assessment	1	0
MMPI/MMPI-2	1	0
neuropsychological assessment	1	0
nicotine dependence/withdrawal	1	1
personal meaning-making processes	1	0
single subject design, time series regression, dynamic factor analysis	1	0
Spanish-speaking families	1	1
suicide	1	0
teachers' evaluations of children's problems	2	0
trauma	2	0

Clinical opportunities
Extensive opportunities with diverse populations are available.

University of Toledo

Department of Psychology
2801 West Bancroft Street
Toledo, OH 43606-3390
phone#: (419) 530-2721
e-mail: mtaylor2@pop3.utoledo.edu
Web address:
http://psychology.utoledo.edu/default.asp?id=56

1	2	3	**4**	5	6	7

Clinically oriented   Equal emphasis   Research oriented

What percentage of your faculty subscribes to or practices in each of the following orientations?

Psychodynamic/Psychoanalytic	25%
Applied behavioral analysis/Radical behavioral	0%
Family systems/Systems	13%
Existential/Phenomenological/Humanistic	13%
Cognitive/Cognitive-behavioral	13%
Neuropsychology	13%

What percentage of students applying for internship last year was accepted into APPIC-member internships?
Data not available

What courses are required for incoming students to have completed prior to enrolling?
Psychology major, including experimental, statistics

Are there courses you recommend that are not mandatory?
Topical seminars

GRE mean
Data not available

GPA mean
Psychology GPA 3.5

Number of applications/admission offers/incoming students in 2003
85 applied/10 admission offers/6 incoming

% of students receiving:
Tuition waiver only: 0%
Assistantship/fellowship only: 0%
Both tuition waiver & assistantship/fellowship: 100%

Approximate percentage of incoming students who entered with a B.A./B.S. only: 90%   **Master's:** 10%

Approximate percentage of students who are Women: 75%   **Ethnic Minority:** 25%
International: Data not available

Average years to complete the doctoral program (including internship): 5.5 years

Personal interview
Preferred in person but telephone acceptable

Research areas	# Faculty	# Grants
ADHD/LD	2	0
child/adolescent psychopathology	3	1
chronic mental illness	1	1
neuropsychology	1	0
posttraumatic stress syndrome	1	0
psychotherapy research	2	0
qualitative research	1	0

Clinical opportunities
child abuse/neglect
college adjustment problems
family/conjoint therapy
neuropsychology
process-experimental therapy

University of Tulsa

Department of Psychology
Tulsa, OK 74104
phone#: (918) 631-2248
e-mail: sandra-barney@utulsa.edu
Web address: http://www.cas.utulsa.edu/psych/

1	2	3	4	**5**	6	7

Clinically oriented   Equal emphasis   Research oriented

What percentage of your faculty subscribes to or practices in each of the following orientations?

Psychodynamic/Psychoanalytic	0%
Applied behavioral analysis/Radical behavioral	0%
Family systems/Systems	0%
Existential/Phenomenological/Humanistic	0%
Cognitive/Cognitive-behavioral	100%

What percentage of students applying for internship last year was accepted into APPIC-member internships? 100%

What courses are required for incoming students to have completed prior to enrolling?
18 hours of psychology including abnormal psychology, statistics or research methods, and basic core psychology courses

Are there courses you recommend that are not mandatory?
Advanced courses in psychology core areas

GRE mean
Verbal 559   Quantitative 658
Analytical Writing Data not available

GPA mean
GPA 3.89

Number of applications/admission offers/incoming students in 2005
55 applied/9 admission offers/5 incoming

% of students receiving:
Tuition waiver only: 0%
Assistantship/fellowship only: 13%
Both tuition waiver & assistantship/fellowship: 40%

Approximate percentage of incoming students who entered with a B.A./B.S. only: 65%   **Master's:** 35%

Approximate percentage of students who are Women: 78%   **Ethnic Minority:** 15%   **International:** 1%

Average years to complete the doctoral program (including internship): 5 years

Personal interview
Preferred in person but telephone acceptable

Research areas	# Faculty	# Grants
clinical gerontology	1	0
life-span development	2	0
neuropsychology	1	1
personality disorders	2	0
posttraumatic stress disorder	2	2
stress	3	1

Clinical opportunities
Practicum program is community-based with access to 18 general and specialty clinics.

Uniformed Services University of Health Sciences

4301 Jones Bridge Road
Bethesda, MD 20814-4799
phone#: (301) 295-3270
e-mail: mfeuerstein@usuhs.mil
Web address:
http://www.usuhs.mil/mps/Psychology/index.html

1	2	3	**4**	5	6	7
Clinically oriented		Equal emphasis			Research oriented	

What percentage of your faculty subscribes to or practices in each of the following orientations?

Psychodynamic/Psychoanalytic	10%
Applied behavioral analysis/Radical behavioral	0%
Family systems/Systems	10%
Existential/Phenomenological/Humanistic	10%
Cognitive/Cognitive-behavioral	80%

What percentage of students applying for internship last year was accepted into APPIC-member internships?
Data not available

What courses are required for incoming students to have completed prior to enrolling?
None

Are there courses you recommend that are not mandatory?
Basic undergraduate sequence of courses in psychology, course work related to the biological sciences (e.g. biology, chemistry) and research design/statistics.

GRE mean
Verbal 560   Quantitative 605
Analytical Writing Data not available

GPA mean
GPA 3.55

Number of applications/admission offers/incoming students in 2003
43 applied/2 admission offers/2 incoming

% of students receiving:
Tuition waiver only: 0%
Assistantship/fellowship only: 0%
Both tuition waiver & assistantship/fellowship: 100%

Approximate percentage of incoming students who entered with a B.A./B.S. only: 50%   **Master's:** 50%

Approximate percentage of students who are Women: 54%   **Ethnic Minority:** 27%
International: Data not available

Average years to complete the doctoral program (including internship): 5 years

Personal interview
Preferred in person but telephone acceptable

Research areas	# Faculty	# Grants
drug abuse and behavioral toxicology	1	3
mood disorders	1	2
neuropsychology	1	1

241

obesity and eating disorders	1	1
occupational health psychology	1	3
stress and pain in the workplace		
sexual dysfunction	1	0
stress and animal models	1	3
stress and cardiovascular disease	2	4

Clinical opportunities
children and adolescent
employee assistance program
forensic psychology
medical center
military teaching hospitals
occupational health (for police, fire fighters, secret service)
substance abuse
VA hospitals

University of Utah

Department of Psychology
380 S 1530 E, Room 502
Salt Lake City, UT 84112
phone#: (801) 581-6126
e-mail: Catalan@psych.utah.edu
Web address:
http://www.psych.utah.edu/clinical/clinical.html

1	2	3	**4**	5	6	7

Clinically oriented	Equal emphasis	Research oriented

What percentage of your faculty subscribes to or practices in each of the following orientations?

Psychodynamic/Psychoanalytic	30%
Applied behavioral analysis/Radical behavioral	0%
Family systems/Systems	40%
Existential/Phenomenological/Humanistic	0%
Cognitive/Cognitive-behavioral	50%

What percentage of students applying for internship last year was accepted into APPIC-member internships?
Data not available

What courses are required for incoming students to have completed prior to enrolling?
Undergraduate degree in psychology or its equivalent, including statistics, research design and abnormal psychology

Are there courses you recommend that are not mandatory?
Advanced statistics and research design

GRE mean
Verbal 593 Quantitative 629
Advanced Psychology 671
Analytical Writing Data not available

GPA mean
Junior/Senior GPA 3.67

Number of applications/admission offers/incoming students in 2003
110 applied/15 admission offers/7 incoming

% of students receiving:
Tuition waiver only: 0%
Assistantship/fellowship only: 0%
Both tuition waiver & assistantship/fellowship: 100%

Approximate percentage of incoming students who entered with a B.A./B.S. only: 80%   **Master's:** 20%

Approximate percentage of students who are Women: 75%   **Ethnic Minority:** 12%   **International:** Data not available

Average years to complete the doctoral program (including internship): 6.5 years

Personal interview
Required in person

Research areas	# Faculty	# Grants
adolescent/child psychology	3	1
adult psychopathology	3	1
behavioral medicine/health psychology	2	3
developmental issues	4	2
family/couple research	4	2
forensic	1	1
minority mental health	2	0
neuropsychology	1	0
pediatric psychology	1	1
personality assessment	2	0
personality disorders	2	0
sexuality	1	1
stress and coping	2	2

Clinical opportunities
adolescent/child assessment and psychotherapy
behavioral medicine/ health psychology
family therapy
forensic psychology
homeless/disadvantaged population
inpatient psychiatry
interpersonal psychotherapy
minority mental health
pediatric psychology
personality disorders
rational-emotive therapy
sex therapy/sexuality
substance abuse treatment

Vanderbilt University–Department of Psychology and Human Development**

111 21st Avenue South
Nashville, TN 37203
phone#: (615) 322-0080
e-mail: burnspm@ctruax.vanderbilt.edu
Web address: http://sitemason.vanderbilt.edu/site/cUBtpC/clinicalsciences

**Authors' Note: The clinical programs at Vanderbilt (Peabody College/Department of Psychology and Human Development and College of Arts & Sciences/Department of Psychology) have merged into a single program with two tracks: generalist and child, adolescent, and family.

	1	2	3	4	5	**6**	7
Clinically oriented			Equal emphasis			Research oriented	

What percentage of your faculty subscribes to or practices in each of the following orientations?

Psychodynamic/Psychoanalytic	0%
Applied behavioral analysis/Radical behavioral	5%
Family systems/Systems	5%
Existential/Phenomenological/Humanistic	0%
Cognitive/Cognitive-behavioral	90%

What percentage of students applying for internship last year was accepted into APPIC-member internships? 100%

What courses are required for incoming students to have completed prior to enrolling?
None

Are there courses you recommend that are not mandatory?
introduction to psychology; abnormal or psychopathology; biological bases of behavior; research methods; statistics

GRE mean
Verbal 670   Quantitative 720
Analytical Writing Data not available

GPA mean
Overall GPA 3.70   Psychology GPA 3.80

Number of applications/admission offers/incoming students in 2004
375 applied/17 admission offers/8 incoming

% of students receiving:
Tuition waiver only: 0%
Assistantship/fellowship only: 0%
Both tuition waiver & assistantship/fellowship: 100%

Approximate percentage of incoming students who entered with a B.A./B.S. only: 95%   **Master's:** 5%

Approximate percentage of students who are Women: 75%   **Ethnic Minority:** 19%   **International:** 3%

Average years to complete the doctoral program (including internship): 6.5 years

Personal interview
Preferred in person but telephone acceptable

Research areas	# Faculty	# Grants
autism	1	1
depression	4	4
eating	1	0
emotion	4	2
gender issues	1	1
health disparities	2	2
health psychology	3	3
neuroimaging	3	3
neuropsychology	2	2
prevention	2	2
psychopathology	6	6
psychophysiology	2	0
schizophrenia	1	1
statistics	2	1
therapy process and outcome	2	2
vocal communication	1	1

Clinical opportunities
affective disorders
aggression/impulse control
anxiety disorders
behavioral medicine
clinical child and family
neuropsychology
pediatric psychology
personality disorders
schizophrenia

University of Vermont

Department of Psychology
John Dewey Hall
Burlington, VT 05405
phone#: (802) 656-2670
e-mail: esther.rothblum@uvm.edu
Web address: http://www.uvm.edu/~psych/
?Page=programs/graduate/clinical/
clinical_overview.html&SM=gradmenu.html

	1	2	3	**4**	5	6	7
Clinically oriented			Equal emphasis			Research oriented	

What percentage of your faculty subscribes to or practices in each of the following orientations?

Psychodynamic/Psychoanalytic	0%
Applied behavioral analysis/Radical behavioral	10%
Family systems/Systems	10%
Existential/Phenomenological/Humanistic	0%
Cognitive/Cognitive-behavioral	90%

What percentage of students applying for internship last year was accepted into APPIC-member internships? 100%

What courses are required for incoming students to have completed prior to enrolling?
Psychology major or equivalent including general psychology, statistics, research design, and at least 3 other psychology courses

Are there courses you recommend that are not mandatory?
No

GRE mean
Verbal 560   Quantitative 650
Advanced Psychology 635

GPA mean
Overall GPA 3.53

Number of applications/admission offers/incoming students in 2003
150 applied/8 admission offers/6 incoming

% of students receiving:
Tuition waiver only: 0%
Assistantship/fellowship only: 80%
Both tuition waiver & assistantship/fellowship: 20%

Approximate percentage of incoming students who entered with a B.A./B.S. only: 86%   **Master's:** 14%

Approximate percentage of students who are Women: 75%   **Ethnic Minority:** 10%   **International:** 8%

Average years to complete the doctoral program (including internship): 5 years

Personal interview
Telephone required

Research areas	# Faculty	# Grants
adolescent treatment	2	1
anxiety disorders	1	3
child psychopathology	3	2
health psychology/behavioral medicine	2	2
lesbian/gay issues	1	1
prevention	2	1
sex offenders/abuse	1	1

Clinical opportunities
adolescent psychotherapy
anxiety disorders
behavioral medicine
childhood disorders
chronically mentally ill
depression
eating disorders
family therapy
HIV/AIDS
mental retardation
neuropsychology
prevention
substance abuse

University of Victoria
Department of Psychology
Victoria, British Columbia V8W 3P5, Canada
phone#: (250) 721-7525
e-mail: ptaylor@uvic.ca
Web address: http://www.uvic.ca/psyc/clinical/

1	2	3	**4**	5	6	7
Clinically oriented		Equal emphasis			Research oriented	

What percentage of your faculty subscribes to or practices in each of the following orientations?

Psychodynamic/Psychoanalytic	22%
Applied behavioral analysis/Radical behavioral	0%
Family systems/Systems	33%
Existential/Phenomenological/Humanistic	15%
Cognitive/Cognitive-behavioral	44%

What percentage of students applying for internship last year was accepted into APPIC accredited internships? 100%

What courses are required for incoming students to have completed prior to enrolling?
"A"-level grades for 1 full year of course work in 4 areas: social psychology, biological psychology, cognitive psychology, developmental, or abnormal psychology

Are there courses you recommend that are not mandatory?
Additional special topics in clinical psychology selections

GRE mean
Verbal 550   Quantitative 700
Analytical Writing 5.0

GPA mean
Overall GPA 7.5   Psychology GPA 7.5

Number of applications/admission offers/incoming students in 2005
101 applied/7 admission offers/3 incoming

% of students receiving:
Tuition waiver only: 0%
Assistantship/fellowship only: 95%
Both tuition waiver & assistantship/fellowship: 0%

Approximate percentage of incoming students who entered with a B.A./B.S. only: 85%   **Master's:** 15%

Approximate percentage of students who are Women: 79%   **Ethnic Minority:** 19%   **International:** 9%

Average years to complete the doctoral program (including internship): 6.5 years

Personal interview
Preferred in person but telephone acceptable

Research areas	# Faculty	# Grants
addictions	1	1
attention-deficit disorder	1	1
childhood sexual abuse	1	0
cognitive disorders in the elderly	1	1
cross-cultural psych	1	1
epilepsy	1	1
families and disabilities	1	1
families and divorce	1	1
fetal alcohol syndrome	1	1
traumatic brain injury	2	2

Clinical opportunities
adolescent and adult forensic
adult psychiatric
adult rehabilitation
child and adult mental health
child inpatient
pediatric and adult neuropsychology

University of Virginia–Department of Human Services

Curry School of Education
P.O. Box 400270
Charlottesville, VA 22904-4270
phone#: (434) 924-7472
e-mail: clin-psych@virginia.edu
Web address: http://curry.edschool.virginia.edu/
go/clinpsych/

	1	2	3	**4**	5	6	7

Clinically oriented   Equal emphasis   Research oriented

What percentage of your faculty subscribes to or practices in each of the following orientations?

Psychodynamic/Psychoanalytic	0%
Applied behavioral analysis/Radical behavioral	0%
Family systems/Systems	63%
Existential/Phenomenological/Humanistic	0%
Cognitive/Cognitive-behavioral	63%

What percentage of students applying for internship last year was accepted into APPIC-member internships? 100%

What courses are required for incoming students to have completed prior to enrolling?
None

Are there courses you recommend that are not mandatory?
Undergraduate statistics, child development, learning, abnormal psychology, physiological psychology/biopsychology, social psychology

GRE mean
Verbal 619   Quantitative 671
Advanced Psychology 628
Analytical Writing Data not available

GPA mean
Overall GPA 3.6   Psychology GPA 3.8
Junior/Senior GPA 3.7

Number of applications/admission offers/incoming students in 2005
183 applied/9 admission offers/6 incoming

% of students receiving:
Tuition waiver only: 0%
Assistantship/fellowship only: 0%
Both tuition waiver & assistantship/fellowship: 100%

Approximate percentage of incoming students who entered with a B.A./B.S. only: 74%   **Master's:** 26%

Approximate percentage of students who are Women: 82%   **Ethnic Minority:** 18%   **International:** 3%

Average years to complete the doctoral program (including internship): 5.4 years

Personal interview
Preferred in person but telephone acceptable

Research areas	# Faculty	# Grants
adolescent suicide	2	1
child clinical	1	0
cognitive/learning disorders	1	0
forensic psychology	2	3
incarcerated populations	2	2
multicultural	3	1
multiproblem families	1	0
parenting behavior	3	1
school interventions	4	1
test development	3	0
youth mentoring	4	4
youth violence	2	1

Clinical opportunities
adult psychotherapy
child and family assessment and intervention
couples therapy
crisis intervention
developmental psychopathology
family therapy
forensic psychology
medical consultation
neuropsychology
parenting/parent–child interaction
school interventions
school psychology
systems consultation
youth and adult correctional facilities
youth and adult inpatient facilities

University of Virginia–Department of Psychology

College of Arts and Sciences
102 Gilmer Hall
Charlottesville, VA 22903-2477
phone#: (804) 982-4750
Web address: http://www.virginia.edu/psychology/
research/areas.php#clinical

	1	2	3	4	5	**6**	7

Clinically oriented   Equal emphasis   Research oriented

What percentage of your faculty subscribes to or practices in each of the following orientations?

Psychodynamic/Psychoanalytic	25%
Applied behavioral analysis/Radical behavioral	0%
Family systems/Systems	25%
Existential/Phenomenological/Humanistic	0%
Cognitive/Cognitive-behavioral	50%

What percentage of students applying for internship last year was accepted into APPIC-member internships? 100%

What courses are required for incoming students to have completed prior to enrolling?
B.A. in psychology or equivalent

Are there courses you recommend that are not mandatory?
Abnormal psychology, statistics

GRE mean
Verbal 620   Quantitative 620   Analytical 620
Advanced Psychology 620
Analytical Writing Data not available

GPA mean
Overall GPA 3.5

Number of applications/admission offers/incoming students in 2003
250 applied/8 admission offers/5 incoming

% of students receiving:
Tuition waiver only: 0%
Assistantship/fellowship only: 0%
Both tuition waiver & assistantship/fellowship: 100%

Approximate percentage of incoming students who entered with a B.A./B.S. only: 70%   Master's: 30%

Approximate percentage of students who are
Women: 75%   Ethnic Minority: 25%   International: 5%

Average years to complete the doctoral program (including internship): 6 years

Personal interview
Preferred in person but telephone acceptable

Research areas	# Faculty	# Grants
adult psychopathology	3	3
anxiety/obsessive–compulsive disorders	1	0
behavioral genetics	2	1
child clinical/psychopathology	5	5
community psychology	3	3
developmental adolescence	3	3
epidemiology	2	1
family research/systems	2	2
minority mental health	2	2
neuropsychology	1	0
personality disorders	2	1
prevention	3	2
schizophrenia/psychosis	2	0
violence/abuse/victim–offender	4	2

Clinical opportunities
anxiety disorders
behavioral medicine
community psychology
depression
family therapy
forensic psychology
marital/couples therapy
neuropsychology
obsessive–compulsive disorder
pediatric psychology
psychology/law
schizophrenia/psychosis
victim/battering/abuse

Virginia Commonwealth University
Department of Psychology
808 West Franklin Street
Richmond, VA 23284-2018
phone#: (804) 828-1158 (admissions)
e-mail: clin-psy@vcu.edu
Web address: http://www.has.vcu.edu/psy/clinical/clinical_welcome.shtml

1	2	3	4	**5**	6	7
Clinically oriented		Equal emphasis			Research oriented	

What percentage of your faculty subscribes to or practices in each of the following orientations?
Psychodynamic/Psychoanalytic	0%
Applied behavioral analysis/Radical behavioral	0%
Family systems/Systems	10%
Existential/Phenomenological/Humanistic	0%
Cognitive/Cognitive-behavioral	75%
Interpersonal	15%

What percentage of students applying for internship last year was accepted into APPIC-member internships?
Data not available

What courses are required for incoming students to have completed prior to enrolling?
18 hours of psychology including general psychology, history and systems, experimental psychology, statistics

Are there courses you recommend that are not mandatory?
We recommend additional psychology, statistics, and other science courses.

GRE mean
Verbal 610   Quantitative 640
Advanced Psychology Not required
Analytical Writing Data not available

GPA mean
Overall GPA 3.4

Number of applications/admission offers/incoming students in 2003
186 applied/12 admission offers/8 incoming

% of students receiving:
Tuition waiver only: 0%
Assistantship/fellowship only: 0%
Both tuition waiver & assistantship/fellowship: 100%

Approximate percentage of incoming students who entered with a B.A./B.S. only: 65%   Master's: 35%

Approximate percentage of students who are
Women: 70%   Ethnic Minority: 25%
International: Data not available

Average years to complete the doctoral program (including internship): 5.8 years

Personal interview
Preferred in person but telephone acceptable

Research areas	# Faculty	# Grants
adolescent	4	3
anxiety	2	0
behavioral medicine	4	3
child clinical/pediatric	4	3
community	3	2
emotion	1	0
divorce	1	0
forensic psychology	1	0
minority/cross-cultural	2	1
pregnancy issues	1	1
psychopathology	1	1
psychophysiology	2	0
psychotherapy	1	1
stress and coping	3	0
substance abuse	2	1

Clinical opportunities

assessment and testing
behavioral medicine
child and adult anxiety
child pediatric
children of divorce
chronic mental illness
community psychology
correctional psychology
inpatient
neuropsychology
pain management
school
substance abuse
unipolar mood disorder

Virginia Consortium Program in Clinical Psychology (Psy.D.)

College of William & Mary, Eastern Virginia Medical School, Norfolk State University, and Old Dominion University Administrative Office
Virginia Beach Higher Education Center/Suite 259
1881 University Drive
Virginia Beach, VA 23453
phone#: (757) 368-1820
e-mail: rlewis@odu.edu
Web address: http://www.sci.odu.edu/vcpcp

1	2	**3**	4	5	6	7
Clinically oriented		Equal emphasis			Research oriented	

What percentage of your faculty subscribes to or practices in each of the following orientations?

Psychodynamic/Psychoanalytic	31%
Applied behavioral analysis/Radical behavioral	13%
Family systems/Systems	28%
Existential/Phenomenological/Humanistic	7%
Cognitive/Cognitive-behavioral	31%

What percentage of students applying for internship last year was accepted into APPIC-member internships? 90%

What courses are required for incoming students to have completed prior to enrolling?
B.A. in psychology or equivalent

Are there courses you recommend that are not mandatory?
Strong background in psychology

GRE mean
Verbal 614   Quantitative 637
Advanced Psychology 654
Analytical Writing 4.5

GPA mean
Undergraduate GPA 3.45

Number of applications/admission offers/incoming students in 2005
172 applied/19 admission offers/10 incoming

% of students receiving:
Tuition waiver only: 0%
Assistantship/fellowship only: 0%
Both tuition waiver & assistantship/fellowship: 100%
(significant tuition reduction but not a complete waiver)

Approximate percentage of incoming students who entered with a B.A./B.S. only: 60%   Master's: 40%

Approximate percentage of students who are
Women: 75%   Ethnic Minority: 29%   International: 2%

Average years to complete the doctoral program (including internship): 4.4 years

Personal interview
Required in person

Research areas	# Faculty	# Grants
ADHD	1	2
anxiety issues	2	0
attachment	1	0
attention disorders	1	0
behavior therapy	1	0
biofeedback	1	0
body image	1	0
child/clinical	1	0
childhood assessment	5	0
childhood trauma	1	0
community	1	1
competency	1	0
couples	2	0
depression	2	1
developmental psychopathology	3	0
eating disorders	1	0
family	2	0
gay and lesbian issues	1	0
gender issues	3	0
humor	1	0
intimacy	2	0
learning & learning disabilities	2	0
marital therapy	2	0
neuropsychology	1	2
organizations	1	1
parent–child interactions	2	0

parents' training	1	1
pediatric psychology	1	0
personal constructs	1	0
prevention	1	3
psychoanalysis	1	0
psychotherapy	2	0
psychotic disorders	1	1
rehabilitation psychology	1	0
relationships	1	0
religion	1	0
schizophrenia	1	0
self-discrepancy	1	0
social behavior	1	0
stereotypes	1	0
substance abuse	1	3
women's issues	2	0

Clinical opportunities

The Virginia Consortium Program in Clinical Psychology is a unified program sponsored by the College of William and Mary, Eastern Virginia Medical School, Norfolk State University, and Old Dominion University. Clinical training is provided in over 30 public and private agencies that serve adults, adolescents, and children. During the first 2 years in the program, the student develops skills in diagnostic interviewing, assessment, and therapy in a sequence of practicum experiences that leads to advanced training in the third year. The sequence of practicum experiences closely parallels the course work and is designed to provide students with the clinical work that best suits the student's professional development. Early practica involve role induction, specific skills training, and directive supervision, whereas later practica rely heavily on self-awareness and a less directive, more exploratory focus on therapy and supervision processes. Intensive advanced training is available in neuropsychology, and individual therapy. Students may develop other advanced training plans using resources as approved by the council.

Virginia Polytechnic Institute and State University

Department of Psychology
5088 Derring Hall
Blacksburg, VA 24061-0436
phone#: (540) 231-6275
e-mail: rswinett@vt.edu
Web address:
http://www.psyc.vt.edu/?p=grad2&content=clinical

1	2	3	4	5	**6**	7
Clinically oriented		Equal emphasis			Research oriented	

What percentage of your faculty subscribes to or practices in each of the following orientations?

Psychodynamic/Psychoanalytic	0%
Applied behavioral analysis/Radical behavioral	5%
Family systems/Systems	20%
Existential/Phenomenological/Humanistic	0%
Cognitive/Cognitive-behavioral	100%

What percentage of students applying for internship last year was accepted into APPIC-member internships?
Data not available

What courses are required for incoming students to have completed prior to enrolling?
Introductory psychology, research methods, statistics, learning, electives

Are there courses you recommend that are not mandatory?
Abnormal psychology, social psychology, developmental psychology, personality

GRE mean
Verbal 1225   Quantitative 1250
Analytical Writing Data not available

GPA mean
Overall GPA 3.6   Psychology GPA 3.7
Junior/Senior GPA 3.8

Number of applications/admission offers/incoming students in 2003
125 applied/12 admission offers/8 incoming

% of students receiving:
Tuition waiver only: 0%
Assistantship/fellowship only: 0%
Both tuition waiver & assistantship/fellowship: 100%

Approximate percentage of incoming students who entered with a B.A./B.S. only: 80%   **Master's:** 20%

Approximate percentage of students who are Women: 75%   **Ethnic Minority:** 15%
International: Data not available

Average years to complete the doctoral program (including internship): 6.1 years

Personal interview
Preferred in person but telephone acceptable

Research areas	# Faculty	# Grants
AIDS	2	0
affective disorders/depression	2	0
anxiety disorders	3	1
attention-deficit disorder	1	0
autism	1	0
behavioral medicine	3	2
child clinical	3	2
eating disorders	1	0
gender roles	1	0
hypnosis	1	1
marriage/couples	1	0
minority mental health	2	1
neuropsychology	2	0
pain management	2	0
parent–child interaction	2	1
pediatric psychology	1	1
prevention	4	3
psychotherapy outcome	2	1
shyness	1	0
social skills	3	0
stress and coping	1	0
substance abuse	2	3

Clinical opportunities
ADHD
AIDS
affective disorders
anxiety disorders
behavioral medicine
child clinical
conduct disorder
consultation
data management systems
gerontology
marital/couples therapy
neuropsychology
prevention in the community
substance abuse
systems management

University of Washington

Department of Psychology
Seattle, WA 98195
Web address:
http://web.psych.washington.edu/graduate/apply.html

1	2	3	4	5	**6**	7
Clinically oriented		Equal emphasis			Research oriented	

What percentage of your faculty subscribes to or practices in each of the following orientations?

Psychodynamic/Psychoanalytic	10%
Applied behavioral analysis/Radical behavioral	10%
Family systems/Systems	20%
Existential/Phenomenological/Humanistic	0%
Cognitive/Cognitive-behavioral	60%

What percentage of students applying for internship last year was accepted into APPIC-member internships? 100%

What courses are required for incoming students to have completed prior to enrolling?
None

Are there courses you recommend that are not mandatory?
Abnormal/psychopathology, biological bases of behavior, developmental, statistics, learning & motivation, social psychology

GRE median
Verbal 645 Quantitative 620
Analytical Writing Not required

GPA mean
Overall GPA 3.68

Number of applications/admission offers/incoming students in 2005
340 applied/13 admission offers/11 incoming

% of students receiving:
Tuition waiver only: 0%
Assistantship/fellowship only: 0%
Both tuition waiver & assistantship/fellowship: 100%

Approximate percentage of incoming students who entered with a B.A./B.S. only: 100% **Master's:** 0%

Approximate percentage of students who are
Women: 82% **Ethnic Minority:** 21% **International:** 0.1%

Average years to complete the doctoral program (including internship): 6 years

Personal interview
Interview not required

Research areas	# Faculty	# Grants
anxiety disorders	3	1
autism	1	1
child emotional development	3	3
cognitive therapy	4	2
depression	3	1
minority	5	4
psychology process	1	1
sport psychology	2	1
spouse abuse	2	1
substance abuse	3	3
suicide	1	1

Clinical opportunities
anxiety disorders
autism
community psychology
couples
family
minority
neuropsychology
pediatric psychology
personality disorders
psychoeducational (coping skills) training
rehabilitation medicine
substance abuse

Washington State University

Department of Psychology
P.O. Box 644820
Pullman, WA 99164-4820
phone#: (509) 335-2631
Web address: http://www.wsu.edu/psychology/2005/Graduate/Clinical.html

1	2	3	**4**	5	6	7
Clinically oriented		Equal emphasis			Research oriented	

What percentage of your faculty subscribes to or practices in each of the following orientations?

Psychodynamic/Psychoanalytic	23%
Applied behavioral analysis/Radical behavioral	0%
Family systems/Systems	23%
Existential/Phenomenological/Humanistic	8%
Cognitive/Cognitive-behavioral	100%

What percentage of students applying for internship last year was accepted into APPIC-member internships? 100%

What courses are required for incoming students to have completed prior to enrolling?
None

Are there courses you recommend that are not mandatory?
Abnormal, social, developmental, personality, statistics, research methods

GRE mean
Verbal + Quantitative 1150
Analytical Writing Not required

GPA mean
Overall GPA 3.6

Number of applications/admission offers/incoming students in 2005
156 applied/8 admission offers/6 incoming

% of students receiving:
Tuition waiver only: 0%
Assistantship/fellowship only: 0%
Both tuition waiver & assistantship/fellowship: 100%

Approximate percentage of incoming students who entered with a B.A./B.S. only: 69% **Master's:** 31%

Approximate percentage of students who are Women: 71% **Ethnic Minority:** 24% **International:** 12%

Average years to complete the doctoral program (including internship): 6 years

Personal interview
Preferred in person but telephone acceptable

Research areas	# Faculty	# Grants
adult psychopathology	5	6
behavioral medicine/health psychology	5	8
child clinical	4	4
neuropsychology	1	1

Clinical opportunities
adult and child inpatient
adult and child neuropsychological assessment
adult and child psychotherapy
health psychology

Washington University

Department of Psychology
Campus Box 1125
One Brookings Drive
St. Louis, MO 63130-4899
phone#: (314) 935-6520
e-mail: toltmann@artsci.wustl.edu
Web address: http://www.psych.wustl.edu/clinical/

1	2	3	4	5	6	**7**
Clinically oriented		Equal emphasis			Research oriented	

What percentage of your faculty subscribes to or practices in each of the following orientations?

Psychodynamic/Psychoanalytic	10%
Applied behavioral analysis/Radical behavioral	0%
Family systems/Systems	0%
Existential/Phenomenological/Humanistic	0%
Cognitive/Cognitive-behavioral	80%

What percentage of students applying for internship last year was accepted into APPIC-member internships? 100%

What courses are required for incoming students to have completed prior to enrolling?
24 credits of psychology and 30 credits in the physical, biological, and social sciences; courses in experimental psychology (with laboratory), and a course in quantitative methods

Are there courses you recommend that are not mandatory?
History and systems

GRE mean
Verbal 620   Quantitative 690   Analytical 710
Advanced Psychology 680
Analytical Writing 4.8

GPA mean
Overall GPA 3.65   Psychology GPA 3.8
Junior/Senior GPA 3.8

Number of applications/admission offers/incoming students in 2005
163 applied/8 admission offers/6 incoming

% of students receiving:
Tuition waiver only: 0%
Assistantship/fellowship only: 0%
Both tuition waiver & assistantship/fellowship: 100%

Approximate percentage of incoming students who entered with a B.A./B.S. only: 80% **Master's:** 20%

Approximate percentage of students who are Women: 70% **Ethnic Minority:** 33% **International:** 17%

Average years to complete the doctoral program (including internship): 6 years

Personal interview
Required in person

Research areas	# Faculty	# Grants
aging/gerontology	2	5
hypnosis	1	0
neuropsychology	2	3
psychopathology	3	4
psychological treatment	3	4

Clinical opportunities
A psychological services center, as well as a wide range of other practicum agencies throughout the St. Louis area, are used. The student's particular interests, as well as the need for diverse training, are considered in placement at these various agencies.

University of Waterloo

Department of Psychology
Waterloo, Ontario N2L 3G1 Canada
phone#: (519) 885-1211, ext. #3140
e-mail: ewoody@uwaterloo.ca
Web address: http://www.psychology.uwaterloo.ca/
gradprog/programs/phd/clinical/index.html

1	2	3	4	5	**6**	7
Clinically oriented		Equal emphasis			Research oriented	

What percentage of your faculty subscribes to or practices in each of the following orientations?

Psychodynamic/Psychoanalytic	40%
Applied behavioral analysis/Radical behavioral	20%
Family systems/Systems	20%
Existential/Phenomenological/Humanistic	20%
Cognitive/Cognitive-behavioral	100%

What percentage of students applying for internship last year was accepted into APPIC-member internships? 100%

What courses are required for incoming students to have completed prior to enrolling?
Basic statistics, research design, research courses, undergraduate thesis or equivalent

Are there courses you recommend that are not mandatory?
History of psychology

GRE mean
Verbal 628   Quantitative 674   Analytical 730
Advanced Psychology 702
Analytical Writing Data not available

GPA mean
Overall GPA 80

Number of applications/admission offers/incoming students in 2005
85 applied/8 admission offers/2 incoming

% of students receiving:
Tuition waiver only: 0%
Assistantship/fellowship only: 100%
Both tuition waiver & assistantship/fellowship: 0%

Approximate percentage of incoming students who entered with a B.A./B.S. only: 75%   **Master's:** 25%

Approximate percentage of students who are Women: 80%   **Ethnic Minority:** 13%   **International:** 5%

Average years to complete the doctoral program (including internship): 6.5 years

Personal interview
Preferred in person but telephone acceptable

Research areas	# Faculty	# Grants
depression	1	1
hypnosis	1	1
obsessive–compulsive disorder	2	2
relatedness, authenticity, and well-being	1	0
social anxiety and other anxiety disorders	1	1

Clinical opportunities
child/adolescent/adult
hypnosis
neuropsychology
school/educational

Wayne State University

Department of Psychology
5057 Woodward Avenue, 7th Floor
Detroit, MI 48202
phone#: (313) 577-2800
e-mail: aallen@wayne.edu
Web address: http://www.psych.wayne.edu/graduate/
gradclinpsych.htm

1	2	3	4	**5**	6	7
Clinically oriented		Equal emphasis			Research oriented	

What percentage of your faculty subscribes to or practices in each of the following orientations?

Psychodynamic/Psychoanalytic	10%
Applied behavioral analysis/Radical behavioral	0%
Family systems/Systems	20%
Existential/Phenomenological/Humanistic	0%
Cognitive/Cognitive-behavioral	60%

What percentage of students applying for internship last year was accepted into APPIC-member internships? 100%

What courses are required for incoming students to have completed prior to enrolling?
12 semester hour) in psychology, including experimental psychology (with laboratory experience) and statistical methods

Are there courses you recommend that are not mandatory?
Undergraduate courses in mathematics and life sciences

GRE mean
Verbal 600   Quantitative 680
Analytical Writing 5.5

GPA mean
Overall GPA 3.75

Number of applications/admission offers/incoming students in 2005
130 applied/18 admission offers/7 incoming

% of students receiving:
Tuition waiver only: 10%
Assistantship/fellowship only: 50%
Both tuition waiver & assistantship/fellowship: 33% (1st-year students: 100%)

Approximate percentage of incoming students who entered with a B.A./B.S. only: 90%   **Master's:** 10%

Approximate percentage of students who are
Women: 70% **Ethnic Minority:** 10% **International:** 10%

Average years to complete the doctoral program (including internship): 6.5 years

Personal interview
Required in person

Research areas	# Faculty	# Grants
behavioral medicine	2	2
community psychology	2	2
neuropsychology	2	2
risk factors/family	1	2
schizophrenia	1	0

Clinical opportunities
behavioral medicine
community psychology
neuropsychology
schizophrenia

West Virginia University

Department of Psychology
1126 Life Sciences Building
Morgantown, WV 26506-6040
phone#: (304) 293-2003, ext. # 31628
e-mail: debra.swinney@mail.wvu.edu
Web address:
http://www.as.wvu.edu/psyc/Programs/AC/index.htm

1	2	3	4	**5**	6	7
Clinically oriented		Equal emphasis			Research oriented	

What percentage of your faculty subscribes to or practices in each of the following orientations?
Psychodynamic/Psychoanalytic — 0%
Applied behavioral analysis/Radical behavioral — 50%
Family systems/Systems — 0%
Existential/Phenomenological/Humanistic — 0%
Cognitive/Cognitive-behavioral — 50%

What percentage of students applying for internship last year was accepted into APPIC-member internships? 100%

What courses are required for incoming students to have completed prior to enrolling?
None

Are there courses you recommend that are not mandatory?
Psychology major or related field, research, clinical experience

GRE mean
Verbal + Quantitative 1249
Advanced Psychology 681
Analytical Writing Data not available

GPA mean
Overall GPA 3.75

Number of applications/admission offers/incoming students in 2005
149 applied/9 admission offers/8 incoming

% of students receiving:
Tuition waiver only: 0%
Assistantship/fellowship only: 0%
Both tuition waiver & assistantship/fellowship: 100%

Approximate percentage of incoming students who entered with a B.A./B.S. only: 62% **Master's:** 38%

Approximate percentage of students who are
Women: 74% **Ethnic Minority:** 1% **International:** 0.2%

Average years to complete the doctoral program (including internship): 5 years

Personal interview
Preferred in person but telephone acceptable

Research areas	# Faculty	# Grants
ADHD	2	1
anxiety disorders	2	0
behavioral dentistry	1	0
behavioral medicine	4	2
cardiovascular reactivity	1	0
child behavior disorders	1	0
developmental disabilities	1	0
ethnic minority issues	1	0
forensics	1	0
gerontology	1	0
hypertension	1	2
pain	1	0
pediatric psychology	2	3
posttraumatic stress disorder	1	0

Clinical opportunities
anxiety disorders (adults and children)
behavioral dentistry
behavioral medicine (adults and children)
burn trauma
developmental disabilities
eating disorders
forensic psychology
gerontology
parent training
school interventions
victim/battering/abuse

Western Michigan University

Department of Psychology
Kalamazoo, MI 49008
phone#: (269) 387-4330
e-mail: donna.areaux@wmich.edu
Web address:
http://www.wmich.edu/psychology/grad/clinical.html

1	2	3	**4**	5	6	7
Clinically oriented		Equal emphasis			Research oriented	

What percentage of your faculty subscribes to or practices in each of the following orientations?

Psychodynamic/Psychoanalytic	0%
Applied behavioral analysis/Radical behavioral	71%
Family systems/Systems	14%
Existential/Phenomenological/Humanistic	0%
Cognitive/Cognitive-behavioral	43%

What percentage of students applying for internship last year was accepted into APPIC-member internships?
Data not available

What courses are required for incoming students to have completed prior to enrolling?
Psychology major at an accredited institution

Are there courses you recommend that are not mandatory?
Basic course in behavioral principles/theory

GRE mean
Data not available

GPA mean
Psychology GPA 3.4

Number of applications/admission offers/incoming students in 2003
89 applied/8 admission offers/6 incoming

% of students receiving:
Tuition waiver only: 0%
Assistantship/fellowship only: 0%
Both tuition waiver & assistantship/fellowship: 100%

Approximate percentage of incoming students who entered with a B.A./B.S. only: 83% **Master's:** 17%

Approximate percentage of students who are Women: 79% **Ethnic Minority:** 6%
International: Data not available

Average years to complete the doctoral program (including internship): 5.5 years

Personal interview
Preferred in person but telephone acceptable

Research areas	# Faculty	# Grants
aging	1	1
AIDS prevention/education	1	1
anxiety disorders/PTSD	1	0
autism/developmental disabilities	1	1
behavioral medicine	1	1
behavioral neuroscience	1	0
conceptual analysis of behavior therapy	2	0
depression	2	0
habit behaviors (tics, trichotilamania)	1	0
interpersonal victimization	1	0
program evaluation	1	0
psychotherapy outcome	4	0
sexual deviations and dysfunctions	1	1

Clinical opportunities
forensic mental health
function-based treatment
posttraumatic stress disorder
refugee mental health
school refusal

University of Western Ontario

Department of Psychology
London, Ontario N6A 5C2, Canada
phone#: (519) 661-2064
e-mail: vmvandom@uwo.ca
Web address: http://www.ssc.uwo.ca/psychology/clinical

1	2	3	4	5	**6**	7
Clinically oriented		Equal emphasis			Research oriented	

What percentage of your faculty subscribes to or practices in each of the following orientations?

Psychodynamic/Psychoanalytic	35%
Applied behavioral analysis/Radical behavioral	5%
Family systems/Systems	10%
Existential/Phenomenological/Humanistic	5%
Cognitive/Cognitive-behavioral	45%

What percentage of students applying for internship last year was accepted into APPIC-member internships?
Data not available

What courses are required for incoming students to have completed prior to enrolling?
—

Are there courses you recommend that are not mandatory?
Abnormal psychology, statistics, history and systems of psychology

GRE mean
Verbal 621 Quantitative 663
Advanced Psychology 704

GPA mean
Overall GPA A Psychology GPA A

Number of applications/admission offers/incoming students in 2003
104 applied/4 admission offers/3 incoming

% of students receiving:
Tuition waiver only: 0%
Assistantship/fellowship only: 0%
Both tuition waiver & assistantship/fellowship: 100%

Approximate percentage of incoming students who entered with a B.A./B.S. only: 80% **Master's:** 20%

Approximate percentage of students who are Women: 81% **Ethnic Minority:** Data not available
International: Data not available

Average years to complete the doctoral program (including internship): 7 years

Personal interview
Preferred in person but telephone acceptable

Research areas	# Faculty	# Grants
applied assessment	1	0
attachment in infancy	2	1
cognitive deficits in schizophrenia	1	1
depression	1	1

drug addiction	1	1
emotion and cognition	1	0
family violence	1	1
health psychology	4	2
humor	2	0
medical treatment decisions	2	3
menopause	1	1
pain	1	1
physical and sexual abuse	1	1
psychology of physical symptoms	1	1
psychopharmacology	1	0
stress and coping	5	0

Clinical opportunities
anxiety disorders
behavioral medicine
career counseling and development
child behavior and emotion
child forensics
inpatient psychiatry
mood disorders
outpatient psychiatry
pediatric health psychology
rehabilitation

Wheaton College (Psy.D.)

Department of Psychology
Wheaton, IL 60187-5593
phone#: (630) 752-7053
e-mail: Robert.J.Gregory@wheaton.edu
Web address: http://www.wheaton.edu/psychology/
graduate/overview/index.html

1	2	**3**	4	5	6	7
Clinically oriented		Equal emphasis			Research oriented	

What percentage of your faculty subscribes to or practices in each of the following orientations?

Psychodynamic/Psychoanalytic	25%
Applied behavioral analysis/Radical behavioral	0%
Family systems/Systems	33%
Existential/Phenomenological/Humanistic	0%
Cognitive/Cognitive-behavioral	42%

What percentage of students applying for internship last year was accepted into APPIC-member internships?
Data not available

What courses are required for incoming students to have completed prior to enrolling?
Introduction to psychology, theories of personality, physiological psychology, abnormal psychology, research/statistics

Are there courses you recommend that are not mandatory?
Developmental, cognition, social

GRE mean
Verbal 500   Quantitative 550   Analytical 550
Advanced Psychology 560

Analytical Writing Data not available

GPA mean
Overall GPA 3.0

Number of applications/admission offers/incoming students in 2005
80 applied/34 admission offers/19 incoming

% of students receiving:
Tuition waiver only: 0%
Assistantship/fellowship only: 0%
Both tuition waiver & assistantship/fellowship: 0%

Approximate percentage of incoming students who entered with a B.A./B.S. only: 65%   **Master's:** 35%

Approximate percentage of students who are Women: 52%   **Ethnic Minority:** 25%
International: Data not available

Average years to complete the doctoral program (including internship): 5 years

Personal interview
Required in person

Research areas	# Faculty	# Grants
church–psychology collaboration	3	1
family transitions	1	0
gender research	1	1
geropsychology issues	1	0
meta-analysis	1	0
parent training (Hispanic and African American)	1	1
rural psychology	2	0
spirituality and psychology	2	0

Clinical opportunities
Chicago and suburban area has great variety of offerings.

Widener University (Psy.D.)

Institute for Graduate Clinical Psychology
One University Place
Graduate Clinical Psychology
Chester, PA 19013
phone#: (610) 499-1208
e-mail: ellen.t.madison@widener.edu
Web address: http://www.widener.edu/Academics/
Schools_amp_Colleges/School_of_Human_Service_
Professions_/Institute_for_Graduate_Clinical_Psychology/
PsyD_Program_Overview/391

1	2	3	4	5	6	7
Clinically oriented		Equal emphasis			Research oriented	

What percentage of your faculty subscribes to or practices in each of the following orientations?

Psychodynamic/Psychoanalytic	40%
Applied behavioral analysis/Radical behavioral	0%
Family systems/Systems	20%
Existential/Phenomenological/Humanistic	10%
Cognitive/Cognitive-behavioral	30%

What percentage of students applying for internship last year was accepted into APPIC-member internships? 100%

What courses are required for incoming students to have completed prior to enrolling?
Introduction to psychology, statistics

Are there courses you recommend that are not mandatory?
Research design, abnormal psychology, developmental psychology

GRE mean
Verbal 564   Quantitative 637
Analytical Writing 4.9

GPA mean
Overall GPA 3.53

Number of applications/admission offers/incoming students in 2003
285 applied/59 admission offers/34 incoming

% of students receiving:
Tuition waiver only: 42%
Assistantship/fellowship only: 0%
Both tuition waiver & assistantship/fellowship: 42%

Approximate percentage of incoming students who entered with a B.A./B.S. only: 72%   **Master's:** 18%

Approximate percentage of students who are Women: 70%   **Ethnic Minority:** 29%   **International:** 2%

Average years to complete the doctoral program (including internship): 5 years

Personal interview
Required in person

Research areas	# Faculty	# Grants
assessment/diagnosis	1	0
early childhood	1	0
learning disabilities	1	0
problem solving	2	0
stress and coping	2	0

Clinical opportunities
assessment
brief intervention
couples therapy
diversity
family therapy
forensic psychology
group therapy
neuropsychology
organizational psychology
psychoanalytic/psychodynamic therapy
school psychology certification—state level
sex therapy

University of Windsor
Department of Psychology
Windsor, Ontario N9B 3P4, Canada
phone#: (519) 253-3000
fax#: (519) 973-7021
e-mail: bzakoor@uwindsor.ca
Web address:
http://web4.uwindsor.ca/units/psychology/clinical.nsf/
831fc2c71873e46285256d6e006c367a/76637c78d4470b
818525691a0063cdfc!OpenDocument

1	2	**3**	4	5	6	7
Clinically oriented		Equal emphasis			Research oriented	

What percentage of your faculty subscribes to or practices in each of the following orientations?

Psychodynamic/Psychoanalytic	45%
Applied behavioral analysis/Radical behavioral	15%
Family systems/Systems	15%
Existential/Phenomenological/Humanistic	30%
Cognitive/Cognitive-behavioral	25%

What percentage of students applying for internship last year was accepted into APPIC-member internships?
Data not available

What courses are required for incoming students to have completed prior to enrolling?
Statistics, experimental method, human learning, abnormal, honors thesis or equivalent

Are there courses you recommend that are not mandatory?
No

GRE mean
Data not available

GPA mean
Data not available

Number of applications/admission offers/incoming students in 2003
162 applied/42 admission offers/22 incoming

% of students receiving:
Tuition waiver only: 20%
Assistantship/fellowship only: 95%
Both tuition waiver & assistantship/fellowship: 20%

Approximate percentage of incoming students who entered with a B.A./B.S. only: 87%   **Master's:** 13%

Approximate percentage of students who are Women: 60%   **Ethnic Minority:** 10%
International: Data not available

Average years to complete the doctoral program (including internship): 6 years

Personal interview
Telephone required

Research areas	# Faculty	# Grants
addiction	2	1
child research	3	2
community psychology	2	2

255

eating disorders	2	1
gambling behavior	1	1
neuropsychological	4	4
psychotherapy research	3	1

Clinical opportunities

We have a Psychological Service Center, which serves the campus and general community. Extensive training in psychotherapy is available at the PSC. In addition we have numerous training sites for practica and internships in the Detroit area. We current;y have students placed in 7 sites in the Detroit Medical Center consortium. These training sites offer exceptional training in all aspects of clinical psychology. In total we have students train in more than 40 internship and practica sites in Canada and the U.S.A.

University of Wisconsin–Madison

Department of Psychology
W. J. Brogden Psychology Building
1202 West Johnson Street
Madison, WI 53706
phone#: (608) 262-2079
e-mail: tbb@ctri.medicinejpnewman@facstaff.wisc.edu
Web address:
http://psych.wisc.edu/gradstudies/clinical.html

1	2	3	4	5	6	**7**

Clinically oriented	Equal emphasis	Research oriented

What percentage of your faculty subscribes to or practices in each of the following orientations?

Psychodynamic/Psychoanalytic	16%
Applied behavioral analysis/Radical behavioral	0%
Family systems/Systems	8%
Existential/Phenomenological/Humanistic	0%
Cognitive/Cognitive-behavioral	92%
Motivational/Interviewing	25%
Child	16%

Note: Some faculty endorsed more than one orientation, some only one, and some endorsed none.

What percentage of students applying for internship last year was accepted into APPIC-member internships? 100%

What courses are required for incoming students to have completed prior to enrolling?

Psychology major or related field training

Are there courses you recommend that are not mandatory?

No

GRE mean

Verbal + Quantitative 1290
Analytical Writing Data not available

GPA mean

GPA 3.73

Number of applications/admission offers/incoming students in 2005

179 applied/13 admission offers/7 incoming

% of students receiving:

Tuition waiver only: 0%
Assistantship/fellowship only: 0%
Both tuition remission (out of state portion only) & assistantship/fellowship: 100%

Approximate percentage of incoming students who entered with a B.A./B.S. only: 100%   Master's: 0%

Approximate percentage of students who are Women: 78%   Ethnic Minority: 13%   International: 4%

Average years to complete the doctoral program (including internship): 7 years

Personal interview

Preferred in person but telephone acceptable

Research areas	# Faculty	# Grants
affective disorders	5	8
developmental psychopathology	4	15
health	3	3
personality disorders: psychopathy	1	2
schizophrenia and other psychotic disorders	2	3
self-concept	1	1
sleep research	1	3
substance abuse	3	9

Clinical opportunities

addictive disorders
assessment (IQ, objective, psychophysiological, neuropsychological)
assessment of forensic populations
assessment of schizophrenia, 1st-degree relatives of schizophrenics, and at-risk populations
brief dynamic psychotherapy
cognitive therapy for affective and anxiety disorders
families/couples therapy
inpatient therapy
self-concept
sleep disorders
therapy with criminal offenders

University of Wisconsin–Milwaukee

Department of Psychology
P.O. Box 413
Milwaukee, WI 53201
phone#: (414) 224-5521
e-mail: makovsky@uwm.edu
Web address: http://www.uwm.edu/Dept/Psychology/clinical/index.html

1	2	3	**4**	5	6	7

Clinically oriented	Equal emphasis	Research oriented

What percentage of your faculty subscribes to or practices in each of the following orientations?

Psychodynamic/Psychoanalytic	0%
Applied behavioral analysis/Radical behavioral	30%
Family systems/Systems	20%
Existential/Phenomenological/Humanistic	0%
Cognitive/Cognitive-behavioral	50%

What percentage of students applying for internship last year was accepted into APPIC-member internships? 100%

What courses are required for incoming students to have completed prior to enrolling?
B.A.or B.S. in psychology or equivalent

Are there courses you recommend that are not mandatory?
B.A.or B.S. in psychology or undergraduate courses in psychological statistics, a laboratory course in research methodology, and an advanced laboratory course in psychology

GRE mean
Verbal 561   Quantitative 652
Verbal + Quantitative 1213
Advanced Psychology 651
Analytical Writing Data not available

GPA mean
Overall GPA 3.59   Psychology GPA 3.71
Junior/Senior GPA 3.70

Number of applications/admission offers/incoming students in 2005
92 applied/9 admission offers/5 incoming

% of students receiving:
Tuition waiver only: 0%
Assistantship/fellowship only: 0%
Both tuition waiver & assistantship/fellowship: 100%

Approximate percentage of incoming students who entered with a B.A./B.S. only: 79%   **Master's:** 21%

Approximate percentage of students who are Women: 50%   **Ethnic Minority:** 21.4%   **International:** 4%

Average years to complete the doctoral program (including internship): 6.5 years

Personal interview
Preferred in person but telephone acceptable

Research areas	# Faculty	# Grants
alcohol and substance abuse	1	0
anxiety/impulse control disorders	2	1
attachment	2	0
child psychology	5	5
developmental disabilities	1	1
emotion regulation	1	0
health psychology/behavioral medicine	2	0
learning disabilities	1	0
mood disorders	1	1
multicultural issues	1	0
neuropsychology	2	1
psychotherapy/behavior therapy research	3	4

Clinical opportunities
acceptance and commitment therapy
behavior therapy
behavioral medicine
child and adult neuropsychology
child development
couples therapy
developmental
disabilities/autism
family violence
functional analytic psychotherapy
inpatient psychiatric
learning disability
OC spectrum disorders
premature infants and their families—stress

The Wright Institute (Psy.D.)
2728 Durant Avenue
Berkeley, CA 94704
phone#: (510) 841-9230
e-mail: info@wrightinst.edu
Web address: http://www.wrightinst.edu

1	**2**	3	4	5	6	7

Clinically oriented   Equal emphasis   Research oriented

What percentage of your faculty subscribes to or practices in each of the following orientations?
Psychodynamic/Psychoanalytic	40%
Applied behavioral analysis/Radical behavioral	0%
Family systems/Systems	20%
Existential/Phenomenological/Humanistic	10%
Cognitive/Cognitive-behavioral	30%

What percentage of students applying for internship last year was accepted into APPIC-member internships?
Data not available

What courses are required for incoming students to have completed prior to enrolling?
None

Are there courses you recommend that are not mandatory?
Human development or personality theory, abnormal psychology, statistics

GRE mean
Do not use GRE scores in admission decisions

GPA mean
Overall GPA 3.3   Psychology GPA 3.3

Number of applications/admission offers/incoming students in 2005
315 applied/100 admission offers/57 incoming

% of students receiving:
Tuition waiver only: 0%
Assistantship/fellowship only: 18%
Both tuition waiver & assistantship/fellowship: 0%

Approximate percentage of incoming students who entered with a B.A./B.S. only: 60%   **Master's:** 40%

Approximate percentage of students who are Women: 75%   **Ethnic Minority:** 20%
International: Data not available

Average years to complete the doctoral program (including internship): 5.5 years

Personal interview
Preferred in person but telephone acceptable

Research areas	# Faculty	# Grants
chronic illness	1	0
cross-cultural psychology	3	0
evolutionary psychology	1	1
gender studies	3	0
infant/parent psychotherapy outcome	3	0
jail and prison facilities	1	0
neurogerontology	1	0
parenting	3	0
step-families	1	0
stress-related somatic difficulties	1	0
substance abuse	2	0

Clinical opportunities
AIDS/HIV
affect disorders
assessment
brief and long-term therapy
child/adolescent assessment
child/adolescent psychopathology
couples therapy
crisis intervention
empirically supported treatments
ethnic minority
family therapy
forensic populations
geropsychology
GLBT
group therapy
men's issues
neuropsychology
pediatric/developmental
personality disorders
program development/evaluation
psychodynamic
public policy/advocacy
rehabilitation psychology
schizophrenia
substance abuse
university counseling
women's issues

Wright State University (Psy.D.)

School of Professional Psychology
3640 Colonel Glenn Highway
Dayton, OH 45435
phone#: (937) 775-3492
e-mail: sopp1@wright.edu
Web address: http://www.wright.edu/sopp/

1	**2**	3	4	5	6	7
Clinically oriented		Equal emphasis			Research oriented	

What percentage of your faculty subscribes to or practices in each of the following orientations?
Psychodynamic/Psychoanalytic	30%
Applied behavioral analysis/Radical behavioral	0%
Family systems/Systems	35%
Existential/Phenomenological/Humanistic	25%
Cognitive/Cognitive-behavioral	35%

What percentage of students applying for internship last year was accepted into APPIC-member internships?
Data not available

What courses are required for incoming students to have completed prior to enrolling?
Introductory psychology, introductory statistics, abnormal psychology, developmental psychology, physiological psychology, research methods

Are there courses you recommend that are not mandatory?
Learning, tests and measurements, multicultural issues, gender issues, personality theory, social psychology

GRE mean
Verbal + Quantitative 1000
Analytical Writing Data not available

GPA mean
Data not available

Number of applications/admission offers/incoming students in 2003
130 applied/44 admission offers/25 incoming

% of students receiving:
Tuition waiver only: 10%
Assistantship/fellowship only: 10%
Both tuition waiver & assistantship/fellowship: 5%

Approximate percentage of incoming students who entered with a B.A./B.S. only: 80%   **Master's:** 20%

Approximate percentage of students who are Women: 80%   **Ethnic Minority:** 20%   **Disabled:** 5%
International: Data not available

Average years to complete the doctoral program (including internship): 5 years

Personal interview
Required in person

Research areas	# Faculty	# Grants
domestic violence	4	1
family therapy	1	1
gender issues	5	1
health psychology	3	1
hearing impaired	1	1
managed care	1	0
minority mental health	5	1
multicultural issues	5	2
peace psychology	1	0
professional issues	4	0
violence reduction	6	2

Clinical opportunities
brief therapy/cognitive-behavioral therapy
children/adolescent
crisis intervention
mental health and deafness
family systems
forensic psychology
health psychology

258

marital/couples
multicultural issues
multidisciplinary teams
neuropsychology
victim/battering/abuse
violence reduction

University of Wyoming

Department of Psychology
Box 3415 University Station
Laramie, WY 82071
phone#: (307) 766-6303
e-mail: psyc.uw@uwyo.edu
Web address: http://uwadmnweb.uwyo.edu/psychology/
clinicalpsychology.asp

1	2	3	4	**5**	6	7

Clinically oriented   Equal emphasis   Research oriented

What percentage of your faculty subscribes to or practices in each of the following orientations?

Psychodynamic/Psychoanalytic	0%
Applied behavioral analysis/Radical behavioral	40%
Family systems/Systems	0%
Existential/Phenomenological/Humanistic	0%
Cognitive/Cognitive-behavioral	60%

What percentage of students applying for internship last year was accepted into APPIC-member internships? 100%

What courses are required for incoming students to have completed prior to enrolling?
None

Are there courses you recommend that are not mandatory?
Statistics, 30–45 psychology credits, research experience

GRE mean
Verbal + Quantitative 1290
Advanced Psychology 670
Analytical Writing 5.0

GPA mean
Overall GPA 3.62   Psychology GPA 3.8
Junior/Senior GPA 3.85

Number of applications/admission offers/incoming students in 2005
71 applied/6 admission offers/4 incoming

% of students receiving:
100% of students in years 1–3 receive full assistantship plus tuition waiver

Approximate percentage of incoming students who entered with a B.A./B.S. only: 75%   **Master's:** 25%

Approximate percentage of students who are Women: 70%   **Ethnic Minority:** 5%   **International:** 0%

Average years to complete the doctoral program (including internship): 6.5 years

Personal interview
Preferred in person but telephone acceptable

Research areas	# Faculty	# Grants
applied social psychology	3	2
child abuse/delinquency prevention	2	2
depression	2	1
HIV/AIDS prevention	1	3
mental retardation	2	1
Native American mental health	1	1
primary care	3	1
psychology and the law	2	3
self-regulation/self-efficacy	2	0
substance abuse	1	2
trauma/posttraumatic stress disorder	1	1

Clinical opportunities
adult/child inpatient and residential
bereavement
developmental disabilities
empirically supported psychotherapies
mood/anxiety disorders
primary/interdisciplinary care
rural/community health care

Xavier University (Psy.D.)

Department of Psychology
3800 Victory Parkway
Cincinnati, OH 45207-6511
phone#: (513) 745-3533
e-mail: maybury@xavier.edu
Web address:
http://www.xavier.edu/psychology_doctorate/

1	2	**3**	4	5	6	7

Clinically oriented   Equal emphasis   Research oriented

What percentage of your faculty subscribes to or practices in each of the following orientations?

Psychodynamic/Psychoanalytic	40%
Applied behavioral analysis/Radical behavioral	0%
Family systems/Systems	20%
Existential/Phenomenological/Humanistic	0%
Cognitive/Cognitive-behavioral	60%

What percentage of students applying for internship last year was accepted into APPIC-member internships?
Data not available

What courses are required for incoming students to have completed prior to enrolling?
Minimum 18 semester hours including the following: introductory psychology, psychology statistics, research methods, abnormal psychology, psychology testing, social development.

Are there courses you recommend that are not mandatory?
Anatomy and physical science, calculus.

GRE mean
Data not available

GPA mean
Data not available

Number of applications/admission offers/incoming students in 2003
118 applied/38 offers/ 22 incoming

% of students receiving:
Tuition waiver only: 0%
Assistantship/fellowship only: 42% (includes partial tuition remission)
Both tuition waiver & assistantship/fellowship: 0%

Approximate percentage of incoming students who entered with a B.A./B.S. only: 91%   **Master's:** 9%

**Approximate percentage of students who are
Women:** 82%   **Ethnic Minority:** 7%
International: Data not available

Average years to complete the doctoral program (including internship): 5 years

Personal interview
Interview not required

Research areas	# Faculty	# Grants
cognitive/behavioral	5	0
geropsychology	2	0
psychoanalytic	4	0
social/experimental	1	0
statistician	2	0

Clinical opportunities
college-related concerns
Xavier University Psychology Services Center

Yale University

Department of Psychology
P.O. Box 208205
New Haven, CT 06520-8205
phone#: (203) 432-4505
e-mail: kelly.brownell@yale.edu,
william.corbin@yale.edu, alan.kazdin@yale.edu,
doug.mennin@yale.edu, mitch.prinstein@yale.edu,
teresa.treat@yale.edu
Web address:
http://www.yale.edu/psychology/clinical.html

1	2	3	4	5	6	**7**
Clinically oriented		Equal emphasis			Research oriented	

What percentage of your faculty subscribes to or practices in each of the following orientations?

Psychodynamic/Psychoanalytic	0%
Applied behavioral analysis/Radical behavioral	0%
Family systems/Systems	0%
Existential/Phenomenological/Humanistic	16%
Cognitive/Cognitive-behavioral	100%
Evidence-based Treatment	100%

What percentage of students applying for internship last year was accepted into APPIC-member internships? 100%

What courses are required for incoming students to have completed prior to enrolling?
None

Are there courses you recommend that are not mandatory?
Broad psychology background, undergraduate psychology major

GRE mean
Verbal 653   Quantitative 712
Analytical Writing 5.54

GPA mean
Overall GPA 3.83

Number of applications/admission offers/incoming students in 2005
309 applied/4 admission offers/4 incoming

% of students receiving:
Tuition waiver only: 0%
Assistantship/fellowship only: 0%
Both tuition waiver & assistantship/fellowship: 100%

Approximate percentage of incoming students who entered with a B.A./B.S. only: 100%   **Master's:** 0%

**Approximate percentage of students who are
Women:** 85%   **Ethnic Minority:** 20%
International: Data not available

Average years to complete the doctoral program (including internship): 5.61 years

Personal interview
No preference given

Research areas	# Faculty	# Grants
adult psychopathology	5	1
alcohol use/dependence	1	2
anxiety disorders	2	0
cognitive processes	2	0
depression/suicidality	1	1
developmental psychopathology	1	2
eating disorders	2	2
health psychology	2	1

Clinical opportunities
adolescents
anxiety and mood disorders
child psychotherapy
conduct disorders
eating and weight disorders
health psychology
substance abuse

Yeshiva University (Psy.D.)

Department of Psychology
Ferkauf Graduate School of Psychology
1300 Morris Park Avenue
Bronx, NY 10461
phone#: (718) 430-3850
e-mail: gill@aecom.yu.edu
Web address:
http://www.yu.edu/ferkauf/index_sub.asp?504

1	**2**	3	4	5	6	7
Clinically oriented		Equal emphasis			Research oriented	

What percentage of your faculty subscribes to or practices in each of the following orientations?

Psychodynamic/Psychoanalytic	40%
Applied behavioral analysis/Radical behavioral	5%
Family systems/Systems	10%
Existential/Phenomenological/Humanistic	5%
Cognitive/Cognitive-behavioral	40%

What percentage of students applying for internship last year was accepted into APPIC-member internships? 98%

What courses are required for incoming students to have completed prior to enrolling?
Introductory psychology, statistics, abnormal psychology, experimental psychology, physiological psychology, personality

Are there courses you recommend that are not mandatory?
No

GRE mean
Verbal 550 Quantitative 600
Analytical Writing Data not available

GPA mean
Overall GPA 3.5 Psychology GPA 3.5

Number of applications/admission offers/incoming students in 2005
300 applied/79 admission offers/25 incoming

% of students receiving:
Tuition waiver only: 0%
Assistantship/fellowship only: 70%
Both tuition waiver & assistantship/fellowship: 0%

Approximate percentage of incoming students who entered with a B.A./B.S. only: 85% **Master's:** 15%

Approximate percentage of students who are Women: 73% **Ethnic Minority:** 15%
International: Data not available

Average years to complete the doctoral program (including internship): 5 years

Personal interview
Required in person

Research areas	# Faculty	# Grants
anxiety disorders	1	0
depression	2	0
early childhood intervention	1	0
ethnicity and identity	2	0
family therapy	1	0
forensics	1	0
gero-psychology	1	1
parenting styles	1	0
psychoanalytic therapy	5	0
psychotherapy process and outcome	3	0
sleep disorders/nightmares	1	0
stress and coping	4	1
trauma	2	0

Clinical opportunities
anxiety disorders
cognitive behavior therapy
depression
family therapy
geriatrics
interpersonal therapy
marital/couples
parent training
psychodynamic therapy
psychoeducational assessment

York University–Adult Clinical Program

Department of Psychology
Toronto, Ontario M3J 1P3, Canada
phone#: (416) 736-2100, ext. 22444
e-mail: jirvine@yorku.ca
Web address: http://www.psych.yorku.ca/grad/
index.php?option=com_content&task=view&id=
19&Itemid=33

1	2	3	**4**	5	6	7
Clinically oriented		Equal emphasis			Research oriented	

What percentage of your faculty subscribes to or practices in each of the following orientations?

Psychodynamic/Psychoanalytic	25%
Applied behavioral analysis/Radical behavioral	0%
Family systems/Systems	6%
Existential/Phenomenological/Humanistic	38%
Cognitive/Cognitive-behavioral	31%

What percentage of students applying for internship last year was accepted into APPIC-member internships? 50%

What courses are required for incoming students to have completed prior to enrolling?
Introductory psychology, physical/neuropsychology, organizational/social/groups, research design and statistics analysis, learning/perception/emotion/motivation, personality/abnormal/individual differences

Are there courses you recommend that are not mandatory?
Multicultural psychology, sex-roles, tests and measurements

GRE mean
Verbal 562 Quantitative 630
Advanced Psychology 600
Analytical Writing Data not available

GPA mean
Overall GPA A–

Number of applications/admission offers/incoming students in 2004
185 applied/10 admission offers/9 incoming

% of students receiving:
Tuition waiver only: N/A
Assistantship/fellowship only: 100% incoming students; 35% all other
Both tuition waiver & assistantship/fellowship: N/A

Approximate percentage of incoming students who entered with a B.A./B.S. only: 100%   **Master's:** 0%

Approximate percentage of students who are Women: 89%   **Ethnic Minority:** Data not available
International: Data not available

Average years to complete the doctoral program (including internship): 6 years

Personal interview
Preferred in person but telephone acceptable

Research areas	# Faculty	# Grants
alcohol and substance abuse	1	3
anxiety/stress/coping	1	1
depression	1	2
eating disorders	1	2
emotional and attentional processes	1	2
forgiveness	1	1
grief and trauma	1	0
health—cardiovascular disease	1	4
interpersonal processes/family and groups	1	2
memory and cognition/brain injury/ dementia/Alzheimer's	1	2
narrative processes	1	2
neuropsychology	2	2
pain	1	2
perfectionism	1	1
personality factors in mental, physical, and neuropsychological health	2	2
pyschotherapy process and outcome	4	3
schizophrenia	1	1

Clinical opportunities
alcohol and substance abuse
anxiety disorders
depression
eating disorders
forensic
geriatric
health psychology
neuropsychological assessment/rehab

York University–
Clinical–Developmental Area

Department of Psychology
Toronto, Ontario M3J 1P3, Canada
phone#: (416) 736-2100
e-mail: cdarea@yorku.ca
Web address: http://www.psych.yorku.ca/grad/index.php?option=com_content&task=view&id=15&Itemid=34

1	2	3	**4**	5	6	7
Clinically oriented		Equal emphasis			Research oriented	

What percentage of your faculty subscribes to or practices in each of the following orientations?
Psychodynamic/Psychoanalytic   10%
Applied behavioral analysis/Radical behavioral   10%
Family systems/Systems   75%
Existential/Phenomenological/Humanistic   0%
Cognitive/Cognitive-behavioral   75%

What percentage of students applying for internship last year was accepted into APPIC-member internships?
Data not available

What courses are required for incoming students to have completed prior to enrolling?
Honors degree in psychology

Are there courses you recommend that are not mandatory?
—

GRE mean
Verbal 600   Quantitative 735
Advanced Psychology 670
Analytical Writing Data not available

GPA mean
Data not available

Number of applications/admission offers/incoming students in 2003
115 applied/10 admission offers/8 incoming

% of students receiving:
Tuition waiver only: 0%
Assistantship/fellowship only: 100%
Both partial tuition waiver & assistantship/fellowship: 100%

Approximate percentage of incoming students who entered with a B.A./B.S. only: 90%   **Master's:** 10%

Approximate percentage of students who are Women: 80%   **Ethnic Minority:** 18%
International: Data not available

Average years to complete the doctoral program (including internship): 6.5 years

Personal interview
Preferred in person but telephone acceptable

Research areas	# Faculty	# Grants
adolescent peer relations	3	3
aggression—child and adolescence	3	3
autism, developmental disability	2	2

bullying and victimization	2	1
child abuse	3	2
child testimony	1	2
cognitive and language development	2	1
history of psychology	1	0
problem-solving/emotion	1	0
stress and coping	1	0
teen violence	2	2
underachievement	1	1

Clinical opportunities
children's rehabilitation center
dual diagnosis clinic
gender disorder clinic
learning disability clinic
mental health centers
psychiatric clinics
school boards

Clinical Psychology Programs That Have Been Discontinued

New York University (accredited, inactive)

The Wright Institute (accredited, inactive)

REPORTS ON INDIVIDUAL COUNSELING PSYCHOLOGY PROGRAMS

University of Akron

Department of Psychology and
Department of Counseling
Akron, OH 44325-4301
phone#: (330) 972-7280 or (330) 972-7777
e-mail: dmt5@uakron.edu
Web address:
http://www3.uakron.edu/psychology/counseling

1	2	3	**4**	5	6	7
Clinically oriented		Equal emphasis			Research oriented	

What percentage of your faculty subscribes to or practices in each of the following orientations?

Psychodynamic/Psychoanalytic	10%
Applied behavioral analysis/Radical behavioral	0%
Family systems/Systems	10%
Existential/Phenomenological/Humanistic	20%
Cognitive/Cognitive-behavioral	60%

What percentage of students applying for internship last year was accepted into APPIC-member internships? 100%

What courses are required for incoming students to have completed prior to enrolling?
The program has 2 tracks: 1 track (Department of Psychology) admits students with a bachelor's degree in psychology; the other track (Department of Counseling and Special Education) admits students with a master's degree in counseling.

Are there courses you recommend that are not mandatory?
No

GRE mean
1100 recommended
Analytical Writing Data not available

GPA mean
Overall GPA 3.25

Number of applications/admission offers/incoming students in 2003
80 applied/14 admission offers/11 incoming

% of students receiving:
Tuition waiver only: 10%
Assistantship/fellowship only: 0%
Both tuition waiver & assistantship/fellowship: 90%

Approximate percentage of incoming students who entered with a B.A./B.S. only: 50% **Master's:** 50%

Approximate percentage of students who are Women: 80% **Ethnic Minority:** 10%
International: Data not available

Average years to complete the doctoral program (including internship): 6 years

Personal interview
No preference given

Research areas	# Faculty	# Grants
multicultural issues	2	0
personality assessment	2	0
suicide	2	0
vocational counseling	2	0
women's issues	3	0

Clinical opportunities
clinic for child study and family therapy
community mental health center
VA medical center

University at Albany/ State University of New York

Division of Counseling Psychology
Department of Education and Counseling Psychology
ED 220
Albany, NY 12222
phone#: (518) 442-5040
e-mail: mfriedlander@uamail.albany.edu
Web address: http://www.albany.edu/counseling_psych

1	2	3	**4**	5	6	7
Clinically oriented		Equal emphasis			Research oriented	

What percentage of your faculty subscribes to or practices in each of the following orientations?

Psychodynamic/Psychoanalytic	15%
Applied behavioral analysis/Radical behavioral	0%
Family systems/Systems	15%
Existential/Phenomenological/Humanistic	20%
Cognitive/Cognitive-behavioral	50%

What percentage of students applying for internship last year was accepted into APPIC-member internships? 85%

What courses are required for incoming students to have completed prior to enrolling?
Undergraduate/graduate preparation in basic psychology (18 credits minimum including statistics)

Are there courses you recommend that are not mandatory?
abnormal, developmental or personality

GRE mean
Verbal + Quantitative 1200
Analytical and Advanced Psychology not considered
Analytical Writing not considered

GPA mean
Overall GPA 3.6 Psychology GPA 3.8

Number of applications/admission offers/incoming students in 2005
111 applied/17 admission offers/8 incoming

% of students receiving:
Tuition waiver only: 8%
Assistantship/fellowship only: 0%
Both tuition waiver & assistantship/fellowship: 92%

Approximate percentage of incoming students who entered with a B.A./B.S. only: 50% **Master's:** 50%

Approximate percentage of students who are
Women: 75%   **Ethnic Minority:** 22%   **International:** 15%

Average years to complete the doctoral program (including internship): 6 years

Personal interview
Preferred in person but telephone acceptable

Research areas	# Faculty	# Grants
alcoholism	1	3
career development	1	0
cross-cultural	2	2
family dynamics	1	0
family therapy	1	1
methodology	2	2
psychotherapy process	1	1
social phobia	1	0
sports psychology	1	0
supervision	2	0
women's issues	2	0

Clinical opportunities
adolescent residential treatment centers
college and university counseling centers (large and small, public and private)
community agencies
county mental health clinics including general and substance abuse clinics and adolescent units
inpatient and outpatient units at state psychiatric center and private hospitals
neuropsychology rehabilitation center
various units at VA hospitals, including primary care, outpatient, day treatment, substance abuse, inpatient psychiatry

Arizona State University

Division of Psychology and Education
Arizona State University
Tempe, AZ 85287-0611
phone#: (480) 965-6339
e-mail: dpe@asu.edu
Web address: http://coe.asu.edu/psyched/

1	2	3	**4**	5	6	7
Clinically oriented		Equal emphasis			Research oriented	

What percentage of your faculty subscribes to or practices in each of the following orientations?
Psychodynamic/Psychoanalytic   20%
Applied behavioral analysis/Radical behavioral   0%
Family systems/Systems   10%
Existential/Phenomenological/Humanistic   30%
Cognitive/Cognitive-behavioral   40%

What percentage of students applying for internship last year was accepted into APPIC-member internships? 80%

What courses are required for incoming students to have completed prior to enrolling?
No specific courses

Are there courses you recommend that are not mandatory?
Psychology or related background.

GRE mean
Verbal 510   Quantitative 550
Analytical Writing Data not available

GPA mean
Overall GPA 3.26   Junior/Senior GPA 3.67

Number of applications/admission offers/incoming students in 2005
120 applied/16 admission offers/12 incoming

% of students receiving:
Tuition waiver only: 0%
Assistantship/fellowship only: 58%
Both tuition waiver & assistantship/fellowship: 42%

Approximate percentage of incoming students who entered with a B.A./B.S. only: 35%   **Master's:** 65%

Approximate percentage of students who are
Women: 75%   **Ethnic Minority:** 50%
International: Data not available

Average years to complete the doctoral program (including internship): 5 years

Personal interview
Preferred in person but telephone acceptable

Research areas	# Faculty	# Grants
career development and counseling	3	0
cognitive appraisal	1	0
cognitive-behavioral interventions	1	0
consultation	2	0
counseling process	4	0
counseling the gifted and talented	2	1
counseling women and minorities	5	1
culture sensitivity training and counselor's race ethics	4	0
experimental methodology	2	0
family enrichment	1	0
gender issues in counseling	2	0
group counseling	1	0
health psychology	1	0
HIV	1	0
international issues	1	0
interpersonal models of personality and therapy	3	0
psychology of women	2	0
social psychological approaches to counseling	2	0
suicidology	1	0
training and supervision	4	0
values and decision making	1	0

Clinical opportunities
Varied

Auburn University

Department of Counseling and Counseling Psychology
Auburn, AL 36849-5218
phone#: (334) 844-5160
e-mail: ccp@mail.auburn.edu
Web address: http://www.auburn.edu/ccp

1	2	3	**4**	5	6	7
Clinically oriented		Equal emphasis			Research oriented	

What percentage of your faculty subscribes to or practices in each of the following orientations?

Psychodynamic/Psychoanalytic	33%
Applied behavioral analysis/Radical behavioral	0%
Family systems/Systems	0%
Existential/Phenomenological/Humanistic	33%
Cognitive/Cognitive-behavioral	33%

What percentage of students applying for internship last year was accepted into APPIC-member internships? 100%

What courses are required for incoming students to have completed prior to enrolling?
None

Are there courses you recommend that are not mandatory?
No

GRE mean
Cases considered individually.
Advanced Psychology not required
Analytical Writing not required

GPA mean
Overall GPA 3.6

Number of applications/admission offers/incoming students in 2005
86 applied/6 admission offers/4 incoming

% of students receiving:
Tuition waiver only: 0%
Assistantship/fellowship only: 20%
Both tuition waiver & assistantship/fellowship: 80%

Approximate percentage of incoming students who entered with a B.A./B.S. only: 75% **Master's:** 25%

Approximate percentage of students who are Women: 75% **Ethnic Minority:** 25% **International:** 10%

Average years to complete the doctoral program (including internship): 5.5 years

Personal interview
Preferred in person but telephone acceptable

Research areas	# Faculty	# Grants
alternative methods	1	0
gay/lesbian/bisexual themes	2	0
professional issues/ethics	3	0
psychometrics	2	0
substance abuse prevention	3	1

Clinical opportunities
mental health center (outpatient)
substance abuse unit (inpatient and outpatient)
university counseling center

Ball State University

Department of Counseling Psychology and Guidance Services
Muncie, IN 47306
phone#: (765) 285-8040
fax#: (765) 285-2067
e-mail: SBOWMAN@BSU.EDU
Web address: http://www.bsu.edu/web/counselingpsych/

1	2	3	**4**	5	6	7
Clinically oriented		Equal emphasis			Research oriented	

What percentage of your faculty subscribes to or practices in each of the following orientations?

Psychodynamic/Psychoanalytic	15%
Applied behavioral analysis/Radical behavioral	0%
Family systems/Systems	35%
Existential/Phenomenological/Humanistic	20%
Cognitive/Cognitive-behavioral	30%

What percentage of students applying for internship last year was accepted into APPIC-member internships? 100%

What courses are required for incoming students to have completed prior to enrolling?
Counseling theories, counseling techniques (pre-practicum), practicum, one other counseling course

Are there courses you recommend that are not mandatory?
No

GRE mean
Verbal + Quantitative 1115
Analytical Writing not required

GPA mean
Overall master's GPA 3.8

Number of applications/admission offers/incoming students in 2005
50 applied/13 admission offers/8 incoming

% of students receiving:
Tuition waiver only: 0%
Assistantship/fellowship only: 0%
Both tuition waiver & assistantship/fellowship: 100%

Approximate percentage of incoming students who entered with a B.A./B.S. only: 0% **Master's:** 100%

Approximate percentage of students who are Women: 67% **Ethnic Minority:** 28% **International:** 23%

Average years to complete the doctoral program (including internship): 4.6 years

Personal interview
Preferred in person but telephone acceptable

269

Research areas	# Faculty	# Grants
behavioral medicine/wellness	1	0
career/vocational	4	0
child/adolescent	2	0
clinical judgment	1	0
multicultural	3	1
organizational/EAP	1	0
social psychology applications	2	0
vocational rehabilitation	2	1
women's identity	2	0

Clinical opportunities
departmental mental health clinic
gerontology
oncology
university counseling center

Boston College

Department of Counseling, Developmental
and Educational Psychology
School of Education
Chestnut Hill, MA 02167
phone#: (617) 552-4710 or (617) 552-4214
e-mail: gsoe@bc.edu
Web address: http://www.bc.edu/bc_org/avp/soe/
academics/grad/doctoral/counseling_psych/default.html

1	2	3	4	**5**	6	7

Clinically oriented	Equal emphasis	Research oriented

What percentage of your faculty subscribes to or practices in each of the following orientations?

Psychodynamic/Psychoanalytic	40%
Applied behavioral analysis/Radical behavioral	0%
Family systems/Systems	30%
Existential/Phenomenological/Humanistic	10%
Cognitive/Cognitive-behavioral	10%

What percentage of students applying for internship last year was accepted into APPIC-member internships? 100%

What courses are required for incoming students to have completed prior to enrolling?
For applicants without a master's degree (i.e., direct admits), we require that students complete at least 18 credit hours of undergraduate psychology, including courses such as statistics, abnormal psychology, developmental psychology, theories of personality. These course are strongly recommended, but not necessarily required.

Are there courses you recommend that are not mandatory?
See comments above.

GRE mean
Verbal 566   Quantitative 629
Analytical Writing 5.5

GPA mean
Overall GPA 3.67

Number of applications/admission offers/incoming students in 2005
249 applied/12 admission offers/7 incoming

% of students receiving:
Tuition waiver only: 0%
Assistantship/fellowship only: 0%
Both tuition waiver & assistantship/fellowship: 100%

Approximate percentage of incoming students who entered with a B.A./B.S. only: 0%   **Master's:** 100%
Note. We are now expanding our applicant pool to include students without a master's degree as well as students with master's degrees in counseling or related areas. Therefore, the statistics represented above will change in subsequent years.

Approximate percentage of students who are
Women: 86%   **Ethnic Minority:** 29%   **International:** 14%

Average years to complete the doctoral program (including internship): 5.6 years

Personal interview
Preferred in person but telephone acceptable

Research areas	# Faculty	# Grants
adolescent development	2	0
career development	1	1
gender roles	2	0
integrative services in schools and agencies	4	6
mentoring in adolescence	1	1
multicultural issues	3	1
risk and resilience	4	3
violence prevention (community and marital)	3	2

Clinical opportunities
acute psychiatric
college counseling center
community mental health
inpatient adult unit
inpatient child
school based mental health clinic
violence prevention/intervention

Brigham Young University

Department of Counseling Psychology and Special
Education
Provo, UT 84602-5093
phone#: (801) 422-3859
e-mail: aaron_jackson@byu.edu
Web address: http://education.byu.edu/cpse/index.html

1	2	3	**4**	5	6	7

Clinically oriented	Equal emphasis	Research oriented

What percentage of your faculty subscribes to or practices in each of the following orientations?

Psychodynamic/Psychoanalytic	10%
Applied behavioral analysis/Radical behavioral	0%
Family systems/Systems	5%
Existential/Phenomenological/Humanistic	30%
Cognitive/Cognitive-behavioral	55%

What percentage of students applying for internship last year was accepted into APPIC-member internships? 86%

What courses are required for incoming students to have completed prior to enrolling?
Introductory undergraduate psychology courses, including abnormal, personality, developmental and research methods.

Are there courses you recommend that are not mandatory?
Statistics

GRE mean
Verbal 597   Quantitative 620
Analytical Writing 5.2

GPA mean
Overall GPA 3.8

Number of applications/admission offers/incoming students in 2005
58 applied/13 admission offers/10 incoming

% of students receiving:
Tuition waiver only: 0%
Assistantship/fellowship only: 10%
Both tuition waiver & assistantship/fellowship: 90%

Approximate percentage of incoming students who entered with a B.A./B.S. only: 100%   **Master's:** 0%

Approximate percentage of students who are Women: 66%   **Ethnic Minority:** 33%   **International:** 8%

Average years to complete the doctoral program (including internship): 5.5 years

Personal interview
Preferred in person but telephone acceptable

Research areas	# Faculty	# Grants
crisis intervention	1	1
mental health and spirituality	6	3
mental health in schools	2	1
multicultural counseling	2	2
Native American vocational development	2	3
outcome research	3	2
women's issues	2	1

Clinical opportunities
eating disorders
family clinic

University of British Columbia
Department of Educational and Counseling Psychology, and Special Education
2125 Main Mall
Vancouver, British Columbia V6T 1Z4, Canada
phone#: (604) 822-5259
e-mail: Karen Yan: karen.yan@ubc.ca
Web address: http://ecps.educ.ubc.ca/

1	2	3	**4**	5	6	7

Clinically oriented	Equal emphasis	Research oriented

What percentage of your faculty subscribes to or practices in each of the following orientations?

Psychodynamic/Psychoanalytic	5%
Applied behavioral analysis/Radical behavioral	0%
Family systems/Systems	30%
Existential/Phenomenological/Humanistic	45%
Cognitive/Cognitive-behavioral	20%

What percentage of students applying for internship last year was accepted into APPIC-member internships? 0%

What courses are required for incoming students to have completed prior to enrolling?
Ph.D. applicants are required to have completed courses equivalent to the M.A. in Counseling offered by the department. Please check the Web site.

Are there courses you recommend that are not mandatory?
No

GRE mean
Data not available

GPA mean
Data not available

Number of applications/admission offers/incoming students in 2003
24 applied/10 admission offers/9 incoming

% of students receiving:
Tuition waiver only: 100%
Assistantship/fellowship only: 0%
Both tuition waiver & assistantship/fellowship: 80%

Approximate percentage of incoming students who entered with a B.A./B.S. only: 0%   **Master's:** 100%

Approximate percentage of students who are Women: 70%   **Ethnic Minority:** 20%   **International:** 10%

Average years to complete the doctoral program (including internship): 4-5 years

Personal interview
Preferred in person but telephone acceptable; telephone required

Research areas	# Faculty	# Grants
aboriginal approaches to healing	2	1
anxiety issues in other cultures	1	2
Asian approaches to counseling	1	0
assessment issues in rehabilitation	1	1
counseling process and research	1	0
ethics	1	0
issues in career development	3	4
issues related to infertility	1	0
stress and coping	1	2
trauma	2	1
women's sexuality and reproductive health	1	0

Clinical opportunities
—

Colorado State University

Department of Psychology
Fort Collins, CO 80523
phone#: (970) 491-6363
e-mail: jmoran@lamar.colostate.edu
Web address: http://www.colostate.edu/Depts/
Psychology/counseling/index.htm

1	2	**3**	4	5	6	7

Clinically oriented	Equal emphasis	Research oriented

What percentage of your faculty subscribes to or practices in each of the following orientations?

Psychodynamic/Psychoanalytic	0%
Applied behavioral analysis/Radical behavioral	0%
Family systems/Systems	0%
Existential/Phenomenological/Humanistic	0%
Cognitive/Cognitive-behavioral	80%

What percentage of students applying for internship last year was accepted into APPIC-member internships? 100%

What courses are required for incoming students to have completed prior to enrolling?
None

Are there courses you recommend that are not mandatory?
Learning, personality, history and systems, developmental, abnormal, statistics

GRE mean
Verbal 603   Quantitative 657
Advanced Psychology no longer required
Analytical Writing not required

GPA mean
Overall GPA 3.61

Number of applications/admission offers/incoming students in 2005
210 applied/15 admission offers/9 incoming

% of students receiving:
Tuition waiver only: 0%
Assistantship/fellowship only: 0%
Both tuition waiver & assistantship/fellowship: 100%

Approximate percentage of incoming students who entered with a B.A./B.S. only: 90%   **Master's:** 10%

Approximate percentage of students who are Women: 80%   **Ethnic Minority:** 30%   **International:** 0%

Average years to complete the doctoral program (including internship): 5 years

Personal interview
No interviews

Research areas	# Faculty	# Grants
ADHD	7	0
adolescent issues	3	5
aggression (anger research and reduction)	1	1
aging/geriatrics	3	2
anxiety (reduction)	1	1

assessment (including ethnic/ minority issues)	3	1
behavioral medicine	3	3
body image beating disturbances	1	0
child issues (behavior problems and custody)	3	0
cognitive issues	2	0
college teaching	1	0
educational outcomes	1	1
emotional disorders	1	0
ethics	1	0
health psychology	5	3
interpersonal relationships	1	0
learning disabilities	1	0
men's issues	1	0
multicultural issues	6	3
parent–child interaction	1	0
psychopathology (including child)	3	0
psychotherapy process (behavior therapy)	1	0
stress and coping processes	2	0
substance abuse	4	3
supervision and training	2	0
violence/abuse	2	0
vocational psychology	2	0
women's issues	3	0

Clinical opportunities
family stress center
inpatient psychiatry
university counseling center

Columbia University, Teachers College (Ph.D.)

Program in Counseling Psychology
New York, NY 10027
phone#: (212) 678-3257
e-mail: miville@exchange.tc.columbia.edu
Web address: http://devweb.tc.columbia.edu/academic/
CCP/CounPsych/proginfo.asp?Id=Counseling+
Psychology+%28Ph%2ED%2E%29+Home&Info=
Degree+Requirements

1	2	3	4	**5**	6	7

Clinically oriented	Equal emphasis	Research oriented

What percentage of your faculty subscribes to or practices in each of the following orientations?

Psychodynamic/Psychoanalytic	5%
Applied behavioral analysis/Radical behavioral	10%
Family systems/Systems	40%
Existential/Phenomenological/Humanistic	35%
Cognitive/Cognitive-behavioral	25%
Multicultural/Diversity	75%

What percentage of students applying for internship last year was accepted into APPIC-member internships? 100%

What courses are required for incoming students to have completed prior to enrolling?
Bachelor's, but master's degree preferred

Are there courses you recommend that are not mandatory?
Yes

GRE mean
Verbal 570   Quantitative 570
Analytical Writing Data not available

GPA mean
Overall GPA 3.75

Number of applications/admission offers/incoming students in 2003
160 applied/7 admission offers/5 incoming

% of students receiving:
Tuition waiver only: 100%
Assistantship/fellowship only: 25%
Both tuition waiver & assistantship/fellowship: 75%

Approximate percentage of incoming students who entered with a B.A./B.S. only: 10%   Master's: 90%

**Approximate percentage of students who are Women: 100%   Ethnic Minority: 80%
International: Data not available**

Average years to complete the doctoral program (including internship): 6.5 years

Personal interview
Required in person

Research areas	# Faculty	# Grants
cognition and stereotypes		
cultural competence		
immigration issues		
multicultural counseling and therapy		
prevention in counseling psychology		
racism and racial identity	2	0
sexual harassment	1	0
women and leadership	1	0

Clinical opportunities
—

University of Denver

College of Education
Denver, CO 80208
phone#: (303) 871-2484
e-mail: mriva@du.edu
Web address:
http://www.du.edu/education/academicPrograms/cnp/

1	2	3	**4**	5	6	7

Clinically oriented   Equal emphasis   Research oriented

What percentage of your faculty subscribes to or practices in each of the following orientations?

Psychodynamic/Psychoanalytic	25%
Applied behavioral analysis/Radical behavioral	0%
Family systems/Systems	15%
Existential/Phenomenological/Humanistic	25%
Cognitive/Cognitive-behavioral	35%

What percentage of students applying for internship last year was accepted into APPIC-member internships? 100%

What courses are required for incoming students to have completed prior to enrolling?
None

Are there courses you recommend that are not mandatory?
Learning, personality theory, statistics

GRE mean
Verbal 550   Quantitative 550
Analytical Writing 4.7

GPA mean
Overall GPA 3.5

Number of applications/admission offers/incoming students in 2005
90 applied/12 admission offers/7 incoming

% of students receiving:
Tuition waiver only: 30%
Assistantship/fellowship only: 60%
Both tuition waiver & assistantship/fellowship: 10%

Approximate percentage of incoming students who entered with a B.A./B.S. only: 0%   Master's: 100%

Approximate percentage of students who are Women: 80%   Ethnic Minority: 20%   International: 5%

Average years to complete the doctoral program (including internship): 5 years

Personal interview
Preferred in person but telephone acceptable

Research areas	# Faculty	# Grants
ethics	1	0
group counseling	1	0
health psychology	1	0
multicultural counseling	1	1
social support and caregivers	1	1
worker job satisfaction	1	1

Clinical opportunities
Numerous and diverse opportunities
conducting counseling groups
counseling centers
hospital settings
mental health centers
placements working with racial and ethnic minorities
psychological assessments/neuropsychological assessments
veteran administration hospital

University of Florida

Department of Psychology
Gainesville, FL 32611
phone#: (352) 392-0601
e-mail: kgr1@UFL.EDU
Web address: http://www.psych.ufl.edu/

1	2	3	4	5	**6**	7
Clinically oriented		Equal emphasis			Research oriented	

What percentage of your faculty subscribes to or practices in each of the following orientations?

Psychodynamic/Psychoanalytic   0%
Applied behavioral analysis/Radical behavioral   0%
Family systems/Systems   29%
Existential/Phenomenological/Humanistic   14%
Cognitive/Cognitive-behavioral   57%

What percentage of students applying for internship last year was accepted into APPIC-member internships? 100%

What courses are required for incoming students to have completed prior to enrolling?
Undergraduate 4-year degree in psychology or related field

Are there courses you recommend that are not mandatory?
Statistics, research design/methods, personality, abnormal

GRE mean
Verbal 600   Quantitative 720
Advanced Psychology and Analytical Writing are not used

GPA mean
Overall GPA 3.80
Psychology GPA 3.90
Junior/Senior GPA 3.80

Number of applications/admission offers/incoming students in 2005
136 applied/11 admission offers/10 incoming

% of students receiving:
Tuition waiver only: 0%
Assistantship/fellowship only: 0%
Both tuition waiver & assistantship/fellowship: 100%
All students are currently funded by grants, teaching assistantships, or campus placements.

Approximate percentage of incoming students who entered with a B.A./B.S. only: 50%   **Master's:** 50%

Approximate percentage of students who are Women: 55%   **Ethnic Minority:** 36%
International: Data not available

Average years to complete the doctoral program (including internship): 6 years

Personal interview
Preferred in person but telephone acceptable

Research areas	# Faculty	# Grants
behavioral medicine/health psychology	2	1
constructivist psychology	1	0
discrimination/stigma	1	0
eating disorders	1	0
elderly	1	0
gender and emotion	1	0
mental health of minority populations	1	0
personality and mental health	1	0
psychology and law	1	1
sexual orientation issues	1	0
sleep disorders	1	1
women's issues	1	0

Clinical opportunities
assessment (inpatient psychiatric)
career counseling center
community mental health
crisis intervention center
domestic violence clinic
family medical practice clinic
forensics hospital/prison
hospice
nursing facility
pediatric/psychiatric assessment and treatment
rural health care clinic
sexual offender assessment and treatment
substance abuse clinic
university counseling center

Fordham University

Division of Psychological and Educational Services
New York, NY 10023
phone#: (212) 636-6460
e-mail: Jponterott@aol.com
Web address: http://www.fordham.edu/images/
Academics/Education/popups/gse_pes_course_desript
.html#DoctorofPhilosophyPhDinCounselingPsychology

1	2	3	**4**	5	6	7
Clinically oriented		Equal emphasis			Research oriented	

What percentage of your faculty subscribes to or practices in each of the following orientations?

Psychodynamic/Psychoanalytic   25%
Applied behavioral analysis/Radical behavioral   20%
Family systems/Systems   16%
Existential/Phenomenological/Humanistic   50%
Cognitive/Cognitive-behavioral   100%

What percentage of students applying for internship last year was accepted into APPIC-member internships? 100%

What courses are required for incoming students to have completed prior to enrolling?
Should have 5 undergraduate psychology courses completed before enrollment

Are there courses you recommend that are not mandatory?
Qualitative research methods

GRE mean
Verbal 600   Quantitative 600
Analytical Writing Data not available

GPA mean
Overall GPA 3.54

Number of applications/admission offers/incoming students in 2003
128 applied/18 admission offers/10 incoming

% of students receiving:
Tuition waiver only: 0%
Assistantship/fellowship only: 0%
Both tuition waiver & assistantship/fellowship: 32%

Approximate percentage of incoming students who entered with a B.A./B.S. only: 50%   **Master's:** 50%

**Approximate percentage of students who are
Women:** 75%   **Ethnic Minority:** 25%
International: Data not available

Average years to complete the doctoral program (including internship): 5 years

Personal interview
Preferred in person but telephone acceptable

Research areas	# Faculty	# Grants
career development	2	1
criminal behavior	1	0
health psychology	2	1
multicultural counseling	4	0
supervision	2	0

Clinical opportunities
College counseling centers, community mental health centers, and hospitals where students complete practica

University of Georgia
Department of Counseling and Human Development Services
Athens, GA 30602
phone#: (706) 542-1812
e-mail: bglaser@coe.uga.edu
Web address: http://www.coe.uga.edu/chds/counselingpsych/index.html

1	2	3	**4**	5	6	7
Clinically oriented		Equal emphasis			Research oriented	

What percentage of your faculty subscribes to or practices in each of the following orientations?

Psychodynamic/Psychoanalytic	20%
Applied behavioral analysis/Radical behavioral	0%
Family systems/Systems	20%
Existential/Phenomenological/Humanistic	10%
Cognitive/Cognitive-behavioral	50%

What percentage of students applying for internship last year was accepted into APPIC-member internships? 100%

What courses are required for incoming students to have completed prior to enrolling?
Research methods, descriptive statistics, interpersonal relationships, individual assessment, vocational development, theories of counseling, individual counseling practicum, group counseling or group process, multicultural counseling (master's degree required)

Are there courses you recommend that are not mandatory?
No

GRE mean
Verbal + Quantitative 1100
Analytical Writing Data not available

GPA mean
Overall GPA undergraduate 3.0   Graduate 3.5

Number of applications/admission offers/incoming students in 2003
87 applied/12 admission offers/9 incoming

% of students receiving:
Tuition waiver only: 0% (out-of-state)
Assistantship/fellowship only: 0%
Both tuition waiver & assistantship/fellowship: 100%

Approximate percentage of incoming students who entered with a B.A./B.S. only: 0%   **Master's:** 100%

**Approximate percentage of students who are
Women:** 75%   **Ethnic Minority:** 40%
International: Data not available

Average years to complete the doctoral program (including internship): 4 years

Personal interview
Preferred in person but telephone acceptable

Research areas	# Faculty	# Grants
accident trauma	1	0
attributions and therapy	2	0
empowering schools/developmental	2	1
juvenile delinquency/aggression	2	2
men's development/gender	1	0
minority male adolescent development	1	1
multicultural development and counseling	2	0
preventing violence and aggression in schools	2	3
school counselor education	2	0
substance abuse	1	0
young adult development	2	0

Clinical opportunities
adolescents including minority youth
college instruction
college students
departmental captive clinic
homeless shelter
juvenile offenders (males and females)
life-span
preparing future faculty
school-age children and supervision

Georgia State University

Department of Counseling and Psychological Services
Atlanta, GA 30303
phone#: (404) 651-2550
e-mail: cpsrec@langate.gsu.edu
Web address: http://education.gsu.edu/cps/
Ph.D.%20Counseling%20Psychology.htm

1	2	3	**4**	5	6	7
Clinically oriented		Equal emphasis			Research oriented	

What percentage of your faculty subscribes to or practices in each of the following orientations?

Psychodynamic/Psychoanalytic	12%
Applied behavioral analysis/Radical behavioral	0%
Family systems/Systems	13%
Existential/Phenomenological/Humanistic	50%
Cognitive/Cognitive-behavioral	25%

What percentage of students applying for internship last year was accepted into APPIC-member internships? 100%

What courses are required for incoming students to have completed prior to enrolling?
M.A. in counseling or clinical psychology

Are there courses you recommend that are not mandatory?
No

GRE mean
Verbal 640   Quantitative 600   Analytical 630
Advanced Psychology 625
Analytical Writing Data not available

GPA mean
Overall GPA 3.42

Number of applications/admission offers/incoming students in 2003
65 applied/8 admission offers/6 incoming

% of students receiving:
Tuition waiver only: 0%
Assistantship/fellowship only: 0%
Both tuition waiver & assistantship/fellowship: 100%

Approximate percentage of incoming students who entered with a B.A./B.S. only: 0%   **Master's:** 100%

Approximate percentage of students who are Women: 70%   **Ethnic Minority:** 35%
International: Data not available

Average years to complete the doctoral program (including internship): 5 years

Personal interview
Preferred in person but telephone acceptable

Research areas	# Faculty	# Grants
career development	1	0
cognitive structures	2	0
multicultural counseling	2	1
stress/coping	3	0
traumatology	2	0

Clinical opportunities
behavioral medicine
college counseling
forensic
multicultural counseling
stress managment

University of Houston

Department of Educational Psychology
Houston, TX 77004-5874
phone#: (713) 743-5019
e-mail: EPSY@UH.EDU
Web address: http://www.coe.uh.edu/degrees.cfm?ID=28

1	2	3	4	**5**	6	7
Clinically oriented		Equal emphasis			Research oriented	

What percentage of your faculty subscribes to or practices in each of the following orientations?

Psychodynamic/Psychoanalytic	30%
Applied behavioral analysis/Radical behavioral	0%
Family systems/Systems	30%
Existential/Phenomenological/Humanistic	0%
Cognitive/Cognitive-behavioral	30%

What percentage of students applying for internship last year was accepted into APPIC-member internships? 90%

What courses are required for incoming students to have completed prior to enrolling?
None

Are there courses you recommend that are not mandatory?
No

GRE mean
Verbal 530   Quantitative 620   Analytical 640
Analytical Writing 4.5
These scores represent the departmental guidelines; however, exceptions to the cutoff scores have been made when an applicant provides clear evidence of academic potential.

GPA mean
Overall master's GPA 3.5 (on last 60 hours, including graduate work)

Number of applications/admission offers/incoming students in 2005
62 applied/9 admission offers/9 incoming

% of students receiving:
Tuition waiver only: 0%
Assistantship/fellowship only: 10%
Both tuition waiver & assistantship/fellowship: 90%

Approximate percentage of incoming students who entered with a B.A./B.S. only: 20%   **Master's:** 80%

Approximate percentage of students who are Women: 85%   **Ethnic Minority:** 41%   **International:** 0%

Average years to complete the doctoral program (including internship): 5 years

Personal interview
Preferred in person but telephone acceptable

Research areas	# Faculty	# Grants
adult attachment/adult survivors of childhood trauma	2	1
career counseling/cross-cultural counseling	2	0
children and adolescents with behavioral disorders	1	1
gender identity and psychological well-being in men	1	0
mental health policy	1	0
telehealth	2	0

Clinical opportunities
Child guidance center; family therapy; crisis intervention program for children and their families; university counseling center; VA hospital with a variety of rotations including substance abuse, gerontology, family therapy, chronic inpatient, behavioral medicine, forensic, postttraumatic stress disorder, school districts; medical schools; pediatric hospitals.

Howard University
Counseling Psychology Program
School of Education
2441 Fourth Street, NW
Washington DC 20059
phone#: (202) 806-7351 or
(202) 806-7350
e-mail: Fibrahim2@howard.edu
Web address: http://www.howard.edu/schooleducation/
Departments/HDPES/CPsychology/index.htm

1	2	3	**4**	5	6	7

Clinically oriented   Equal emphasis   Research oriented

What percentage of your faculty subscribes to or practices in each of the following orientations?
Psychodynamic/Psychoanalytic	0%
Applied behavioral analysis/Radical behavioral	0%
Family systems/Systems	0%
Existential/Phenomenological/Humanistic	50%
Cognitive/Cognitive-behavioral	50%

What percentage of students applying for internship last year was accepted into APPIC-member internships? 75%

What courses are required for incoming students to have completed prior to enrolling?
Equivalent of Howard University Counseling Psychology master's (48–52 credit hours) or undergraduate degree in psychology.

Are there courses you recommend that are not mandatory?
Evaluated on a case-by-case basis based on above criteria.

GRE mean
Verbal 477.5   Quantitative 535   Analytical 506.5 (M)
Analytical Writing Data not available

GPA mean
Overall master's GPA 3.8

Number of applications/admission offers/incoming students in 2003
12 applied/5 admission offers/4 incoming

% of students receiving:
Tuition waiver only: 2%
Assistantship/fellowship only: 2%
Both tuition waiver & assistantship/fellowship: 2%

Approximate percentage of incoming students who entered with a B.A./B.S. only: 0%   Master's: 100%

Approximate percentage of students who are
Women: 95%   Ethnic Minority: 100%
International: Data not available

Average years to complete the doctoral program (including internship): 5 years

Personal interview
Required in person; but telephone acceptable *for overseas candidates*

Research areas	# Faculty	# Grants
drug and alcohol use/addiction among African American and Bedouin Arabs	3	1
hope in counseling interventions	1	0
multicultural competencies	1	1
racism stress	1	1
role of spirituality in counseling	2	0
using videotapes in training	1	1
worldview, racial identity and self-efficacy of diverse African and African Americans	1	0

Clinical opportunities
Howard University (HU) Cancer Center
HU Center on Sickle Cell Anemia
HU Genome Center
HU Student Counseling Center (APA accredited)

University of Illinois at Urbana–Champaign
Department of Educational Psychology
Champaign, IL 61820
phone#: (888) 843-3779
Web address:
http://www.ed.uiuc.edu/edpsy/programs/phd.html

1	2	3	4	5	**6**	7

Clinically oriented   Equal emphasis   Research oriented

What percentage of your faculty subscribes to or practices in each of the following orientations?
Psychodynamic/Psychoanalytic	0%
Applied behavioral analysis/Radical behavioral	0%
Family systems/Systems	0%
Existential/Phenomenological/Humanistic	0%

Cognitive/Cognitive-behavioral	0%
Eclectic	100%

What percentage of students applying for internship last year was accepted into APPIC-member internships? 100%

What courses are required for incoming students to have completed prior to enrolling?
None

Are there courses you recommend that are not mandatory?
Undergraduate psychology degree

GRE mean
Verbal 549   Quantitative 667
Analytical Writing Data not available

GPA mean
Overall GPA 3.81

Number of applications/admission offers/incoming students in 2003
83 applied/10 admission offers/9 incoming

% of students receiving:
Tuition waiver only: 0%
Assistantship/fellowship only: 0%
Both tuition waiver & assistantship/fellowship: 100%

Approximate percentage of incoming students who entered with a B.A./B.S. only: 56%   **Master's:** 44%

Approximate percentage of students who are Women: 66%   **Ethnic Minority:** 22%
International: Data not available

Average years to complete the doctoral program (including internship): 5.5 years

Personal interview
Preferred in person but telephone acceptable

Research areas	# Faculty	# Grants
adolescent aggression	1	0
breast and cervical cancer control	1	1
cancer survivorship	1	1
eating disorders	1	0
ethnic/racial identity	2	0
medically underserved Latina populations	1	1
personality assessment	1	1
racial and sexual violence	2	0
racism	2	2
vocational psychology	2	1
women's career development	1	0

Clinical opportunities
child/adolescent
health psychology
mental health counseling
rehabilitation counseling
undergraduate counseling center
VA medical center

Indiana University
Department of Counseling and Educational Psychology
Wright Education Building, Room 4003
Bloomington, IN 47405
phone#: (812) 856-8300
e-mail: chatomp@indiana.edu
Web address:
http://www.indiana.edu/~counsel/cphdhome.html

1	2	3	**4**	5	6	7

Clinically oriented   Equal emphasis   Research oriented

What percentage of your faculty subscribes to or practices in each of the following orientations?

Psychodynamic/Psychoanalytic	0%
Applied behavioral analysis/Radical behavioral	10%
Family systems/Systems	30%
Existential/Phenomenological/Humanistic	30%
Cognitive/Cognitive-behavioral	30%

What percentage of students applying for internship last year was accepted into APPIC-member internships? 90%

What courses are required for incoming students to have completed prior to enrolling?
We look at overall preparation without concern for specific courses

Are there courses you recommend that are not mandatory?
Statistics and research methods

GRE mean
Verbal 527   Quantitative 642
Analytical Writing 4.81

GPA mean
Overall Undergraduate GPA 3.55
Overall Graduate GPA 3.86

Number of applications/admission offers/incoming students in 2005
100 applied/15 admission offers/9 incoming

% of students receiving:
Tuition waiver only: 0%
Assistantship/fellowship only: 0%
Both tuition waiver & assistantship/fellowship: 100%

Approximate percentage of incoming students who entered with a B.A./B.S. only: 22%   **Master's:** 78%

Approximate percentage of students who are Women: 78%   **Ethnic Minority:** 11%   **International:** 22%

Average years to complete the doctoral program (including internship): 4 years

Personal interview
Preferred in person but telephone acceptable

Research areas	# Faculty	# Grants
at-risk youth	1	2
counselor training	5	0
elementary school counseling	2	1
group counseling	2	0
human sexuality	3	0

marriage and family counseling	3	3
multicultural counseling	2	0
women's vocational behavior	1	0

Clinical opportunities
—

Indiana State University

Department of Counseling
Terre Haute, IN 47809
phone#: (812) 237-2832
e-mail: egshuff@isugw.indstate.edu
Web address:
http://counseling.indstate.edu/dcp/default.htm

1	2	**3**	4	5	6	7
Clinically oriented		Equal emphasis			Research oriented	

What percentage of your faculty subscribes to or practices in each of the following orientations?

Psychodynamic/Psychoanalytic	0%
Applied behavioral analysis/Radical behavioral	0%
Family systems/Systems	40%
Existential/Phenomenological/Humanistic	40%
Cognitive/Cognitive-behavioral	40%

What percentage of students applying for internship last year was accepted into APPIC-member internships? 83%

What courses are required for incoming students to have completed prior to enrolling?
Bachelor's degree and master's degree in counseling/psychology, including graduate courses in techniques of counseling, practicum, psychological assessment, and career development

Are there courses you recommend that are not mandatory?
Yes

GRE mean
Data not available

GPA mean
Data not available

Number of applications/admission offers/incoming students in 2003
36 applied/13 admission offers/8 incoming

% of students receiving:
Tuition waiver only: 0%
Assistantship/fellowship only: 0%
Both tuition waiver & assistantship/fellowship: 100%

Approximate percentage of incoming students who entered with a B.A./B.S. only: 0%   **Master's:** 100%

Approximate percentage of students who are Women: 67%   **Ethnic Minority:** 10%
International: Data not available

Average years to complete the doctoral program (including internship): 5 years

Personal interview
Preferred in person but telephone acceptable

Research areas	# Faculty	# Grants
AIDS/HIV	1	0
career development/assessment	2	0
counseling/supervision process	3	0
family therapy	3	1
health psychology	1	0
men's studies	2	0
personality assessment	1	0
program evaluation	1	0
psychology philosophy	1	0
school counseling	1	1
values/learning skills	1	0

Clinical opportunities
community mental health centers
local hospitals and community medical health centers
marriage and family therapy clinic
prison/penitentiary population
university counseling center
VA medical center

University of Iowa

Division of Psychological and Quantitative Foundations
Iowa City, IA 52242
phone#: (319) 335-5639
e-mail: daniel-clay@uiowa.edu
Web address: http://www.education.uiowa.edu/counspsy/program.htm#gradstudy

1	2	3	**4**	5	6	7
Clinically oriented		Equal emphasis			Research oriented	

What percentage of your faculty subscribes to or practices in each of the following orientations?

Psychodynamic/Psychoanalytic	25%
Applied behavioral analysis/Radical behavioral	0%
Family systems/Systems	25%
Existential/Phenomenological/Humanistic	0%
Cognitive/Cognitive-behavioral	50%

What percentage of students applying for internship last year was accepted into APPIC-member internships? 100%

What courses are required for incoming students to have completed prior to enrolling?
None are required but we encourage as much core psychology as possible

Are there courses you recommend that are not mandatory?
See above

GRE mean
Verbal 519   Quantitative 625   Analytical 650
Analytical Writing 5.06

GPA mean
Overall GPA 3.58

Number of applications/admission offers/incoming students in 2005
91 applied/11 admission offers/9 incoming

% of students receiving:
Tuition waiver only: 0%
Assistantship/fellowship only: 40%
Both tuition waiver & assistantship/fellowship: 60%

Approximate percentage of incoming students who entered with a B.A./B.S. only: 78%   **Master's:** 22%

Approximate percentage of students who are
Women: 67%   **Ethnic Minority:** 35%   **International:** 2%

Average years to complete the doctoral program (including internship): 7 years

Personal interview
Interview not required

Research areas	# Faculty	# Grants
child and adolescent health psychology	1	1
college student suicide	1	0
ethics	2	1
multicultural issues	2	1
psychosocial oncology	2	1
public health	3	2

Clinical opportunities
community mental health
hospitals
individualized specialty settings
prisons
public schools
university counseling centers
VA medical center
women's center

Iowa State University

Department of Psychology
Ames, IA 50011-3180
phone#: (515) 294-1743
e-mail: dle@iastate.edu
Web address:
http://www.psychology.iastate.edu/grad/counseling.htm

1	2	3	4	**5**	6	7
Clinically oriented		Equal emphasis			Research oriented	

What percentage of your faculty subscribes to or practices in each of the following orientations?

Psychodynamic/Psychoanalytic	0%
Applied behavioral analysis/Radical behavioral	0%
Family systems/Systems	20%
Existential/Phenomenological/Humanistic	20%
Cognitive/Cognitive-behavioral	60%

What percentage of students applying for internship last year was accepted into APPIC-member internships? 100%

What courses are required for incoming students to have completed prior to enrolling?
A minimum of 15 credits in psychology including statistics, psychological measurement, psychopathology, developmental psychology, counseling or psychotherapy, research methods

Are there courses you recommend that are not mandatory?
psychology, learning/memory/cognition, most successful applicants have a diversified psychology major (30–40 semester hours)

GRE mean
Verbal 614   Quantitative 666
Advanced Psychology 663
Analytical Writing 5.0

GPA mean
Overall GPA 3.68   Psychology GPA 3.8
Junior/Senior GPA 3.77

Number of applications/admission offers/incoming students in 2005
55 applied/8 admission offers/6 incoming

% of students receiving:
Tuition waiver only: 0%
Assistantship/fellowship only: 0%
Both tuition waiver & assistantship/fellowship: 100%

Approximate percentage of incoming students who entered with a B.A./B.S. only: 84%   **Master's:** 16%

Approximate percentage of students who are
Women: 73%   **Ethnic Minority:** 8%   **International:** 12%

Average years to complete the doctoral program (including internship): 6 years

Personal interview
Preferred in person but telephone acceptable

Research areas	# Faculty	# Grants
attachment and adjustment of international students	1	0
attachment and discrimination	1	0
ethics and legal issues in counseling	1	0
gender roles	1	1
multicultural	1	0
psychology and religion (forgiveness)	1	0
risk assessment with sex offenders	1	1
social support in intimate relationships	1	1
vocational development of women in science	1	1
vocational interest assessment	2	0

Clinical opportunities
ADHD assessment clinic in private practice
community mental health center
mental health unit in general medical hospital
private psychological group practices
university counseling center
VA medical center

University of Kansas

Department of Psychology and Research in Education
Counseling Psychology Program
Lawrence, KS 66045
phone#: (785) 864-3931
e-mail: preadmit@ku.edu
Web address:
http://www.soe.ku.edu/depts/pre/cpsy/index.php

1	2	3	**4**	5	6	7
Clinically oriented		Equal emphasis			Research oriented	

What percentage of your faculty subscribes to or practices in each of the following orientations?

Psychodynamic/Psychoanalytic 30%
Applied behavioral analysis/Radical behavioral 0%
Family systems/Systems 20%
Existential/Phenomenological/Humanistic 40%
Cognitive/Cognitive-behavioral 60%

What percentage of students applying for internship last year was accepted into APPIC-member internships? 100%

What courses are required for incoming students to have completed prior to enrolling?
None

Are there courses you recommend that are not mandatory?
Basic courses in psychology (e.g., social psychology, personality, abnormal psychology, experimental psychology)

GRE mean
Verbal 560   Quantitative 650   Analytical 590
Advanced Psychology not required
Analytical Writing 4.6

GPA mean
Overall GPA 3.5

Number of applications/admission offers/incoming students in 2005
58 applied/12 admission offers/6 incoming

% of students receiving:
Tuition waiver only: 16%
Assistantship/fellowship only: 33%
Both tuition waiver & assistantship/fellowship: 50%

Approximate percentage of incoming students who entered with a B.A./B.S. only: 50%   **Master's:** 50%

Approximate percentage of students who are Women: 75%   **Ethnic Minority:** 25%   **International:** 5%

Average years to complete the doctoral program (including internship): 5.5 years

Personal interview
No preference given

Research areas	# Faculty	# Grants
creativity	1	1
health psychology	1	0
positive psychology	3	1
therapy outcome and process	1	0
vocational decision making	1	0

Clinical opportunities
—

University of Kentucky

Department of Educational and Counseling Psychology
Lexington, KY 40506
phone#: (606) 257-7881
e-mail: westil3@pop.uky.edu
Web address:
http://www.uky.edu/Education/EDP/counphd.html

1	2	3	4	5	**6**	7
Clinically oriented		Equal emphasis			Research oriented	

What percentage of your faculty subscribes to or practices in each of the following orientations?

Psychodynamic/Psychoanalytic 0%
Applied behavioral analysis/Radical behavioral 30%
Family systems/Systems 20%
Existential/Phenomenological/Humanistic 10%
Cognitive/Cognitive-behavioral 40%

What percentage of students applying for internship last year was accepted into APPIC-member internships? 100%

What courses are required for incoming students to have completed prior to enrolling?
None

Are there courses you recommend that are not mandatory?
Prefer master's degree in behavioral science

GRE mean
Verbal + Quantitative 1100
Analytical Writing Not enough to determine an average

GPA mean
Overall GPA 3.4   Psychology GPA 3.6
Junior/Senior GPA 3.5

Number of applications/admission offers/incoming students in 2005
45 applied/8 admission offers/5 incoming

% of students receiving:
Tuition waiver only: 0%
Assistantship/fellowship only: 45%
Both tuition waiver & assistantship/fellowship: 25%

Approximate percentage of incoming students who entered with a B.A./B.S. only: 0%   **Master's:** 100%

Approximate percentage of students who are Women: 60%   **Ethnic Minority:** 25%   **International:** 0%

Average years to complete the doctoral program (including internship): 5.1 years

Personal interview
Preferred in person but telephone acceptable

Research areas	# Faculty	# Grants
behavioral	2	1
family	2	0
gender	2	1
multicultural	2	0

Clinical opportunities
community mental health center
counseling center
federal medical center (prison)
residential treatment facility
rural mental health centers
VA hospital

Lehigh University

Education and Human Services
Bethlehem, PA 18015-4792
phone#: (610) 758-3250
Web address: http://www.lehigh.edu/collegeofeducation/
degree_programs/counseling_psych/degrees/phd/
phd_philosophy.htm

1	2	3	4	**5**	6	7

Clinically oriented   Equal emphasis   Research oriented

What percentage of your faculty subscribes to or practices in each of the following orientations?
Psychodynamic/Psychoanalytic	25%
Applied behavioral analysis/Radical behavioral	0%
Family systems/Systems	25%
Existential/Phenomenological/Humanistic	25%
Cognitive/Cognitive-behavioral	25%

What percentage of students applying for internship last year was accepted into APPIC-member internships? 100%

What courses are required for incoming students to have completed prior to enrolling?
None

Are there courses you recommend that are not mandatory?
Psychology related

GRE mean
Verbal 550   Quantitative 550
Analytical Writing Data not available

GPA mean
Overall GPA 3.7

Number of applications/admission offers/incoming students in 2003
95 applied/9 admission offers/5 incoming

% of students receiving:
Tuition waiver only: 0%
Assistantship/fellowship only: 20%
Both tuition waiver & assistantship/fellowship: 80%

Approximate percentage of incoming students who entered with a B.A./B.S. only: 50%   **Master's:** 50%

**Approximate percentage of students who are
Women:** 70%   **Ethnic Minority:** 40%
International: Data not available

Average years to complete the doctoral program (including internship): 6 years

Personal interview
Preferred in person but telephone acceptable

Research areas	# Faculty	# Grants
cross-cultural	1	1
family systems	1	1
supervision/training	1	1
vocational psychology	1	1

Clinical opportunities
—

Louisiana Tech University

Department of Psychology
P.O. Box 10048
Ruston, LA 71272
phone#: (318) 257-4315
e-mail: Buboltz@latech.edu
Web address:
http://www.latech.edu/tech/education/cphd/

1	2	3	4	**5**	6	7

Clinically oriented   Equal emphasis   Research oriented

What percentage of your faculty subscribes to or practices in each of the following orientations?
Psychodynamic/Psychoanalytic	20%
Applied behavioral analysis/Radical behavioral	0%
Family systems/Systems	20%
Existential/Phenomenological/Humanistic	10%
Cognitive/Cognitive-behavioral	50%

What percentage of students applying for internship last year was accepted into APPIC-member internships? 100%

What courses are required for incoming students to have completed prior to enrolling?
None

Are there courses you recommend that are not mandatory?
No

GRE mean
Verbal 540   Quantitative 620
Analytical Writing Not used for admission purposes

GPA mean
Overall GPA 3.6

Number of applications/admission offers/incoming students in 2005
36 applied/10 admission offers/5 incoming

% of students receiving:
Tuition waiver only: 0%
Assistantship/fellowship only: 100%
Both tuition waiver & assistantship/fellowship: 0%

Approximate percentage of incoming students who entered with a B.A./B.S. only: 40%   **Master's:** 60%

Approximate percentage of students who are Women: 85%   **Ethnic Minority:** 15%   **International:** 0%

Average years to complete the doctoral program (including internship): 5–6 years

Personal interview
Preferred in person but telephone acceptable

Research areas	# Faculty	# Grants
career development issues and relation to family issues	1	0
family therapy and child custody	1	0
lesbian/gay/bisexual issues	1	0
psychological reactance theory	1	0
sleep and academic performance and health	1	0

Clinical opportunities
children's home
community health centers
developmental center
in-house clinic
medical center
prison settings
university counseling center
VA medical centers

University of Louisville

Department of Educational and Counseling Psychology
Louisville, KY 40292
phone#: (502) 852-6884
e-mail: daya.sandhu@louisville.edu
Web address: http://www.louisville.edu/edu/ecpy/
programs/phd_cp/index.html

1	2	3	**4**	5	6	7

Clinically oriented   Equal emphasis   Research oriented

What percentage of your faculty subscribes to or practices in each of the following orientations?

Psychodynamic/Psychoanalytic	67%
Applied behavioral analysis/Radical behavioral	40%
Family systems/Systems	10%
Existential/Phenomenological/Humanistic	0%
Cognitive/Cognitive-behavioral	100%

What percentage of students applying for internship last year was accepted into APPIC-member internships? 100%

What courses are required for incoming students to have completed prior to enrolling?
30 hours M.A. in counseling psychology or psychology plus abnormal psychology, human or life-span development, statistics or methodology, social psychology

Are there courses you recommend that are not mandatory?
Psycholinguistics, sociology, anthropology, psychology (general and clinical)

GRE mean
Data not available

GPA mean
Overall master's GPA 3.9

Number of applications/admission offers/incoming students in 2003
20 applied/8 admission offers/8 incoming

% of students receiving:
Tuition waiver only: 0%
Assistantship/fellowship only: 0%
Both tuition waiver & assistantship/fellowship: 35%

Approximate percentage of incoming students who entered with a B.A./B.S. only: 0%   **Master's:** 100%

Approximate percentage of students who are Women: 70%   **Ethnic Minority:** 17%   **International:** 0%

Average years to complete the doctoral program (including internship): 6 to 7 years

Personal interview
No preference given

Research areas	# Faculty	# Grants
divorce adjustment	1	2
drug and alcohol abuse	2	1
evolutionary psychology	2	0
GBLT issues	1	1
school adjustment of special populations	1	0
school violence	1	2
stress and parenting	1	0

Clinical opportunities
child developmental disabilities
child treatment center
prison settings
sex offender treatment

Loyola University of Chicago

Department of Leadership, Foundations, and Counseling Psychology
820 North Michigan Avenue
Chicago, IL 60611
phone#: (312) 915-6311
e-mail: SBROWN@LUC.EDU
Web address: http://www.luc.edu/schools/education/
degree/doctorate/counselingpsych/

1	2	3	**4**	5	6	7

Clinically oriented   Equal emphasis   Research oriented

What percentage of your faculty subscribes to or practices in each of the following orientations?

Psychodynamic/Psychoanalytic	0%
Applied behavioral analysis/Radical behavioral	0%
Family systems/Systems	25%
Existential/Phenomenological/Humanistic	25%
Cognitive/Cognitive-behavioral	50%

What percentage of students applying for internship last year was accepted into APPIC-member internships? 100%

What courses are required for incoming students to have completed prior to enrolling?

Master's degree in counseling, psychology, or related field

Are there courses you recommend that are not mandatory?

No

GRE mean

Verbal 620   Quantitative 560
Advanced Psychology 500
Analytical Writing Data not available

GPA mean

Overall GPA 3.4   Psychology GPA 3.8
Junior/Senior GPA 3.8

Number of applications/admission offers/incoming students in 2005

78 applied/7 admission offers/5 incoming

% of students receiving:

Tuition waiver only: 0%
Assistantship/fellowship only: 0%
Both tuition waiver & assistantship/fellowship: 98%

Approximate percentage of incoming students who entered with a B.A./B.S. only: 0%   **Master's:** 100%

Approximate percentage of students who are
Women: 60%   **Ethnic Minority:** 40%   **International:** 2%

Average years to complete the doctoral program (including internship): 5 years

Personal interview

Required in person

Research areas	# Faculty	# Grants
adolescent risk behavior	1	1
child/adolescent development	2	0
counseling process	1	0
counseling supervision	1	0
multicultural counseling	2	0
vocational psychology	1	1

Clinical opportunities

Opportunities in the greater Chicago area include hospitals, clinics, and universities.

Marquette University

Department of Counseling and Educational Psychology
146 Schroeder Complex
Milwaukee, WI 53201
phone#: (414) 288-7379
E-mail: tim.melchert@marquette.edu
Web address: www.marquette.edu/coep

1	2	3	**4**	5	6	7
Clinically oriented			Equal emphasis			Research oriented

What percentage of your faculty subscribes to or practices in each of the following orientations?

Psychodynamic/Psychoanalytic	14.3%
Applied behavioral analysis/Radical behavioral	0%
Family systems/Systems	14.3%
Existential/Phenomenological/Humanistic	28.6%
Cognitive/Cognitive-behavioral	42.9%

What courses are required for incoming students to have completed prior to enrolling?

None are specified

Are there courses you recommend that are not mandatory?

None are specified, though applicants need background in the field.

GRE mean

Verbal 629   Quantitative 685   Analytical 780
Psychology advanced test not required
Analytical Writing 5.33

GPA mean

Overall GPA 3.71

Number of applications/admission offers/incoming students in 2005

61 applied/14 admission offers/8 incoming

% of students receiving:

Tuition waiver only: 37.5% (partial)
Assistantship/fellowship only: 0%
Both tuition waiver & assistantship/fellowship: 62.5% (partial)

Approximate percentage of incoming students who entered with a B.A./B.S. only: 37.5%   **Master's:** 62.5%

Approximate percentage of students who are
Women: 50%   **Ethnic Minority:** 0%   **International:** 0%

Average years to complete the doctoral program (including internship): 5.7 years

Personal interview

Preferred in person but telephone acceptable

Research areas	# Faculty	# Grants
addictions	1	2
child maltreatment	1	0
multicultural issues	3	0
parenting	1	1
program evaluation in education	2	1
psychotherapy process	2	0
strengths, optimal functioning	3	0

Clinical opportunities
childhood disorders
medical psychology
neuropsychology
obsessive–compulsive disorder
substance abuse
university counseling centers

University of Maryland

Department of Psychology and Department of
Counseling and Personnel Services
College Park, MD 20742
Web address: http://www.bsos.umd.edu/psyc/
counsel2.htm

1	2	3	4	**5**	6	7
Clinically oriented		Equal emphasis			Research oriented	

What percentage of your faculty subscribes to or practices in each of the following orientations?

Psychodynamic/Psychoanalytic	25%
Applied behavioral analysis/Radical behavioral	0%
Family systems/Systems	0%
Existential/Phenomenological/Humanistic	12%
Cognitive/Cognitive-behavioral	12%
Interpersonal	19%
Feminist	19%
Integrative	12%

What percentage of students applying for internship last year was accepted into APPIC-member internships? 100%

What courses are required for incoming students to have completed prior to enrolling?
No specific courses but we require that students have a minimum of 15 credits of coursework in psychology

Are there courses you recommend that are not mandatory?
—

GRE mean
Verbal 577   Quantitative 617
Analytical Writing N/A

GPA mean
Overall Undergraduate GPA 3.50
Junior/Senior GPA 3.5   Overall master's GPA 3.62

Number of applications/admission offers/incoming students in 2005
133 applied/13 admission offers/6 incoming

% of students receiving:
Tuition waiver only: 0%
Assistantship/fellowship only: 0%
Both tuition waiver & assistantship/fellowship: 100%

Approximate percentage of incoming students who entered with a B.A./B.S. only: 75%   **Master's:** 25%

Approximate percentage of students who are
Women: 67%   **Ethnic Minority:** 15%   **International:** 5%

Average years to complete the doctoral program (including internship): 6 years

Personal interview
Telephone required

Research areas	# Faculty	# Grants
AIDS/HIV	1	0
career counseling	4	2
career/vocational psychology	4	2
counseling process	3	0
counseling relationship	2	0
countertransference	2	0
domestic violence	1	0
dreams (their use in therapy)	1	0
health issues	2	0
interpersonal relationships	1	0
multicultural issues	3	0
supervision/training	3	0

Clinical opportunities
multicultural, group, individual, consultation, career, and supervision practica

McGill University

Department of Educational and Counseling Psychology
Faculty of Education
3700 McTavish Street
Montreal, Quebec H3A 1Y2, Canada
phone#: (514) 398-4245
e-mail: ted.maroun@mcgill.ca (program director)
diane.bernier@mcgill.ca (program coordinator)
Web address:
http://www.mcgill.ca/edu-ecp/programs/counselling/phd/

1	2	**3**	4	5	6	7
Clinically oriented		Equal emphasis			Research oriented	

What percentage of your faculty subscribes to or practices in each of the following orientations?

Psychodynamic/Psychoanalytic	75%
Applied behavioral analysis/Radical behavioral	65%
Family systems/Systems	35%
Existential/Phenomenological/Humanistic	0%
Cognitive/Cognitive-behavioral	55%

What courses are required for incoming students to have completed prior to enrolling?
Undergraduate degree in psychology. Master's degree in either Counseling Psychology or Clinical Psychology with and internship component as well as a practicum course. Courses in theories of counseling, testing, psychometry are also required.

Are there courses you recommend that are not mandatory?
Yes—otherwise the applicant will have to be accepted at the Ph.D. 1 level and do these courses concurrently with the doctoral program.

GRE mean
Data not available

GPA mean
B.A. 3.0 M.A. 3.5

Number of applications/admission offers/incoming students in 2003
8 applied/4 admission offers/3 incoming

% of students receiving:
Tuition waiver only: 30%
Assistantship/fellowship only: 75%
Both tuition waiver & assistantship/fellowship: 10%

Approximate percentage of incoming students who entered with a B.A./B.S. only: 0% **Master's:** 100%

Approximate percentage of students who are Women: 95% **Ethnic Minority:** 5%
International: Data not available

Average years to complete the doctoral program (including internship): 7 years

Personal interview
Preferred in person but telephone acceptable

Research areas	# Faculty	# Grants
development and training of researchers	1	0
feminism pedagogy and multicultural pedagogy	1	0
psychotherapy	2	1
training paraprofessional helper	1	0
working alliance in therapy	1	1

Clinical opportunities
behavioral therapy clinic
children's behavior clinic
eating disorders
psychiatry clinic
psychotherapy clinic

University of Memphis
Department of Counseling, Educational Psychology and Research
Ball Education Building, Room 100
Memphis, TN 38152
phone#: (901) 678-2841
e-mail: slease@memphis.edu
Web address:
http://www.people.memphis.edu/~coe_cepr/

1	2	3	**4**	5	6	7
Clinically oriented		Equal emphasis			Research oriented	

What percentage of your faculty subscribes to or practices in each of the following orientations?
Psychodynamic/Psychoanalytic — 17%
Applied behavioral analysis/Radical behavioral — 17%
Family systems/Systems — 67%
Existential/Phenomenological/Humanistic — 50%
Cognitive/Cognitive-behavioral — 83%
Feminist — 33%
Constructivist — 33%
Social learning — 50%

What percentage of students applying for internship last year was accepted into APPIC-member internships? 90%

What courses are required for incoming students to have completed prior to enrolling?
Master's degree in counseling, psychology, or related mental health area. Must have theories of counseling, group counseling, career counseling, statistics/research, introduction to assessment, practicum.

Are there courses you recommend that are not mandatory?
Psychological assessment, psychopathology

GRE mean
Verbal 563 Quantitative 520
Analytical Writing Not used for admission purposes

GPA mean
Overall GPA 3.89

Number of applications/admission offers/incoming students in 2005
41 applied/14 admission offers/8 incoming

% of students receiving:
Tuition waiver only: 0%
Assistantship/fellowship only: 0%
Both tuition waiver & assistantship/fellowship: 96%

Approximate percentage of incoming students who entered with a B.A./B.S. only: 0% **Master's:** 100%

Approximate percentage of students who are Women: 68% **Ethnic Minority:** 23% **International:** 10%

Average years to complete the doctoral program (including internship): 4.5 years

Personal interview
Preferred in person but telephone acceptable

Research areas	# Faculty	# Grants
AIDS/HIV counseling and education	1	1
at-risk families and children	2	1
consultation	2	1
counseling gays, lesbians, and bisexuals	3	1
crisis/trauma	2	0
disabled persons	4	3
international psychology	2	2
multicultural counseling and supervision	5	1
professional development	2	0
psychological resources (e.g., resilience)	2	0
vocational psychology	2	1

Clinical opportunities
adolescents/children
assessment
couples/families
domestic violence
forensic psychology
inpatients/outpatients
rehabilitation

substance abuse unit
university students

University of Miami

Department of Educational and Psychological Studies
P.O. Box 248065
Coral Gables, FL 33124-2040
phone#: (305) 284-3001
e-mail: blewis@miami.edu
Web address: http://www.education.miami.edu/program/
Programs.asp?Program_ID=47

1	2	3	**4**	5	6	7

Clinically oriented   Equal emphasis   Research oriented

What percentage of your faculty subscribes to or practices in each of the following orientations?

Psychodynamic/Psychoanalytic	10%
Applied behavioral analysis/Radical behavioral	0%
Family systems/Systems	60%
Existential/Phenomenological/Humanistic	40%
Cognitive/Cognitive-behavioral	70%

What percentage of students applying for internship last year was accepted into APPIC-member internships? 100%

What courses are required for incoming students to have completed prior to enrolling?
Standard curriculum for master's in counseling

Are there courses you recommend that are not mandatory?
No

GRE mean
Verbal 610   Quantitative 600
Analytical Writing Data not available

GPA mean
Overall GPA 3.4   Psychology GPA 3.9

Number of applications/admission offers/incoming students in 2005
65 applied/8 admission offers/6 incoming

% of students receiving:
Tuition waiver only: 0%
Assistantship/fellowship only: 0%
Both tuition waiver & assistantship/fellowship: 100%

Approximate percentage of incoming students who entered with a B.A./B.S. only: 25%   **Master's:** 75%

Approximate percentage of students who are Women: 60%   **Ethnic Minority:** 30%
International: Data not available

Average years to complete the doctoral program (including internship): 6 years

Personal interview
Preferred in person but telephone acceptable

Research areas	# Faculty	# Grants
couple violence	1	0
ethnic minorities	1	0
families	2	1
health psychology	2	1

Clinical opportunities
Tailor to students' interests

University of Minnesota–Department of Educational Psychology

129 Burton Hall
Minneapolis, MN 55455
phone#: (612) 624-6827
e-mail: cspp-adm@umn.edu
Web address:
http://www.education.umn.edu/edpsych/cspp/PhD.html

1	2	3	**4**	5	6	7

Clinically oriented   Equal emphasis   Research oriented

What percentage of your faculty subscribes to or practices in each of the following orientations?

Psychodynamic/Psychoanalytic	25%
Applied behavioral analysis/Radical behavioral	10%
Family systems/Systems	30%
Existential/Phenomenological/Humanistic	60%
Cognitive/Cognitive-behavioral	60%

What percentage of students applying for internship last year was accepted into APPIC-member internships? 100%

What courses are required for incoming students to have completed prior to enrolling?
None

Are there courses you recommend that are not mandatory?
Foundational courses in undergraduate psychology

GRE mean
Verbal 533   Quantitative 612
Analytical Writing 4.5

GPA mean
Overall GPA 3.5

Number of applications/admission offers/incoming students in 2005
49 applied/13 admission offers/10 incoming

% of students receiving:
Tuition waiver only: 0%
Assistantship/fellowship only: 10%
Both tuition waiver & assistantship/fellowship: 90%

Approximate percentage of incoming students who entered with a B.A./B.S. only: 30%   **Master's:** 70%

Approximate percentage of students who are Women: 70%   **Ethnic Minority:** 20%   **International:** 0%

Average years to complete the doctoral program (including internship): 5 years

Personal interview
Interview not required

Research areas	# Faculty	# Grants
burnout prevention	2	0
career development	2	2
genetic counseling	1	1
high-risk adolescents	2	1
international counseling	4	0
master therapist	1	0
multicultural counseling	4	0
multicultural integrative therapy	1	0
prevention	1	0
school counseling	3	0
supervision	2	1
therapist/counselor development	1	0
therapy outcome	1	0

Clinical opportunities
Multiple practicum sites in the Twin Cities

University of Minnesota– Department of Psychology

75 East River Road
Minneapolis, MN 55455
phone#: (612) 625-3873
e-mail: counpsy@umn.edu
Web address:
http://www.psych.umn.edu/areas/counseling/index.htm

1	2	3	4	5	6	**7**
Clinically oriented		Equal emphasis			Research oriented	

What percentage of your faculty subscribes to or practices in each of the following orientations?

Psychodynamic/Psychoanalytic	33%
Applied behavioral analysis/Radical behavioral	0%
Family systems/Systems	0%
Existential/Phenomenological/Humanistic	0%
Cognitive/Cognitive-behavioral	66%

What percentage of students applying for internship last year was accepted into APPIC-member internships? 100%

What courses are required for incoming students to have completed prior to enrolling?
Prefer applicants with a broad base of scientific or empirical training in psychology with a background in statistics

Are there courses you recommend that are not mandatory?
See above

GRE mean
Verbal 630   Quantitative 731
Analytical and Advanced Psychology not required
Analytical Writing 5.25

GPA mean
Overall GPA 3.52   Psychology GPA 3.58

Number of applications/admission offers/incoming students in 2005
82 applied/8 admission offers/4 incoming

% of students receiving:
Tuition waiver only: 0%
Assistantship/fellowship only: 0%
Both tuition waiver & assistantship/fellowship: 100%

Approximate percentage of incoming students who entered with a B.A./B.S. only: 50%   **Master's:** 50%

Approximate percentage of students who are Women: 69%   **Ethnic Minority:** 15%   **International:** 15%

Average years to complete the doctoral program (including internship): 6 years

Personal interview
Interview not required

Research areas	# Faculty	# Grants
Asian American identity and family	1	1
career development and choice	1	1
coping with stressful life events	1	0
interest measurement	1	1
interpersonal relations	1	1
issues related to organ transplants	1	0
multicultural counseling	1	0
occupational health psychology	1	0
personality and adjustment	1	0
posttraumatic growth	1	0
rape interventions	1	0
sexual assault recovery	1	0
values and work adjustment	1	0

Clinical opportunities
We use about 30 locations as practica and advanced practica locations. The sites are matched with students' interests and with the goal of providing them with diversity in experience over a 3- to 4-year period.

University of Missouri–Columbia

Department of Educational and Counseling Psychology
Columbia, MO 65211-2130
phone#: (573) 882-7731
e-mail: ecpgrad@tiger.coe.missouri.edu
Web address:
http://escp.coe.missouri.edu/counseling/description.html

1	2	3	**4**	5	6	7
Clinically oriented		Equal emphasis			Research oriented	

What percentage of your faculty subscribes to or practices in each of the following orientations?

Psychodynamic/Psychoanalytic	30%
Family systems/Systems	30%
Existential/Phenomenological/Humanistic	50%
Cognitive/Cognitive-behavioral	50%
Integrative	30%
Interpersonal	30%
Feminist	30%

What percentage of students applying for internship last year was accepted into APPIC-member internships? 90%

What courses are required for incoming students to have completed prior to enrolling?
If entering without a master's degree, an applicant either must have completed or plan to complete 15 hours of prerequisite course work as indicated below:
Statistics: A course in statistics covering descriptive statistics, correlation, *t*-tests, and Chi-square.
Psychological theory: 2 courses in psychological theory (not including the introductory course in psychology) for example, personality, social, developmental or learning.
Additional courses: 2 additional courses in education, psychology and/or sociology.
However, if applicants are deficient in 1 or more of these areas, they may still be admitted with the provision that they make up any deficiencies during graduate enrollment.

Are there courses you recommend that are not mandatory?
No

GRE mean
Verbal 540   Quantitative 610
Analytical Writing N/A

GPA mean
Overall GPA 3.5

Number of applications/admission offers/incoming students in 2005
100 applied/9 admission offers/7 incoming

% of students receiving:
Tuition waiver only: 0%
Assistantship/fellowship only: 0%
Both tuition waiver & assistantship/fellowship: 100%

Approximate percentage of incoming students who entered with a B.A./B.S. only: 57%   **Master's:** 43%

Approximate percentage of students who are Women: 74%   **Ethnic Minority:** 36%   **International:** 23%

Average years to complete the doctoral program (including internship): 6.5 years

Personal interview
Preferred in person but telephone acceptable

Research areas	# Faculty	# Grants
addictions	2	0
African American adolescents	1	2
career development	5	2
counseling process	3	2
counseling supervision	2	1
counseling/therapy integration	1	0
disability issues	1	0
eating disorders	1	1
gender issues	2	0
group process	2	1
health psychology	2	1
identity development	1	0
multicultural counseling	5	2
perfectionism	1	0
problem solving	3	2
rape	1	1
scale construction	4	3

Clinical opportunities
family counseling center
intensive cognitive-behavioral outpatient center
learning disabilities clinic
local and rural community mental health centers
psychiatric clinic
psychology clinic
Rusk Rehabilitation Center
state hospital
state prison
university and college counseling centers
university career planning and placement center
university medical clinics
VA hospital
women's center
women's shelters

University of Missouri–Kansas City

Division of Counseling, Educational Psychology, and Exercise Science
School of Education, Room 215
5100 Rockhill Road
Kansas City, MO 64110
phone#: (816) 235-2722
e-mail: umkccepsy@umkc.edu
Web address:
http://education.umkc.edu/CEP/phd/index.asp

1	2	3	**4**	5	6	7
Clinically oriented		Equal emphasis			Research oriented	

What percentage of your faculty subscribes to or practices in each of the following orientations?

Psychodynamic/Psychoanalytic	10%
Applied behavioral analysis/Radical behavioral	5%
Family systems/Systems	20%
Existential/Phenomenological/Humanistic	25%
Cognitive/Cognitive-behavioral	40%

What percentage of students applying for internship last year was accepted into APPIC-member internships? 100%

What courses are required for incoming students to have completed prior to enrolling?
Undergraduate psychology major or master's degree in counseling or psychology

Are there courses you recommend that are not mandatory?
No

GRE mean
Data not available

GPA mean
Data not available

Number of applications/admission offers/incoming students in 2003
90 applied/8 admission offers/8 incoming

% of students receiving:
Tuition waiver only: 0%
Assistantship/fellowship only: 0%
Both tuition waiver & assistantship/fellowship: 62.5% (3 chose not to accept support)

Approximate percentage of incoming students who entered with a B.A./B.S. only: 62.5% **Master's:** 25% (12.5% doctoral respecialization)

Approximate percentage of students who are Women: 75% **Ethnic Minority:** 37.5%
International: Data not available

Average years to complete the doctoral program (including internship): 6 years

Personal interview
Preferred in person but telephone acceptable

Research areas	# Faculty	# Grants
AIDS	1	1
behavioral medicine	4	3
cross-cultural perspectives of counseling	4	2
family systems theory	1	0
health psychology	3	0
interpersonal relations	3	0
professional issues	3	0
psychopathology prevention	3	0
psychotherapy process	3	0
sports psychology	1	0
stress and coping	1	0
substance abuse	1	0
supervision	2	0
vocational interests	1	0

Clinical opportunities
—

University of Nebraska–Lincoln

Department of Educational Psychology
38 Teachers College Hall
Lincoln, NE 68588-0345
phone#: (402) 472-2223
e-mail: mscheel2@unl.edu
Web address:
http://cehs.unl.edu/edpsych/graduate/copsych.shtml

1	2	3	**4**	5	6	7

Clinically oriented · Equal emphasis · Research oriented

What percentage of your faculty subscribes to or practices in each of the following orientations?
Psychodynamic/Psychoanalytic 20%
Applied behavioral analysis/Radical behavioral 0%
Family systems/Systems 20%
Existential/Phenomenological/Humanistic 20%
Cognitive/Cognitive-behavioral 40%

What percentage of students applying for internship last year was accepted into APPIC-member internships? 100%

What courses are required for incoming students to have completed prior to enrolling?
Bachelor's in a closely related area or master's in counseling or closely related field

Are there courses you recommend that are not mandatory?
—

GRE mean
Verbal 550   Quantitative 550

GPA mean
Overall GPA 3.5

Number of applications/admission offers/incoming students in 2003
42 applied/8 admission offers/6 incoming

% of students receiving:
Tuition waiver only: 0%
Assistantship/fellowship only: 0%
Both tuition waiver & assistantship/fellowship: 100%

Approximate percentage of incoming students who entered with a B.A./B.S. only: 20% **Master's:** 80%

Approximate percentage of students who are Women: 70% **Ethnic Minority:** 36%
International: Data not available

Average years to complete the doctoral program (including internship): 5 years

Personal interview
Preferred in person but telephone acceptable

Research areas	# Faculty	# Grants
family counseling	1	0
multicultural issues	1	0
psychological assessment	1	0
vocational	1	0

Clinical opportunities
couple and family counseling
health psychology
multicultural counseling
psychological assessment
vocational counseling

New Mexico State University

Department of Counseling and Educational Psychology
MSC 3CEP
P.O. Box 30001
Las Cruces, NM 88003-8001
phone#: (505) 646-2121
e-mail: eadams@nmsu.edu
Web address:
http://education.nmsu.edu/cep/phd/index.html

1	2	3	**4**	5	6	7

Clinically oriented · Equal emphasis · Research oriented

What percentage of your faculty subscribes to or practices in each of the following orientations?

Psychodynamic/Psychoanalytic	22%
Applied behavioral analysis/Radical behavioral	0%
Family systems/Systems	11%
Existential/Phenomenological/Humanistic	33%
Cognitive/Cognitive-behavioral	22%

What percentage of students applying for internship last year was accepted into APPIC-member internships? 100%

What courses are required for incoming students to have completed prior to enrolling?
None

Are there courses you recommend that are not mandatory?
Counseling Practicum, human development, multicultural psychology, counseling theory and techniques, family therapy, group work, career/life planning, counseling research, diagnosis and treatment planning, addictions counseling

GRE mean
Verbal + Quantitative 1000
Analytical Writing 4.5

GPA mean
master's GPA 3.76

Number of applications/admission offers/incoming students in 2005
35 applied/19 admission offers/7 incoming

% of students receiving:
Tuition waiver only: 0%
Assistantship/fellowship only: 70%
Both tuition waiver & assistantship/fellowship: 30%

Approximate percentage of incoming students who entered with a B.A./B.S. only: 0%   **Master's:** 100%

**Approximate percentage of students who are
Women:** 54%   **Ethnic Minority:** 46%   **International:** 4%

Average years to complete the doctoral program (including internship): 5 years

Personal interview
Preferred in person but telephone acceptable

Research areas	# Faculty	# Grants
acculturation	3	0
Adlerian psychology	1	0
career	2	0
family systems	1	0
gender	3	0
identity/phenotype	3	0
multicultural curriculum development	1	0
relationship enhancement	1	1

Clinical opportunities
community organizations
departmental training center
families
groups
low income
medically underserved
minorities
rural
substance abuse
university counseling center
vocational career development

New York University

School of Education
Counseling Psychology
Department of Applied Psychology
East Building, 4th Floor
239 Greene Street
New York, NY 10003
phone#: (212) 998-5559
Web address: http://education.nyu.edu/education/appsych/index.php/program/24/

1	2	3	**4**	5	6	7
Clinically oriented		Equal emphasis			Research oriented	

What percentage of your faculty subscribes to or practices in each of the following orientations?

Psychodynamic/Psychoanalytic	50%
Applied behavioral analysis/Radical behavioral	0%
Family systems/Systems	13%
Existential/Phenomenological/Humanistic	25%
Cognitive/Cognitive-behavioral	13%

What percentage of students applying for internship last year was accepted into APPIC-member internships? 100%

What courses are required for incoming students to have completed prior to enrolling?
18 credits of prerequisites in psychology at undergraduate or graduate level. Not necessary to complete prerequisites before enrollment.

Are there courses you recommend that are not mandatory?
In general, basic areas in psychology course work are recommended

GRE mean
Data not available

GPA mean
Data not available

Number of applications/admission offers/incoming students in 2003
120 applied/4 admission offers/4 incoming

% of students receiving:
Tuition waiver only: 0%
Assistantship/fellowship only: 5%
Both tuition waiver & assistantship/fellowship: 50%

Approximate percentage of incoming students who entered with a B.A./B.S. only: 25%   **Master's:** 75%

**Approximate percentage of students who are
Women:** 80%   **Ethnic Minority:** 10%   **International:** 4%

Average years to complete the doctoral program (including internship): 7 years

Personal interview
Required in person

Research areas	# Faculty	# Grants
group process	1	0
multicultural counseling and assessment	2	0
psychoanalytic constructs	1	0
psychopathology and differential diagnosis	2	0
religion and spirituality	1	1
women's development	2	2
work as a developmental context	1	0

Clinical opportunities
Wide range of specialized practica and externship sites are available in the New York metropolitan area.

University of North Dakota

Department of Counseling
Box 8255
Grand Forks, ND 58202-8255
phone#: (701) 777-2729
fax#: (701) 777-3184
e-mail: michael.loewy@und.edu
Web address: http://www.counseling.und.edu/
docbrochure_brokendown/phdcoverpage.htm

1	2	3	**4**	5	6	7
Clinically oriented		Equal emphasis			Research oriented	

What percentage of your faculty subscribes to or practices in each of the following orientations?

Psychodynamic/Psychoanalytic	40%
Applied behavioral analysis/Radical behavioral	0%
Family systems/Systems	20%
Existential/Phenomenological/Humanistic	40%
Cognitive/Cognitive-behavioral	50%
Feminist	50%

What percentage of students applying for internship last year was accepted into APPIC-member internships? 83%

What courses are required for incoming students to have completed prior to enrolling?
20 semester hours of undergraduate psychology including statistics, research methods, abnormal psychology, developmental psychology, personality theory and general psychology.

Are there courses you recommend that are not mandatory?
Research methods, master's level practicum, 60 hours supervised practice (for post-master's applicants)

GRE mean
Verbal 545   Quantitative 590   Analytical 665
Advanced Psychology 607
Analytical Writing 4.8

GPA mean
Overall undergraduate GPA 3.5
Junior/Senior GPA 3.5
Overall master's GPA 3.95

Number of applications/admission offers/incoming students in 2005
22 applied/10 admission offers/7 incoming

% of students receiving:
Tuition waiver only: 0%
Assistantship/fellowship only: 0%
Both tuition waiver & assistantship/fellowship: 100%

Approximate percentage of incoming students who entered with a B.A./B.S. only: 43%   **Master's:** 57%

Approximate percentage of students who are Women: 57%   **Ethnic Minority:** 0%   **International:** 0%

Average years to complete the doctoral program (including internship): 4.5 years

Personal interview
Preferred in person but telephone acceptable

Research areas	# Faculty	# Grants
body image	1	0
career development	2	0
domestic violence	1	0
gay, lesbian, bisexual issues	2	1
gender and intimacy	1	1
geriatric psychology	2	1
group identity development	1	0
healthy relationships	1	0
HIV prevention	1	1
immigrant and refugee mental health and adjustment	1	0
multicultural counseling	1	0
Native American career development	1	0
psychological implication in study of poverty	1	0
resiliency in adolescence	1	0
rural mental health	2	0
sizism	1	0
social support and chronic illness	1	0
student self-efficacy	1	0
supervisor strategies	2	0
vocational interests testing	1	1
white privilege	1	0
women/career development	1	0

Clinical opportunities
Fieldwork placements at a variety of community and academic settings

University of North Texas

Department of Psychology
NT Box 13587
Denton, TX 76203-3587
phone#: (940) 565-2671
e-mail: AMYG@UNT.EDU
Web address:
http://www.psyc.unt.edu/gradcounseling.shtml

1	2	3	**4**	5	6	7
Clinically oriented		Equal emphasis			Research oriented	

What percentage of your faculty subscribes to or practices in each of the following orientations?

Psychodynamic/Psychoanalytic	35%
Applied behavioral analysis/Radical behavioral	0%
Family systems/Systems	45%
Existential/Phenomenological/Humanistic	20%
Cognitive/Cognitive-behavioral	45%

What percentage of students applying for internship last year was accepted into APPIC-member internships? 100%

What courses are required for incoming students to have completed prior to enrolling?
Statistics and three of the following: experimental (or research methods), cognition, learning, perception (sensory processes), motivation, physiological psychology (biological psychology), psychological measurement, or research thesis

Are there courses you recommend that are not mandatory?
Social psychology, physiological psychology, tests and measurements

GRE mean
Applicants undergo holistic review. Verbal, quantitative, and analytical scores must be submitted.
Verbal 500 Quantitative 500 Analytic 500
Analytical Writing 4

GPA mean
Overall GPA 3.0 or 3.5 on last 60 hours for bachelor's
Or overall GPA 3.5 for master's Psychology GPA 3.5

Number of applications/admission offers/incoming
students in 2005
84 applied/22 admission offers/12 incoming

% of students receiving:
Tuition waiver only: 0%
Assistantship/fellowship only: 50%
Both tuition waiver & assistantship/fellowship: 0%

Approximate percentage of incoming students who entered with a B.A./B.S. only: 75% **Master's:** 25%

Approximate percentage of students who are Women: 73% **Ethnic Minority:** 2% **International:** 1%

Average years to complete the doctoral program (including internship): 7.7 years

Personal interview
Preferred in person but telephone acceptable

Research areas

Research areas	# Faculty	# Grants
counseling and therapy	6	0
eating disorders	3	0
gerontology	1	1
marriage and family	3	2
minority and cross-cultural	2	1
professional issues	4	0
sports psychology	2	1
vocational development	3	1

Clinical opportunities
external agencies after completing required on-campus
  practica
psychology clinic
university counseling and testing center

University of Northern Colorado (Psy.D.)

Division of Professional Psychology
Greeley, CO 80639
phone#: (970) 351-2209
e-mail: david.gonzalez@unco.edu
Web address:
http://www.unco.edu/cebs/counspsych/index.html

1	2	**3**	4	5	6	7
Clinically oriented		Equal emphasis			Research oriented	

What percentage of your faculty subscribes to or practices in each of the following orientations?

Psychodynamic/Psychoanalytic	0%
Applied behavioral analysis/Radical behavioral	10%
Family systems/Systems	30%
Existential/Phenomenological/Humanistic	30%
Cognitive/Cognitive-behavioral	30%

What percentage of students applying for internship last year was accepted into APPIC-member internships? 100%

What courses are required for incoming students to have completed prior to enrolling?
A master's degree is required in a related field of applied psychology. It is particularly important that students have completed a counseling practicum.

Are there courses you recommend that are not mandatory?
No

GRE mean
Verbal 550 Quantitative 550
Recommended GRE total 1000
Analytical Writing 5.0

GPA mean
Overall GPA in master's program 3.8

Number of applications/admission offers/incoming
students in 2005
40 applied/7 admission offers/6 incoming

% of students receiving:
Tuition waiver only: 0%
Assistantship/fellowship only: 50%
Both tuition waiver & assistantship/fellowship: 25%

Approximate percentage of incoming students who entered with a B.A./B.S. only: 0%   **Master's:** 100%

Approximate percentage of students who are Women: 70%   **Ethnic Minority:** 10%   **International:** 10%

Average years to complete the doctoral program (including internship): 4–5 years

Personal interview
Preferred in person but telephone acceptable

Research areas	# Faculty	# Grants
child psychology	8	0
college student adjustment	2	2
counseling process	1	0
eating disorders	2	0
family dynamics	4	1
multicultural	6	0

Clinical opportunities
clinical hypnosis
cognitive/academic
individual therapy
marriage and family therapy
neuropsychological assessment
personality/behavioral assessment
play therapy
supervision

University of Notre Dame

Department of Psychology
Notre Dame, IN 46556
phone#: (574) 631-6650
fax#: (574) 631-8883
e-mail: JudyA.Spiro.2@nd.edu
Web address:
http://www.nd.edu/%7Epsych/counseling/index.htm

1	2	3	4	5	**6**	7

Clinically oriented   Equal emphasis   Research oriented

What percentage of your faculty subscribes to or practices in each of the following orientations?

Psychodynamic/Psychoanalytic	20%
Applied behavioral analysis/Radical behavioral	10%
Family systems/Systems	20%
Existential/Phenomenological/Humanistic	30%
Cognitive/Cognitive-behavioral	20%

What percentage of students applying for internship last year was accepted into APPIC-member internships? 100%

What courses are required for incoming students to have completed prior to enrolling?
Undergraduate psychology major, statistics, methodology, and some research experience

Are there courses you recommend that are not mandatory?
No

GRE mean
Verbal + Quantitative 1250
Analytical Writing Data not available

GPA mean
Overall GPA 3.8   Psychology GPA 3.8

Number of applications/admission offers/incoming students in 2003
136 applied/3 admission offers/3 incoming

% of students receiving:
Tuition waiver only: 0%
Assistantship/fellowship only: 0%
Both tuition waiver & assistantship/fellowship: 100%

Approximate percentage of incoming students who entered with a B.A./B.S. only: 90%   **Master's:** 10%

Approximate percentage of students who are Women: 65%   **Ethnic Minority:** 34%
International: Data not available

Average years to complete the doctoral program (including internship): 6 years

Personal interview
Preferred in person but telephone acceptable

Research areas	# Faculty	# Grants
behavioral medicine	1	1
health psychology	1	1
marital therapy	1	1
multicultural counseling	2	1
narrative psychology	1	1
social/clinical psychology interface	2	0
social phobia	2	2

Clinical opportunities
juvenile justice center
local community mental health center
local community outpatient hospital
university counseling center

Ohio State University

Department of Psychology
Columbus, OH 43210
Ohio State University remains fully accredited by the APA. However, the program is no longer accepting new applications.

University of Oklahoma

Department of Educational Psychology
Norman, OK 73019-0260
phone#: (405) 325-5974
e-mail: cstoltenberg@ou.edu or gpoedpsych@ou.edu
Web address:
http://www.ou.edu/education/cpp/CP/descCP.htm

1	2	3	**4**	5	6	7
Clinically oriented		Equal emphasis			Research oriented	

What percentage of your faculty subscribes to or practices in each of the following orientations?

Psychodynamic/Psychoanalytic	57%
Applied behavioral analysis/Radical behavioral	14%
Family systems/Systems	71%
Existential/Phenomenological/Humanistic	57%
Cognitive/Cognitive-behavioral	86%
Narrative	28%
Feminist	28%
Integrative	71%

What percentage of students applying for internship last year was accepted into APPIC-member internships? 100%

What courses are required for incoming students to have completed prior to enrolling?
College algebra (or equivalent), 2 semesters of English grammar and composition, 18 semester hours in psychology or related area

Are there courses you recommend that are not mandatory?
No

GRE mean
Verbal 550 Quantitative 600
Analytical Writing Data not available

GPA mean
Data not available

Number of applications/admission offers/incoming students in 2003
65 applied/8 admission offers/8 incoming

% of students receiving:
Tuition waiver only: 0%
Assistantship/fellowship only: 0%
Both tuition waiver & assistantship/fellowship: 80%

Approximate percentage of incoming students who entered with a B.A./B.S. only: 25% **Master's:** 87.5%

Approximate percentage of students who are Women: 60% **Ethnic Minority:** 20%
International: Data not available

Average years to complete the doctoral program (including internship): 5 years

Personal interview
Preferred in person but telephone acceptable

Research areas	# Faculty	# Grants
American Indian issues	3	0
assessment	3	0
career issues	2	0
child treatment	4	0
clinical supervision	3	0
counseling process and outcomes	5	0
ecopsychology	2	0
gender issues	4	0
health psychology	3	0
marriage and family issues	4	0
multicultural counseling	4	0
narrative issues	1	0
relational health	2	0
trauma/violence	2	0

Clinical opportunities
child abuse and neglect clinics
child study center
community mental health clinics
correctional facilities
health sciences center/medical clinics/children's
hospital/schools
Indian health service clinic
psychiatric hospitals
rehabilitation clinics
university counseling center
VA hospital

Oklahoma State University

School of Applied Health and Educational Psychology
Stillwater, OK 74078
phone#: (405) 744-6040
e-mail: carvin@okstate.edu
Web address:
http://www.okstate.edu/education/sahep/cpsy/index.html

1	2	3	**4**	5	6	7
Clinically oriented		Equal emphasis			Research oriented	

What percentage of your faculty subscribes to or practices in each of the following orientations?

Psychodynamic/Psychoanalytic	20%
Applied behavioral analysis/Radical behavioral	0%
Family systems/Systems	30%
Existential/Phenomenological/Humanistic	30%
Cognitive/Cognitive-behavioral	70%

What percentage of students applying for internship last year was accepted into APPIC-member internships? 100%

What courses are required for incoming students to have completed prior to enrolling?
Bachelor's or master's degree in psychology or related area

Are there courses you recommend that are not mandatory?
Introductory psychology courses, statistics, research design.

GRE mean
We don't use cutoff scores. We recommend 500 for Verbal and 500 for Quantitative
Analytical Writing 4.5

GPA mean
Data not available

Number of applications/admission offers/incoming students in 2005
65 applied/8 admission offers/8 incoming

% of students receiving:
Tuition waiver only: 10%
Assistantship/fellowship only: 0%
Both tuition waiver & assistantship/fellowship: 95%

Approximate percentage of incoming students who entered with a B.A./B.S. only: 27%   **Master's:** 73%

Approximate percentage of students who are
Women: 60%   **Ethnic Minority:** 30%   **International:** 5%

Average years to complete the doctoral program (including internship): 4–5 years

Personal interview
Preferred in person but telephone acceptable

Research areas	# Faculty	# Grants
American Indian issues	3	3
at-risk youth	2	1
career issues	4	1
health psychology	2	1
LGBT issues	1	0
multicultural issues	4	5
professional issues	2	1
psychological assessment	1	0
rural mental health	1	0
sports psychology	1	0
supervision	3	0
women/gender issues	2	0

Clinical opportunities
domestic violence center
correctional psychology unit
hospitals (inpatient, outpatient, both)
Indian health services
marriage and family clinic
rural mental health clinic
university counseling centers
youth and family services

University of Oregon
Counseling Psychology Program
5251 University of Oregon
Eugene, OR 97403-5251
phone#: (541) 346-2456
e-mail: cpsy@uoregon.edu
Web address:
http://counpsych.uoregon.edu/programdescription.htm

1	2	3	4	**5**	6	7
Clinically oriented		Equal emphasis			Research oriented	

What percentage of your faculty subscribes to or practices in each of the following orientations?

Psychodynamic/Psychoanalytic	0%
Applied behavioral analysis/Radical behavioral	0%
Family systems/Systems	50%
Existential/Phenomenological/Humanistic	25%
Cognitive/Cognitive-behavioral	100%

What percentage of students applying for internship last year was accepted into APPIC-member internships? 100%

What courses are required for incoming students to have completed prior to enrolling?
No specific courses required

Are there courses you recommend that are not mandatory?
Psychology

GRE mean
Verbal 550   Quantitative 550
Analytical Writing N/A

GPA mean
Overall 3.5

Number of applications/admission offers/incoming students in 2005
119 applied/10 admission offers/9 incoming

% of students receiving:
Tuition waiver only: 0%
Assistantship/fellowship only: 0%
Both tuition waiver & assistantship/fellowship: 100% (less UO Fees)

Approximate percentage of incoming students who entered with a B.A./B.S. only: 80%   **Master's:** 20%

Approximate percentage of students who are
Women: 75%   **Ethnic Minority:** 47%   **International:** 5%

Average years to complete the doctoral program (including internship): 5.5 years

Personal interview
Preferred in person but telephone acceptable

Research areas	# Faculty	# Grants
child and family psychology	3	2
college student development	2	0
domestic violence	1	0
multicultural issues	4	1
prevention research	4	2
social support and interactions	3	0
treatment outcomes	4	1
vocational psychology	2	0

Clinical opportunities
child–family
community prevention
counseling centers
inpatient settings
VA

Our Lady of the Lake University (Psy.D.)

Graduate Admissions Office
School of Education and Clinical Studies
411 SW 24th Street
San Antonio, TX 78207-4689
phone#: (210) 431-3914
e-mail: BOBEM@lake.ollusa.edu
Web address: http://www.ollusa.edu/ACADEMIC/
SECS/psychology/PSY_PsyDinCounseling.htm

1	**2**	3	4	5	6	7

Clinically oriented   Equal emphasis   Research oriented

What percentage of your faculty subscribes to or practices in each of the following orientations?

Psychodynamic/Psychoanalytic	20%
Applied behavioral analysis/Radical behavioral	0%
Family systems/Systems	80%
Existential/Phenomenological/Humanistic	0%
Cognitive/Cognitive-behavioral	0%

What percentage of students applying for internship last year was accepted into APPIC-member internships? 100%

What courses are required for incoming students to have completed prior to enrolling
Master's or bachelor's degree in psychology or closely related area

Are there courses you recommend that are not mandatory?
Yes, At least 18 undergraduate semester hours in psychology is required including courses in: statistics, research methods, social psychology, developmental, abnormal, counseling skills or personality theories for applicants without a master's in psychology.

GRE mean
Verbal 560 Quantitative 550
Analytical Writing Not used at this time

GPA mean
Overall GPA 3.67

Number of applications/admission offers/incoming students in 2005
45 applied/12 admission offers/6 incoming

% of students receiving:
Tuition waiver only: 10%
Assistantship/fellowship only: 0%
Both tuition waiver & assistantship/fellowship: 25%

Approximate percentage of incoming students who entered with a B.A./B.S. only: 0% **Master's:** 100%

Approximate percentage of students who are Women: 86% **Ethnic Minority:** 43% **International:** 3%

Average years to complete the doctoral program (including internship): 5.5 years

Personal interview
Required in person

Research areas	# Faculty	# Grants
brief therapy	3	2
ethics	1	0
reimbursement issues	1	0

Clinical opportunities
community counseling service
health psychology
school-age population
Spanish-speaking population

Pennsylvania State University

Department of Counselor Education, Counseling Psychology, and Rehabilitation Services
University Park, PA 16802
phone#: (814) 865-8304
e-mail: CnPsydoc@psu.edu
Web address: http://www.ed.psu.edu/cnpsy/

1	2	3	**4**	5	6	7

Clinically oriented   Equal emphasis   Research oriented

What percentage of your faculty subscribes to or practices in each of the following orientations?

Psychodynamic/Psychoanalytic	30%
Applied behavioral analysis/Radical behavioral	0%
Family systems/Systems	30%
Existential/Phenomenological/Humanistic	30%
Cognitive/Cognitive-behavioral	0%
Other	10%

What percentage of students applying for internship last year was accepted into APPIC-member internships? 100%

What courses are required for incoming students to have completed prior to enrolling?
Recommended: theories of counseling/psychotherapy, assessment/testing, statistics/research design, career counseling, multicultural counseling, group counseling/ psychotherapy, counselor skills training/prepracticum counseling practicum

Are there courses you recommend that are not mandatory?
Human development, core courses in psychology

GRE mean
Verbal 520 Quantitative 577 Analytical 628
Analytical Writing N/A

GPA mean
Overall master's GPA 3.8

Number of applications/admission offers/incoming students in 2005
54 applied/8 admission offers/6 incoming

% of students receiving:
Tuition waiver only: 0%
Assistantship/fellowship only: 0%
Both tuition waiver & assistantship/fellowship: 100%

Approximate percentage of incoming students who entered with a B.A./B.S. only: 0% **Master's:** 100%

Approximate percentage of students who are Women: 74% **Ethnic Minority:** 38% **International:** 8%

Average years to complete the doctoral program (including internship): 5 years

Personal interview
Preferred in person but telephone acceptable

Research areas	# Faculty	# Grants
family systems	2	0
lesbian/gay/bisexual issues	1	0
perfectionism	1	0
psychotherapy	1	0

Clinical opportunities
—

Purdue University

Department of Educational Studies
BRNG Hall, 100 N. University St.,
West Lafayette, IN 47907-2098
phone#: (765) 494-9748 (Secretary: Ros Bol)
e-mail: pistole@purdue.edu
Web address: http://www.edst.purdue.edu/cd/
psychology/main.html

1	2	3	4	5	**6**	7

Clinically oriented   Equal emphasis   Research oriented

What percentage of your faculty subscribes to or practices in each of the following orientations?

Psychodynamic/Psychoanalytic	25%
Applied behavioral analysis/Radical behavioral	0%
Family systems/Systems	25%
Existential/Phenomenological/Humanistic	0%
Cognitive/Cognitive-behavioral	75%

What percentage of students applying for internship last year was accepted into APPIC-member internships? No applications in Fall 2004 because new program

What courses are required for incoming students to have completed prior to enrolling?
None

Are there courses you recommend that are not mandatory?
Statistics, research design recommended

GRE mean
Verbal 547 Quantitative 624
Analytical and Advanced Psychology not typically used as indicators
Analytical Writing 4.6

GPA mean
Overall GPA 3.5

Number of applications/admission offers/incoming students in 2003
50 applied/10 admission offers/7 incoming

% of students receiving:
Tuition waiver only: 0%
Assistantship/fellowship only: 0%
Both tuition waiver & assistantship/fellowship: 100%

Approximate percentage of incoming students who entered with a B.A./B.S. only: 23% **Master's:** 77%

Approximate percentage of students who are Women: 70% **Ethnic Minority:** 9% **International:** 21%

Average years to complete the doctoral program (including internship): 5 years

Personal interview
Preferred in person but telephone acceptable

Research areas	# Faculty	# Grants
adult attachment theory in romantic relationships and counseling	1	0
career and talent development	1	0
grief and bereavement/adolescent development/loss as a therapeutic model	1	0
problem solving/coping/psychological adjustment/procrastination	1	0

Clinical opportunities
In-house clinic for community and university clients

University of St. Thomas (Psy.D.)

Graduate Department of Professional Psychology
TMH451, 1000 La Salle Avenue
Minneapolis, MN 55403-2005
phone#: (651) 962-4650
e-mail: GradPsych@St.Thomas.Edu
Web address:
http://www.stthomas.edu/gradpsych/psyd.cfm

1	**2**	3	4	5	6	7

Clinically oriented   Equal emphasis   Research oriented

What percentage of your faculty subscribes to or practices in each of the following orientations?

Psychodynamic/Psychoanalytic	10%
Applied behavioral analysis/Radical behavioral	0%
Family systems/Systems	20%
Existential/Phenomenological/Humanistic	10%
Cognitive/Cognitive-behavioral	40%

What percentage of students applying for internship last year was accepted into APPIC-member internships? 29%

What courses are required for incoming students to have completed prior to enrolling?
Students must complete a 45-credit M.A. program in counseling psychology or equivalent

Are there courses you recommend that are not mandatory?
Abnormal psychology, psychological statistics, research design, personality theory, developmental psychology

GRE mean
Verbal 500 Quantitative 500
Analytical Writing 3.5

GPA mean
Overall GPA 3.2

Number of applications/admission offers/incoming students in 2005
37 applied/16 admission offers/15 incoming

% of students receiving:
Tuition waiver only: 0%
Assistantship/fellowship only: 12%
Both tuition waiver & assistantship/fellowship: 0%

Approximate percentage of incoming students who entered with a B.A./B.S. only: 0% **Master's:** 100%

Approximate percentage of students who are Women: 80% **Ethnic Minority:** 13% **International:** 6%

Average years to complete the doctoral program (including internship): 5.0 years

Personal interview
Preferred in person

Research areas	# Faculty	# Grants
counseling process	3	0
cultural sensitive therapy	2	0
disorders	2	0
interprofessional ethics	1	0
licensure and regulatory boards	1	0
master therapists	1	0
religion and psychotherapy	1	0

Clinical opportunities
Clinical opportunities include the full range of diagnostic disorders in a variety of clinical settings

Seton Hall University

Counseling Psychology Program
College of Education
400 South Orange Avenue
South Orange, NJ 07079
phone#: (973) 275-2740
e-mail: palmerla@shu.edu
Web address: http://education.shu.edu/
academicprograms/profpsych/phd_counsel/index.html

1	2	3	**4**	5	6	7

Clinically oriented Equal emphasis Research oriented

What percentage of your faculty subscribes to or practices in each of the following orientations?

Psychodynamic/Psychoanalytic	25%
Applied behavioral analysis/Radical behavioral	0%
Family systems/Systems	0%
Existential/Phenomenological/Humanistic	25%
Cognitive/Cognitive-behavioral	50%

What percentage of students applying for internship last year was accepted into APPIC-member internships? 100%

What courses are required for incoming students to have completed prior to enrolling?
Group counseling, abnormal psychology, test and measurement, counseling skills

Are there courses you recommend that are not mandatory?
No

GRE mean
Verbal 490 Quantitative 520 Analytical 510
Analytical Writing N/A

GPA mean
Overall GPA 3.3

Number of applications/admission offers/incoming students in 2005
80 applied/7 admission offers/5 incoming

% of students receiving:
Tuition waiver only: 0%
Assistantship/fellowship only: 100%
Both tuition waiver & assistantship/fellowship: 0%

Approximate percentage of incoming students who entered with a B.A./B.S. only: 0% **Master's:** 100%

Approximate percentage of students who are Women: 72% **Ethnic Minority:** 44% **International:** 8%

Average years to complete the doctoral program (including internship): 5 years

Personal interview
Preferred in person but telephone acceptable

Research areas	# Faculty	# Grants
career development	1	0
multicultural counseling	3	0
neuropsychology	1	0
psychological trauma	1	0
resiliency	1	0
student well-being	1	0

Clinical opportunities
The university does not run any specialty clinics. The program has developed an extensive offering of diverse clinical training opportunities in the greater New York area.

Southern Illinois University

Department of Psychology
Carbondale, IL 62901
phone#: (618) 453-3564
e-mail: gradpsyc@siu.edu (graduate secretary)
chwalisz@siu.edu (program director)
Web address:
http://www.psychology.siu.edu/counseling/index.html

1	2	3	**4**	5	6	7

Clinically oriented Equal emphasis Research oriented

What percentage of your faculty subscribes to or practices in each of the following orientations?

Psychodynamic/Psychoanalytic	0%
Applied behavioral analysis/Radical behavioral	0%
Family systems/Systems	0%
Existential/Phenomenological/Humanistic	67%
Cognitive/Cognitive-behavioral	33%

What percentage of students applying for internship last year was accepted into APPIC-member internships? 100%

What courses are required for incoming students to have completed prior to enrolling?
—

Are there courses you recommend that are not mandatory?
At least 1 basic statistics course; if student was not an undergraduate psychology major, we look for coursework in core areas of psychology (e.g., history and systems, abnormal, personality, cognitive, social, physiological)

GRE mean
Verbal 603 Quantitative 621
Analytical Writing Data not available

GPA mean
Overall GPA 3.60

Number of applications/admission offers/incoming students in 2003
92 applied/9 admission offers/7 incoming

% of students receiving:
Tuition waiver only: 0%
Assistantship/fellowship only: 0%
Both tuition waiver & assistantship/fellowship: 100%

Approximate percentage of incoming students who entered with a B.A./B.S. only: 100%   **Master's:** 0%

Approximate percentage of students who are Women: 80%   **Ethnic Minority:** 35%   **International:** 8%

Average years to complete the doctoral program (including internship): 5.5 years

Personal interview
Preferred in person but telephone acceptable

Research areas	# Faculty	# Grants
academic disidentification	1	0
academic self-concept, achievement and motivation	1	0
adjustment to brain injury/disability	1	0
career assessment and counseling	1	1
career choice and development	1	1
caregiver burden	1	1
counseling supervision	2	0
disaster management/crisis intervention	1	0
expectations about counseling	2	0
gender and cultural influences on therapy	3	0
health psychology	1	0
human sexual behavior	1	0
occupational stress and health	1	0
personality assessment	1	0
psychological measurement	1	0
psychological student development	1	0
qualitative research methodology	1	0
racial/ethnic identity	2	0
self-efficacy	1	0
sexual harassment	1	0
spiritual/religious issues	1	0
stress and coping	2	0
women in management	1	0
workplace violence	1	0

Clinical opportunities
career development services
clinical center, marriage and family practicum
local community mental health centers (rural mental health)
partial hospitalization program
psychiatric (inpatient) hospital
state correctional system (medium security facility; youth facility)
student health service
university counseling center
VA hospital
vocational rehabilitation assessment center
wellness center: substance abuse unit, stress management unit, sexuality counseling unit
women's shelter

University of Southern Mississippi

Department of Psychology
Hattiesburg, MS 39406-5012
phone#: (601) 266-4602
Web address:
http://www.usm.edu/psy/counseling/home.htm

1	2	3	4	**5**	6	7

Clinically oriented   Equal emphasis   Research oriented

What percentage of your faculty subscribes to or practices in each of the following orientations?
Psychodynamic/Psychoanalytic   0%
Applied behavioral analysis/Radical behavioral   0%
Family systems/Systems   20%
Existential/Phenomenological/Humanistic   30%
Cognitive/Cognitive-behavioral   50%

What percentage of students applying for internship last year was accepted into APPIC-member internships? 100%

What courses are required for incoming students to have completed prior to enrolling?
None

Are there courses you recommend that are not mandatory?
Undergraduate statistics, personality theory, human growth and development, testing and assessment

GRE mean
Verbal 600 Quantitative 600
Analytical Writing Data not available

GPA mean
Overall GPA 3.50 Overall master's GPA 3.80

Number of applications/admission offers/incoming students in 2003
50 applied/10 admission offers/7 incoming

% of students receiving:
Tuition waiver only: 0%
Assistantship/fellowship only: 0%
Both tuition waiver & assistantship/fellowship: 100%

Approximate percentage of incoming students who entered with a B.A./B.S. only: 25%   Master's: 75%

**Approximate percentage of students who are Women: 75%   Ethnic Minority: 10%
International:** Data not available

Average years to complete the doctoral program (including internship): 4 years

Personal interview
Preferred in person but telephone acceptable

Research areas	# Faculty	# Grants
anger	1	0
attachment	3	0
body image	1	0
children and adolescents	2	0
constructivist assessment and therapy	1	0
eating disorders	1	0
empirically supported treatments	2	0
forgiveness	1	0
minority/multicultural	3	0
tobacco cessation	2	2
spirituality	1	0

Clinical opportunities
community alcohol and drug treatment center
community mental health center
counseling program assessment center
counseling program training clinic
university counseling center
university medical center (Jackson, MS)
VA hospital (Biloxi, MS)

Temple University

Counseling Psychology Program
Temple University remains fully accredited by APA. However, the program is no longer accepting new applications.

University of Tennessee

Department of Psychology
311 Austin Peay Building
Knoxville, TN 37996-0900
phone#: (423) 974-3728
e-mail: fleong@utk.edu
Web address:
http://psychology.utk.edu/gradstudy/cpphd.html

1	2	3	**4**	5	6	7

Clinically oriented   Equal emphasis   Research oriented

What percentage of your faculty subscribes to or practices in each of the following orientations?

Psychodynamic/Psychoanalytic	20%
Applied behavioral analysis/Radical behavioral	0%
Family systems/Systems	14%
Existential/Phenomenological/Humanistic	29%
Cognitive/Cognitive-behavioral	43%

What percentage of students applying for internship last year was accepted into APPIC-member internships? 60%

What courses are required for incoming students to have completed prior to enrolling?
None

Are there courses you recommend that are not mandatory?
No

GRE mean
Verbal 497   Quantitative 614
Analytical Writing 4.4

GPA mean
Overall GPA 3.67

Number of applications/admission offers/incoming students in 2005
56 applied/6 admission offers/6 incoming

% of students receiving:
Tuition waiver only: 0%
Assistantship/fellowship only: 0%
Both tuition waiver & assistantship/fellowship: 94%

Approximate percentage of incoming students who entered with a B.A./B.S. only: 67%   Master's: 33%

Approximate percentage of students who are Women: 58%   Ethnic Minority: 13%   International: 2%

Average years to complete the doctoral program (including internship): 6 years

Personal interview
Interview not required

Research areas	# Faculty	# Grants
careers	3	0
counseling process	3	0

Clinical opportunities
Assistantship available in department's psychological clinic

Tennessee State University

Department of Psychology
Nashville, TN 37209-1561
phone#: (615) 963-5141
e-mail: cblazina@tnstate.edu
Web address:
http://www.tnstate.edu/interior.asp?ptid=1&mid=878

1	2	3	**4**	5	6	7

Clinically oriented   Equal emphasis   Research oriented

What percentage of your faculty subscribes to or practices in each of the following orientations?

Psychodynamic/Psychoanalytic	60%
Applied behavioral analysis/Radical behavioral	0%
Family systems/Systems	20%
Existential/Phenomenological/Humanistic	17%
Cognitive/Cognitive-behavioral	20%

What percentage of students applying for internship last year was accepted into APPIC-member internships? 100%

What courses are required for incoming students to have completed prior to enrolling?
Learning; statistics and research methodology; counseling; intellectual assessment, personality theory, developmental or psychometrics (2 out of 3); master's-level practicum; history & systems of psychology

Are there courses you recommend that are not mandatory?
No

GRE mean
Verbal 500   Quantitative 500
Analytical Writing N/A

GPA mean
Overall GPA 3.25

Number of applications/admission offers/incoming students in 2006
28 applied/15 admission offers/11 incoming

% of students receiving:
Tuition waiver only: 0%
Assistantship/fellowship only: 10%
Both tuition waiver & assistantship/fellowship: 100%

Approximate percentage of incoming students who entered with a B.A./B.S. only: 0%   **Master's:** 100%

**Approximate percentage of students who are
Women:** 66.6%   **Ethnic Minority:** 33.3%   **International:** 1%

Average years to complete the doctoral program (including internship): 4 years

Personal interview
Preferred in person but telephone acceptable

Research areas	# Faculty	# Grants
decision making	1	0
eating disorders	2	1
men's issues	1	0
multicultural concerns	2	1
teaching of psychology	1	0

Clinical opportunities
adult, child, and adolescent psychiatry
behavioral health
forensics
university counseling center

Texas A&M University

Department of Educational Psychology
College Station, TX 77843
phone#: (409) 845-1833
e-mail: rnutt@mail.twu.edu
Web address:
http://www.twu.edu/as/psyphil/Counseling_Doctoral.htm

1	2	**3**	4	5	6	7

Clinically oriented   Equal emphasis   Research oriented

What percentage of your faculty subscribes to or practices in each of the following orientations?

Psychodynamic/Psychoanalytic	10%
Applied behavioral analysis/Radical behavioral	10%
Family systems/Systems	50%
Existential/Phenomenological/Humanistic	100%
Cognitive/Cognitive-behavioral	40%

What percentage of students applying for internship last year was accepted into APPIC-member internships? 100%

What courses are required for incoming students to have completed prior to enrolling?
Introduction to general psychology, life span development, statistics, learning, experimental psychology

Are there courses you recommend that are not mandatory?
No

GRE mean
Verbal 560   Quantitative 560
Analytical Writing Data not available

GPA mean
Overall GPA 3.8   Psychology GPA 3.5
Junior/Senior GPA 3.5

Number of applications/admission offers/incoming students in 2005
62 applied/11 admission offers/6 incoming

% of students receiving:
Tuition waiver only: 0%
Assistantship/fellowship only: 20%
Both tuition waiver & assistantship/fellowship: 20%

Approximate percentage of incoming students who entered with a B.A./B.S. only: 50%   **Master's:** 50%

**Approximate percentage of students who are
Women:** 89%   **Ethnic Minority:** 34%   **International:** 5%

Average years to complete the doctoral program (including internship): 6 years

Personal interview
Preferred in person but telephone acceptable

Research areas	# Faculty	# Grants
career development	3	1
ethics and regulation	2	0
gender issues	4	1
infidelity	1	1
marital issues	3	0
sexual harassment	3	1

Clinical opportunities
15 agency settings in the Dallas–Forth Worth metropolitan area

University of Texas at Austin

Department of Educational Psychology
D 5800
Austin, TX 78712
phone#: (512) 471-4409
e-mail: bennie.crum@mail.utexas.edu
Web address: http://edpsych.edb.utexas.edu/admissions/counseling.htm

1	2	3	4	**5**	6	7
Clinically oriented		Equal emphasis			Research oriented	

What percentage of your faculty subscribes to or practices in each of the following orientations?

Psychodynamic/Psychoanalytic	25%
Applied behavioral analysis/Radical behavioral	0%
Family systems/Systems	12.5%
Existential/Phenomenological/Humanistic	12.5%
Cognitive/Cognitive-behavioral	25%

What percentage of students applying for internship last year was accepted into APPIC-member internships? 95%

What courses are required for incoming students to have completed prior to enrolling?
6 hours in psychology

Are there courses you recommend that are not mandatory?
No

GRE mean
Verbal + Quantitative 1280
Analytical Writing Data not available

GPA mean
Overall GPA 3.5

Number of applications/admission offers/incoming students in 2005
150 applied/12 admission offers/10 incoming

% of students receiving:
Tuition waiver only: 0%
Assistantship/fellowship only: 20%
Both tuition waiver & assistantship/fellowship: 20%

Approximate percentage of incoming students who entered with a B.A./B.S. only: 70% **Master's:** 30%

Approximate percentage of students who are Women: 70% **Ethnic Minority:** 20% **International:** 5%

Average years to complete the doctoral program (including internship): 5.5 years

Personal interview
Preferred in person but telephone acceptable

Research areas

	# Faculty	# Grants
depression (cognitive-behavioral methods)	1	0
family issues	1	0
multicultural/cross-cultural issues	2	1
psychoanalysis	1	0
psychology of women	1	0

Clinical opportunities
adolescent and adult inpatient and outpatient
community practicum
immigrant/refugee clinic
inpatient units at state and VA hospitals
long-term outpatient psychotherapy clinic
university counseling centers

Texas Tech University

Department of Psychology
Lubbock, TX 79409
phone#: (806) 742-3711, ext. 231
e-mail: robert.morgan@ttu.edu
Web address: http://www.depts.ttu.edu/psy/psy.php?page=graduate/counseling/counseling

1	2	3	**4**	5	6	7
Clinically oriented		Equal emphasis			Research oriented	

What percentage of your faculty subscribes to or practices in each of the following orientations?

Psychodynamic/Psychoanalytic	20%
Applied behavioral analysis/Radical behavioral	0%
Family systems/Systems	10%
Existential/Phenomenological/Humanistic	35%
Cognitive/Cognitive-behavioral	35%

What percentage of students applying for internship last year was accepted into APPIC-member internships? 100%

What courses are required for incoming students to have completed prior to enrolling?
18 undergraduate hours in psychology and 1 statistics course

Are there courses you recommend that are not mandatory?
No

GRE mean
Verbal 529 Quantitative 627
Analytical Writing 5.0

GPA mean
Overall GPA 3.68

Number of applications/admission offers/incoming students in 2005
48 applied/10 admission offers/8 incoming

% of students receiving:
Tuition waiver only: 0%
Assistantship/fellowship only: 0%
Both tuition waiver & assistantship/fellowship: 100%

Approximate percentage of incoming students who entered with a B.A./B.S. only: 80% **Master's:** 20%

Approximate percentage of students who are Women: 100% **Ethnic Minority:** 38% **International:** 0%

Average years to complete the doctoral program (including internship): 6 years

Personal interview
Required in person

Research areas	# Faculty	# Grants
Asian Americans	1	0
behavioral addictions	1	0
cardiac rehabilitation	1	0
coping and stress	2	0
cultural differences in the self	1	0
depression	1	0
family	2	0
forensic/correctional	1	0
gender and women	2	0
group therapy	1	0
health psychology	4	0
multicultural counseling	1	0
positive psychology	1	0
professional issues	1	0
relationships	1	0
religion	1	0
sexual behavior	1	0
vocational	2	0

Clinical opportunities
child advocacy center
community mental health center and acute inpatient
    psychiatric unit
community outpatient psychology clinic
departmental outpatient psychology clinic
health sciences center
K–12 public school district
neuropsychological and personality assessment practice
psychiatric prison unit
university counseling center

Texas Woman's University

Department of Psychology and Philosophy
P.O. Box 425470
Denton, TX 76204
phone#: (940) 898-2303
e-mail: RNutt@twu.edu
Web address:
http://www.twu.edu/as/psyphil/Counseling_Doctoral.htm

1	2	**3**	4	5	6	7

Clinically oriented	Equal emphasis	Research oriented

What percentage of your faculty subscribes to or practices in each of the following orientations?

Psychodynamic/Psychoanalytic	10%
Applied behavioral analysis/Radical behavioral	10%
Family systems/Systems	50%
Existential/Phenomenological/Humanistic	100%
Cognitive/Cognitive-behavioral	40%

What percentage of students applying for internship last year was accepted into APPIC-member internships? 100%

What courses are required for incoming students to have completed prior to enrolling?
Introduction to general psychology, life span development, statistics, learning, experimental psychology

Are there courses you recommend that are not mandatory?
No

GRE mean
Verbal 560 Quantitative 560
Analytical Writing Data not available

GPA mean
Psychology GPA 3.7 Junior/Senior GPA 3.5

Number of applications/admission offers/incoming students in 2005
80 applied/9 admission offers/7 incoming

% of students receiving:
Tuition waiver only: 0%
Assistantship/fellowship only: 20%
Both tuition waiver & assistantship/fellowship: 0%

Approximate percentage of incoming students who entered with a B.A./B.S. only: 50% **Master's:** 50%

Approximate percentage of students who are Women: 80% **Ethnic Minority:** 38% **International:** 4%

Average years to complete the doctoral program (including internship): 6 years

Personal interview
Preferred in person but telephone acceptable

Research areas	# Faculty	# Grants
career development	3	1
ethics and regulation	2	0
gender issues	4	1
infidelity	1	1
marital issues	3	0
sexual harassment	3	1

Clinical opportunities
12 agency settings in the Dallas–Fort Worth metropolitan area, including:
university counseling center,
community mental health centers
domestic violence agencies
hospitals

University of Utah

Department of Educational Psychology
1705E Campus Center Drive, Room 327
Salt Lake City, UT 84112-9255
phone#: (801) 581-7148
e-mail: morrow@ed.utah.edu
Web address:
http://www.ed.utah.edu/psych/programs/CP/index.htm

1	2	3	**4**	5	6	7

Clinically oriented   Equal emphasis   Research oriented

What percentage of your faculty subscribes to or practices in each of the following orientations?

Psychodynamic/Psychoanalytic	13%
Applied behavioral analysis/Radical behavioral	0%
Ecological	4%
Family systems/Systems	0%
Existential/Phenomenological/Humanistic	0%
Cognitive/Cognitive-behavioral	25%
Feminist/Multicultural	9%
Multicultural	9%
Integrative	27%
Interpersonal	9%
Experiential	2%

What percentage of students applying for internship last year was accepted into APPIC-member internships? 100%

What courses are required for incoming students to have completed prior to enrolling?
Undergraduate and/or previous graduate preparation in psychology is required but no specific courses are required.

Are there courses you recommend that are not mandatory?
General/experimental psychology, personality, developmental, physiological, normal and abnormal behavior, elementary statistics, research methods, social psychology, and learning

GRE mean
Verbal 550   Quantitative 608   Analytical N/A
Advanced Psychology not required
Analytical Writing 4.44

GPA mean
Overall GPA 3.83

Number of applications/admission offers/incoming students in 2005
60 applied/13 admission offers/5 incoming

% of students receiving:
Tuition waiver only: 0%
Assistantship/fellowship only: 0%
Both tuition waiver & assistantship/fellowship: 100%
[reduced tuition (1/2)]

Approximate percentage of incoming students who entered with a B.A./B.S. only: 60%   **Master's:** 40%

**Approximate percentage of students who are
Women:** 80%   **Ethnic Minority:** 0%   **International:** 0%

Average years to complete the doctoral program (including internship): 6.5 years

Personal interview
Interview not required

Research areas	# Faculty	# Grants
abuse	2	1
adolescent mood disorders	1	0
applied gerontology	1	0
children and adolescents	3	2
gender and women's issues	2	0
human emotion	1	0
ethical issues	1	0
lesbian, gay, bisexual, transgender	2	0
multicultural counseling	3	0
professional education, training, & supervision	1	0
psychotherapy process and outcome, therapist factors	1	0
substance abuse prevention & treatment	1	1
women's career development: multiple role planning	1	0

Clinical opportunities
community mental health center
drug and alcohol treatment clinic
ethnic student center
family medicine health services center (outpatient medical)
gerontology services center
sexual abuse treatment unit (victims and perpetrators)
university counseling center
VA medical center (inpatient)
women's resource center

Virginia Commonwealth University

Department of Psychology
Richmond, VA 23284-2018
phone#: (804) 828-1193
Web address: http://www.has.vcu.edu/psy/counseling/
counseling_welcome.shtml

1	2	3	4	**5**	6	7

Clinically oriented   Equal emphasis   Research oriented

What percentage of your faculty subscribes to or practices in each of the following orientations?

Psychodynamic/Interpersonal	30%
Applied behavioral analysis/Radical behavioral	0%
Family systems/Systems	10%
Existential/Phenomenological/Humanistic	8%
Cognitive-behavioral/Feminist	28%
Life developmental/Life skills	8%
Eclectic/Integrative/Emotion-focused	16%

What percentage of students applying for internship last year was accepted into APPIC-member internships? 100%

What courses are required for incoming students to have completed prior to enrolling?
18 undergraduate credit hours in psychology, including statistics, experimental methods, and introductory psychology

Are there courses you recommend that are not mandatory?
No

GRE mean
Verbal 570 Quantitative 610
Analytical Writing 5.0

GPA mean
Overall GPA 3.54

Number of applications/admission offers/incoming students in 2005
143 applied/14 admission offers/9 incoming

% of students receiving:
Tuition waiver only: 0%
Assistantship/fellowship only: 0%
Both tuition waiver & assistantship/fellowship: 100%

Approximate percentage of incoming students who entered with a B.A./B.S. only: 83%   **Master's:** 17%

Approximate percentage of students who are
Women: 86%   **Ethnic Minority:** 26%   **International:** 7%

Average years to complete the doctoral program (including internship): 6.0 years

Personal interview
Preferred in person but telephone acceptable

Research areas	# Faculty	# Grants
career intervention, decision making and forensics	1	2
cultural factors in minority mental health	3	0
forgiveness/religious values	2	0
health psychology (cancer, obesity, stress & coping, eating disorders, child health, etc.)	5	5
interventions	1	1
leadership and group dynamics	1	0
marital and family enrichment	2	0
teaching of life skills/community psychology	1	1

Clinical opportunities
on-campus community mental health center
university counseling center
opportunities at external agencies (after completing required on-campus practica) include:
child treatment center
community mental health center
federal correctional center
rehabilitation medicine unit
state juvenile correctional system
state psychiatric hospital
substance abuse treatment facility
VA hospital

Washington State University

Department of Educational Leadership and Counseling Psychology
Pullman, WA 99164
phone#: (509) 335-7016
e-mail: church@mail.wsu.edu
Web address: http://www.educ.wsu.edu/elcp/documents/PhD_CounPsy.html

1	2	3	**4**	5	6	7
Clinically oriented		Equal emphasis			Research oriented	

What percentage of your faculty subscribes to or practices in each of the following orientations?

Psychodynamic/Psychoanalytic	0%
Applied behavioral analysis/Radical behavioral	0%
Family systems/Systems	10%
Existential/Phenomenological/Humanistic	40%
Cognitive/Cognitive-behavioral	50%

What percentage of students applying for internship last year was accepted into APPIC-member internships? 100%

What courses are required for incoming students to have completed prior to enrolling?
None

Are there courses you recommend that are not mandatory?
No

GRE mean
Verbal 500 Quantitative 560 Analytical 554
Analytical Writing Data not available

GPA mean
Overall GPA 3.57
Overall master's GPA 3.85

Number of applications/admission offers/incoming students in 2005
89 applied/12 admission offers/5 incoming

% of students receiving:
Tuition waiver only: 0%
Assistantship/fellowship only: 0%
Both tuition waiver & assistantship/fellowship: 75%

Approximate percentage of incoming students who entered with a B.A./B.S. only: 70%   **Master's:** 30%

Approximate percentage of students who are
Women: 58%   **Ethnic Minority:** 63%   **International:** 7%

Average years to complete the doctoral program (including internship): 6.0 years

Personal interview
Interview not required

Research areas	# Faculty	# Grants
acculturation/ethnic identity	3	0
cross-cultural/multicultural	3	1
disabilities	1	1
eating disorders	1	0
hypnosis and attentional processes	2	1
measurement/assessment	3	1

personality	1	0
resiliency	1	0
social influence	1	0
supervision	1	0
vocational	2	0

Clinical opportunities
—

West Virginia University

Department of Counseling, Rehabilitation Counseling,
and Counseling Psychology
P.O. Box 6122
Morgantown, WV 26506-6122
phone#: (304) 293-3807 x1209
e-mail: sherry.cormier@mail.wvu.edu
Web address: http://www.hre.wvu.edu/crc/
counseling_psychology/index.htm

| 1 | 2 | **3** | 4 | 5 | 6 | 7 |

Clinically oriented   Equal emphasis   Research oriented

What percentage of your faculty subscribes to or practices in each of the following orientations?

Psychodynamic/Psychoanalytic	20%
Applied behavioral analysis/Radical behavioral	0%
Family systems/Systems	20%
Existential/Phenomenological/Humanistic	40%
Cognitive/Cognitive-behavioral	20%

What percentage of students applying for internship last year was accepted into APPIC-member internships? 100%

What courses are required for incoming students to have completed prior to enrolling?
Master's degree in counseling or clinical psychology or a related field

Are there courses you recommend that are not mandatory?
Supervised field experience
Intellectual Assessment

GRE mean
Verbal 590   Quantitative 560
Analytical Writing Data not available

GPA mean
Overall GPA 3.25
Overall Graduate GPA 3.75

Number of applications/admission offers/incoming students in 2003
45 applied/9 admission offers/9 incoming

% of students receiving:
Tuition waiver only: 1%
Assistantship/fellowship only: 0%
Both tuition waiver & assistantship/fellowship: 99%

Approximate percentage of incoming students who entered with a B.A./B.S. only: 0%   **Master's:** 100%

Approximate percentage of students who are
Women: 55%   **Ethnic Minority:** 11%
International: Data not available

Average years to complete the doctoral program (including internship): 5 years

Personal interview
Required in person

Research areas	# Faculty	# Grants
clinical models of supervision	1	0
consulting models	1	0
group counseling	1	0
injured athletes	1	0
personality assessment	1	0
premature termination from counseling	1	0
psychiatric rehabilitation	1	0
psychology and mental health	3	0
psychology of disability	1	0
psychotherapeutic techniques	3	0
rehab counseling and psychology	3	0
self-efficacy and health	2	0
vocational counseling	4	0

Clinical opportunities
community agencies
correctional facilities
counseling centers
VA hospital

Western Michigan University

Department of Counselor Education
and Counseling Psychology
3102 Sangren Hall
Kalamazoo, MI 49008-5195
phone#: (616) 387-5100
Web address:
http://www.wmich.edu/cecp/programs/#doctoral

| 1 | 2 | 3 | 4 | **5** | 6 | 7 |

Clinically oriented   Equal emphasis   Research oriented

What percentage of your faculty subscribes to or practices in each of the following orientations?

Psychodynamic/Psychoanalytic	13%
Applied behavioral analysis/Radical behavioral	0%
Family systems/Systems	20%
Existential/Phenomenological/Humanistic	88%
Cognitive/Cognitive-behavioral	88%

What percentage of students applying for internship last year was accepted into APPIC-member internships? 100%

What courses are required for incoming students to have completed prior to enrolling?
—

307

Are there courses you recommend that are not mandatory?
Psychology or social science major

GRE mean
Verbal + Quantitative 1000
Analytical Writing Data not available

GPA mean
Overall Graduate GPA 3.25
Overall Undergraduate GPA 3.0

Number of applications/admission offers/incoming students in 2003
50 applied/12 admission offers/8 incoming

% of students receiving:
Tuition waiver only: 0%
Assistantship/fellowship only: 60%
Both tuition waiver & assistantship/fellowship: 40%

Approximate percentage of incoming students who entered with a B.A./B.S. only: 20%   **Master's:** 90%

Approximate percentage of students who are Women: 70%   **Ethnic Minority:** 30%
International: Data not available

Average years to complete the doctoral program (including internship): 5 years

Personal interview
Required in person

Research areas	# Faculty	# Grants
families		
group work		
multicultural concerns		
psychological assessment		
treatment issues		

Clinical opportunities
In house clinic and in local hospitals, agencies and schools.

University of Wisconsin–Madison

Department of Counseling Psychology
321 Education Building, 1000 Bascom Mall
Madison, WI 53706
phone#: (608) 263-2746
e-mail: counpsych@education.wisc.edu
Web address:
http://www.education.wisc.edu/CP/doctoralprogram.htm

1	2	3	4	**5**	6	7

Clinically oriented   Equal emphasis   Research oriented

What percentage of your faculty subscribes to or practices in each of the following orientations?

Psychodynamic/Psychoanalytic	30%
Applied behavioral analysis/Radical behavioral	0%
Family systems/Systems	10%
Existential/Phenomenological/Humanistic	40%
Cognitive/Cognitive-behavioral	30%
Multicultural	100%

What percentage of students applying for internship last year was accepted into APPIC-member internships? 60%

What courses are required for incoming students to have completed prior to enrolling?
Master's degree in counseling or admitted with deficiencies, including multicultural counseling and career psychology

Are there courses you recommend that are not mandatory?
No

GRE mean
Data not available

GPA mean
Junior/Senior GPA 3.6

Number of applications/admission offers/incoming students in 2003
79 applied/16 admission offers/8 incoming

% of students receiving:
Tuition waiver only: 0%
Assistantship/fellowship only: 10%
Both tuition waiver & assistantship/fellowship: 30%

Approximate percentage of incoming students who entered with a B.A./B.S. only: 0%   **Master's:** 95%

Approximate percentage of students who are Women: 75%   **Ethnic Minority:** 25%
International: Data not available

Average years to complete the doctoral program (including internship): 6 years

Personal interview
Telephone required

Research areas	# Faculty	# Grants
academic retention	2	0
career development	2	0
clinical supervision	1	1
corporate systems	1	0
ethnic identity	4	2
gender	4	0
group	1	0
multidisciplinary environments	2	1
multiethnic/cultural environments	5	3
process-outcome	3	0
school counseling	2	2
other	1	1

Clinical opportunities
counseling psychology

University of Wisconsin–Milwaukee

Urban Education Doctoral Program
P.O. Box 413
Milwaukee, WI 53201
Nadya Fouad, Training Director
phone#: (414) 229-4729
e-mail: nadya@uwm.edu
Web address: http://www.soe.uwm.edu/pages/
welcome/Departments/Urban_Education/Specializations/
Counseling_Psychology

1	2	3	4	5	**6**	7

Clinically oriented	Equal emphasis	Research oriented

What percentage of your faculty subscribes to or practices in each of the following orientations?

Psychodynamic/Psychoanalytic	0%
Applied behavioral analysis/Radical behavioral	0%
Developmental Systems	20%
Interpersonal	20%
Existential/Phenomenological/Humanistic	0%
Cognitive/Cognitive-behavioral	60%

What percentage of students applying for internship last year was accepted into APPIC-member internships? 66%

What courses are required for incoming students to have completed prior to enrolling?
Group counseling, listening skills, statistics, multicultural counseling, theories of counseling, cognition, career development, personality
Note: These are required master's courses; if students do not have these courses, they can complete when in the doctoral program.

Are there courses you recommend that are not mandatory?
Cognition and personality

GRE mean
Verbal 482   Quantitative 525   Analytical 532
Analytical Writing 4.2

GPA mean
Overall GPA 3.8

Number of applications/admission offers/incoming students in 2005
25 applied/8 admission offers/6 incoming

% of students receiving:
Tuition waiver only: 0%
Assistantship/fellowship only: 0%
Both tuition waiver & assistantship/fellowship: 80%

Approximate percentage of incoming students who entered with a B.A./B.S. only: 15%   **Master's:** 85%

**Approximate percentage of students who are
Women:** 75%   **Ethnic Minority:** 25%   **International:** 8%

Average years to complete the doctoral program (including internship): 5 years

Personal interview
Preferred in person but telephone acceptable

Research areas	# Faculty	# Grants
action research to improve outcomes of youth addictions	1	2
barriers for women in math/science	1	1
belongingness and academic achievement	1	1
hypnosis and hypnotizability	1	0
international research	1	2
intervention programming	1	1
masculinity, male gender role, and counseling training	1	0
multicultural counseling	2	2
pediatric behavioral health	1	0
vocational development	2	2

Clinical opportunities
children's hospital
community mental health agencies
counseling center
family services
inpatient psychiatric hospital
medical college
Veteran's administration

Counseling Psychology Programs That Have Been Discontinued

Michigan State University (accredited, inactive)

Northwestern University (accredited, inactive)

Ohio State University (accredited, inactive)

University of Pittsburgh (accredited, inactive)

University of Southern California (accredited, inactive)

Stanford University (accredited, inactive)

Temple University (accredited, inactive)

APPENDIX A
TIME LINE

Freshman and Sophomore Years

1. Take the core psychology courses—introduction, statistics, research methods, abnormal, physiological.
2. Find out about faculty interests and research.
3. Make preliminary contact with faculty members whose research interests you.
4. Explore volunteer opportunities in clinical settings.
5. Investigate various career choices.
6. Join psychology student organizations and become an active member.
7. Attend departmental colloquia and social gatherings.
8. Enroll in courses helpful for graduate school, including biological sciences, mathematics, writing, and public speaking.
9. Learn to use library and electronic resources, such as scholarly journals and PsycLit.
10. Consider participating in your university's honors program, if you qualify.
11. Begin a career folder and place activities, honors, and other valuable reminders in it.

Junior Year

1. Take more advanced psychology courses, for example, cognitive, developmental, psychological testing.
2. Begin clinical work, both volunteer and practicum.
3. Volunteer for research with faculty and begin researching a potential honors thesis/independent project.

4. Continue contact with faculty and upperclassmen.
5. Enroll in professional organizations, for example, student affiliate of American Psychological Association or American Psychological Society.
6. Apply for membership in your local Psi Chi chapter.
7. Draft a curriculum vitae to determine your strengths and weaknesses.
8. Attend a state or regional psychology convention.
9. Peruse graduate school bulletins to acquaint yourself with typical requirements, offerings, and policies.
10. Surf the Web. Become comfortable with leading Web sites on graduate school admissions.
11. Update your folder by putting your curriculum vita/resume and reminders of your activities and accomplishments in it.
12. Try to focus your interests in particular research areas, theoretical orientations, and clinical populations.
13. Consider serving as an officer in one of the student organizations on campus.

Application Year

June–August

1. Continue to acquire research competencies, clinical experiences—about 20 to 40.
2. Surf the Web and begin to gather information from program Web sites.
3. Begin to narrow down potential schools to 20–40.
4. Prepare for the GREs.
5. Consider taking the GRE General Test if you are prepared; this will afford ample time to retake them in the fall if necessary.

6. Investigate financial aid opportunities for graduate students.
7. Set aside money for the cost of the GREs and applications.

August–September

1. Download program information and applications from program Web sites and/or write to schools for applications.
2. Receive information packets and read through them.
3. Consult with advisors regarding graduate programs, application procedures, faculty of interest, etc.
4. Continue to study diligently for the GREs.
5. Update your curriculum vitae.
6. Investigate possible financial aid opportunities.
7. Begin a file in your institution's Office of Career Services/Planning.
8. Gather applications for salient fellowships and scholarships.

September–October

1. Take the GRE General Test.
2. Register for the GRE Psychology Subject Test administered in November and December.
3. Create a short list of schools using the worksheets.
4. Record the deadlines for submitting each application.
5. Choose the faculty at each school that most interest you.
6. Research your area of interest, focusing on the work of faculty with whom you would like to work.
7. Write to graduate faculty expressing interest in their work (if appropriate).
8. Request a copy of your own transcript and inspect it for any errors or omissions.
9. Begin first drafts of your personal statement.
10. Update your CV or resume.

October–November

1. Take the GRE Psychology Subject Test.
2. Take the MAT (only if necessary).

3. Prepare letters to your recommenders, including a complete vitae or resume.
4. Request letters of recommendation.
5. Arrange for the registrar to send your transcripts to schools.
6. Gather information on financial aid and loans available to graduate students.
7. Finalize your personal statements.

November–December

1. Complete applications.
2. Maintain a photocopy of each application for your records.
3. If the opportunity arises, visit professors with whom you have been in contact.
4. Submit applications.
5. Verify that the applications and all necessary materials have been received.
6. Request ETS forward your GRE scores to the appropriate institutions.

January–March

1. Wait patiently.
2. Insure that all of your letters of recommendation have been sent.
3. Be prepared for surprise telephone interviews.
4. Practice and prepare for interviews.
5. Travel to interviews as invited.
6. Develop contingency plans if not accepted into any programs.

April–May

1. If other programs make early offers, call your top choices to determine the current status of your application.
2. Accept an offer of admission and promptly turn down less-preferred offers.
3. Send official transcripts with Spring term grades to the program you plan to attend.
4. If not accepted to any schools, refer to Chapter 7.

A P P E N D I X   B

WORKSHEET FOR CHOOSING SCHOOLS

| Area of Interest | School | Research | | | Clinical | | | Self-Rating |
		# Faculty	Funded	Rank	Orienta-tion	Res/Clin	Rank	

Area of Interest	School	Research			Clinical			
		# Faculty	Funded	Rank	Orienta-tion	Res/Clin	Rank	Self-Rating

APPENDIX C

WORKSHEET FOR ASSESSING PROGRAM CRITERIA

School	Self-Rating	Courses	GRE-V	GRE-Q	GRE-S	GPA	Research	Clinical	Compete	**Total**

APPENDIX D

WORKSHEET
FOR MAKING
FINAL CHOICES

School	School Criteria	Research	Clinical	Theoretical Orientation	Financial Aid	Quality of Life

A P P E N D I X   E

RESEARCH AREAS

	# Faculty	# Grants

Acquired Immune Deficiency Syndrome/HIV

Arizona State University (Co)	1	0
Azusa Pacific University (Cl)	1	0
Binghamton University/State University of New York (Cl)	1	1
Colorado State University (Co)	1	0
DePaul University (Cl)	1	3
George Washington University (Ph.D.) (Cl)	1	2
Georgia State University (Cl)	1	1
Indiana State University (Co)	1	0
Jackson State University (Cl)	3	3
Kent State University (Cl)	1	1
Loyola University–Chicago (Cl)	2	1
San Diego State University/University of California–San Diego (Cl)	7	1
Southern Illinois University (Cl)	1	0
Syracuse University (Cl)	2	2
University of Georgia (Cl)	1	0
University of Illinois at Chicago (Cl)	1	1
University of Maryland (Co)	1	0
University of Memphis (Co)	1	1
University of Miami (Cl)	6	2+
University of Missouri–Kansas City (Co)	1	1
University of North Dakota (Co)	1	1
University of North Texas (Cl)	1	0
University of Wyoming (Cl)	1	3
Virginia Polytechnic Institute and State University (Cl)	2	0
Western Michigan University (Cl)	1	1

Adjustment

Biola University (Ph.D.) (Cl)	4	0
Biola University (Psy.D.) (Cl)	4	0
Bowling Green State University (Cl)	2	0
Regent University (Cl)	1	0
St. Louis University (Cl)	2	0
University of Massachusetts at Amherst (Cl)	1	0

University of Minnesota (Co)	1	0
Yale University (Cl)	1	1

Adolescent/At-Risk Adolescent

Alliant International University–Fresno (Psy. D.) (Cl)	1	2
Alliant International University–Los Angeles (Psy.D.) (Cl)	2	0
Alliant International University–San Diego (Ph.D. & Psy.D.) (Cl)	5	0
Argosy University, Atlanta (Psy.D.)	1	1
Argosy University, Chicago (Psy.D.)	1	1
Ball State University (Co)	2	0
Carlos Albizu University–Miami Campus (Cl)	3	0
Carlos Albizu University–San Juan (Ph.D.) (Cl)	3	1
Catholic University of America (Cl)	3	1
Colorado State University (Co)	3	5
Dalhousie University (Cl)	1	1
Emory University (Cl)	2	0
Florida State University (Cl)	4	5
George Fox University (Cl)	1	1
George Washington University (Ph.D.) (Cl)	2	2
Immaculata College (Cl)	2	0
Indiana University (Co)	1	2
Loyola University–Chicago (Cl)	3	4
Loyola University–Chicago (Co)	1	1
Northern Illinois University (Cl)	3	0
Northwestern University, Feinberg School of Medicine (Cl)	3	3
Nova Southeastern University (Ph.D. & Psy.D.) (Cl)	5	0
Oklahoma State University (Co)	2	1
Rosalind Franklin University of Medicine (Cl)	1	0
Rutgers University (Psy.D.) (Cl)	4	1
St. Louis University (Cl)	2	0
Suffolk University (Cl)	2	0

Note. Cl, Clinical; Co, Counseling; Cm, combined professional–scientific psychology programs.

	# Faculty	# Grants
Southern Illinois University (Cl)	2	0
Temple University (Cl)	2	9
Texas Tech University (Cl)	1	0
University of Cincinnati	2	1
University of Denver (Ph.D.) (Cl)	2	2
University of Georgia (Cl)	1	1
University of Hartford (Cl)	1	0
University of Houston (Co)	1	1
University of Kentucky (Cl)	1	0
University of Minnesota—Department of Educational Psychology (Co)	2	1
University of Missouri–Columbia (Co)	1	2
University of Nebraska–Lincoln (Cl)	2	1
University of North Carolina at Chapel Hill (Cl)	1	1
University of North Carolina at Greensboro (Cl)	1	0
University of Northern Colorado (Co)	2	2
University of Pittsburgh (Cl)	7	10
University of South Florida (Cl)	2	0
University of Southern California (Cl)	1	0
University of Toledo (Cl)	2	0
University of Utah (Cl)	1	0
University of Vermont (Cl)	2	1
University of Virginia—Department of Human Services (Cl)	3	3
University of Wisconsin–Milwaukee (Co)	1	1
University of Wyoming (Cl)	2	2
Utah State University (Cm)	2	1
Virginia Commonwealth University (Cl)	4	3
Yeshiva University (Cm)	2	0
York University—Clinical-Developmental Area (Cl)	3	3

Affective Disorders/Depression/ Mood Disorders

	# Faculty	# Grants
Alliant International University– San Diego (Ph.D. & Psy.D.) (Cl)	5	0
American University (Cl)	1	0
Baylor University (Psy.D.) (Cl)	3	0
Binghamton University/State University of New York (Cl)	1	1
Boston University (Cl)	2	2
Carlos Albizu University–Miami Campus (Cl)	3	0
Catholic University of America (Cl)	2	0
Clark University (Cl)	1	1
Colorado State University (Co)	1	0
Dalhousie University (Cl)	2	5
Duke University (Cl)	3	2
Fairleigh Dickinson University (Cl)	1	0
Florida State University (Cl)	3	3
Forest Institute of Professional Psychology (Cl)	2	1
Fuller Theological Seminary (Ph.D. & Psy.D.) (Cl)	1	0
Gallaudet University (Cl)	1	1
George Washington University (Ph.D.) (Cl)	1	1
Georgia State University (Cl)	1	0

	# Faculty	# Grants
Hofstra University (Cm)	1	0
Illinois Institute of Technology (Cl)	1	1
Indiana State University (Cl)	2	0
Jackson State University (Cl)	1	0
James Madison University (Cm)	1	0
Kent State University (Cl)	1	0
Louisiana State University (Cl)	1	1
Loyola University–Chicago (Cl)	1	0
Marquette University (Cl)	1	0
McGill University (Cl)	2	2
Northwestern University (Cl)	2	0
Ohio State University (Cl)	3	1
Pennsylvania State University (Cl)	2	0
Purdue University (Cl)	1	0
Rutgers University (Ph.D.) (Cl)	1	0
St. Louis University (Cl)	2	0
San Diego State University/University of California–San Diego (Cl)	3	2
Simon Fraser University (Cl)	2	1
Southern Illinois University (Cl)	2	0
Stony Brook University/State University of New York (Cl)	1	1
Temple University (Cl)	1	2
Texas Tech University (Cl)	1	1
Texas Tech University (Co)	1	0
Uniformed Services University of Health Sciences (Cl)	1	2
University of Alabama (Cl)	1	1
University of Arizona (Cl)	2	1
University of Arkansas (Cl)	2	0
University at Buffalo/State University of New York (Cl)	1	1
University of California–Los Angeles (Cl)	1	2
University of Colorado (Cl)	3	2
University of Georgia (Cl)	3	0
University of Hawaii at Manoa (Cl)	2	0
University of Houston (Cl)	3	1
University of Illinois at Chicago (Cl)	1	0
University of Iowa (Cl)	2	2
University of Maine (Cl)	1	0
University of Miami (Cl)	3	1
University of Minnesota (Cl)	3	1
University of Missouri–Columbia (Cl)	1	1
University of Montana (Cl)	1	0
University of Nevada–Reno (Cl)	1	0
University of North Carolina at Greensboro (Cl)	1	0
University of North Dakota (Co)	3	1
University of Oregon (Cl)	3	2
University of Pennsylvania (Cl)	3	4
University of Pittsburgh (Cl)	5	7
University of South Dakota (Cl)	2	0
University of South Florida (Cl)	1	0
University of Texas at Austin (Co)	1	1
University of Texas Southwestern Medical Center at Dallas (Cl)	5	4
University of Washington (Cl)	3	1
University of Waterloo (Cl)	1	1
University of Western Ontario (Cl)	1	1
University of Wisconsin–Madison (Cl)	5	8
University of Wisconsin-Milwaukee (Cl)	1	1
University of Wyoming (Cl)	2	1
Vanderbilt University (Cl)	4	4

	# Faculty	# Grants
Virginia Consortium Program in Clinical Psychology (Cl)	2	1
Virginia Polytechnic Institute and State University (Cl)	2	0
Washington State University (Cl)	1	0
Western Michigan University (Cl)	2	0
Yale University (Cl)	1	1
Yeshiva University (Psy.D.) (Cl)	2	0
York University—Adult Clinical Program (Cl)	1	2

Aging/Gerontology/Adult Development

Adelphi University (Cl)	1	1
Adler School of Professional Psychology (Cl)	1	0
Argosy University, Atlanta (Ph.D.) (Cl)	2	0
Arizona State University (Cl)	3	3
Boston University (Cl)	2	2
Carlos Albizu University–Miami Campus (Cl)	1	0
Carlos Albizu University–San Juan (Psy.D.) (Cl)	2	0
Carlos Albizu University–San Juan (Ph.D.) (Cl)	1	1
Case Western Reserve University (Cl)	2	1
Colorado State University (Co)	3	2
Columbia University, Teachers College (Cl)	1	1
Florida Institute of Technology (Cl)	2	0
Idaho State University (Cl)	1	0
Kent State University (Cl)	1	0
Long Island University (Cl)	1	1
Loyola College in Maryland (Cl)	2	0
Marquette University (Cl)	2	0
McGill University (Cl)	2	1
Michigan State University (Cl)	1	0
Nova Southeastern University (Ph.D. & Psy.D.) (Cl)	2	0
Rosalind Franklin University of Medicine (Cl)	1	1
San Diego State University/University of California–San Diego (Cl)	14	1
Texas A&M University (Cl)	2	1
University of Alabama (Cl)	3	3
University of Alabama at Birmingham (Cl)	3	6
University of California–Berkeley (Cl)	1	1
University of Connecticut (Cl)	1	0
University of Florida (Co)	1	0
University of Georgia (Cl)	1	1
University of Louisville (Cl)	2	0
University of Massachusetts at Amherst (Cl)	2	0
University of Missouri–St. Louis (Cl)	1	4
University of Nevada–Reno (Cl)	2	3
University of North Carolina at Chapel Hill (Cl)	2	1
University of North Texas (Cl)	1	1
University of North Texas (Co)	1	1
University of St. Thomas (Co)	1	0

University of Southern California (Cl)	3	3
University of Texas Southwestern Medical Center at Dallas (Cl)	1	1
University of Tulsa (Cl)	1	0
University of Utah (Co)	1	2
University of Victoria (Cl)	1	1
Washington University (Cl)	2	5
West Virginia University (Cl)	1	0
Western Michigan University (Cl)	1	1
Wheaton College (Cl)	1	0
Wright Institute (Cl)	1	0
Xavier University (Cl)	2	0
Yeshiva University (Psy.D.) (Cl)	1	1
York University—Adult Clinical Program (Cl)	1	2

Aggression/Anger Control

Carlos Albizu University–San Juan (Ph.D.) (Cl)	1	3
Central Michigan University (Cl)	1	0
Colorado State University (Co)	1	1
Hofstra University (Cm)	2	0
Kent State University (Cl)	1	1
Long Island University–C.W. Post Campus (Cl)	1	0
McGill University (Cl)	1	1
Northern Illinois University (Cl)	1	0
University of Arkansas (Cl)	3	1
University of Georgia (Cl)	1	1
University of Georgia (Co)	2	2
University of Illinois at Urbana–Champaign (Co)	1	0
University of Kentucky (Cl)	2	2
University of Southern Mississippi (Co)	1	0
York University—Clinical-Developmental Area (Cl)	5	4

Anxiety Disorders/Panic Disorders

American University (Cl)	1	0
Auburn University (Cl)	2	1
Binghamton University/State University of New York (Cl)	2	1
Boston University (Cl)	7	5
Catholic University of America (Cl)	3	0
Central Michigan University (Cl)	1	1
Colorado State University (Co)	1	1
Concordia University (Cl)	2	3
Dalhousie University (Cl)	2	6
Drexel University (Cl)	1	0
Florida State University (Cl)	3	3
George Washington University (Ph.D.) (Cl)	1	0
Georgia State University (Cl)	1	1
Indiana State University (Psy.D.) (Cl)	1	0
Indiana University–Purdue University Indianapolis (Cl)	2	1
Kent State University (Cl)	2	0
Loma Linda University (Ph.D. & Psy.D.) (Cl)	1	0
Louisiana State University (Cl)	1	1

	# Faculty	# Grants
Loyola College in Maryland (Cl)	1	0
Miami University (Cl)	3	0
Michigan State University (Cl)	1	2
Northern Illinois University (Cl)	3	0
Northwestern University (Cl)	2	1
Nova Southeastern University (Ph.D. & Psy.D.) (Cl)	1	0
Ohio State University (Cl)	2	1
Oklahoma State University (Cl)	1	0
Ontario Institute for Studies in Education (Cm)	2	2
Pacific University (Cl)	2	0
Pennsylvania State University (Cl)	7	3
Purdue University (Cl)	1	0
Rosalind Franklin University of Medicine (Cl)	1	1
Rutgers University (Psy.D.) (Cl)	3	1
St. John's University (Cl)	2	0
San Diego State University/University of California–San Diego (Cl)	4	1
Southern Illinois University (Cl)	3	0
Temple University (Cl)	1	2
Texas A&M University (Cl)	3	1
Texas Tech University (Cl)	1	1
University of Arkansas (Cl)	2	0
University at Albany/State University of New York (Cl)	1	0
University at Albany/State University of New York (Co)	1	0
University at Buffalo/State University of New York (Cl)	3	2
University of British Columbia (Cl)	3	5
University of California–Los Angeles (Cl)	1	3
University of Connecticut (Cl)	1	0
University of Delaware (Cl)	2	1
University of Florida (Cl)	2	3
University of Georgia (Cl)	1	0
University of Hawaii at Manoa (Cl)	1	1
University of Houston (Cl)	3	1
University of Illinois at Chicago (Cl)	1	0
University of Iowa (Co)	1	0
University of Louisville (Cl)	3	1
University of Maine (Cl)	2	0
University of Manitoba (Cl)	4	0
University of Maryland (Cl)	2	2
University of Minnesota (Cl)	3	1
University of Missouri–Columbia (Cl)	1	1
University of Nebraska–Lincoln (Cl)	2	2
University of Nevada–Reno (Cl)	2	0
University of North Dakota (Cl)	1	0
University of Oregon (Cl)	2	2
University of Pennsylvania (Cl)	2	5
University of St. Thomas (Co)	2	1
University of Texas at Austin (Cl)	1	0
University of Vermont (Cl)	1	3
University of Virginia—Department of Psychology (Cl)	1	0
University of Washington (Cl)	3	1
University of Waterloo (Cl)	1	1
University of Wisconsin–Milwaukee (Cl)	2	1
Virginia Commonwealth University (Cl)	2	0
Virginia Consortium Program in Clinical Psychology (Cl)	2	0
Virginia Polytechnic Institute and State University (Cl)	3	1
West Virginia University (Cl)	2	0
Western Michigan University (Cl)	1	0
Yale University (Cl)	2	0
Yeshiva University (Psy.D.) (Cl)	1	0
York University—Adult Clinical Program (Cl)	1	1

Assessment/Diagnosis

	# Faculty	# Grants
Alliant International University–San Diego (Psy.D.) (Cl)	1	0
Binghamton University/State University of New York (Cl)	4	0
Brigham Young University (Cl)	2	0
Catholic University of America (Cl)	2	0
Central Michigan University (Cl)	1	0
Clark University (Cl)	1	0
Colorado State University (Co)	3	1
Fairleigh Dickinson University (Cl)	6	2
Fordham University (Cl)	3	0
Gallaudet University (Cl)	1	1
George Fox University (Cl)	1	1
George Washington University (Psy.D.) (Cl)	3	0
Indiana State University (Cl)	2	0
Indiana State University (Psy.D.) (Cl)	1	0
Jackson State University (Cl)	6	0
McGill University (Cl)	2	0
New School University (Cl)	2	1
New York University (Co)	2	2
Ohio State University (Co)	3	0
Oklahoma State University (Co)	1	0
Pacific Graduate School of Psychology (Cl)	5	1
Rutgers University (Psy.D.) (Cl)	2	0
St. Louis University (Cl)	3	0
Suffolk University (Cl)	1	0
San Diego State University/University of California–San Diego (Cl)	4	0
Southern Illinois University (Cl)	8	0
Texas A&M University (Cl)	3	0
Texas Tech University (Cl)	2	0
University of Alabama (Cl)	1	0
University of Colorado (Cl)	2	2
University of Detroit–Mercy (Cl)	1	0
University of Iowa (Cl)	1	0
University of Kentucky (Cl)	3	0
University of Mississippi (Cl)	2	0
University of Montana (Cl)	1	0
University of Nebraska–Lincoln (Co)	1	0
University of Nevada–Reno (Cl)	3	0
University of North Carolina at Chapel Hill (Cl)	1	0
University of North Carolina at Greensboro (Cl)	1	0
University of Oklahoma (Co)	3	0

	# Faculty	# Grants
University of Southern California (Cl)	2	0
Virginia Consortium Program in Clinical Psychology (Cl)	5	0
University of Western Ontario (Cl)	1	0
Washington State University (Co)	3	1
Western Michigan University (Co)		
Widener University (Cl)	1	0
Yeshiva University (Cm)	2	0

Attachment

Alliant International University–Fresno (Ph.D.) (Cl)	1	0
Catholic University of America (Cl)	2	0
City University of New York at City College (Cl)	3	1
Iowa State University (Co)	1	0
James Madison University (Cm)	1	0
Long Island University–C.W. Post Campus (Cl)	1	0
Purdue University (Co)	1	0
Stony Brook University/State University of New York (Cl)	1	1
University of Delaware (Cl)	2	2
University of Houston (Co)		
University of Southern Mississippi (Co)	3	0
University of Wisconsin–Milwaukee (Cl)	2	0
Virginia Consortium Program in Clinical Psychology (Cl)		
Yeshiva University (Cm)	3	0

Attention-Deficit/Hyperactivity Disorder

Argosy University, Chicago Northwest (Psy.D.)	1	0
Argosy University–Pheonix (Cl)	1	0
Carlos Albizu University–San Juan (Ph.D.) (Cl)	1	0
Colorado State University (Co)	1	0
Emory University (Cl)	1	1
Illinois Institute of Technology (Cl)	1	0
Marquette University (Cl)	1	0
McGill University (Cl)	1	1
Michigan State University (Cl)	1	3
Nova Southeastern University (Ph.D. & Psy.D.) (Cl)	3	0
Ontario Institute for Studies in Education (Cm)	4	9
Pepperdine University (Cl)	1	2
Purdue University (Cl)	1	3
Regent University (Cl)	1	0
University at Buffalo/State University of New York (Cl)	3	8
University of British Columbia (Cl)	1	2
University of California–Berkeley (Cl)	1	2
University of Houston (Co)	1	1
University of Montana (Cl)	1	0
University of North Carolina at Greensboro (Cl)	1	2
University of Pittsburgh (Cl)	2	2

University of Rochester (Cl)	1	1
University of Texas at Austin (Cl)	1	1
University of Toledo (Cl)	2	0
University of Victoria (Cl)	1	1
Utah State University (Cm)	1	0
Virginia Consortium Program in Clinical Psychology (Cl)	1	0
Virginia Polytechnic Institute and State University (Cl)	1	0
Washington State University (Co)	2	1
West Virginia University (Cl)	2	1
Yeshiva University (Cm)	2	0

Attitudes, Beliefs, and Values

Arizona State University (Co)	1	0
Hofstra University (Cm)	2	0
Immaculata College (Cl)	1	0
Indiana State University (Co)	1	0
James Madison University (Cm)	3	0
Southern Illinois University (Cl)	1	0

Autism/Pervasive Developmental Disorder

Louisiana State University (Cl)	1	1
Rutgers University (Ph.D.) (Cl)	1	1
Rutgers University (Psy.D.) (Cl)	1	1
San Diego State University/University of California–San Diego (Cl)	2	0
St. John's University (Cl)	1	1
University at Albany/State University of New York (Cl)	1	1
University at Buffalo/State University of New York (Cl)	1	1
University of California–Santa Barbara (Cm)	1	2
University of Connecticut (Cl)	1	3
University of Illinois at Chicago (Cl)	1	4
University of Pittsburgh (Cl)	2	3
Vandrerbilt University (Cl)	1	1
Virginia Polytechnic Institute and State University (Cl)	1	0
University of Rochester (Cl)	2	2
University of Texas at Austin (Cl)	1	1
University of Wisconsin–Milwaukee (Cl)	1	1
Western Michigan University (Cl)	1	1
York University—Clinical-Developmental Area (Cl)	2	2

Behavior Therapy/Applied Behavioral Analysis

Hofstra University (Cm)	3	0
McGill University (Cl)	1	0
Nova Southeastern University (Ph.D. & Psy.D.) (Cl)	8	0
Rutgers University (Ph.D.) (Cl)	2	0
Rutgers University (Psy.D.) (Cl)	1	1
San Diego State University/University of California–San Diego (Cl)	4	0
University of Denver (Psy.D.) (Cl)	1	0

	# Faculty	# Grants
University of Georgia (Cl)	1	0
University of Kentucky (Co)	2	1
University of Manitoba (Cl)	3	2
University of Nevada–Reno (Cl)	3	0
University of North Carolina at Greensboro (Cl)	1	0
University of North Dakota (Cl)	2	0
University of Wisconsin–Milwaukee (Cl)	3	4
Virginia Consortium Program in Clinical Psychology (Cl)	1	0
Yeshiva University (Cl)	1	0
Yeshiva University (Cm)	2	0

Behavioral Genetics

Boston University (Cl)	1	1
Emory University (Cl)	2	1
Indiana University (Cl)	4	2
McGill University (Cl)	1	1
Northwestern University (Cl)	1	0
Southern Illinois University (Cl)	1	0
University of Denver (Ph.D.) (Cl)	1	1
University of Illinois at Urbana–Champaign (Cl)	1	0
University of Minnesota (Cl)	4	4
University of Pittsburgh (Cl)	3	4
University of Virginia (Cl)	2	1

Behavioral Medicine/Health Psychology

Adelphi University (Cl)	1	1
Alliant International University–Fresno (Psy.D.) (Cl)	1	0
Alliant International University–Los Angeles (Ph.D. & Psy.D.) (Cl)	9	2
Alliant International University–San Diego (Ph.D. & Psy.D.) (Cl)	8	3
Alliant International University–San Francisco (Ph.D.) (Cl)	5	2
Alliant International University–San Francisco (Psy.D.) (Cl)	4	0
Antioch/New England Graduate School (Cl)	1	1
Argosy University, Atlanta (Psy.D.)	3	0
Argosy University, Chicago (Psy.D.)	3	0
Argosy University–Honolulu Campus (Cl)	3	0
Arizona State University (Cl)	11	10
Arizona State University (Co)	1	0
Ball State University (Co)	1	0
Baylor University (Cl)	1	0
Binghamton University/State University of New York (Cl)	1	1
Bowling Green State University (Cl)	2	1
Brigham Young University (Cl)	2	1
Carlos Albizu University–San Juan (Psy.D.) (Cl)	1	0
Case Western Reserve University (Cl)	1	0
Central Michigan University (Cl)	1	1
Chicago School of Professional Psychology (Cl)	2	0

Colorado State University (Co)	3	3
Concordia University (Cl)	2	2
Drexel University (Cl)	2	0
Duke University (Cl)	4	6
Fairleigh Dickinson University (Cl)	3	1
Fielding Graduate Institute (Cl)	—	—
Florida Institute of Technology (Cl)	3	2
Fordham University (Cl)	1	0
Fordham University (Co)	2	1
Fuller Theological Seminary (Ph.D. & Psy.D.) (Cl)	3	0
George Washington University (Ph.D.) (Cl)	2	0
Howard University (Cl)	3	3
Illinois Institute of Technology (Cl)	1	1
Indiana State University (Cl)	3	1
Indiana State University (Co)	1	0
Indiana University (Cl)	5	4
Indiana University of Pennsylvania (Cl)	1	0
Indiana University–Purdue University Indianapolis (Cl)	3	1
Loma Linda University (Ph.D. & Psy.D.) (Cl)	4	2
Long Island University (Cl)	1	1
Loyola College in Maryland (Cl)	3	0
McGill University (Cl)	4	4
Nova Southeastern University (Ph.D. & Psy.D.) (Cl)	7	2
Ohio State University (Cl)	5	7
Ohio State University (Co)	2	0
Ohio University (Cl)	3	4
Oklahoma State University (Cl)	2	0
Oklahoma State University (Co)	2	1
Pacific Graduate School of Psychology (Cl)	2	1
Pacific University (Cl)	1	0
Pennsylvania State University (Cl)	2	0
Rosalind Franklin University of Medicine (Cl)	2	0
Rutgers University (Ph.D.) (Cl)	5	6
Rutgers University (Psy.D.) (Cl)	1	0
St. John's University (Cl)	3	1
San Diego State University/University of California–San Diego (Cl)	22	3
Simon Fraser University (Cl)	1	0
Southern Illinois University (Cl)	2	0
Southern Illinois University (Co)	1	0
Spalding University (Cl)	2	1
St. John's University (Cl)	2	1
Suffolk University (Cl)	1	0
Texas A&M University (Cl)	2	1
Texas Tech University (Cl)	3	1
Texas Tech University (Co)	4	0
Uniformed Services University of Health Sciences (Cl)	2	5
University of Alabama (Cl)	3	1
University of Alabama at Birmingham (Cl)	2	2
University at Albany/State University of New York (Cl)	2	0
University at Buffalo/State University of New York (Cl)	1	1

	# Faculty	# Grants
University at Buffalo/State University of New York (Cl)	4	0
University of Arizona (Cl)	6	6
University of British Columbia (Cl)	1	2
University of California–Los Angeles (Cl)	6	7
University of Cincinnati (Cl)	5	2
University of Connecticut (Cl)	3	2
University of Denver (Psy.D.) (Cl)	1	0
University of Denver (Co)	1	0
University of Florida (Cl)	3	3
University of Florida (Co)	2	1
University of Georgia (Cl)	2	0
University of Georgia (Co)	1	0
University of Hawaii at Manoa (Cl)	1	0
University of Illinois at Chicago (Cl)	4	1
University of Iowa (Cl)	3	3
University of Iowa (Co)	6	4
University of Kansas (Cl)	2	1
University of Kansas (Co)	1	0
University of Kentucky (Cl)	2	1
University of Kentucky (Co)	2	0
University of Louisville (Cl)	2	1
University of Maine (Cl)	1	0
University of Manitoba (Cl)	2	1
University of Maryland–Baltimore County (Cl)	5	4
University of Maryland (Co)	2	0
University of Memphis (Cl)	4	7
University of Miami (Cl)	14	2
University of Miami (Co)	2	1
University of Michigan (Cl)	2	0
University of Minnesota—Department of Psychology (Co)	2	0
University of Mississippi (Cl)	1	0
University of Missouri–Columbia (Cl)	3	2
University of Missouri–Columbia (Co)	2	1
University of Missouri–Kansas City (Co)	4	3
University of Missouri–Kansas City (Co)	1	1
University of Montana (Cl)	3	1
University of Nevada–Reno (Cl)	2	0
University of New Mexico (Cl)	3	0
University of North Carolina at Chapel Hill (Cl)	1	2
University of North Dakota (Cl)	2	0
University of North Dakota (Co)	1	0
University of Notre Dame (Co)	1	1
University of Oklahoma (Co)	3	0
University of Ottawa (Cl)	3	5
University of Pittsburgh (Cl)	20	44
University of Rhode Island (Cl)	3	10
University of Saskatchewan (Cl)	3	3
University of South Dakota (Cl)	2	0
University of South Florida (Cl)	7	10
University of Southern California (Cl)	3	5
University of Tennessee (Cl)	1	1
University of Texas at Austin (Cl)	1	1
University of Texas Southwestern Medical Center at Dallas (Cl)	4	4
University of Utah (Cl)	2	3
University of Vermont (Cl)	2	2

	# Faculty	# Grants
University of Western Ontario (Cl)	4	2
University of Wisconsin–Madison (Cl)	3	3
University of Wisconsin–Milwaukee (Cl)	2	0
Utah State University (Cm)	2	1
Vanderbilt University (Cl)	5	5
Virginia Commonwealth University (Cl)	4	3
Virginia Commonwealth University (Co)	5	5
Virginia Polytechnic Institute and State University (Cl)	3	2
Washington State University (Cl)	5	8
Wayne State University (Cl)	2	2
West Virginia University (Cl)	6	4
West Virginia University (Co)	2	0
Western Michigan University (Cl)	1	1
Wright State University (Cl)	3	1
Yale University (Cl)	2	1
York University—Adult Clinical Program (Cl)	1	4

Biofeedback/Relaxation

	# Faculty	# Grants
Fuller Theological Seminary (Ph.D. & Psy.D.) (Cl)	1	0
George Washington University (Ph.D.) (Cl)	1	0
Hofstra University (Cm)	1	0
Loyola University–Chicago (Cl)	2	0
Nova Southeastern University (Ph.D. & Psy.D.) (Cl)	2	0
Pennsylvania State University (Cl)	2	1
San Diego State University/University of California–San Diego (Cl)	1	0
Virginia Consortium Program in Clinical Psychology (Cl)	1	0

Biopsychology

	# Faculty	# Grants
Fuller Theological Seminary (Ph.D. & Psy.D.) (Cl) (biopsychosocial)	3	2
Indiana University–Purdue University Indianapolis (Cl)	3	6
Loma Linda University (Ph.D. & Psy.D.) (Cl)	2	0

Brain Injury/Head Injury

	# Faculty	# Grants
Georgia State University (Cl)	3	0
James Madison University (Cm)	1	0
Regent University (Cl)	1	1
San Diego State University/University of California–San Diego (Cl)	2	0
Southern Illinois University (Co)	1	0
University of Montana (Cl)	1	0
University of Victoria (Cl)	2	2

Child Abuse/Neglect/Sexual Abuse

	# Faculty	# Grants
Alliant International University–San Diego (Psy.D.) (Cl)	2	1
Clark University (Cl)	1	1

	# Faculty	# Grants
Columbia University, Teachers College (Cl)	1	1
DePaul University (Cl)	1	1
Drexel University (Cl)	1	0
Loma Linda University (Ph.D. & Psy.D.) (Cl)	2	0
Marquette University (Co)	1	0
Northern Illinois University (Cl)	1	2
Ontario Institute for Studies in Education (Cm)	2	1
St. John's University (Cl)	1	2
Southern Illinois University (Cl)	1	0
State University of New York at Buffalo (Cl)	1	1
Texas Tech University (Cl)	1	0
University of Iowa (Cl)	2	2
University of Michigan (Cl)	1	0
University of Missouri–St. Louis (Cl)	1	1
University of Nebraska–Lincoln (Cl)	2	2
University of Rochester (Cl)	1	4
University of Saskatchewan (Cl)	1	1
University of Southern California (Cl)	3	2
University of Victoria (Cl)	1	0
University of Wyoming (Cl)	2	2
Virginia Consortium Program in Clinical Psychology (Cl)	1	0
York University—Clinical-Developmental Area (Cl)	3	2

Child/Child Clinical/Pediatric

	# Faculty	# Grants
Adler School of Professional Psychology (Cl)	2	0
Alliant International University–Los Angeles (Ph.D.) (Cl)	2	0
Alliant International University–San Diego (Ph.D.) (Cl)	3	2
Alliant International University–San Francisco (Ph.D.) (Cl)	6	0
Alliant International University–San Francisco (Psy.D.) (Cl)	5	2
American University (Cl)	1	0
Antioch/New England Graduate School (Cl)	2	0
Argosy University, Atlanta (Ph.D.) (Cl)	2	0
Argosy University, Atlanta (Ph.D.) (Cl)	2	0
Arizona State University (Cl)	5	5
Auburn University (Cl)	2	0
Ball State University (Co)	2	0
Binghamton University/State University of New York (Cl)	3	3
Bowling Green State University (Cl)	5	1
Carlos Albizu University–Miami Campus (Cl)	3	0
Catholic University of America (Cl)	4	1
Central Michigan University (Cl)	1	2
Chicago School of Professional Psychology (Cl)	2	0
Clark University (Cl)	2	1
Drexel University (Cl)	5	2
Fairleigh Dickinson University (Cl)	4	2

	# Faculty	# Grants
Fordham University (Cl)	1	0
Fuller Theological Seminary (Ph.D. & Psy.D.) (Cl)	3	1
George Washington University (Ph.D. & Psy.D.) (Cl)	2	1
Hofstra University (Cm)	2	0
Illinois Institute of Technology (Cl)	4	2
Immaculata College (Cl)	2	0
Indiana State University (Cl)	1	0
Indiana University (Cl)	3	4
Jackson State University (Cl)	1	0
Loma Linda University (Ph.D. & Psy.D.) (Cl)	1	2
Long Island University (Cl)	4	1
Loyola University–Chicago (Cl)	5	4
Marquette University (Cl)	4	1
McGill University (Cl)	1	1
Miami University (Cl)	1	0
New School University (Cl)	1	1
Nova Southeastern University (Ph.D. & Psy.D.) (Cl)	5	0
Ohio State University (Cl)	1	0
Ohio University (Cl)	3	0
Oklahoma State University (Cl)	2	0
Ontario Institute for Studies in Education (Cm)	2	1
Pace University (Psy.D.) (Cm)	2	0
Pennsylvania State University (Cl)	3	2
St. Louis University (Cl)	2	0
San Diego State University/University of California–San Diego (Cl)	5	0
Simon Fraser University (Cl)	3	3
Southern Illinois University (Cl)	3	0
Temple University (Cl)	1	3
Texas A&M University (Cl)	4	3
Texas Tech University (Cl)	2	2
University of Alabama (Cl)	3	1
University at Albany/State University of New York (Cl)	3	1
University of Arkansas (Cl)	2	0
University at Buffalo/State University of New York (Cl)	3	1
University of California–Santa Barbara (Cm)	4	4
University of Central Florida (Cl)	1	0
University of Cincinnati (Cl)	3	2
University of Colorado (Cl)	3	2
University of Delaware (Cl)	4	5
University of Florida (Cl)	3	4
University of Georgia (Cl)	3	0
University of Hawaii at Manoa (Cl)	3	4
University of Houston (Cl)	3	2
University of Illinois at Urbana–Champaign (Cl)	6	2
University of Kentucky (Cl)	3	1
University of Maine (Cl)	1	0
University of Massachusetts at Amherst (Cl)	4	2
University of Memphis (Co)	2	1
University of Miami (Cl)	6	2+
University of Michigan (Cl)	8	5
University of Mississippi (Cl)	3	0
University of Missouri–St. Louis (Cl)	2	0

	# Faculty	# Grants
University of Nebraska–Lincoln (Cl)	3	1
University of New Mexico (Cl)	1	0
University of North Carolina at Chapel Hill (Cl)	2	2
University of North Carolina at Greensboro (Cl)	1	0
University of North Texas (Cl)	1	1
University of Northern Colorado (Co)	8	0
University of Oklahoma (Co)	4	0
University of Oregon (Co)	3	1
University of Ottawa (Cl)	3	1
University of Pittsburgh (Cl)	12	18
University of Rhode Island (Cl)	1	0
University of South Dakota (Cl)	3	0
University of South Florida (Cl)	4	2
University of Southern Mississippi (Co)	2	1
University of Texas Southwestern Medical Center at Dallas (Cl)	1	0
University of Utah (Cl)	3	1
University of Utah (Co)	3	2
University of Virginia—Department of Human Services (Cl)	1	0
University of Virginia—Department of Psychology (Cl)	5	5
University of Windsor (Cl)	2	2
University of Wisconsin–Milwaukee	5	5
Utah State University (Cm)	1	1
Virginia Commonwealth University (Cl)	4	3
Virginia Consortium Program in Clinical Psychology (Cl)	1	0
Virginia Polytechnic Institute and State University (Cl)	4	2
Washington State University (Cl)	4	4
West Virginia University (Cl)	2	3
Widener University (Cl)	1	0
Yeshiva University (Cm)	1	0

Chronic Illness

	# Faculty	# Grants
Northwestern University, Feinberg School of Medicine (Cl)	1	0
University of Illinois at Urbana–Champaign (Co)	1	1
University of Kansas (Cl)	2	1
University of Miami (Cl)	4	1
University of Michigan (Cl)	1	0
University of Manitoba (Cl)	1	1
University of Pittsburgh (Cl)	3	4
Wright Institute (Cl)	1	0

Chronic/Severe Mental Illness

	# Faculty	# Grants
Case Western Reserve University (Cl)	1	0
Illinois Institute of Technology (Cl)	2	1
Indiana University–Purdue University Indianapolis (Cl)	2	3–4
Nova Southeastern University (Ph.D. & Psy.D.) (Cl)	2	0
Rutgers University (Psy.D.) (Cl)	2	1
University of Cincinnati (Cl)	3	2
University of Houston (Cl)	3	1

	# Faculty	# Grants
University of Louisville (Cl)	1	0
University of Maryland (Cl)	2	2
University of Massachusetts at Boston (Cl)	2	1
University of Nebraska–Lincoln (Cl)	1	1
University of South Carolina (Cl)	1	0
University of South Dakota (Cl)	2	0
University of Toledo (Cl)	1	1

Clinical Judgment/Decision Making

	# Faculty	# Grants
Ball State University (Co)	1	0
Indiana State University (Cl)	1	0
Indiana University of Pennsylvania (Cl)	1	0
James Madison University (Psy.D.) (Cm)	3	0
Loma Linda University (Ph.D. & Psy.D.) (Cl)	1	0
San Diego State University/University of California–San Diego (Cl)	1	0
Southern Illinois University (Cl)	1	0
Tennessee State University (Co)	1	0
University of Alabama (Cl)	2	0
University of Detroit–Mercy (Cl)	1	0
University of Rhode Island (Cl)	1	0

Cognition/Social Cognition

	# Faculty	# Grants
Alliant International University–Los Angeles (Psy.D.) (Cl)	1	0
Argosy University–Washington, DC Campus (Cl)	1	0
Arizona State University (Co)	1	0
Binghamton University/State University of New York (Cl)	1	0
Case Western Reserve University (Cl)	2	0
Catholic University of America (Cl)	3	0
Colorado State University (Co)	2	0
Columbia University (Ph.D.) (Co)		
Concordia University (Cl)	4	5
Duke University (Cl)	2	2
Fuller Theological Seminary (Ph.D. & Psy.D.) (Cl)	1	0
Gallaudet University (Cl)	1	1
George Fox University (Cl)	1	1
George Mason University (Cl)	4	0
Georgia State University (Co)	2	0
Indiana University (Cl)	1	0
Marquette University (Cl)	1	0
McGill University (Cl)	3	1
Michigan State University (Cl)	2	1
New School University (Cl)	2	1
Northeastern University (Cm)	2	0
Northwestern University (Cl)	1	1
Nova Southeastern University (Ph.D. & Psy.D.) (Cl)	1	0
Ontario Institute for Studies in Education (Cm)	3	2
Pennsylvania State University (Cl)	2	0
Rutgers University (Psy.D.) (Cl)	1	1
San Diego State University/University of California–San Diego (Cl)	17	0
Simon Fraser University (Cl)	6	4

	# Faculty	# Grants
Suffolk University (Cl)	1	0
Texas Tech University (Cl)	1	0
University of Denver (Co)	1	1
University of Denver (Psy.D.) (Cl)	1	0
University of Hawaii at Manoa (Cl)	2	0
University of Indianapolis (Cl)	1	0
University of Pittsburgh (Cl)	4	6
University of Rochester (Cl)	3	2
University of Virginia—Department of Human Services (Cl)	1	0
University of Western Ontario (Cl)	2	1
Washington State University (Co)	2	1
Yale University (Cl)	2	0

Cognitive Therapy/Cognitive-Behavioral Therapy

Arizona State University (Co)	1	0
Baylor University (Cl)	3	0
Brigham Young University (Cl)	1	1
George Fox University (Cl)	2	6
Georgia State University (Cl)	1	1
Ontario Institute for Studies in Education (Cm)	2	2
Pacific University (Cl)	7	0
San Diego State University/University of California–San Diego (Cl)	2	0
Texas Tech University (Cl)	3	0
University of Southern California (Cl)	5	3
University of Washington (Cl)	4	2
University of Wisconsin–Milwaukee (Cl)	3	0
Western Michigan University (Cl)	2	0
Xavier University (Cl)	5	0
York Univeristy—Clinical-Developmental Area (Cl)	1	0

Community Psychology

Alliant International University–San Francisco (Ph.D.) (Cl)	6	2
Antioch/New England Graduate School (Cl)	2	2
Arizona State University (Cl)	6	5
Boston University (Cl)	2	0
Bowling Green State University (Cl)	1	1
Catholic University of America (Cl)	1	1
Fairleigh Dickinson University (Cl)	3	0
Florida State University (Cm)	2	1
George Washington University (Ph.D.) (Cl)	2	1
George Washington University (Psy.D.) (Cl)	3	1
Loyola University–Chicago (Cl)	3	0
Miami University (Cl)	2	1
Nova Southeastern University (Ph.D. & Psy.D.) (Cl)	4	0
Pace University (Psy.D.) (Cm)	1	0
Regent University (Cl)	4	3
Rutgers University (Psy.D.) (Cl)	2	1
St. Louis University (Cl)	1	0
San Diego State University/University of California–San Diego (Cl)	1	0

Southern Illinois University (Cl)	1	0
Texas Tech University (Cl)	1	0
University of Denver (Ph.D.) (Cl)	1	1
University of Hartford (Cl)	1	0
University of Illinois at Chicago (Cl)	2	1
University of Illinois at Urbana–Champaign (Cl)	5	1
University of La Verne (Psy.D.) (Cl)	12	0
University of Manitoba (Cl)	1	0
University of Maryland–Baltimore County (Cl)	4	2
University of Mississippi (Cl)	2	0
University of North Dakota (Cl)	2	0
University of Pennsylvania (Cl)	1	0
University of Rhode Island (Cl)	1	4
University of South Carolina (Cl)	2	1
University of South Dakota (Cl)	6	1
University of Texas Southwestern Medical Center at Dallas (Cl)	1	0
University of Virginia—Department of Psychology (Cl)	3	3
University of Windsor (Cl)	3	2
Virginia Commonwealth University (Cl)	3	2
Virginia Consortium Program in Clinical Psychology (Cl)	1	1
Wayne State University (Cl)	2	2

Conduct Disorder

Dalhousie University (Cl)	2	3
Florida State University (Cl)	1	1
Georgia State University (Cl)	2	1
Miami University (Cl)	3	1
Duke University (Cl)	2	3
Purdue University (Cl)	1	1
Temple University (Cl)	1	0
University of Maryland–Baltimore County (Cl)	1	1
University of North Carolina at Greensboro (Cl)	1	0
University of South Carolina (Cl)	1	1

Conflict Mediation/Resolution

Loma Linda University (Ph.D. & Psy.D.) (Cl)	1	0
University at Albany/State University of New York (Co)	1	0
University of North Dakota (Co)	1	0

Consultation

Arizona State University (Co)	2	0
Northeastern University (Cm)	1	1
Regent University (Cl)	4	2
University of Memphis (Co)	1	1

Crisis Intervention

Brigham Young University (Co)	1	1
Southern Illinois University (Co)	1	0
University of Detroit–Mercy (Cl)	2	0

	# Faculty	# Grants

Deafness/Hearing Impairment

Gallaudet University (Cl)	9	2
University of Iowa (Cl)	1	0
Wright State University (Cl)	1	1

Death and Dying/Bereavement

Biola University (Ph.D.) (Cl)	1	0
Biola University (Psy.D.) (Cl)	1	0
Drexel University (Cl)	2	2
Indiana University of Pennsylvania (Cl)	1	0
Loyola University–Chicago (Cl)	1	0
San Diego State University/University of California–San Diego (Cl)	2	0
University at Buffalo/State University of New York (Co)	1	0
University of Michigan (Cl)	2	2
University of Missouri–St. Louis (Cl)	1	1
University of Saskatchewan (Cl)	1	0

Developmental (Child and Adolescent)

Adelphi University (Cl)	1	1
Boston College (Co)	1	1
Brigham Young University (Cl)	3	1
Concordia University (Cl)	8	10
Colorado State University (Co)	1	1
Fordham University (Cl)	1	0
Fuller Theological Seminary (Ph.D. & Psy.D.) (Cl)	3	1
George Washington University (Psy.D.) (Cl)	2	2
Hofstra University (Cm)	1	0
Howard University (Cl)	3	2
George Washington University (Ph.D.) (Cl)	3	3
Idaho State University (Cl)	1	1
Immaculata College (Cl)	3	0
Long Island University (Cl)	1	1
Loyola University–Chicago (Co)	2	0
McGill University (Cl)	1	1
New School University (Cl)	1	0
Pacific Graduate School of Psychology (Cl)	4	0
Pennsylvania State University (Cl)	2	1
Purdue University (Cl)	1	0
Simon Fraser University (Cl)	6	6
Spalding University (Cl)	2	0
Stony Brook University/State University of New York (Cl)	1	1
Suffolk University (Cl)	5	0
University of Central Florida (Cl)	2	0
University of Cincinnati (Cl)	1	1
University of Colorado (Cl)	2	2
University of Georgia (Co)	1	1
University of Kentucky (Cl)	2	1
University of Ottawa (Cl)	3	2
University of Pittsburgh (Cl)	8	18

University of South Florida (Cl)	4	2
University of Texas Southwestern Medical Center at Dallas (Cl)	1	1
University of Tulsa (Cl)	2	0
University of Utah (Cl)	4	2
University of Virginia (Cl)	3	3
University of Washington (Cl)	3	3
University of Wisconsin–Milwaukee (Cl)	2	0
Virginia Commonwealth University (Cl)	2	2
Yale University (Cl)	1	1

Developmental Disabilities/ Mental Retardation

Auburn University (Cl)	1	0
Binghamton University/State University of New York (Cl)	1	2
Case Western Reserve University (Cl)	1	1
George Washington University (Psy.D.) (Cl)	2	2
Georgia State University (Cl)	1	4
Long Island University–C.W. Post Campus (Cl)	1	0
Louisiana State University (Cl)	1	1
Ontario Institute for Studies in Education (Cm)	1	1
Pennsylvania State University (Cl)	3	1
Purdue University (Cl)	1	0
Rutgers University (Psy.D.) (Cl)	4	3
Stony Brook University/State University of New York (Cl)	1	1
University of Alabama at Birmingham (Cl)	6	16
University at Albany/State University of New York (Cl)	1	2
University of Denver (Ph.D.) (Cl)	1	2
University of Illinois at Chicago (Cl)	1	0
University of Manitoba (Cl)	3	0
University of Wyoming (Cl)	2	1
Virginia Consortium Program in Clinical Psychology (Cl)	1	0
West Virginia University (Cl)	1	0
York University—Clinical-Developmental Area (Cl)	2	1

Disabilities/Disabled Persons

DePaul University (Cl)	2	2
Loyola University–Chicago (Cl)	1	2
University of Memphis (Co)	4	3
University of Missouri–Columbia (Co)	1	0
Washington State University (Co)	1	1

Disaster/Trauma

Alliant International University– Los Angeles (Ph.D.) (Cl)	1	0
Chicago School of Professional Psychology (Cl)	2	0
Columbia University, Teachers College (Cl)	2	2
Fairleigh Dickinson University (Cl)	2	0
Georgia State University (Co)	2	2

	# Faculty	# Grants
Idaho State University (Cl)	2	1
Long Island University (Cl)	1	1
Miami University (Cl)	2	0
Nova Southeastern University (Ph.D. & Psy.D.) (Cl)	7	0
Seton Hall University (Co)	1	0
Temple University (Cl) (rape)	2	0
Texas Tech University (Cl)	2	0
University of British Columbia (Co)	2	1
University of Denver (Ph.D.) (Cl)	3	1
University of Denver (Psy.D.) (Cl)	1	0
University of Georgia (Co)	1	0
University of Houston (Co)	2	1
University of Kansas (Cl)	2	1
University of Manitoba (Cl)	3	0
University of Massachusetts at Boston (Cl)	4	1
University of Memphis (Co)	2	0
University of Miami (Cl)	4	2+
University of Minnesota–Department of Psychology (Co)	1	0
University of Mississippi (Cl)	2	0
University of Missouri–Columbia (Co) (rape)	1	1
University of Missouri–Kansas City (Cl)	1	1
University of Connecticut (Cl)	3	0
University of North Dakota (Co)	2	0
University of North Texas (Cl)	2	0
University of Pittsburgh (Cl)	1	1
University of South Dakota (Cl)	5	2
University of Wyoming (Cl)	1	0
Yeshiva University (Psy.D.) (Cl)	2	0
York University—Adult Clinical Program (Cl)	1	0

Divorce/Child Custody

	# Faculty	# Grants
Colorado State University (Co)	3	0
Drexel University (Cl)	1	1
Louisiana Tech University (Co)	1	0
University of Louisville (Co)	1	2
University of Michigan (Cl)	1	1
University of Victoria (Cl)	1	1
Virginia Commonwealth University (Cl)	1	0

Dreams

	# Faculty	# Grants
Miami University (Cl)	1	0
University of Maryland (Co)	1	0
University of Michigan (Cl)	1	0

Eating Disorders/Body Image

	# Faculty	# Grants
American University (Cl)	1	0
Argosy University, Atlanta (Psy.D.)	1	0
Argosy University, Chicago (Psy.D.) (Cl)	1	0
Brigham Young University (Cl)	1	1
Colorado State University (Co)	1	0
Duke University (Cl)	1	0
Emory University (Cl)	1	0

	# Faculty	# Grants
Fairleigh Dickinson University (Cl)	1	0
Florida Institute of Technology (Cl)	1	0
Florida State University (Cl)	3	3
Georgia State University (Cl)	1	1
Hofstra University (Cm)	2	0
Indiana State University (Cl)	2	1
Kent State University (Cl)	1	0
Louisiana State University (Cl)	1	1
Miami University (Cl)	1	0
McGill University (Cl)	1	1
Michigan State University (Cl)	1	2
Northeastern University (Cm)	1	1
Rutgers University (Ph.D.) (Cl)	1	1
Rutgers University (Psy.D.) (Cl)	1	1
Suffolk University (Cl)	1	0
Tennessee State University (Co)	2	1
Texas Tech University (Cl)	1	0
Uniformed Services University of Health Sciences (Cl)	1	1
University of Alabama at Birmingham (Cl)	1	1
University at Albany/State University of New York (Cl)	1	0
University of Arkansas (Cl)	1	0
University of Central Florida (Cl)	2	0
University of Colorado (Cl)	1	0
University of Detroit–Mercy (Cl)	2	0
University of Florida (Co)	1	1
University of Hawaii at Manoa (Cl)	2	0
University of Iowa (Cl)	1	1
University of Kentucky (Cl)	1	1
University of Illinois at Chicago (Cl)	1	0
University of Illinois at Urbana–Champaign (Co)	1	0
University of Iowa (Cl)	1	1
University of Manitoba (Cl)	2	0
University of Minnesota (Cl)	2	1
University of Missouri–Columbia (Cl)	1	1
University of Missouri–Columbia (Co)	1	1
University of New Mexico (Cl)	1	1
University of North Dakota (Co)	1	0
University of North Texas (Cl)	3	0
University of Northern Colorado (Co)	2	3
University of Pittsburgh (Cl)	1	3
University of St. Thomas (Co)	2	0
University of South Florida (Cl)	2	1
University of Southern Mississippi (Co)	2	0
University of Windsor (Cl)	2	1
Vanderbilt University (Cl)	1	0
Virginia Consortium Program in Clinical Psychology (Cl)	1	0
Virginia Polytechnic Institute and State University (Cl)	1	0
Washington State University (Co)	1	0
Yale University (Cl)	2	2
York University—Adult Clinical Program (Cl)	1	2

Emotion

	# Faculty	# Grants
Boston University (Cl)	3	1
Catholic University of America (Cl)	2	0
George Mason University (Cl)	4	0

	# Faculty	# Grants
Georgia State University (Cl)	3	0
Hofstra University (Cm)	1	0
Idaho State University (Cl)	1	0
Long Island University (Cl) (socio-emotional development)	1	0
Loyola University–Chicago (Cl)	3	1
McGill University (Cl)	1	1
Michigan State University (Cl)	1	0
New School University (Cl)	1	0
Ontario Institute for Studies in Education (Cm)	3	3
Pennsylvania State University (Cl)	5	1
Suffolk University (Cl)	3	0
Temple University (Cl)	1	1
University of Arkansas (Cl)	3	0
University of California–Berkeley (Cl)	1	1
University of Delaware (Cl)	4	1
University of Florida (Cl)	1	3
University of Florida (Co)	1	0
University of Georgia (Cl)	1	1
University of Illinois at Urbana–Champaign (Cl)	5	2
University of Mississippi (Cl)	2	1
University of Montana (Cl)	1	1
University of North Texas (Cl)	1	0
University of Pittsburgh (Cl)	3	4
University of South Florida (Cl)	2	0
University of Utah (Co)	1	0
University of Western Ontario (Cl)	1	0
University of Wisconsin–Milwaukee (Cl)	1	0
Vanderbilt University (Cl)	4	2
Virginia Commonwealth University (Cl)	1	0
York University—Clincal-Developmental Area (Cl)	1	2

Epidemiology

Alliant International University–Fresno (Ph.D.) (Cl)	1	0
University of Kansas (Co)	1	1
University of Texas at Austin (Cl)	1	0
University of Virginia (Cl)	2	1

Ethical Issues

Arizona State University (Co)	1	0
Boston College (Co)	1	1
Colorado State University (Co)	1	0
Fairleigh Dickinson University (Cl)	2	0
Gallaudet University (Cl)	1	0
Indiana University of Pennsylvania (Cl)	1	0
Iowa State University (Co)	1	0
Loma Linda University (Ph.D. & Psy.D.) (Cl)	1	0
Loyola College in Maryland (Cl)	2	0
Loyola University–Chicago (Cl)	1	0
Our Lady of the Lake University (Co)	1	0
Rutgers University (Ph.D.) (Cl)	1	0
Rutgers University (Psy.D.) (Cl)	1	0
St. Louis University (Cl)	3	0

Texas A&M University (Co)	2	0
Texas Tech University (Cl)	1	0
Texas Woman's University (Co)	2	
University of British Columbia (Co)	1	0
University of Denver (Co)	1	0
University of Iowa (Co)	2	1
University of St. Thomas (Co)	1	0
University of South Dakota (Cl)	1	0
University of Tennessee (Co)	1	0

Family/Family Therapy/ Systems

Alliant International University–Los Angeles (Psy.D.) (Cl)	1	0
Alliant International University–San Francisco (Ph.D.) (Cl)	6	0
Argosy University, Chicago Northwest (Psy.D.)	1	0
Arizona State University (Cl)	4	4
Arizona State University (Co)	1	0
Boston University (Cl)	2	1
Bowling Green State University (Cl)	2	0
Catholic University of America (Cl)	2	1
Clark University (Cl)	3	2
Colorado State University (Co)	1	0
Drexel University (Cl)	4	1
Florida Institute of Technology (Cl)	2	0
Fordham University (Cl)	1	0
Fuller Theological Seminary (Ph.D. & Psy.D.) (Cl)	2	1
George Washington University (Cl)	1	1
Georgia State University (Cl)	1	4
Hofstra University (Cm)	1	0
Howard University (Cl)	2	0
Illinois Institute of Technology (Cl)	1	0
Indiana State University (Co)	3	1
Indiana University (Cl)	1	1
Indiana University (Co)	3	3
Indiana University of Pennsylvania (Cl)	3	0
James Madison University (Cm)	2	0
Kent State University (Cl)	2	2
Lehigh University (Co)	1	1
Louisiana Tech University (Co)	1	0
Marquette University (Cl)	2	1
McGill University (Cl)	2	1
Miami University (Cl)	1	0
New Mexico State University (Co)	1	0
Ohio University (Cl)	3	1
Pennsylvania State University (Cl)	2	1
Pennsylvania State University (Co)	2	0
Pepperdine University (Cl)	0	0
Purdue University (Cl)	2	1
Rutgers University (Psy.D.) (Cl)	4	2
St. Louis University (Cl)	3	0
San Diego State University/University of California–San Diego (Cl)	5	0
Simon Fraser University (Cl)	3	3
Southern Illinois University (Cl)	1	0
Suffolk University (Cl)	3	0
Syracuse University (Cl)	1	1
Texas A&M University (Cl)	5	3
Texas Tech University (Co)	2	0

	# Faculty	# Grants
University at Albany/State University of New York (Co)	1	1
University of Arizona (Cl)	2	4
University of Arkansas (Cl)	2	0
University at Buffalo/State University of New York (Cm)	1	0
University of California–Berkeley (Cl)	1	1
University of California–Los Angeles (Cl)	3	3
University of California–Santa Barbara (Cm)	4	4
University of Colorado (Cl)	1	1
University of Denver (Ph.D.) (Cl)	3	1
University of Denver (Psy.D.) (Cl)	2	0
University of Detroit–Mercy (Cl)	2	0
University of Georgia (Cl)	1	1
University of Houston (Cl)	3	2
University of Illinois at Urbana–Champaign (Cl)	5	1
University of Indianapolis (Cl)	1	1
University of Kentucky (Co)	2	0
University of Maryland–Baltimore County (Cl)	1	1
University of Massachusetts at Amherst (Cl)	2	2
University of Massachusetts at Boston (Cl)	3	2
University of Memphis (Co)	2	1
University of Miami (Cl)	1	1
University of Miami (Co)	2	1
University of Michigan (Cl)	6	3
University of Missouri–Kansas City (Co)	1	0
University of New Mexico (Cl)	2	3
University of North Carolina at Chapel Hill (Cl)	1	2
University of North Texas (Co)	3	0
University of Northern Colorado (Co)	4	1
University of Oklahoma (Co)	4	0
University of Oregon (Co)	3	2
University of Ottawa (Cl)	1	1
University of Pennsylvania (Cl)	1	0
University of Pittsburgh (Cl)	8	18
University of Rhode Island (Cl)	1	0
University of South Florida (Cl)	1	0
University of Southern California (Cl)	6	2
University of Texas at Austin (Co)	1	0
University of Utah (Cl)	4	2
University of Victoria (Cl)	1	1
University of Virginia (Cl)	2	2
University of Virginia–Department of Human Services (Cl)	1	0
Virginia Commonwealth University (Co)	2	0
Virginia Consortium Program in Clinical Psychology (Cl)	2	0
Wayne State University (Cl)	1	2
Western Michigan University (Co)		
Wheaton College (Cl)	1	0
Wright Institute (Cl)	1	0
Wright State University (Cl)	1	1
Yeshiva University (Cm)	2	0
Yeshiva University (Cl)	4	0
York University—Adult Clinical Program (Cl)	1	2

Forensic

	# Faculty	# Grants
Alliant International University–San Diego (Ph.D. & Psy.D.) (Cl)	2	0
Argosy University–Pheonix (Cl)	2	0
Azusa Pacific University (Cl)	2	1
Carlos Albizu University–Miami Campus (Cl)	1	0
Chicago School of Professional Psychology (Cl)	3	0
Colorado State University (Co)	2	1
Dalhousie University (Cl)	1	3
Fairleigh Dickinson University (Cl)	2	0
George Mason University (Cl)	1	1
Long Island University (Cl)	3	0
Northeastern University (Cm)	1	1
Nova Southeastern University (Ph.D. & Psy.D.) (Cl)	3	2
Pacific University (Cl)	2	0
Simon Fraser University (Cl)	4	4
Texas Tech University (Co)	1	0
University of Alabama (Cl)	3	0
University of Denver (Psy.D.) (Cl)	2	0
University of La Verne (Psy.D.) (Cl)	2	0
University of Louisville (Cl)	1	0
University of Maine (Cl)	3	0
University of Nebraska–Lincoln (Cl)	2	2
University of North Texas (Cl)	2	1
University of Ottawa (Cl)	1	0
University of Saskatchewan (Cl)	3	2
University of Utah (Cl)	1	1
University of Virginia—Department of Human Services (Cl)	2	3
Virginia Commonwealth University (Cl)	1	0
Virginia Consortium Program in Clinical Psychology (Cl)	1	0
West Virginia University (Cl)	1	0
Yeshiva University (Psy.D.) (Cl)	1	0

Forgiveness

	# Faculty	# Grants
University of Southern Mississippi (Co)	2	0
Virginia Commonwealth University (Co)	1	0

Gay/Lesbian/Bisexuality

	# Faculty	# Grants
Alliant International University–Los Angeles (Ph.D.) (Cl)	1	0
Argosy University, Atlanta (Psy.D.)	2	0
Argosy University, Chicago (Psy.D.) (Cl)	2	0
Argosy University–Honolulu Campus (Cl)	1	0
Auburn University (Co)	2	0
Gallaudet University (Cl)	1	0
George Mason University (Cl)	1	0
Louisiana Tech University (Co)	1	0
Loyola College in Maryland (Cl)	1	0
Oklahoma State University (Co)	1	0
Pennsylvania State University (Co)	1	0

	# Faculty	# Grants
University of California–Santa Barbara (Cm)	1	1
University of Florida (Co)	1	0
University of Houston (Co)	1	0
University of Houston (Cl)	2	1
University of Louisville (Co)	1	1
University of Memphis (Co)	3	1
University of North Dakota (Co)	2	1
University of Utah (Co)	2	0
University of Vermont (Cl)	1	1

Gender Roles/Sex Differences

	# Faculty	# Grants
Alliant International University–San Francisco (Ph.D.) (Cl)	6	0
Alliant International University–San Francisco (Psy.D.) (Cl)	3	0
Arizona State University (Cl)	2	1
Arizona State University (Co)	2	0
Biola University (Psy.D.) (Cl)	2	1
Boston College (Co)	2	0
Boston University (Cl)	1	0
Brigham Young University (Cl)	2	1
Clark University (Cl)	1	0
Colorado State University (Co)	1	0
Concordia University (Cl)	2	1
Georgia State University (Cl)	1	1
Immaculata College (Cl)	3	0
Indiana State University (Co)	2	0
Indiana State University (Cl)	3	0
Indiana University of Pennsylvania (Cl)	1	0
Iowa State University (Co)	2	1
McGill University (Cl)	1	1
New Mexico State University (Co)	3	0
Nova Southeastern University (Ph.D. & Psy.D.) (Cl)	1	0
Oklahoma State University (Co)	2	0
Ontario Institute for Studies in Education (Cm)	1	1
Pace University (Psy.D.) (Cm)	2	0
Rutgers University (Psy.D.) (Cl)	1	0
St. John's University (Cl)	2	0
San Diego State University/University of California–San Diego (Cl)	2	0
Simon Fraser University (Cl)	2	1
Southern Illinois University (Cl)	2	0
Southern Illinois University (Co)	3	0
Suffolk University (Cl)	1	0
Texas A&M University (Co)	4	1
Texas Tech University (Co)	2	0
Texas Woman's University (Co)	4	1
University of Florida (Co)	1	0
University of Georgia (Co)	1	0
University of Houston (Co)	1	0
University of Kentucky (Co)	2	1
University of La Verne (Psy.D.) (Cl)	2	0
University of Missouri–Columbia (Co)	2	0
University of Montana (Co)	2	1
University of North Dakota (Cl)	2	0
University of North Dakota (Co)	4	0

	# Faculty	# Grants
University of Oklahoma (Co)	4	0
University of Wisconsin–Madison (Co)	4	0
University of Wisconsin–Milwaukee (Co)	1	0
Vanderbilt University (Cl)	1	1
Virginia Consortium Program in Clinical Psychology (Cl)	3	0
Virginia Polytechnic Institute and State University (Cl)	1	0
Wheaton College (Cl)	1	1
Wright Institute (Cl)	3	0
Wright State University (Cl)	5	1

Group Process and Therapy

	# Faculty	# Grants
Adelphi University (Cl)	2	0
Antioch/New England Graduate School (Cl)	1	0
Arizona State University (Co)	1	0
Baylor University (Cl)	1	0
Brigham Young University (Cl)	3	1
Fuller Theological Seminary (Ph.D. & Psy.D.) (Cl)	1	0
George Washington University (Psy.D.) (Cl)	3	0
Indiana University (Co)	2	0
New York University (Co)	1	0
Ohio State University (Co)	2	0
Texas Tech University (Co)	1	0
University of Denver (Co)	1	0
University of Hartford (Cl)	1	0
University of Missouri–Columbia (Co)	2	1
University of North Dakota (Co)	1	0
University of Tennessee (Co)	1	0
University of Wisconsin–Madison (Co)	1	0
Virginia Commonwealth University (Co)	1	0
Washington State University (Co)	1	0
West Virginia University (Co)	1	0
Western Michigan University (Co)		
York University—Adult Clinical Program (Cl)	1	2

Homelessness

	# Faculty	# Grants
Azusa Pacific University (Cl)	1	0
Drexel University (Cl)	1	0
University of Cincinnati (Cl)	2	1
University of Denver (Ph.D.) (Cl)	1	0
University of Michigan (Cl)	1	0

Hypnosis

	# Faculty	# Grants
Binghamton University/State University of New York (Cl)	1	1
Pennsylvania State University (Cl)	1	0
University of Manitoba (Cl)	1	0
University of Waterloo (Cl)	1	1
University of Wisconsin–Milwaukee (Co)	1	0
Virginia Polytechnic Institute and State University (Cl)	1	1
Washington State University (Cl)	2	1
Washington University (Cl)	1	0

	# Faculty	# Grants

Infancy

	# Faculty	# Grants
Alliant International University–Fresno (Ph.D.) (Cl)	1	1
Alliant International University–Los Angeles (Ph.D.) (Cl)	1	1
Concordia University (Cl)	4	4
Emory University (Cl)	1	2
George Washington University (Psy.D.) (Cl)	1	1
Pace University (Psy.D.) (Cm)	3	0
University of Western Ontario (Cl)	2	1

Interpersonal Relations/Processes

	# Faculty	# Grants
Adelphi University (Cl)	1	1
Alliant International University–Los Angeles (Ph.D. & Psy.D) (Cl)	2	0
Arizona State University (Cl)	1	1
Arizona State University (Co)	3	0
Catholic University of America (Cl)	2	0
Colorado State University (Co)	1	0
Dalhousie University (Cl)	2	2
Fairleigh Dickinson University (Cl)	4	0
Indiana State University (Cl)	1	0
Indiana University (Cl)	3	1
James Madison University (Cm)	4	0
McGill University (Cl)	2	2
New Mexico State University (Co)	1	1
Ontario Institute for Studies in Education (Cm)	2	2
San Diego State University/University of California–San Diego (Cl)	1	0
Southern Illinois University (Cl)	2	0
Texas Tech University (Co)	1	0
University of Arkansas (Cl)	3	1
University of Cincinnati (Cl)	2	0
University of Denver (Ph.D.) (Cl)	2	2
University of Georgia (Cl)	1	1
University of Hartford (Cl)	1	0
University of Indianapolis (Cl)	2	0
University of Kansas (Co)	1	1
University of Maryland (Co)	1	0
University of Maryland–Baltimore County (Cl)	1	0
University of Michigan (Cl)	1	1
University of Minnesota–Department of Psychology (Co)	1	1
University of Mississippi (Cl)	1	0
University of Missouri–Kansas City (Co)	3	0
University of New Mexico (Cl)	1	2
University of North Carolina at Chapel Hill (Cl)	2	1
University of North Carolina at Greensboro (Cl)	3	2
University of North Dakota (Cl)	1	1
University of Oklahoma (Co)	2	0
University of Oregon (Co)	3	0
University of Waterloo (Cl)	1	0

	# Faculty	# Grants
Virginia Consortium Program in Clinical Psychology (Cl)	2	0
Western Michigan University (Cl)	1	0

Intervention

	# Faculty	# Grants
Chicago School of Professional Psychology (Cl)	1	0
Northeastern University (Cm)	1	1
University of Minnesota—Department of Psychology (Co)	1	1
University of Wisconsin–Milwaukee (Co)	1	1

Learning

	# Faculty	# Grants
Idaho State University (Cl)	1	0
Loyola College in Maryland (Cl)	1	0
Ontario Institute for Studies in Education (Cm)	5	7
Pace University (Psy.D.) (Cm)	1	0
University of Kansas (Co)	1	0
Virginia Consortium Program in Clinical Psychology (Cl)	2	0

Learning Disabilities/Disorders

	# Faculty	# Grants
Argosy University–Phoenix (Cl)	1	0
Binghamton University/State University of New York (Cl)	1	1
Case Western Reserve University (Cl)	1	0
Colorado State University (Co)	1	0
Florida State University (Cl)	2	5
Georgia State University (Cl) (dyslexia)	1	4
Ontario Institute for Studies in Education (Cm)	4	4
Pace University (Psy.D.) (Cm)	1	0
Southern Illinois University (Cl)	2	0
Stony Brook University/State University of New York (Cl)	1	1
Temple University (Cl)	1	1
University of California–Santa Barbara (Cm)	3	0
University of Denver (Ph.D.) (Cl)	1	2
University of Texas Southwestern Medical Center at Dallas (Cl)	1	0
University of Virginia—Department of Human Services (Cl)	1	0
University of Wisconsin–Milwaukee (Cl)	1	0
Virginia Consortium Program in Clinical Psychology (Cl)	2	0
Widener University (Psy.D.) (Cl)	1	0
Yeshiva University (Cm)	3	0
York University—Clinical-Developmental Area (Cl)	1	0

Legal Issues/Law Psychology

	# Faculty	# Grants
Alliant International University–San Diego (Ph.D. & Psy.D.) (Cl)	1	0
George Washington University (Psy.D.) (Cl)	2	0
Iowa State University (Co)	1	0
Loyola College in Maryland (Cl)	1	0

	# Faculty	# Grants
University of Arizona (Cl)	2	2
University of Florida (Co)	1	1
University of Illinois at Urbana–Champaign (Cl)	3	2
University of St. Thomas (Co)	1	0
University of Southern Mississippi (Co)	3	0
University of Wyoming (Cl)	2	3

Malingering/Somatoform Disorders

Alliant International University–San Diego (Ph.D. & Psy.D.) (Cl)	1	0
Rutgers University (Ph.D.) (Cl)	1	1
University of Montana (Cl)	1	1
University of North Texas (Cl)	2	2

Managed Care/Health Care

Jackson State University (Cl)	3	0
Northeastern University (Cm)	1	0
University of Hawaii at Manoa (Cl)	6	2
University of Nevada–Reno (Cl)	1	1
University of Wyoming (Cl)	3	1
Wright State University (Psy.D.) (Cl)	1	0

Marriage/Couples

Adelphi University (Cl)	1	1
Ball State University (Co)	3	0
Binghamton University/State University of New York (Cl)	1	1
Fordham University (Cl)	1	0
Fuller Theological Seminary (Ph.D. & Psy.D.) (Cl)	4	0
George Fox University (Cl)	1	1
Georgia State University (Cl)	2	0
Hofstra University (Cm)	1	0
Illinois Institute of Technology (Cl)	1	1
Indiana University (Cl)	1	1
Indiana University (Co)	3	0
Long Island University–C.W. Post Campus (Cl)	2	0
Purdue University (Co)	1	0
Regent University (Cl)	2	1
Rutgers University (Ph.D.) (Cl)	2	1
Rutgers University (Psy.D.) (Cl)	1	1
San Diego State University/University of California–San Diego (Cl)	5	0
Southern Illinois University (Cl)	1	0
Stony Brook University/State University of New York (Cl)	3	6
Suffolk University (Cl)	1	0
Texas A&M University (Cl)	5	3
Texas A&M University (Co)	4	1
Texas Woman's University (Co)	4	1
University of California–Berkeley (Cl)	2	1
University of California–Los Angeles (Cl)	2	2
University of Colorado (Cl)	1	0
University of Denver (Ph.D.) (Cl)	2	2
University of Denver (Psy.D.) (Cl)	1	0
University of Detroit–Mercy (Cl)	2	0

University of Georgia (Cl)	2	1
University of Houston (Cl)	2	1
University of Illinois at Urbana–Champaign (Cl)	5	1
University of Iowa (Cl)	1	0
University of Indianapolis (Cl)	1	0
University of Nevada–Reno (Cl)	2	0
University of North Carolina at Chapel Hill (Cl)	1	1
University of North Texas (Co)	3	2
University of Notre Dame (Co)	1	1
University of Oklahoma (Co)	4	0
University of Ottawa (Cl)	1	0
University of Rochester (Cl)	1	0
University of South Carolina (Cl)	3	0
University of South Florida (Cl)	1	0
University of Southern California (Cl)	6	2
University of Utah (Cl)	4	2
Virginia Commonwealth University (Co)	2	0
Virginia Consortium Program in Clinical Psychology (Cl)	2	0
Virginia Polytechnic Institute and State University (Cl)	1	0

Minority/Cross-Cultural/Diversity

Alliant International University–Fresno (Ph.D.) (Cl)	1	1
Alliant International University–Fresno (Psy.D.) (Cl)	1	1
Alliant International University–Los Angeles (Ph.D. & Psy.D.) (Cl)	7	1
Alliant International University–Los Angeles (Ph.D.) (Cl)	5	0
Alliant International University–San Diego (Psy.D.) (Cl)	3	2
Alliant International University–San Diego (Ph.D.) (Cl)	3	0
Alliant International University–San Francisco (Ph.D.) (Cl)	6	2
Alliant International University–San Francisco (Psy.D.) (Cl)	5	0
Antioch/New England Graduate School (Cl)	1	0
Argosy University, Atlanta (Ph.D.) (Cl)	3	0
Argosy University, Chicago (Psy.D.)	3	0
Argosy University, Chicago Northwest (Psy.D.)	2	1
Argosy University–Pheonix (Cl)	1	0
Argosy University–Washington, DC Campus (Cl)	1	0
Arizona State University (Cl)	5	4
Arizona State University (Co)	5	4
Ball State University (Co)	3	1
Biola University (Ph.D.) (Cl)	4	0
Biola University (Psy.D.) (Cl)	4	0
Boston College (Co)	1	1
Boston University (Cl)	2	0
Brigham Young University (Co)	2	1
Carlos Albizu University–Miami Campus (Cl)	6	0
Central Michigan University (Cl)	1	0

	# Faculty	# Grants
Chicago School of Professional Psychology (Cl)	2	1
City University of New York at City College (Cl)	2	0
Colorado State University (Co)	6	3
Columbia University, Teachers College (Ph.D.) (Co)	2	0
DePaul University (Cl)	3	1
Fairleigh Dickinson University (Cl)	2	0
Florida Institute of Technology (Cl)	1	0
Fordham University (Co)	4	0
Fuller Theological Seminary (Ph.D. & Psy.D.) (Cl)	2	0
Gallaudet University (Cl)	1	1
George Washington University (Ph.D.) (Cl)	4	3
Hofstra University (Cm)	2	0
Howard University (Cl)	4	4
Howard University (Co)	1	1
Indiana University (Co)	3	0
Indiana University of Pennsylvania (Cl)	3	0
Iowa State University (Co)	1	0
James Madison University (Cm)	4	1
Lehigh University (Co)	1	1
Long Island University (Cl)	4	0
Loyola College in Maryland (Cl)	3	0
Loyola University–Chicago (Cl)	4	3
Loyola University–Chicago (Co)	2	0
Marquette University (Co)	3	0
Miami University (Cl)	2	0
Michigan State University (Cl)	1	2
New Mexico State University (Co)	4	0
New York University (Co)	2	0
Northeastern University (Cm)	1	1
Northwestern University, Feinberg School of Medicine (Cl)	2	2
Nova Southeastern University (Ph.D. & Psy.D.) (Cl)	2	0
Ohio State University (Co)	4	0
Oklahoma State University (Co)	7	8
Ontario Institute for Studies in Education (Cm)	3	3
Pace University (Psy.D.) (Cm)	2	0
Pacific Graduate School of Psychology (Cl)	4	0
Pacific University (Cl)	4	0
Pennsylvania State University (Cl)	2	0
Regent University (Cl)	1	1
Purdue University (Cl)	4	0
Rutgers University (Psy.D.) (Cl)	2	0
St. John's University (Cl)	5	1
San Diego State University/University of California–San Diego (Cl)	10	0
Seton Hall University (Co)	3	0
Southern Illinois University (Co)	2	0
Suffolk University (Cl)	3	0
Tennessee State University (Co)	2	1
Texas Tech University (Cl)	2	3
Texas Tech University (Co)	1	0
University of Akron (Co)	2	0
University of Alabama (Cl)	1	0
University at Albany/State University of New York (Co)	24	2
University of British Columbia (Co)	1	2
University at Buffalo/State University of New York (Cm)	1	0
University of California–Los Angeles (Cl)	3	3
University of California–Santa Barbara (Cm)	4	1
University of Central Florida (Cl)	1	0
University of Connecticut (Cl)	2	1
University of Denver (Ph.D.) (Cl)	3	0
University of Denver (Psy.D.) (Cl)	1	0
University of Denver (Co)	1	1
University of Florida (Co)	1	0
University of Georgia (Cl)	1	0
University of Georgia (Co)	2	0
University of Hawaii at Manoa (Cl)	2	1
University of Houston (Cl)	3	2
University of Houston (Co)	2	0
University of Illinois at Urbana–Champaign (Cl)	5	0
University of Illinois at Urbana–Champaign (Co)	1	1
University of Indianapolis (Cl)	2	1
University of Iowa (Co)	2	1
University of Kansas (Cl)	3	0
University of Kentucky (Co)	2	0
University of La Verne (Psy.D.) (Cl)	7	2
University of Maryland (Co)	3	0
University of Massachusetts at Boston (Cl)	3	0
University of Memphis (Co)	5	1
University of Miami (Co)	1	0
University of Minnesota (Cl)	1	0
University of Minnesota—Department of Educational Psychology (Co)	4	0
University of Minnesota—Department of Psychology (Co)	2	1
University of Mississippi (Cl)	1	0
University of Missouri–Columbia (Co)	5	2
University of Missouri–Kansas City (Co)	4	2
University of Missouri–St. Louis (Cl)	2	1
University of Montana (Cl)	1	0
University of Nebraska–Lincoln (Co)	1	0
University of Nevada–Reno (Cl)	4	2
University of New Mexico (Cl)	3	1
University of North Carolina at Chapel Hill (Cl)	1	0
University of North Dakota (Cl)	4	1
University of North Dakota (Co)	1	0
University of North Texas (Co)	2	1
University of Northern Colorado (Co)	6	0
University of Notre Dame (Co)	1	1
University of Oklahoma (Co)	4	0
University of Oregon (Co)	4	1
University of Rhode Island (Cl)	1	0
University of St. Thomas (Co)	2	0
University of South Carolina (Cl)	6	4
University of South Dakota (Cl)	10	2
University of Southern Mississippi (Co)	3	0
University of Texas at Austin (Cl)	1	0

	# Faculty	# Grants
University of Texas at Austin (Co)	2	1
University of Texas Southwestern Medical Center at Dallas (Cl)	2	0
University of Utah (Cl)	2	0
University of Utah (Co)	3	0
University of Victoria (Cl)	1	1
University of Virginia—Department of Human Services (Cl)	1	1
University of Virginia—Department of Psychology (Cl)	3	1
University of Washington (Cl)	5	4
University of Wisconsin–Madison (Co)	9	5
University of Wisconsin–Milwaukee (Co)	2	2
University of Wisconsin–Milwaukee (Cl)	1	0
University of Wyoming (Cl)	1	1
Utah State University (Cm)	1	0
Virginia Commonwealth University (Cl)	2	1
Virginia Polytechnic Institute and State University (Cl)	2	1
Washington State University (Co)	3	1
West Virginia University (Cl)	1	0
Western Michigan University (Co)		
Wheaton College (Cl)	1	1
Wright Institute (Cl)	3	0
Wright State University (Cl)	5	2
Yeshiva University (Cl)	2	0
Yeshiva University (Cm)	3	0

Moral Development

Azusa Pacific University (Cl)	2	1
New School University (Cl)	1	0
St. John's University (Cl)	3	0
University of La Verne (Psy.D.) (Cl)	2	0

Motivation

Adelphi University (Cl)	1	0
Clark University (Cl)	1	1
James Madison University (Cm)	1	0
University of Rochester (Cl)	4	2

Narrative Psychology/Methodology

Miami University (Cl)	2	0
New School University (Cl)	2	0
Suffolk University (Cl)	1	0
University at Albany/State University of New York (Co)	2	2
University of Notre Dame (Co)	1	1
University of Rochester (Cl)	3	2
University of Saskatchewan (Cl)	1	1
York University—Adult Clinical Program (Cl)	1	2

Neuroimaging/Functional Neuroimaging

Georgia State University (Cl)	3	1
University of Minnesota (Cl)	4	3
Vanderbilt University (Cl)	3	3

Neuropsychology

Alliant International University–Fresno (Ph.D.) (Cl)	1	0
Adler School of Professional Psychology (Cl)	4	1
Argosy University, Atlanta (Ph.D.) (Cl)	3	0
Argosy University, Chicago (Psy.D.) (Cl)	3	0
Argosy University–Honolulu Campus (Cl)	3	0
Argosy University–Phoenix (Cl)	2	0
Binghamton University/State University of New York (Cl)	1	2
Biola University (Ph.D.) (Cl)	1	0
Biola University (Psy.D.) (Cl)	1	1
Boston University (Cl)	3	2
Brigham Young University (Cl)	2	4
Carlos Albizu University–Miami Campus (Cl)	2	0
Central Michigan University (Cl)	1	1
Concordia University (Cl)	9	12
Dalhousie University (Cl)	1	3
Drexel University (Cl)	6	0
Duke University (Cl)	1	0
Emory University (Cl)	1	0
Florida Institute of Technology (Cl)	2	1
Fordham University (Cl)	1	0
Fuller Theological Seminary (Ph.D. & Psy.D.) (Cl)	1	0
Gallaudet University (Cl)	1	1
George Fox University (Cl)	1	0
Howard University (Cl)	2	2
Indiana University–Purdue University Indianapolis (Cl)	2	2
Loma Linda University (Ph.D. & Psy.D.) (Cl)	1	0
Long Island University (Cl)	1	0
Louisiana State University (Cl)	1	0
Loyola College in Maryland (Cl)	2	0
Marquette University (Cl)	2	0
McGill University (Cl)	1	1
Michigan State University (Cl)	2	3
Northeastern University (Cm)	1	0
Northwestern University, Feinberg School of Medicine	3	0
Nova Southeastern University (Ph.D. & Psy.D.) (Cl)	5	2
Ohio State University (Cl)	3	3
Pacific Graduate School of Psychology (Cl)	2	1
Pacific University (Cl)	1	1
Pennsylvania State University (Cl)	2	1
Rosalind Franklin University of Medicine (Cl)	1	2
San Diego State University/University of California–San Diego (Cl)	9	1
Seton Hall University (Co)	1	0
Simon Fraser University (Cl)	4	2
Suffolk University (Cl)	3	0
Temple University (Cl)	1	0
Texas Tech University (Cl)	1	0
Uniformed Services University of Health Sciences (Cl)	1	1
University of Alabama at Birmingham (Cl)	3	2

	# Faculty	# Grants
University at Albany/State University of New York (Cl)	1	1
University of Arizona (Cl)	2	2
University of Arkansas (Cl)	1	0
University of Cincinnati (Cl)	5	2
University of Connecticut (Cl)	3	1
University of Denver (Ph.D.) (Cl)	1	1
University of Florida (Cl)	2	3
University of Georgia (Cl)	1	2
University of Houston (Cl)	3	3
University of Illinois at Urbana–Champaign (Cl)	2	1
University of Kentucky (Cl)	2	1
University of Manitoba (Cl)	2	1
University of Michigan (Cl)	6	0
University of Montana (Cl)	1	0
University of Nebraska–Lincoln (Cl)	1	0
University of New Mexico (Cl)	2	4
University of North Carolina at Chapel Hill (Cl)	2	1
University of North Texas (Cl)	1	0
University of Oklahoma (Co)	1	0
University of Oregon (Cl)	2	2
University of Pittsburgh (Cl)	3	5
University of Saskatchewan (Cl)	1	1
University of South Carolina (Cl)	2	1
University of South Florida (Cl)	1	0
University of Southern California (Cl)	3	1
University of Texas at Austin (Cl)	2	1
University of Texas Southwestern Medical Center at Dallas (Cl)	4	4
University of Toledo (Cl)	1	0
University of Tulsa (Cl)	1	1
University of Utah (Cl)	1	0
University of Virginia (Cl)	1	0
University of Windsor (Cl)	4	4
University of Wisconsin–Milwaukee (Cl)	2	1
Vanderbilt University (Cl)	2	2
Virginia Consortium Program in Clinical Psychology (Cl)	1	2
Virginia Polytechnic Institute and State University (Cl)	2	0
Washington State University (Cl)	1	1
Washington University (Cl)	2	3
Wayne State University (Cl)	2	2
Western Michigan University (Cl)	1	0
York University—Adult Clinical Program (Cl)	2	2

Object Relations

Biola University (Ph.D.) (Cl)	4	0
Biola University (Psy.D.) (Cl)	4	0
City University of New York at City College (Cl)	4	1

Obsessive–Compulsive Disorder

Indiana University (Cl)	2	0
University of Virginia (Cl)	1	0
University of Waterloo (Cl)	2	2

Organizational

Ball State University (Co)	1	0
Indiana State University (Cl)	1	1
Pacific University (Cl)	4	0
Rutgers University (Psy.D.) (Cl)	2	0
Virginia Consortium Program in Clinical Psychology (Cl)	1	1

Pain Management

Binghamton University/State University of New York (Cl)	1	1
Dalhousie University (Cl)	2	9
Forest Institute of Professional Psychology (Cl)	2	1
George Fox University (Cl)	1	1
Jackson State University (Cl)	3	1
Rosalind Franklin University of Medicine (Cl)	1	1
Uniformed Services University of Health Sciences (Cl)	1	4
University of Alabama (Cl)	1	1
University of Florida (Cl)	2	3
University of Georgia (Cl)	1	0
University of Kentucky (Cl)	1	1
University of Manitoba (Cl)	1	0
University of North Dakota (Cl)	1	0
University of Texas Southwestern Medical Center at Dallas (Cl)	1	1
University of Western Ontario (Cl)	1	1
Virginia Polytechnic Institute and State University (Cl)	2	0
West Virginia University (Cl)	1	0
Yeshiva University (Cl)	2	0
York University—Adult Clinical Program (Cl)	1	2

Parent–Child Interactions/Parenting

Biola University (Ph.D.) (Cl)	3	0
Biola University (Psy.D.) (Cl)	3	0
Case Western Reserve University (Cl)	2	0
Catholic University of America (Cl)	2	0
Clark University (Cl)	3	1
Colorado State University (Co)	1	0
DePaul University (Cl)	1	1
Fordham University (Cl)	2	0
Gallaudet University (Cl)	1	1
Georgia State University (Cl)	2	1
Idaho State University (Cl)	1	0
Immaculata College (Cl)	2	0
Indiana University of Pennsylvania (Cl)	1	0
James Madison University (Cm)	2	0
Long Island University–C.W. Post Campus (Cl)	1	0
Louisiana State University (Cl)	1	0
Marquette University (Cl)	3	1
Marquette University (Co)	1	1
Miami University (Cl)	1	1

	# Faculty	# Grants
Ontario Institute for Studies in Education (Cm)	3	3
Pennsylvania State University (Cl)	3	2
Stony Brook University/State University of New York (Cl)	1	2
University of Arkansas (Cl)	1	1
University of Delaware (Cl)	1	2
University of Georgia (Cl)	2	1
University of Houston (Cl)	2	1
University of Indianapolis (Cl)	1	1
University of Louisville (Co)	1	0
University of Virginia—Department of Human Services (Cl)	3	1
Virginia Consortium Program in Clinical Psychology (Cl)	2	0
Virginia Polytechnic Institute and State University (Cl)	2	1
Wheaton College (Cl)	1	0
Wright Institute (Cl)	3	0
Yeshiva University (Cm)	2	0
Yeshiva University (Psy.D.) (Cl)	1	0

Personality Assessment

	# Faculty	# Grants
Argosy University, Atlanta (Ph.D.) (Cl)	4	0
Argosy University, Chicago (Psy.D.) (Cl)	4	0
Argosy University, Chicago Northwest (Psy.D.)	2	0
Arizona State University (Cl)	1	1
Auburn University (Cl)	2	0
Baylor University (Psy.D.) (Cl)	3	0
Florida Institute of Technology (Cl)	3	0
Fordham University (Cl)	1	0
George Washington University (Psy.D.) (Cl)	3	0
Indiana State University (Co)	1	0
Kent State University (Cl)	2	2
Loyola University–Chicago (Cl)	2	0
McGill University (Cl)	1	1
New School University (Cl)	1	0
Northwestern University (Cl)	2	1
Nova Southeastern University (Ph.D. & Psy.D.) (Cl)	1	0
Pennsylvania State University (Cl)	3	1
Regent University (Cl)	1	0
Southern Illinois University (Cl)	4	0
Southern Illinois University (Co)	1	0
Texas Tech University (Cl)	2	0
University of Akron (Co)	2	0
University of Alabama (Cl)	1	0
University of Central Florida (Cl)	1	0
University of Hawaii at Manoa (Cl)	1	0
University of Illinois at Urbana–Champaign	1	1
University of Kentucky (Cl)	3	0
University of Minnesota (Cl)	6	3
University of Missouri–Columbia (Co)	1	0
University of North Dakota (Cl)	2	0
University of South Florida (Cl)	1	0
University of Utah (Cl)	2	0

	# Faculty	# Grants
West Virginia University (Co)	1	0
York University—Adult Clinical Program (Cl)	2	2

Personality Disorders

	# Faculty	# Grants
Argosy University, Atlanta (Psy.D.)	1	0
Argosy University, Chicago (Psy.D.) (Cl)	1	0
Binghamton University/State University of New York (Cl)	1	1
Boston University (Cl)	1	0
Case Western Reserve University (Cl)	1	0
Clark University (Cl)	1	0
Drexel University (Cl)	2	0
Emory University (Cl)	3	2
Fordham University (Cl)	1	0
Indiana State University (Cl)	1	0
Michigan State University (Cl)	1	1
Pennsylvania State University (Cl)	2	0
Rutgers University (Psy.D.) (Cl)	2	0
St. Louis University (Cl)	2	0
University of Colorado (Cl)	1	0
University of Iowa (Cl)	1	1
University of Kentucky (Cl)	2	0
University of Miami (Cl)	1	0
University of Michigan (Cl)	2	0
University of Minnesota (Cl)	5	1
University of North Carolina at Greensboro (Cl)	1	0
University of North Dakota (Cl)	2	0
University of Tulsa (Cl)	2	0
University of Utah (Cl)	2	0
University of Virginia—Department of Psychology (Cl)	2	1
University of Wisconsin–Madison (Cl)	1	2

Personality/Temperament

	# Faculty	# Grants
Case Western Reserve University (Cl)	1	1
Columbia University, Teachers College (Ph.D.) (Co)	1	1
George Mason University (Cl)	1	1
Hofstra University (Cm)	2	0
Loyola University–Chicago (Cl)	2	1
McGill University (Cl)	1	0
Northwestern University (Cl)	2	1
Ohio State University (Cl)	1	0
Pennsylvania State University (Cl)	2	0
Regent University (Cl)	1	1
Simon Fraser University (Cl)	1	0
Southern Illinois University (Cl)	4	0
Suffolk University (Cl)	2	0
University at Albany/State University of New York (Co)	2	1
University of Delaware (Cl)	2	1
University of Florida (Co)	1	0
University of Maryland (Cl)	1	0
University of Minnesota—Department of Psychology (Co)	1	0
Washington State University (Co)	1	0
York University—Adult Clinical Program (Cl)	2	0

	# Faculty	# Grants

Positive Psychology/Resilience

Boston College (Co)	4	3
Carlos Albizu University–Miami Campus (Cl)	1	0
Columbia University, Teachers College (Cl)	2	2
George Mason University (Cl)	3	0
Immaculata College (Cl)	2	0
Marquette University (Co)	3	0
Seton Hall University (Co)	1	0
University of Kansas (Co)	3	1
University of Memphis (Co)	2	0
University of North Dakota (Co)	1	0
Washington State University (Co)	1	0

Posttraumatic Stress Disorder

Argosy University–Honolulu Campus (Cl)	2	1
Binghamton University/State University of New York (Cl)	2	0
Brigham Young University (Cl)	1	1
Duke University (Cl)	2	0
Florida Institute of Technology (Psy.D.) (Cl)	1	1
Fuller Theological Seminary (Ph.D. & Psy.D.) (Cl)	2	0
George Mason University (Cl)	2	0
Howard University (Co)	1	0
Indiana State University (Co)	1	0
Jackson State University (Cl)	1	0
Loma Linda University (Ph.D. & Psy.D.) (Cl)	2	0
Loyola College in Maryland (Cl)	4	0
Nova Southeastern University (Ph.D. & Psy.D.) (Cl)	4	0
Ontario Institute for Studies in Education (Cm)	1	0
Pace University (Psy.D.) (Cm)	1	0
Pacific University (Psy.D.) (Cl)	1	0
Pepperdine University (Cl)	1	2
San Diego State University/University of California–San Diego (Cl)	1	0
Texas Tech University (Co)	1	0
University of Denver (Co)	1	1
University of Detroit–Mercy (Cl)	2	0
University of Indianapolis (Cl)	1	0
University of Mississippi (Cl)	1	0
University of North Texas (Cl)	2	1
University of Pittsburgh (Cl)	1	1
University of Toledo (Cl)	1	0
University of Tulsa (Cl)	2	2
West Virginia University (Cl)	1	0
Western Michigan University (Cl)	1	0
University of Wyoming (Cl)	1	1

Pregnancy

Alliant International University–San Diego (Ph.D. & Psy.D.) (Cl)	1	0

DePaul University (Cl)	2	1
Indiana University of Pennsylvania (Cl)	1	0
Southern Illinois University (Cl)	1	0
Virginia Commonwealth University (Cl)	1	1

Prevention

Arizona State University (Cl)	6	5
Binghamton University/State University of New York (Cl)	3	1
Boston College (Co)	2	1
Clark University (Cl)	3	0
Columbia University (Ph.D.) (Co)		
DePaul University (Cl)		
Fielding Graduate Institute (Cl)	—	—
Fordham University (Cl)	1	0
Hofstra University (Cm)	2	0
Indiana University of Pennsylvania (Cl)	1	0
Loyola University–Chicago (Cl)	3	2
New School University (Cl)	2	1
Northern Illinois University (Cl)	3	2
Rutgers University (Ph.D.)(Cl)	2	1
San Diego State University/University of California–San Diego (Cl)	2	2
University of Central Florida (Cl)	1	0
University of Colorado (Cl)	3	1
University of Denver (Ph.D.) (Cl)	1	1
University of Georgia (Cl)	3	2
University of Minnesota—Department of Educational Psychology (Co)	1	0
University of Nevada–Reno (Cl)	1	1
University of Oregon (Co)	4	2
University of Pittsburgh (Cl)	2	2
University of South Carolina (Cl)	4	0
University of Vermont (Cl)	2	1
University of Virginia (Cl)	3	2
Vanderbilt University (Cl)	2	2
Vanderbilt University, Peabody College (Cl)	2	2
Virginia Consortium Program in Clinical Psychology (Cl)	1	3
Virginia Polytechnic Institute and State University (Cl)	4	3

Problem Solving

San Diego State University/University of California–San Diego (Cl)	4	0
Stony Brook University/State University of New York (Cl)	1	0
University of Missouri–Columbia (Co)	3	2
Widener University (Cl)	2	0
York University—Clinical-Developmental Area (Cl)	1	0

Professional Issues/Training

American University (Cl)	1	1
Antioch/New England Graduate School (Cl)	2	0
Argosy University, Chicago Northwest (Psy.D.)	2	1
Arizona State University (Co)	9	0

	# Faculty	# Grants
Auburn University (Co)	3	0
Azusa Pacific University (Cl)	1	1
Catholic University of America (Cl)	3	0
Chicago School of Professional Psychology (Cl)	5	1
City University of New York at City College (Cl)	1	0
George Fox University (Cl)	1	0
Howard University (Cl)	6	0
Indiana State University (Cl)	1	0
Indiana University (Co)	5	0
Indiana University of Pennsylvania (Cl)	1	0
James Madison University (Cm)	3	0
Long Island University–C.W. Post Campus (Cl)	1	0
McGill University (Co)	1	0
Miami University (Cl)	2	1
Oklahoma State University (Co)	2	1
Our Lady of the Lake University (Co)	1	0
Pacific University (Cl)	3	2
St. Louis University (Cl)	3	0
Texas Tech University (Co)	1	0
University of Alabama (Cl)	2	0
University of Georgia (Co)	4	0
University of Memphis (Co)	2	0
University of Minnesota—Department of Educational Psychology (Co)	1	0
University of Missouri–Kansas City (Co)	3	0
University of North Texas (Co)	4	0
University of St. Thomas (Co)	3	0
University of Tennessee (Co)	1	0
University of Utah (Co)	1	0
University of Wisconsin–Madison (Co)	1	0
Wright State University (Cl)	4	0
Yeshiva University (Cm)	3	0

Program Evaluation

Argosy University, Chicago Northwest (Psy.D.)	1	1
DePaul University (Cl)	3	1
Indiana State University (Co)	1	1
Pepperdine University (Cl)	1	1
Rutgers University (Ph.D.) (Cl)	1	1
Rutgers University (Psy.D.) (Cl)	1	1
Spalding University (Cl)	1	0
Texas Tech University (Co)	1	0

Psychoanalysis/Psychodynamics

Adelphi University (Cl)	8	1
Alliant International University– San Francisco (Psy.D.) (Cl)	5	0
Argosy University, Atlanta (Ph.D.) (Cl)	1	0
Argosy University, Chicago (Psy.D.) (Cl)	1	0
Indiana State University (Co)	1	0
Long Island University (Cl)	1	0
Miami University (Cl)	2	1
New School University (Cl)	2	0
New York University (Co)	1	0

Nova Southeastern University (Ph.D. & Psy.D.) (Cl)	2	0
Pennsylvania State University (Cl)	2	0
Rutgers University (Psy.D.) (Cl)	7	1
University of Maryland (Co)	2	0
University of Pennsylvania (Cl)	2	2
University of Texas at Austin (Co)	1	0
Virginia Consortium Program in Clinical Psychology (Cl)	1	0
Xavier University (Cl)	4	0
Yeshiva University (Cl)	5	0

Psychometrics/Measurement

Auburn University (Co)	2	0
Brigham Young University (Cl)	2	1
Carlos Albizu University–San Juan (Cl)	1	0
Dalhousie University (Cl)	1	1
Hofstra University (Cm)	1	0
Northern Illinois University (Cl)	4	1
Pace University (Psy.D.) (Cm)	3	0
Southern Illinois University (Co)	1	0
Texas Tech University (Cl)	1	0
University of Minnesota—Department of Psychology (Co)	1	1
University of Missouri–Columbia (Co)	6	0
University of Virginia—Department of Human Services (Cl)	3	0

Psychoneuroimmunology

Arizona State University (Cl)	3	3
Forest Institute of Professional Psychology (Cl)	2	1
Ohio State University (Cl)	2	5
University of Iowa (Cl)	1	1
University of Kentucky (Cl)	1	1
University of Manitoba (Cl)	1	0
University of Maryland–Baltimore County (Cl)	1	0
University of Miami (Cl)	6	1
University of Pittsburgh (Cl)	3	5

Psychopathology—Adult Psychopathology

Alliant International University– San Diego (Ph.D.) (Cl)	1	0
Arizona State University (Cl)	3	3
Binghamton University/State University of New York (Cl)	8	2
Brigham Young University (Cl)	2	0
Central Michigan University (Cl)	1	1
Clark University (Cl)	2	1
Colorado State University (Co)	3	0
Concordia University (Cl)	2	1
Florida State University (Cl)	4	2
George Washington University (Psy.D.) (Cl)	4	0
Indiana State University (Cl)	2	0
Indiana University of Pennsylvania (Cl)	1	0
Indiana University–Purdue University Indianapolis (Cl)	2	4
Loyola University–Chicago (Cl)	2	0

	# Faculty	# Grants
McGill University (Cl)	2	2
New School University (Cl)	2	0
New York University (Co)	2	0
Northern Illinois University (Cl)	6	1
Nova Southeastern University (Cl)	2	0
Ohio University (Cl)	2	0
Pacific Graduate School of Psychology (Cl)	7	2
Pennsylvania State University (Cl)	5	1
Purdue University (Cl)	1	0
Rosalind Franklin University of Medicine (Cl)	1	0
Rutgers University (Ph.D.) (Cl)	1	1
Rutgers University (Psy.D.) (Cl)	1	1
San Diego State University/University of California–San Diego (Cl)	3	0
Simon Fraser University (Cl)	8	8
Temple University (Cl)	1	0
Texas A&M University (Cl)	2	1
Texas Tech University (Cl)	1	0
University of Alabama (Cl)	2	0
University at Albany/State University of New York (Cl)	1	0
University of Arkansas (Cl)	2	0
University of Colorado (Cl)	4	2
University of Connecticut (Cl)	5	1
University of Georgia (Cl)	4	1
University of Houston (Cl)	6	3
University of Illinois at Urbana–Champaign (Cl)	5	3
University of Kentucky (Cl)	4	3
University of Manitoba (Cl)	1	0
University of Maryland (Cl)	2	1
University of Massachusetts–Boston (Cl)	2	2
University of Memphis (Cl)	3	0
University of Miami (Cl)	6	2
University of Missouri–Kansas City (Co)	3	0
University of Nebraska–Lincoln (Cl)	3	2
University of North Dakota (Cl)	6	0
University of Ottawa (Cl)	2	3
University of Pittsburgh (Cl)	10	17
University of Southern California (Cl)	6	3
University of Southern Mississippi (Cl)	5	1
University of Tennessee (Cl)	4	1
University of Utah (Cl)	3	1
University of Virginia (Cl)	3	3
Vanderbilt University (Cl)	6	6
Virginia Commonwealth University (Cl)	1	1
Washington State University (Cl)	5	6
Washington University (Cl)	3	4
Yale University (Cl)	5	1

Psychopathology—Child/Developmental

	# Faculty	# Grants
Alliant International University–San Diego (Ph.D. & Psy.D.) (Cl)	6	0
Auburn University (Cl)	2	0
Baylor University (Cl)	2	0
Brigham Young University (Cl)	2	0
Catholic University of America (Cl)	4	1
Clark University (Cl)	2	0
Concordia University (Cl)	3	5
DePaul University (Cl)	2	2
Duke University (Cl)	5	5
Emory University (Cl)	2	1
Florida State University (Cl)	3	3
George Fox University (Cl)	1	0
Idaho State University (Cl)	1	1
Indiana State University (Psy.D.) (Cl)	2	0
Long Island University (Cl)	2	0
Loyola College in Maryland (Cl)	5	0
Loyola University–Chicago (Cl)	5	4
McGill University (Cl)	1	1
Miami University (Cl)	2	0
Northern Illinois University (Cl)	5	1
Northwestern University, Feinberg School of Medicine (Cl)	2	2
Nova Southeastern University (Ph.D. & Psy.D.) (Cl)	2	0
Ohio State University (Cl)	5	8
Ontario Institute for Studies in Education (Cm)	4	5
Pacific University (Cl)	4	6
Pennsylvania State University (Cl)	4	2
Rutgers University (Ph.D.) (Cl)	1	1
San Diego State University/University of California–San Diego (Cl)	3	0
Simon Fraser University (Cl)	3	3
Temple University (Cl)	2	2
Texas Tech University (Cl)	1	0
University of Arkansas (Cl)	1	1
University of Connecticut (Cl)	6	2
University of Delaware (Cl)	4	4
University of Denver (Ph.D.) (Cl)	4	3
University of Georgia (Cl)	5	0
University of Houston (Co)	1	1
University of Iowa (Cl)	1	1
University of Kentucky (Cl)	2	1
University of Manitoba (Cl)	1	0
University of Massachusetts at Amherst (Cl)	1	1
University of Miami (Cl)	7	3+
University of Minnesota (Cl)	5	5
University of Montana (Cl)	1	1
University of Notre Dame (Co)	2	1
University of Oregon (Cl)	2	1
University of Pittsburgh (Cl)	7	18
University of South Florida (Cl)	4	1
University of Southern California (Cl)	4	0
University of Southern Mississippi (Cl)	3	0
University of Tennessee (Cl)	4	2
University of Toledo (Cl)	3	1
University of Vermont (Cl)	3	2
University of Wisconsin–Madison (Cl)	4	15
Utah State University (Cm)	2	1
Virginia Consortium Program in Clinical Psychology (Cl)	3	0
West Virginia University (Cl)	1	0
Yale University (Cl)	1	2

Psychopharmacology

	# Faculty	# Grants
Argosy University–Phoenix (Cl)	1	0
Idaho State University (Cl)	1	2

	# Faculty	# Grants
Indiana University of Pennsylvania (Psy.D.) (Cl)	1	0
McGill University (Cl)	2	1
San Diego State University/University of California–San Diego (Cl)	6	2
University of Georgia (Cl)	1	0
University of Pennsylvania (Cl)	1	1
University of Pittsburgh (Cl)	4	14
University of Western Ontario (Cl)	1	0

Psychophysiology

	# Faculty	# Grants
Binghamton University/State University of New York (Cl)	2	0
Florida State University (Cl)	2	2
Howard University (Cl)	1	0
Indiana University (Cl)	1	2
Louisiana State University (Cl)	1	0
McGill University (Cl)	2	1
Ohio State University (Cl)	2	2
Pennsylvania State University (Cl)	2	0
Rutgers University (Psy.D.) (Cl)	1	0
St. John's University (Cl)	1	1
San Diego State University/University of California–San Diego (Cl)	5	0
Syracuse University (Cl)	2	1
University of Alabama at Birmingham (Cl)	1	1
University of Iowa (Cl)	1	0
Temple University (Cl)	1	1
University of Delaware (Cl)	3	1
University of Illinois at Urbana–Champaign (Cl)	2	1
University of Iowa (Cl)	1	0
University of Kentucky (Cl)	2	1
University of Maryland (Cl)	2	0
University of Minnesota (Cl)	4	3
University of North Dakota (Cl)	1	0
University of Pennsylvania (Cl)	3	3
University of Pittsburgh (Cl)	5	7
Vanderbilt University—Department of Psychology (Cl)	2	0
Virginia Commonwealth University (Cl)	2	0

Psychotherapy Integration

	# Faculty	# Grants
University of Missouri–Columbia (Co)	1	0
Yeshiva University (Cm)	1	0
University of Missouri–Columbia (Cl)	1	1

Psychotherapy/Process and Outcome

	# Faculty	# Grants
Adelphi University (Cl)	3	2
Alliant International University–Los Angeles (Psy.D.) (Cl)	1	0
Alliant International University–San Diego (Psy.D.) (Cl)	1	0
Antioch/New England Graduate School (Cl)	2	0
Argosy University, Chicago Northwest (Psy.D.)	2	1

	# Faculty	# Grants
Argosy University–Twin Cities (Cl)	1	0
Arizona State University (Co)	4	0
Brigham Young University (Co)	3	1
Carlos Albizu University–Miami Campus (Cl)	6	0
Catholic University of America (Cl)	3	0
City University of New York at City College (Cl)	3	0
Clark University (Cl)	1	0
Colorado State University (Co)	1	0
Columbia University, Teachers College (Cl)	3	2
Drexel University (Cl)	5	0
George Mason University (Cl)	1	0
Georgia State University (Cl)	1	0
Hofstra University (Cm)	1	2
Immaculata College (Cl)	1	0
Iowa State University (Co)	2	0
James Madison University (Cm)	1	0
Loma Linda University (Ph.D. & Psy.D.) (Cl)	1	0
Long Island University (Cl)	3	1
Loyola College in Maryland (Cl)	1	0
Loyola University–Chicago (Cl)	4	1
Loyola University–Chicago (Co)	1	0
Marquette University (Cl)	3	0
Marquette University (Co)	2	0
McGill University (Cl)	1	1
McGill University (Co)	2	1
Miami University (Cl)	3	0
New School University (Cl)	3	1
Northwestern University (Cl)	1	0
Northwestern University, Feinberg School of Medicine (Cl)	2	3
Nova Southeastern University (Ph.D. & Psy.D.) (Cl)	3	0
Ohio State University (Co)	2	0
Ohio University (Cl)	2	2
Pacific University (Cl)	2	0
Pennsylvania State University (Cl)	4	3
Pennsylvania State University (Co)	1	0
Pepperdine University (Cl)	6	1
Rutgers University (Ph.D.) (Cl)	5	4
Rutgers University (Psy.D.) (Cl)	5	1
St. John's University (Cl)	1	1
San Diego State University/University of California–San Diego (Cl)	4	0
Southern Illinois University (Co)	3	0
Stony Brook University/State University of New York (Cl)	1	0
Suffolk University (Cl)	2	0
Texas A&M University (Cl)	7	2
University of Alabama (Cl)	2	0
University at Albany/State University of New York (Co)	1	1
University of Arizona (Cl)	4	4
University of British Columbia (Co)	1	0
University of California–Santa Barbara (Cm)	1	1
University of Colorado (Cl)	4	2
University of Delaware (Cl)	1	1
University of Denver (Ph.D.) (Cl)	1	1
University of Detroit–Mercy (Cl)	4	0

	# Faculty	# Grants
University of Georgia (Co)	2	0
University of Hartford (Cl)	4	1
University of Hawaii at Manoa (Cl)	4	4
University of Illinois at Urbana–Champaign (Cl)	1	0
University of Kansas (Co)	1	1
University of La Verne (Psy.D.) (Cl)	3	0
University of Maine (Cl)	3	0
University of Manitoba (Cl)	3	0
University of Maryland (Cl)	3	2
University of Maryland (Co)	3	0
University of Massachusetts at Amherst (Cl)	1	1
University of Memphis (Cl)	3	0
University of Michigan (Cl)	5	0
University of Minnesota—Department of Educational Psychology (Co)	2	0
University of Missouri–Columbia (Co)	3	2
University of Missouri–Kansas City (Co)	3	0
University of Montana (Cl)	2	1
University of North Texas (Co)	6	0
University of Northern Colorado (Co)	1	0
University of Oklahoma (Co)	5	0
University of Oregon (Co)	4	1
University of Ottawa (Cl)	4	0
University of St. Thomas (Co)	1	0
University of Saskatchewan (Cl)	2	1
University of Southern Mississippi (Co)	2	0
University of Tennessee (Co)	2	0
University of Toledo (Cl)	2	0
University of Utah (Co)	1	0
University of Washington (Cl)	1	1
University of Windsor (Cl)	3	1
University of Wisconsin–Milwaukee (Cl)	3	4
Vanderbilt University (Cl)	2	2
Virginia Commonwealth University (Cl)	1	1
Virginia Consortium Program in Clinical Psychology (Cl)	2	0
Virginia Polytechnic Institute and State University (Cl)	2	1
Washington University (Cl)	3	4
West Virginia University (Co)	3	0
Western Michigan University (Cl)	4	0
Wright Institute (Cl)	3	0
Yeshiva University (Psy.D.) (Cl)	3	0
York University—Adult Clinical Program (Cl)	4	3

Rehabilitation

	# Faculty	# Grants
Alliant International University–San Diego (Ph.D.) (Cl)	2	1
Ball State University (Co)	2	1
Illinois Institute of Technology (Cl)	2	1
University of British Columbia (Co)	1	1
University at Buffalo/State University of New York (Cm)	2	0
University of Texas Southwestern Medical Center at Dallas (Cl)	1	1
Virginia Consortium Program in Clinical Psychology (Cl)	1	0
West Virginia University (Co)	4	0

Religion/Spirituality

	# Faculty	# Grants
Azusa Pacific University (Cl)	3	1
Biola University (Ph.D.) (Cl)	4	2
Biola University (Psy.D.) (Cl)	4	2
Bowling Green State University (Cl)	1	1
Brigham Young University (Co)	6	3
Columbia University, Teachers College (Cl)	1	1
Fuller Theological Seminary (Ph.D. & Psy.D.) (Cl)	7	0
George Fox University (Cl)	1	1
Howard University (Co)	2	0
Iowa State University (Co)	1	0
Loma Linda University (Ph.D. & Psy.D.) (Cl)	2	0
Loyola College in Maryland (Cl)	2	0
New York University (Co)	1	1
Regent University (Cl)	4	3
Southern Illinois University (Cl)	1	0
Southern Illinois University (Co)	1	0
Texas Tech University (Co)	1	0
University of Detroit–Mercy (Cl)	3	0
University of Maryland–Baltimore County (Cl)	1	0
University of Southern Mississippi (Co)	1	0
University of St. Thomas (Co)	1	0
Virginia Commonwealth University (Co)	2	0
Virginia Consortium Program in Clinical Psychology (Cl)	1	0
Wheaton College (Cl)	5	1

Research Methodology

	# Faculty	# Grants
Arizona State University (Co)	2	0
Hofstra University (Cm)	2	0
Southern Illinois University (Co)	1	0
Texas Tech University (Cl)	1	0
University at Albany/State University of New York (Co)	2	0
University of Toledo (Cl)	1	0
Wheaton College (Cl)	1	0

Rorschach

	# Faculty	# Grants
Argosy University–Twin Cities (Cl)	2	0
Azusa Pacific University (Cl)	1	0
Immaculata College (Cl)	2	0
Texas Tech University (Cl)	1	1

Rural Mental Health/Psychology

	# Faculty	# Grants
Oklahoma State University (Co)	1	0
Pennsylvania State University (Cl)	1	1
University of Florida (Cl)	1	2
University of Mississippi (Cl)	2	0
University of North Carolina at Chapel Hill (Cl)	1	1
University of North Dakota (Cl)	2	2
University of South Dakota (Cl)	4	0
Utah State University (Cm)	2	1
Wheaton College (Cl)	2	0

	# Faculty	# Grants

Schizophrenia/Psychoses/Severe Mental Illness

	# Faculty	# Grants
Argosy University, Atlanta (Psy.D.)	1	1
Argosy University, Chicago (Psy.D.) (Cl)	1	1
Boston University (Cl)	1	1
Drexel University (Cl)	1	0
Emory University (Cl)	2	1
Hofstra University (Cm)	2	1
Indiana University (Cl)	2	2
Kent State University (Cl)	2	1
Long Island University–C.W. Post Campus (Cl)	1	0
Rosalind Franklin University of Medicine (Cl)	1	0
St. John's University (Cl)	1	0
San Diego State University/University of California–San Diego (Cl)	7	2
University of California–Berkeley (Cl)	1	1
University of California–Los Angeles (Cl)	2	4
University of Central Florida (Cl)	1	0
University of Georgia (Cl)	1	0
University of Hawaii at Manoa (Cl)	5	1
University of Houston (Cl)	2	1
University of Illinois at Chicago (Cl)	1	4
University of Illinois at Urbana–Champaign (Cl)	2	0
University of Manitoba (Cl)	1	0
University of Michigan (Cl)	1	0
University of Minnesota (Cl)	3	0
University of Missouri–Columbia (Cl)	1	0
University of Montana (Cl)	1	0
University of North Carolina at Chapel Hill (Cl)	1	1
University of North Carolina at Greensboro (Cl)	1	1
University of North Texas (Cl)	2	1
University of Pittsburgh (Cl)	1	1
University of Virginia—Department of Psychology (Cl)	2	0
University of Western Ontario (Cl)	1	1
University of Wisconsin–Madison (Cl)	2	3
Vanderbilt University (Cl)	1	1
Virginia Consortium Program in Clinical Psychology (Cl)	1	1
Wayne State University (Cl)	1	0
York University—Adult Clinical Program (Cl)	1	1

School/Education

	# Faculty	# Grants
Argosy University, Atlanta (Psy.D.)	2	1
Argosy University, Chicago (Psy.D.) (Cl)	2	1
Argosy University–Honolulu Campus (Cl)	5	0
Azusa Pacific University (Cl)	2	1
Brigham Young University (Co)	2	1
Colorado State University (Co)	2	1
Duke University (Cl)	5	2
George Fox University (Cl)	1	1
Immaculata College (Cl)	2	0
Indiana State University (Co)	1	1
Indiana University (Co)	2	1
Louisiana Tech University (Co)	1	0
Marquette University (Co)	2	1
Miami University (Cl)	4	2
New Mexico State University (Co)	1	0
Southern Illinois University (Co)	3	0
Suffolk University (Cl)	1	0
Texas Tech University (Cl)	2	0
University of California–Berkeley (Cl)	1	0
University of California–Los Angeles (Cl)	1	1
University of California–Santa Barbara (Cm)	5	3
University of Georgia (Co)	2	1
University of Kansas (Cl)	2	1
University of Kansas (Co)	1	0
University of Louisville (Co)	1	0
University of Minnesota—Department of Educational Psychology (Co)	3	0
University of Oregon (Co)	2	0
University of Virginia–Department of Human Services (Cl)	4	1
University of Wisconsin–Madison (Co)	4	2
University of Wisconsin–Milwaukee (Co)	1	1
Utah State University (Cm)	1	0

Self-Esteem/Self-Efficacy

	# Faculty	# Grants
George Mason University (Cl)	1	0
Southern Illinois University (Co)	1	0
Suffolk University (Cl)	1	0
University of North Carolina at Chapel Hill (Cl)	1	0
University of North Dakota (Co)	1	0
University of Wisconsin–Madison (Cl)	1	1
University of Wyoming (Cl)	2	0
West Virginia University (Cl)	3	0
West Virginia University (Co)	2	0

Sexuality/Dysfunction and Deviation

	# Faculty	# Grants
Argosy University, Atlanta (Ph.D.) (Cl)	2	0
Argosy University, Chicago (Psy.D.) (Cl)	2	0
Argosy University–Pheonix (Cl)	2	0
Auburn University (Cl)	1	0
Brigham Young University (Cl)	1	0
Carlos Albizu University–San Juan (Psy.D.) (Cl)	2	0
Central Michigan University (Cl)	1	0
Colorado State University (Co)	1	0
Hofstra University (Cm)	1	0
Immaculata College (Cl)	2	0
Indiana University (Co)	3	0
Iowa State University (Co)	1	1
Loyola College in Maryland (Cl)	2	0
Loyola University–Chicago (Cl)	1	0
McGill University (Cl)	1	1
Michigan State University (Cl)	1	0
Regent University (Cl)	1	3
San Diego State University/University of California–San Diego (Cl)	1	0
Simon Fraser University (Cl)	2	2

	# Faculty	# Grants
Southern Illinois University (Co)	1	0
Texas Tech University (Co)	1	0
Uniformed Services University of Health Sciences (Cl)	2	4
University of British Columbia (Cl)	1	1
University at Buffalo/State University of New York (Cl)	1	0
University of Florida (Co)	1	0
University of Missouri–Columbia (Cl)	1	0
University of Montana (Cl)	1	0
University of Nevada–Reno (Cl)	1	1
University of Texas at Austin (Cl)	1	1
University of Utah (Cl)	1	1
University of Vermont (Cl)	1	1
Western Michigan University (Cl)	1	1

Sleep Disorders

	# Faculty	# Grants
Dalhousie University (Cl) (in children)	1	1
San Diego State University/University of California–San Diego (Cl)	4	0
University of Arizona (Cl)	1	2
University of Florida (Co)	1	1
University of Texas Southwestern Medical Center at Dallas (Cl)	1	1
University of Wisconsin–Madison (Cl)	1	3
Yeshiva University (Cl)	1	0

Social Anxiety/Phobia

	# Faculty	# Grants
George Mason University (Cl)	1	0
University of Notre Dame (Co)	2	2
University at Albany/State University of New York (Co)	1	0

Social Learning

	# Faculty	# Grants
Rutgers University (Psy.D.) (Cl)	1	1
Clark University (Cl)	1	0
Long Island University (Cl)	1	1
University of Georgia (Cl)	1	0

Social Psychological Approaches

	# Faculty	# Grants
Arizona State University (Co)	2	0
Ball State University (Co)	2	0
Marquette University (Cl)	1	0
Loyola College in Maryland (Cl)	2	3
Ohio State University (Cl)		
University of Maine (Cl)	1	0
University of Notre Dame (Co)	2	0
University of Wyoming (Cl)	3	2
Xavier University (Cl)	1	0

Social Skills/Competence

	# Faculty	# Grants
Binghamton University/State University of New York (Cl)	1	0
Carlos Albizu University–San Juan (Ph.D.) (Cl)	1	0
Concordia University (Cl)	1	1

	# Faculty	# Grants
Drexel University (Cl)	2	2
Duke University (Cl)	3	2
James Madison University (Cm)	—	—
Louisiana State University (Cl)	2	1
Purdue University (Cl)	3	0
San Diego State University/University of California–San Diego (Cl)	1	0
University of Alabama (Cl)	2	0
University of Houston (Cl)	4	2
University of Michigan (Cl)	3	1
University of Mississippi (Cl)	4	0
University of Nevada–Reno (Cl)	3	0
University of Ottawa (Cl)	2	2
Virginia Commonwealth University (Co)	1	1
Virginia Polytechnic Institute and State University (Cl)	3	0
York University—Clinical-Developmental Area (Cl)	3	3

Social Support

	# Faculty	# Grants
DePaul University (Cl)	1	1
Fordham University (Cl)	1	0
Illinois Institute of Technology (Cl)	1	0
Iowa State University (Co)	1	1
San Diego State University/University of California–San Diego (Cl)	2	0
Southern Illinois University (Cl)	1	0
University of Denver (Co)	1	1
University of North Dakota (Co)	1	0
University of Oregon (Co)	3	0
University of Pittsburgh (Cl)	1	2

Speech and Language/Verbal Behavior

	# Faculty	# Grants
Hofstra University (Cm)	1	0
St. John's University (Cl)	2	0
Stony Brook University/State University of New York (Cl)	1	1
University of Nevada–Reno (Cl)	3	0
University of New Mexico (Cl)	1	0
Vanderbilt University (Cl)	1	1
York University—Clinical-Developmental Area (Cl)	2	1

Sports Psychology

	# Faculty	# Grants
Carlos Albizu University–San Juan (Psy.D.) (Cl)	2	0
Catholic University of America (Cl)	1	0
Illinois Institute of Technology (Cl)	1	0
Oklahoma State University (Co)	1	0
Rosalind Franklin University of Medicine (Cl)	1	0
Spalding University (Cl)	2	0
Suffolk University (Cl)	1	0
University at Albany/State University of New York (Co)	1	0
University of Manitoba (Cl)	1	1
University of Missouri–Kansas City (Co)	1	0
University of North Texas (Co)	2	1
University of Washington (Cl)	2	1
West Virginia University (Co)	1	0

	# Faculty	# Grants

Statistics

	# Faculty	# Grants
Arizona State University (Cl)	6	6
Fairleigh Dickinson University (Cl)	2	0
Indiana University (Cl)	2	1
Loma Linda University (Ph.D. & Psy.D.) (Cl)	2	0
San Diego State University/University of California–San Diego (Cl)	4	0
University of Pittsburgh (Cl)	2	2
Vanderbilt University (Cl)	2	1
Xavier University (Cl)	2	0

Stigma

	# Faculty	# Grants
Argosy University, Chicago Northwest (Psy.D.)	1	1
Iowa State University (Co)	1	0
Jackson State University (Cl)	2	0
University of Florida (Co)	1	0

Stress and Coping

	# Faculty	# Grants
American University (Cl)	1	0
Catholic University of America (Cl)	3	1
Colorado State University (Co)	2	0
Columbia University, Teachers College (Cl)	2	2
Drexel University (Cl)	1	1
Duke University (Cl)	6	6
Fairleigh Dickinson University (Cl)	2	1
Fordham University (Cl)	2	0
Forest Institute of Professional Psychology (Cl)	2	1
Fuller Theological Seminary (Ph.D. & Psy.D.) (Cl)	1	0
George Washington University (Ph.D.) (Cl)	2	0
Georgia State University (Cl)	1	0
Georgia State University (Co)	2	0
Howard University (Co)	1	1
Indiana State University (Cl)	2	0
Kent State University (Cl)	4	2
Louisiana State University (Cl)	1	0
McGill University (Cl)	1	1
Purdue University (Co)	1	0
St. John's University (Cl)	1	1
St. Louis University (Cl)	2	0
San Diego State University/University of California–San Diego (Cl)	13	0
Simon Fraser University (Cl)	1	0
Southern Illinois University (Cl)	1	0
Southern Illinois University (Co)	3	0
Texas Tech University (Co)	2	0
Uniformed Services University of Health Sciences (Cl)	3	10
University of British Columbia (Co)	1	2
University of Delaware (Cl)	2	1
University of Denver (Co)	1	1
University of Georgia (Cl)	2	1
University of Kansas (Cl)	2	1
University of Louisville (Cl)	2	0
University of Massachusetts at Amherst (Cl)	1	0
University of Miami (Cl)	9	2
University of Michigan (Cl)	2	0
University of Minnesota (Cl)	2	0
University of Missouri–Kansas City (Co)	1	0
University of North Dakota (Cl)	6	0
University of North Texas (Cl)	2	1
University of Oregon (Cl)	1	0
University of Pittsburgh (Cl)	3	5
University of Texas at Austin (Cl)	1	1
University of Tulsa (Cl)	3	1
University of Utah (Cl)	2	2
University of Western Ontario (Cl)	5	0
Virginia Commonwealth University (Cl)	3	0
Virginia Polytechnic Institute and State University (Cl)	1	0
Widener University (Cl)	2	0
Wright Institute (Cl)	1	0
Yeshiva University (Cl)	4	1
York University—Adult Clinical Program (Cl)	1	1
York University—Clinical-Developmental Area (Cl)	1	0

Substance Abuse/Addictive Behaviors

	# Faculty	# Grants
Alliant International University–San Diego (Psy.D.) (Cl)	1	0
American University (Cl)	2	2
Argosy University, Chicago Northwest (Psy.D.)	1	1
Arizona State University (Cl)	5	5
Auburn University (Co)	3	1
Binghamton University/State University of New York (Cl)	1	1
Boston University (Cl)	1	1
Bowling Green State University (Cl)	1	0
Colorado State University (Co)	4	3
Dalhousie University (Cl)	1	0
DePaul University (Cl)	1	0
Drexel University (Cl)	2	2
Florida Institute of Technology (Cl)	1	1
Florida State University (Cl)	2	1
Fordham University (Cl)	1	0
Fuller Theological Seminary (Ph.D. & Psy.D.) (Cl)	1	0
Hofstra University (Cm)	3	1
Howard University (Co)	3	1
Idaho State University (Cl)	2	0
Indiana State University (Cl)	1	1
Indiana University (Cl)	1	1
Jackson State University (Cl)	2	0
Loyola College in Maryland (Cl)	1	0
Marquette University (Cl)	1	0
Marquette University (Co)	1	2
McGill University (Cl)	1	1
Michigan State University (Cl)	1	1
Nova Southeastern University (Ph.D. & Psy.D.) (Cl)	3	5
Oklahoma State University (Cl)	1	0

Pacific Graduate School of Psychology (Cl)	2	1
Rutgers University (Ph.D.) (Cl)	3	5
Rutgers University (Psy.D.) (Cl)	4	4
St. John's University (Cl)	1	0
San Diego State University/University of California–San Diego (Cl)	19	6
Southern Illinois University (Cl)	1	1
Syracuse University (Cl)	2	4
Texas A&M University (Cl)	1	1
Texas Tech University (Cl)	1	1
Texas Tech University (Co)	1	0
Uniformed Services University of Health Sciences (Cl)	1	3
University of Alabama at Birmingham (Cl)	3	5
University at Albany/State University of New York (Cl)	2	1
University at Buffalo/State University of New York (Cl)	2	2
University of California–Santa Barbara (Cm)	3	4
University of Central Florida (Cl)	1	0
University of Cincinnati (Cl)	5	2
University of Colorado (Cl)	1	1
University of Detroit–Mercy (Cl)	1	1
University of Georgia (Cl)	1	0
University of Hawaii at Manoa (Cl)	1	3
University of Illinois at Chicago (Cl)	4	5
University of Iowa (Cl)	1	0
University of Kentucky (Cl)	4	2
University of Louisville (Cl)	1	0
University of Louisville (Co)	2	1
University of Maryland (Cl)	2	2
University of Maryland–Baltimore County (Cl)	2	2
University of Memphis (Cl)	2	3
University of Michigan (Cl)	2	2
University of Minnesota—Department of Educational Psychology (Co)	1	1
University of Mississippi (Cl)	1	1
University of Missouri–Columbia (Cl)	4	15
University of Missouri–Columbia (Co)	2	0
University of Missouri–Kansas City (Co)	1	0
University of Montana (Cl)	1	1
University of Nevada–Reno (Cl)	2	1
University of New Mexico (Cl)	6	8
University of North Carolina at Chapel Hill (Cl)	1	0
University of North Dakota (Cl)	1	0
University of Pennsylvania (Cl)	1	1
University of Pittsburgh (Cl)	3	5
University of South Dakota (Cl)	1	1
University of South Florida (Cl)	2	5
University of Southern California (Cl)	3	1
University of Southern Mississippi (Co)	2	2
University of Texas at Austin (Cl)	1	1
University of Utah (Co)	1	1
University of Victoria (Cl)	1	1
University of Washington (Cl)	3	3
University of Western Ontario (Cl)	1	1
University of Windsor (Cl)	3	2
University of Wisconsin–Madison (Cl)	3	9

University of Wisconsin–Milwaukee (Cl)	1	2
University of Wisconsin–Milwaukee (Co)	1	2
University of Wyoming (Cl)	1	2
Utah State University (Cm)	1	1
Virginia Commonwealth University (Cl)	2	1
Virginia Consortium Program in Clinical Psychology (Cl)	1	3
Virginia Polytechnic Institute and State University (Cl)	2	3
Wright Institute (Cl)	2	0
Yale University (Cl)	1	2
York University—Adult Clinical Program (Cl)	1	3

Suicide

Arizona State University (Co)	1	0
Catholic University of America (Cl)	2	0
Florida State University (Cl)	1	0
Howard University (Cl)	1	0
James Madison University (Cm)	1	0
Northern Illinois University (Cl)	1	0
Texas Tech University (Cl)	1	0
University of Akron (Co)	2	0
University of Iowa (Co)	1	0
University of Maryland–Baltimore County (Cl)	1	0
University of Nevada–Reno (Cl)	1	0
University of South Florida (Cl)	1	1
University of Washington (Cl)	1	1
Yeshiva University (Cl)	1	0

Supervision/Mentoring

Arizona State University (Co)	4	0
Colorado State University (Co)	2	0
Florida Institute of Technology (Cl)	1	0
Fordham University (Co)	2	0
George Fox University (Cl)	1	0
Indiana State University (Co)	3	0
James Madison University (Cm)	1	0
Lehigh University (Co)	1	1
Loyola University–Chicago (Co)	1	0
Ohio State University (Co)	2	0
Oklahoma State University (Co)	3	0
Pacific University (Cl)	2	0
Southern Illinois University (Co)	2	0
Spalding University (Cl)	1	0
University at Albany/State University of New York (Co)	2	0
University of Manitoba (Cl)	1	0
University of Maryland (Co)	3	0
University of Memphis (Co)	5	1
University of Minnesota—Department of Educational Psychology (Co)	2	1
University of Missouri–Columbia (Co)	2	1
University of Missouri–Kansas City (Co)	2	0
University of North Dakota (Co)	3	0
University of Oklahoma (Co)	3	0
University of Virginia–Department of Human Services (Cl)	6	5

University of Wisconsin–Madison (Co)	1	1
Washington State University (Co)	1	0
West Virginia University (Co)	1	0

Telehealth/Technology

Howard University (Co)	1	1
Ontario Institute for Studies in Education (Cm)	2	1
Suffolk University (Cl)	1	1
University of Florida (Cl)	1	1
University of Houston (Co)	2	0
University of Mississippi (Cl)	1	1

Treatment Cost Effectiveness

American University (Cl)	1	0
University of Nevada–Reno (Cl)	3	1
University of Western Ontario (Cl)	2	3
Western Michigan University (Co)		

Violence/Abuse/Sexual Abuse

Alliant International University– Los Angeles (Psy.D.) (Cl)	2	0
Argosy University, Atlanta (Psy.D.)	1	0
Argosy University, Chicago (Psy.D.) (Cl)	1	0
Argosy University, Chicago Northwest (Psy.D.)	2	0
Boston College (Co)	3	2
Boston University (Cl)	1	0
Catholic University of America (Cl)	1	1
Central Michigan University (Cl)	1	0
Colorado State University (Co)	2	0
Columbia University, Teachers College (Co)	1	0
DePaul University (Cl)		
Drexel University (Cl)	3	3
Duke University (Cl)	2	0
Fairleigh Dickinson University (Cl)	3	0
Fielding Graduate Institute (Cl)	—	—
Idaho State University (Cl)	1	1
Indiana University (Cl)	1	1
Loma Linda University (Ph.D. & Psy.D.) (Cl)	2	0
Long Island University–C.W. Post Campus (Cl)	2	0
Loyola College in Maryland (Cl)	1	0
Miami University (Cl)	1	0
Michigan State University (Cl)	2	1
Northern Illinois University (Cl)	5	5
Nova Southeastern University (Ph.D. & Psy.D.) (Cl)	7	0
Ohio University (Cl)	1	2
Oklahoma State University (Cl)	1	0
Pennsylvania State University (Cl)	2	0
St. John's University (Cl)	1	0
St. Louis University (Cl)	2	1
Simon Fraser University (Cl)	5	5
Southern Illinois University (Cl)	1	0
Southern Illinois University (Co)	2	0
Stony Brook University/State University of New York (Cl)	3	6

Temple University (Cl)	1	1
Texas A&M University (Co)	3	1
Texas Women's University (Co)	3	1
University of Alabama (Cl)	3	1
University of Arkansas (Cl)	3	1
University of California–Santa Barbara (Cm)	3	2
University of Cincinnati (Cl)	2	1
University of Colorado (Cl)	1	0
University of Connecticut (Cl)	2	0
University of Denver (Ph.D.) (Cl)	1	0
University of Georgia (Cl)	6	3
University of Georgia (Co)	4	1
University of Houston (Co)	1	1
University of Illinois at Urbana– Champaign (Co)	2	0
University of Kansas (Cl)	3	1
University of Kentucky (Cl)	2	2
University of Louisville (Co)	1	2
University of Manitoba (Cl)	5	0
University of Maryland (Co)	1	0
University of Maryland–Baltimore County (Cl)	1	1
University of Miami (Co)	1	0
University of Michigan (Cl)	2	2
University of Minnesota—Department of Psychology (Co)	1	0
University of Mississippi (Cl)	2	1
University of Missouri–St. Louis (Cl)	1	1
University of Nebraska–Lincoln (Cl)	2	2
University of Nevada–Reno (Cl)	2	0
University of North Texas (Cl)	2	0
University of Oklahoma (Co)	2	0
University of Oregon (Co)	1	0
University of Pennsylvania (Cm)		
University of South Carolina (Cl)	1	1
University of South Dakota (Cl)	2	0
University of Southern California (Cl)	2	1
University of Utah (Co)	2	1
University of Victoria (Cl)	2	1
University of Virginia—Department of Human Services (Cl)	2	1
University of Virginia—Department of Psychology (Cl)	4	2
University of Washington (Cl)	2	1
University of Western Ontario (Cl)	2	2
Virginia Commonwealth University (Co)	1	0
Wright State University (Cl)	10	3
York University—Clinical-Developmental Area (Cl)	2	2

Vocational Interests/Career Development

Arizona State University (Co)	5	1
Ball State University (Co)	4	0
Boston College (Co)	1	1
Colorado State University (Co)	2	0
Florida State University (Cm)	3	2
Fordham University (Co)	2	1
Georgia State University (Co)	1	0
Indiana State University (Co)	2	0
Indiana University (Co)	1	0

Iowa State University (Co)	3	1
Lehigh University (Co)	1	1
Louisiana Tech University (Co)	1	0
Loyola University–Chicago (Co)	1	1
New Mexico State University (Co)	2	0
New York University (Co)	1	0
Ohio State University (Co)	4	0
Oklahoma State University (Co)	4	1
Seton Hall University (Co)	1	0
Southern Illinois University (Co)	1	1
Texas A&M University (Co)	3	1
Texas Tech University (Co)	2	0
Texas Woman's University (Co)	3	1
University of Akron (Co)	2	0
University at Albany/State University of New York (Co)	1	0
University of British Columbia (Co)	3	4
University at Buffalo/State University of New York (Cm)	1	0
University of California–Santa Barbara (Cm)	2	1
University of Denver (Co)	1	1
University of Houston (Co)	2	0
University of Illinois at Urbana–Champaign (Co)	2	1
University of Kansas (Co)	1	0
University of Maryland (Co)	4	2
University of Memphis (Co)	2	1
University of Minnesota—Department of Educational Psychology (Co)	3	0
University of Minnesota—Department of Psychology (Co)	1	1
University of Missouri–Columbia (Co)	5	2
University of Missouri–Kansas City (Co)	4	0
University of Nebraska–Lincoln (Co)	1	0
University of North Dakota (Co)	2	0
University of North Texas (Co)	3	1
University of Oklahoma (Co)	2	0
University of Oregon (Co)	2	0
University of Tennessee (Co)	2	0
University of Utah (Co)	1	0
University of Wisconsin–Madison (Co)	2	0
University of Wisconsin–Milwaukee (Co)	2	2
Virginia Commonwealth University (Co)	1	2
Washington State University (Co)	2	0
West Virginia University (Co)	4	0
Yeshiva University (Cm)	2	0

Weight Management

University of Florida (Cl)	1	0

Women's Studies/Issues

Alliant International University–Fresno (Psy. D.) (Cl)	1	0
Alliant International University–Los Angeles (Ph.D. & Psy.D.) (Cl)	1	0
Alliant International University–San Diego (Ph.D. & Psy.D.) (Cl)	2	1
Alliant International University–San Francisco (Ph.D.) (Cl)	4	0

Antioch/New England Graduate School (Cl)	2	0
Arizona State University (Co)	5	1
Ball State University (Co)	2	0
Boston University (Cl)	1	0
Brigham Young University (Co)	2	1
Colorado State University (Co)	3	0
Columbia University, Teachers College (Ph.D.) (Co)	1	0
Fairleigh Dickinson University (Cl)	4	0
Indiana State University (Cl)	2	0
Indiana University (Co)	1	0
Indiana University of Pennsylvania (Cl)	3	0
Iowa State University (Co)	1	0
Loyola College in Maryland (Cl)	2	0
New York University (Co)	2	2
Ohio State University (Co)	2	0
Oklahoma State University (Co)	2	0
Pacific University (Cl)	2	0
Southern Illinois University (Co)	1	0
Texas Tech University (Co)	3	0
University at Albany/State University of New York (Co)	2	0
University of Akron (Co)	3	0
University of British Columbia (Co)	1	0
University of Florida (Co)	1	0
University of Georgia (Cl)	2	0
University of Hartford (Cl)	2	0
University of Illinois at Urbana–Champaign (Cl)	3	2
University of Illinois at Urbana–Champaign (Co)	1	0
University of Maine (Cl)	1	0
University of Memphis (Co)	2	0
University of Minnesota—Department of Educational Psychology (Co)	1	0
University of Missouri–St. Louis (Cl)	1	0
University of North Dakota (Cl)	2	0
University of North Dakota (Co)	1	0
University of Texas at Austin (Co)	1	0
University of Utah (Co)	2	0
University of Western Ontario (Cl)	1	0
University of Wisconsin–Milwaukee (Co)	1	1
Virginia Consortium Program in Clinical Psychology (Cl)	2	0

Miscellaneous

aboriginal approaches to healing—University of British Columbia (Co)	2	1
acculturation—Alliant International University–Los Angeles (Ph.D. & Psy.D.) (Cl)	1	0
New Mexico State University (Co)	3	0
action research—Miami University (Cl)	2	1
Adlerian psychology—New Mexico State University (Co)	1	0
adoption—Rutgers University (Psy.D.) (Cl)	1	1
adult survivors of incest—University of Michigan (Cl)	1	0
alternative methods—Alliant International University—Los Angeles (Ph.D.) (Cl)	1	0
Auburn University (Co)	1	0

altruism—Columbia University, Teachers College (Cl)	1	0
behavior control—Emory University (Cl)	1	0
University of Maryland (Cl)	2	1
behavioral dentistry—West Virginia University (Cl)	1	0
brief therapy—Our Lady of the Lake University (Co)	3	2
burnout prevention—University of Minnesota—Department of Educational Psychology (Co)	2	0
caregiver burden—Southern Illinois University (Co)	1	1
change processes—Adelphi University (Cl)	2	0
chaos theory—Marquette University (Cl)	1	1
child testimony—York University—Clinical-Developmental Area (Cl)	1	0
chronic fatigue syndrome—DePaul University (Cl)	1	3
compliance—University of Manitoba (Cl)	2	0
University of Mississippi (Cl)	1	0
conscious/unconscious processes—Drexel University (Cl)	1	0
University of Michigan (Cl)	1	0
constructivist psychology—University of Florida (Co)	1	0
University of Southern Mississippi (Co)	1	0
consumer psychology—Suffolk University (Cl)	1	0
counseling youth/prevention—Florida State University (Cm)	2	1
creativity—Adelphi University (Cl)	1	1
University of Kansas (Co)	1	1
criminal behavior—Florida State University (Cl)	1	0
data-based case management—University of Hawaii at Manoa (Cl)	2	0
dissociative disorders—Central Michigan University (Cl)	1	1
Rutgers University (Psy.D.) (Cl)	1	0
ecopsychology—University of Oklahoma (Co)	2	0
empathy—Suffolk University (Cl)	1	0
epidemiology—Florida State University (Cl)	1	1
epilepsy—University of Victoria (Cl)	1	1
evaluation of counseling services—University of Utah (Co)	1	0
evolutionary psychology—University of Louisville (Co)	2	0
Wright Institute (Cl)	1	1
existential-humanistic—Immaculate College (Cl)	2	0
experiential therapy—Argosy University, Chicago Northwest (Psy.D.)	3	1
extracurricular activities—Loyola University–Chicago (Cl)	1	0
Eye Movement Desensitization and Reprocessing—Central Michigan University (Cl)	1	0
FAS & attention—University of Saskatchewan (Cl)	2	2
feminism pedagogy—McGill University (Co)	1	0
fetal alcohol disorder—Ontario Institute for Studies in Education (Cm)	1	1
University of Victoria (Cl)	1	1
friendship—Marquette University (Cl)	1	0
University of North Dakota (Cl)	2	0
genetic counseling—University of Minnesota—Department of Educational Psychology (Cl)	1	1
gestalt therapy—Pacific University (Cl)	1	0
gifted/talented children—Arizona State University (Co)	2	1
grief counseling—University at Buffalo/State University of New York (Cm)	1	0
Purdue University (Co)	1	0
habit behaviors—Western Michigan University (Cl)	1	0
help-seeking—Marquette University (Cl)	1	1
history of psychology—York University—Clinical-Developmental Area (Cl)	1	0
human error—Hofstra University (Cm)	1	0
humor—San Diego State University/University of California–San Diego (Cl)	1	0
University of Western Ontario (Cl)	2	0
hypothyroidism—Ontario Institute for Studies in Education (Cm)	1	1
identity development—University of Missouri–Columbia (Co)	1	0
University of Detroit–Mercy (Cl)	2	0
identity phenotype—New Mexico State University (Co)	3	0
immigration issues—Columbia University (Ph.D.) (Co)		
incarcerated populations—University of Virginia—Department of Human Services (Cl)	2	2
Wright Institute (Cl)	1	0
infertility—University of British Columbia (Co)	1	0
integrative services—Boston College (Co)	4	6
Pacific University (Cl)	2	0
international student adjustment—University of North Dakota (Cl)	1	0
leadership—Northeastern University (Cm)	3	1
Virginia Commonwealth University (Co)	1	0
media and psychology—University of Massachusetts at Boston (Cl)	1	0
men's issues—Argosy University, Chicago Northwest (Psy.D.)	1	0
Tennessee State University (Co)	1	0
multidisciplinary environments—University of Wisconsin–Madison (Co)	1	1
nightmares—Texas Tech University (Cl)	1	0
nonlinear dynamical systems—University of Montana (Cl)	1	0

nonverbal communication—Loyola College in Maryland (Cl)	1	0
nutrition—San Diego State University/ University of California–San Diego (Cl)	1	0
olfaction—McGill University (Cl)	1	1
peace psychology—Alliant International University–Los Angeles (Ph.D.) (Cl)	1	0
Wright State University (Psy.D.) (Cl)	1	0
perception/eye movement—University of Detroit–Mercy (Cl)	1	1
perfectionism—Pennsylvania State University (Co)	1	0
York University—Adult Clinical Program (Cl)	1	1
personal constructs—Virginia Consortium Program in Clinical Psychology (Cl)	1	0
personal meaning-making processes— Texas Tech University (Cl)	1	0
philosophical issues—Rutgers University (Psy.D.) (Cl)	5	1
Rutgers University (Ph.D.) (Cl)	2	0
policy—University of Houston (Co)	1	0
poverty—University of North Dakota (Co)	1	0
psychiatric diagnosis—Pepperdine University (Cl)	1	1
psychological reactance theory— Louisiana Tech University (Co)	1	0
psychology and the arts—Rutgers (Psy.D.) (Cl)	1	0

psychology of physical symptoms— University of Western Ontario (Cl)	1	1
psychotherapists development— University of Massachusetts at Amherst (Cl)	1	1
rational-emotive therapy—Hofstra University (Cm)	1	0
scale construction—University of Missouri–Columbia (Co)	4	3
self psychology—Case Western Reserve University (Cl)	1	0
shame—George Fox University (Cl)	1	0
shyness—Virginia Polytechnic Institute and State University (Cl)	1	0
sizism—University of North Dakota (Co)	1	0
stereotypes—University of Massachu- setts–Boston (Cl)	1	0
Virginia Consortium Program in Clinical Psychology (Cl)	1	0
stimulus equivalence—University of New Mexico (Cl)	1	0
student well-being—Seton Hall University (Co)	1	0
symbolic play—Yeshiva University (Cm)	1	0
teaching of psychology—Suffolk University (Cl)	1	0
Tennessee State University (Co)	1	0
underachievement—York University— Clinical-Developmental Area (Cl)	1	0
visitor studies—Suffolk University (Cl)	1	0
working alliance in therapy—McGill University (Co)	1	1

APPENDIX F

SPECIALTY CLINICS AND PRACTICA SITES

Acquired Immune Deficiency Syndrome (AIDS)/HIV

Alliant International University–Los Angeles (Ph.D. & Psy.D) (Cl)
Argosy University–Phoenix (Cl)
Argosy University–Twin Cities (Cl)
Azusa Pacific University (Cl)
George Washington University (Ph.D.) (Cl)
Georgia State University (Cl)
University of La Verne (Cl)
Loyola University–Chicago(Cl)
Pacific Graduate School of Psychology (Cl)
Pepperdine University (Cl)
Rutgers University (Psy.D.) (Cl)
University of Illinois at Chicago (Cl)
University of Miami (Cl)
University of Nevada–Reno (Cl)
University of Vermont (Cl)
Virginia Polytechnic Institute and State University (Cl)
Wright Institute (Cl)

Adolescent Psychotherapy/At-Risk Adolescents/Delinquency

Alliant International University–Alameda (Ph.D. & Psy.D.) (Cl)
Alliant International University–Fresno (Ph.D. & Psy.D.) (Cl)
Argosy University–Honolulu Campus (Cl)
Auburn University (Cl)
Binghamton University/State University of New York (Cl)
Boston University (Cl)
Brigham Young University (Cl)
Concordia University (Cl)
Duke University (Cl)
Florida State University (Cl)
George Washington University (Ph.D. & Psy.D.) (Cl)
Georgia School of Professional Psychology (Cl)

Georgia State University (Cl)
Iowa State University (Co)
Marquette University (Co)
Northwestern University, Feinberg School of Medicine (Cl)
Oklahoma State University (Co)
Pepperdine University (Psy.D.) (Cl)
Queen's University (Cl)
Rutgers University (Ph.D.) (Cl)
Rutgers University (Psy.D.) (Cl)
Southern Illinois University (Cl)
Suffolk University (Cl)
Tenessee State University (Co)
Uniformed Services University of Health Sciences (Cl)
University of Akron (Co)
University at Albany/State University of New York (Cl & Co)
University of Denver (Ph.D.) (Cl)
University of Georgia (Co)
University of Indianapolis (Cl)
University of Maine (Cl)
University of Massachusetts at Amherst (Cl)
University of Memphis (Co)
University of Montana (Cl)
University of Pittsburgh (Cl)
University of Saskatchewan (Cl)
University of South Florida (Cl)
University of Utah (Cl)
University of Vermont (Cl)
University of Waterloo (Cl)
Virginia Consortium Program in Clinical Psychology (Cl)
Yale University (Cl)
Yeshiva University (Cl & Cm)

Affective Disorders/Depression/ Mood Disorders

Baylor University (Cl)
Binghamton University/State University of New York (Cl)

Note. Cl, Clinical; Co, Counseling; Cm, combined professional–scientific psychology programs.

351

Boston University (Cl)
Case Western Reserve University (Cl)
Duke University (Cl)
George Washington University (Ph.D.) (Cl)
Georgia State University (Cl)
Illinois Institute of Technology (Cl)
Indiana University (Cl)
Long Island University–C.W. Post Campus (Cl)
Michigan State University (Cl)
Northwestern University (Cl)
Nova Southeastern University (Ph.D. & Psy.D.) (Cl)
Ohio State University (Cl)
Purdue University (Cl)
Rutgers University (Ph.D.) (Cl)
Rutgers University (Psy.D.) (Cl)
University of Arizona (Cl)
University at Buffalo/State University of New York (Cl)
University of California–Los Angeles (Cl)
University of Georgia (Cl)
University of Illinois at Chicago (Cl)
University of Iowa (Cl)
University of Louisville (Cl)
University of Manitoba (Cl)
University of Memphis (Cl)
University of Minnesota (Cl)
University of Nevada–Reno (Cl)
University of North Dakota (Cl)
University of North Texas (Cl)
University of Oregon (Cl)
University of Ottawa (Cl)
University of Pittsburgh (Cl)
University of South Florida (Cl)
University of Texas at Austin (Cl)
University of Texas Southwestern Medical Center at Dallas (Cl)
University of Vermont (Cl)
University of Virginia—Department of Psychology (Cl)
University of Western Ontario (Cl)
University of Wyoming (Cl)
Vanderbilt University—Department of Psychology (Cl)
Virginia Commonwealth University (Cl)
Virginia Polytechnic Institute and State University (Cl)
Wright Institute (Cl)
York University—Adult Clinical Program (Cl)

Aging/Gerontology

Alliant International University–Los Angeles (Ph.D. & Psy.D) (Cl)
Argosy University–Twin Cities (Cl)
Argosy University–Washington, DC Campus (Cl)
Arizona State University (Cl)
Ball State University (Co)
Baylor University (Psy.D.) (Cl)
Boston University (Cl)
Case Western Reserve University (Cl)
Fairleigh Dickinson University (Cl)
Forest Institute of Professional Psychology (Cl)
Fuller Theological Seminary (Ph.D. & Psy.D.) (Cl)
George Fox University (Cl)
Illinois School of Professional Psychology–Chicago Campus (Cl)
Marquette University (Cl)

Michigan State University (Cl)
Nova Southeastern University (Ph.D. & Psy.D.) (Cl)
Ohio State University (Cl)
Pepperdine University (Cl)
Queen's University (Cl)
Rutgers University (Psy.D.) (Cl)
Suffolk University (Cl)
University of Alabama (Cl)
University at Albany/State University of New York (Co)
University of Arizona (Cl)
University of Houston (Co)
University of Louisville (Cl)
University of Massachusetts at Amherst (Cl)
University of Minnesota (Cl)
University of Missouri–St. Louis (Cl)
University of Nevada–Reno (Cl)
University of Southern California (Cl)
University of Utah (Co)
Virginia Polytechnic Institute and State University (Cl)
West Virginia University (Cl)
Wright Institute (Cl)
York University–Adult Clinical Program (Cl)

Anxiety Disorders/Panic Disorders

Alliant International University–Fresno (Ph.D. & Psy.D.) (Cl)
Argosy University–Washington, DC Campus (Cl)
Auburn University (Cl)
Baylor University (Psy.D.) (Cl)
Binghamton University/State University of New York (Cl)
Case Western Reserve University (Cl)
Drexel University (Cl)
Fairleigh Dickinson University (Cl)
Florida State University (Cl)
George Washington University (Ph.D.) (Cl)
Georgia State University (Cl)
Howard University (Cl)
Idaho State University (Cl)
Indiana University (Cl)
Long Island University–C.W. Post Campus (Cl)
Louisiana State University (Cl)
Loyola College in Maryland (Cl)
Northern Illinois University (Cl)
Northwestern University (Cl)
Nova Southeastern University (Ph.D. & Psy.D.) (Cl)
Ohio State University (Cl)
Oklahoma State University (Cl)
Ontario Institute for Studies in Education (Cm)
Purdue University (Cl)
Rosalind Franklin University of Medicine and Science (Cl)
Rutgers University (Ph.D.) (Cl)
Rutgers University (Psy.D.) (Cl)
St. Louis University (Cl)
San Diego State University/University of California–San Diego (Cl)
Syracuse University (Cl)
Temple University (Cl)
University at Albany/State University of New York (Cl)
University at Buffalo/State University of New York (Cl)
University of California–Los Angeles (Cl)
University of Delaware (Cl)
University of Florida (Cl)
University of Hartford (Cl)

University of Houston (Cl)
University of Illinois at Chicago (Cl)
University of Illinois at Urbana–Champaign (Cl)
University of Louisville (Cl)
University of Maine (Cl)
University of Manitoba (Cl)
University of Memphis (Cl)
University of Minnesota (Cl)
University of Montana (Cl)
University of Nebraska–Lincoln (Cl)
University of Nevada–Reno (Cl)
University of North Dakota (Cl)
University of Oregon (Cl)
University of Ottawa (Cl)
University of Pittsburgh (Cl)
University of South Florida (Cl)
University of Texas at Austin (Cl)
University of Vermont (Cl)
University of Virginia—Department of Psychology (Cl)
University of Washington (Cl)
University of Western Ontario (Cl)
University of Wyoming (Cl)
Vanderbilt University—Department of Psychology (Cl)
Virginia Commonwealth University (Cl)
Virginia Polytechnic Institute and State University (Cl)
West Virginia University (Cl)
Yale University (Cl)
Yeshiva University (Cl)
York University—Adult Clinical Program (Cl)

Assessment/Testing

Alliant International University–Fresno (Ph.D. & Psy.D.) (Cl)
Alliant International University–San Diego (Psy.D.) (Cl)
American University (Cl)
Antioch/New England Graduate School (Psy.D.) (Cl)
Argosy University–Atlanta (Cl)
Arizona State University (Cl)
Binghamton University/State University of New York (Cl)
Bowling Green State University (Cl)
Catholic University of America (Cl)
Central Michigan University (Cl)
DePaul University (Cl)
Emory University (Cl)
Fairleigh Dickinson University (Cl)
Fuller Theological Seminary (Ph.D. & Psy.D.) (Cl)
Gallaudet University (Cl)
George Fox University (Cl)
George Mason University (Cl)
George Washington University (Ph.D. & Psy.D.) (Cl)
Georgia School of Professional Psychology (Cl)
Georgia State University (Cl)
Indiana University of Pennsylvania (Cl)
James Madison University (Cm)
Kent State University (Cl)
Long Island University–C.W. Post Campus (Cl)
Loyola University–Chicago (Cl)
Miami University (Cl)
Michigan State University (Cl)
Northern Illinois University (Cl)
Nova Southeastern University (Ph.D. & Psy.D.) (Cl)
Pacific Graduate School of Psychology (Cl)
Pepperdine University (Cl)

Rutgers University (Ph.D.) (Cl)
Rutgers University (Psy.D.) (Cl)
St. Louis University (Cl)
University of British Columbia (Cl)
University of Colorado (Cl)
University of Delaware (Cl)
University of Denver (Psy.D.) (Cl)
University of Denver (Co)
University of Florida (Co)
University of Georgia (Cl)
University of Georgia (Co)
University of Hawaii at Manoa (Cl)
University of Houston (Cl)
University of Illinois at Urbana–Champaign (Cl)
University of Indianapolis (Cl)
University of Kentucky (Cl)
University of Memphis (Co)
University of Mississippi (Cl)
University of Missouri–Columbia (Cl)
University of Montana (Cl)
University of Nebraska–Lincoln (Cl)
University of Nebraska–Lincoln (Co)
University of New Mexico (Cl)
University of North Carolina at Chapel Hill (Cl)
University of North Dakota (Cl)
University of North Texas (Co)
University of Pennsylvania (Cl)
University of Pittsburgh (Cl)
University of South Florida (Cl)
University of Southern Mississippi (Co)
University of Virginia—Department of Human Services (Cl)
University of Wisconsin–Madison (Cl)
Virginia Commonwealth University (Cl)
Virginia Consortium Program in Clinical Psychology (Cl)
Widener University (Cl)
Wright Institute (Cl)

Attention-Deficit/Hyperactivity Disorder

Alliant International University–Fresno (Ph.D. & Psy.D.) (Cl)
Argosy University–Twin Cities (Cl)
Auburn University (Cl)
Case Western Reserve University (Cl)
George Washington University (Ph.D.) (Cl)
Indiana State University (Cl)
Iowa State University (Co)
Long Island University–C.W. Post Campus (Cl)
Miami University (Cl)
Northern Illinois University (Cl)
Ontario Institute for Studies in Education (Cm)
Pepperdine University (Cl)
Purdue University (Cl)
Rutgers University (Psy.D.) (Cl)
St. Louis University (Cl)
University of Arkansas (Cl)
University at Buffalo/State University of New York (Cl)
University of Georgia (Cl)
University of Maine (Cl)
University of Minnesota (Cl)
University of North Texas (Cl)
University of Pittsburgh (Cl)

University of Rochester (Cl)
University of South Florida (Cl)
Virginia Polytechnic Institute and State University (Cl)

Behavioral Medicine/Health Psychology

Alliant International University–Fresno (Ph.D. & Psy.D) (Cl)
Alliant International University–Los Angeles (Ph.D. & Psy.D) (Cl)
Alliant International University–San Diego (Ph.D. & Psy.D.) (Cl)
Antioch/New England Graduate School (Cl)
Argosy University–Atlanta (Cl)
Argosy University–Twin Cities (Cl)
Arizona State University (Cl)
Azusa Pacific University (Cl)
Ball State University (Co)
Baylor University (Cl)
Binghamton University/State University of New York (Cl)
Boston University (Cl)
Bowling Green State University (Cl)
Chicago School of Professional Psychology (Cl)
Drexel University (Cl)
Duke University (Cl)
Emory University (Cl)
Fairleigh Dickinson University (Cl)
Florida Institute of Technology (Cl)
Florida State University (Cl)
Forest Institute of Professional Psychology (Cl)
George Fox University (Cl)
George Washington University (Ph.D.) (Cl)
Georgia School of Professional Psychology (Cl)
Georgia State University (Cl)
Georgia State University (Co)
Howard University (Cl)
Illinois Institute of Technology (Cl)
Illinois School of Professional Psychology–Chicago Campus (Cl)
Illinois School of Professional Psychology–Chicago Northwest (Cl)
Indiana State University (Cl)
Indiana University (Cl)
Indiana University of Pennsylvania (Cl)
Indiana University–Purdue University Indianapolis (Cl)
Iowa State University (Co)
Jackson State University (Cl)
Kent State University (Cl)
Loma Linda University (Ph.D. & Psy.D.) (Cl)
Louisiana State University (Cl)
Louisiana Tech University (Co)
Loyola College in Maryland (Cl)
Loyola University–Chicago (Cl)
Marquette University (Co)
Northwestern University (Cl)
Nova Southeastern University (Ph.D. & Psy.D.) (Cl)
Ohio State University (Cl)
Ohio University (Cl)
Oklahoma State University (Cl)
Our Lady of the Lake University (Co)
Pacific Graduate School of Psychology (Cl)
Pepperdine University (Cl)
Regent University (Cl)

Rosalind Franklin University of Medicine and Science (Cl)
Rutgers University (Ph.D.) (Cl)
Rutgers University (Psy.D.) (Cl)
San Diego State University/University of California–San Diego (Cl)
Spalding University (Cl)
Syracuse University (Cl)
Tennessee State University (Co)
Texas Tech University (Co)
University of Alabama (Cl)
University of Alabama at Birmingham (Cl)
University at Albany/State University of New York (Cl)
University at Albany/State University of New York (Co)
University of Arizona (Cl)
University of British Columbia (Cl)
University of Central Florida (Cl)
University of Cincinnati (Cl)
University of Connecticut (Cl)
University of Denver (Psy.D.) (Cl)
University of Florida (Cl)
University of Florida (Co)
University of Georgia (Cl)
University of Hawaii at Manoa (Cl)
University of Houston (Cl)
University of Houston (Co)
University of Illinois at Chicago (Cl)
University of Illinois at Urbana–Champaign (Co)
University of Indianapolis (Cl)
University of Iowa (Cl)
University of Kentucky (Cl)
University of Louisville (Cl)
University of Manitoba (Cl)
University of Memphis (Cl)
University of Miami (Cl)
University of Mississippi (Cl)
University of Missouri–Columbia (Cl)
University of Missouri–St. Louis (Cl)
University of Nebraska–Lincoln (Co)
University of Nevada–Reno (Cl)
University of New Mexico (Cl)
University of North Carolina at Chapel Hill (Cl)
University of North Dakota (Cl)
University of Oklahoma (Co)
University of Pennsylvania (Cl)
University of Pittsburgh (Cl)
University of Rhode Island (Cl)
University of Saskatchewan (Cl)
University of South Florida (Cl)
University of Texas at Austin (Cl)
University of Texas Southwestern Medical Center at Dallas (Cl)
University of Utah (Cl)
University of Vermont (Cl)
University of Virginia—Department of Human Services (Cl)
University of Virginia—Department of Psychology (Cl)
University of Western Ontario (Cl)
University of Wisconsin–Milwaukee (Cl)
Utah State University (Cm)
Vanderbilt University—Department of Psychology (Cl)
Virginia Commonwealth University (Cl)
Virginia Polytechnic Institute and State University (Cl)
Washington State University (Cl)

Wayne State University (Cl)
West Virginia University (Cl)
Wright State University (Cl)
Yale University (Cl)
Yeshiva University (Cl)
York University—Adult Clinical Program (Cl)

Biofeedback

Alliant International University–San Diego (Psy.D.) (Cl)
Argosy University–Twin Cities (Cl)
Forest Institute of Professional Psychology (Cl)
Nova Southeastern University (Ph.D. & Psy.D.) (Cl)

Child/Pediatric/Developmental

Adelphi University (Cl)
Alliant International University–Alameda (Ph.D. & Psy.D.)
 (Cl)
Alliant International University–Fresno (Ph.D. & Psy.D) (Cl)
Alliant International University–Los Angeles (Ph.D. &
 Psy.D) (Cl)
Antioch/New England Graduate School (Cl)
Argosy University–Atlanta (Cl)
Argosy University–Honolulu Campus(Cl)
Argosy University–Washington, DC Campus (Cl)
Arizona State University (Cl)
Azusa Pacific University (Cl)
Baylor University (Cl)
Binghamton University–State University of New York (Cl)
Boston College (Co)
Biola University (Ph.D.) (Cl)
Biola University (Psy.D.) (Cl)
Bowling Green State University (Cl)
Central Michigan University (Cl)
Carlos Albizu University–Miami Campus (Cl)
Case Western Reserve University (Cl)
Chicago School of Professional Psychology (Cl)
City University of New York at City College (Cl)
Columbia University, Teachers College (Cl)
Concordia University (Cl)
DePaul University (Cl)
Drexel University (Cl)
Duke University (Cl)
Florida State University (Cl)
Forest Institute of Professional Psychology (Cl)
Fuller Theological Seminary (Ph.D. & Psy.D.) (Cl)
George Fox University (Cl)
George Washington University (Ph.D.) (Cl)
Georgia School of Professional Psychology (Cl)
Georgia State University (Cl)
Illinois Institute of Technology (Cl)
Illinois School of Professional Psychology–Chicago
 Campus (Cl)
Illinois School of Professional Psychology–Chicago
Jackson State University (Cl)
Indiana University (Cl)
Kent State University (Cl)
Long Island University (Cl)
Long Island University–C.W. Post Campus (Cl)
Louisiana Tech University (Co)
Loyola College in Maryland (Cl)
Marquette University (Cl)

McGill University (Cl & Co)
Northern Illinois University (Cl)
Northwest (Cl)
Northwestern University, Feinberg School of Medicine (Cl)
Nova Southeastern University (Ph.D. & Psy.D.) (Cl)
Ohio State University (Cl)
Ohio University (Cl)
Ontario Institute for Studies in Education (Cm)
Pace University (Psy.D.) (Cm)
Pacific Graduate School of Psychology (Cl)
Pepperdine University (Cl)
Purdue University (Cl)
Queen's University (Cl)
Regent University (Cl)
St. John's University (Cl)
San Diego State University/University of California–
 San Diego (Cl)
Southern Illinois University (Cl & Co)
Suffolk University (Cl)
Temple University (Cl & Co)
Tennessee State University (Co)
Texas Tech University (Co)
Uniformed Services University of Health Sciences (Cl)
University at Albany–State University of New York (Cl)
University of Arkansas (Cl)
University of British Columbia (Cl)
University at Buffalo/State University of New York (Cl)
University of California–Los Angeles (Cl)
University of Cincinnati (Cl)
University of Connecticut (Cl)
University of Delaware (Cl)
University of Denver (Ph.D.) (Cl)
University of Florida (Cl)
University of Florida (Co)
University of Georgia (Cl)
University of Hawaii at Manoa (Cl)
University of Houston (Cl)
University of Houston (Co)
University of Illinois at Urbana–Champaign (Cl)
University of Illinois at Urbana–Champaign (Co)
University of Indianapolis (Cl)
University of Iowa (Cl)
University of Kansas (Cl)
University of Kentucky (Cl)
University of La Verne (Cl)
University of Louisville (Cl)
University of Louisville (Co)
University of Maine (Cl)
University of Manitoba (Cl)
University of Maryland–Baltimore County (Cl)
University of Massachusetts at Amherst (Cl)
University of Memphis (Co)
University of Miami (Cl)
University of Michigan (Cl)
University of Minnesota (Cl)
University of Mississippi (Cl)
University of Missouri–Columbia (Cl)
University of Missouri–St. Louis (Cl)
University of Montana (Cl)
University of New Mexico (Cl)
University of North Carolina at Chapel Hill (Cl)
University of North Texas (Cl)

University of Oklahoma (Co)
University of Oregon (Cl)
University of Oregon (Co)
University of Ottawa (Cl)
University of Pennsylvania (Cm)
University of Pittsburgh (Cl)
University of Rhode Island (Cl)
University of Rochester (Cl)
University of Saskatchewan (Cl)
University of South Florida (Cl)
University of Southern Mississippi (Cl)
University of Texas at Austin (Cl)
University of Texas at Austin (Co)
University of Texas Southwestern Medical Center at Dallas (Cl)
University of Utah (Cl)
University of Vermont (Cl)
University of Virginia—Department of Human Services (Cl)
University of Virginia—Department of Psychology (Cl)
University of Washington (Cl)
University of Waterloo (Cl)
University of Western Ontario (Cl)
University of Wisconsin–Madison (Cl)
University of Wisconsin–Milwaukee (Cl)
University of Wisconsin–Milwaukee (Co)
Utah State University (Cm)
Vanderbilt University—Department of Psychology (Cl)
Virginia Commonwealth University (Cl)
Virginia Commonwealth University (Co)
Virginia Polytechnic Institute and State University (Cl)
Wright Institute (Cl)
Wright State University (Cl)
Yale University (Cl)
Yeshiva University (Cl & Cm)
York University—Clinical-Developmental Area (Cl)

Chronic/Severe Mental Illness

Alliant International University–Los Angeles (Ph.D. & Psy.D) (Cl)
Azusa Pacific University (Cl)
Fuller Theological Seminary (Ph.D. & Psy.D.) (Cl)
Illinois School of Professional Psychology–Chicago Campus (Cl)
Illinois School of Professional Psychology–Chicago Northwest (Cl)
Indiana University–Purdue University Indianapolis (Cl)
Northeastern University (Cm)
Northwestern University, Feinberg School of Medicine (Cl)
Nova Southeastern University (Ph.D. & Psy.D.) (Cl)
Pepperdine University (Cl)
Southern Illinois University (Cl)
University of Cincinnati (Cl)
University of Connecticut (Cl)
University of Hartford (Cl)
University of Hawaii at Manoa (Cl)
University of Kentucky (Cl)
University of Maryland–Baltimore County (Cl)
University of Mississippi (Cl)
University of Nebraska–Lincoln (Cl)
University of South Dakota (Cl)
University of Vermont (Cl)

Utah State University (Cm)
Virginia Commonwealth University (Cl)

Cognitive/Cognitive-Behavioral Therapy

Alliant International University–San Diego (Ph.D.) (Cl)
American University (Cl)
Antioch/New England Graduate School (Cl)
Arizona State University (Cl) (behavioral analysis)
Central Michigan University (Cl)
Concordia University (Cl)
Duke University (Cl)
Emory University (Cl)
Fielding Graduate Institute (Cl)
George Mason University (Cl)
Georgia State University (Co)
Idaho State University (Cl)
Illinois School of Professional Psychology–Chicago Campus (Cl)
Long Island University (Cl)
McGill University (Co)
Nova Southeastern University (Ph.D. & Psy.D.) (Cl)
Pepperdine University (Cl)
St. John's University (Cl)
San Diego State University/University of California–San Diego (Cl)
University of Colorado (Cl)
University of Denver (Psy.D.) (Cl)
University of Georgia (Cl)
University of Houston (Cl)
University of Iowa (Cl)
University of Kentucky (Cl)
University of Maine (Cl)
University of Manitoba (Cl)
University of Maryland–Baltimore County (Cl)
University of Massachusetts at Amherst (Cl)
University of Minnesota (Cl)
University of Missouri–Columbia (Co)
University of North Carolina at Chapel Hill (Cl)
University of Northern Colorado (Co)
University of Oregon (Cl)
University of Pennsylvania (Cl)
University of Pittsburgh (Cl)
University of Texas Southwestern Medical Center at Dallas (Cl)
University of Wisconsin–Madison (Cl)
Wright State University (Cl)
Yeshiva University (Cl)

Community Psychology

Antioch/New England Graduate School (Cl)
Argosy University–Honolulu Campus (Cl)
Auburn University (Co)
Azusa Pacific University (Cl)
Baylor University (Cl)
Brigham Young University (Cl)
Boston College (Co)
Boston University (Cl)
Bowling Green State University (Cl)
Chicago School of Professional Psychology (Cl)
DePaul University (Cl)
Fairleigh Dickinson University (Cl)
Florida State University (Cm)

Fordham University (Co)
George Fox University (Cl)
George Mason University (Cl)
Georgia State University (Cl)
Howard University (Cl)
Illinois School of Professional Psychology–Chicago Campus (Cl)
Illinois School of Professional Psychology–Chicago Northwest (Cl)
Indiana State University (Co)
Indiana University (Cl)
Iowa State University (Co)
James Madison University (Cm)
Loma Linda University (Ph.D. & Psy.D.) (Cl)
Long Island University (Cl)
Louisiana Tech University (Co)
Miami University (Cl)
Michigan State University (Cl)
New Mexico State University (Co)
Nova Southeastern University (Cl)
Our Lady of the Lake University (Co)
Pacific University (Cl)
Pennsylvania State University (Cl)
Pepperdine University (Cl)
Rutgers University (Ph.D.) (Cl)
Rutgers University (Psy.D.) (Cl)
Stony Brook University/State University of New York (Cl)
Syracuse University (Cl)
Texas A&M University (Cl)
Texas Tech University (Co)
Texas Woman's University (Co)
University of Akron (Co)
University at Albany/State University of New York (Co)
University of Arizona (Cl)
University of Arkansas (Cl)
University of California–Los Angeles (Cl)
University of California–Santa Barbara (Cm)
University of Cincinnati (Cl)
University of Florida (Co)
University of Illinois at Urbana–Champaign (Cl)
University of Iowa (Co)
University of Kansas (Cl)
University of Kentucky (Cl)
University of Kentucky (Co)
University of Maine (Cl)
University of Manitoba (Cl)
University of Maryland (Cl)
University of Minnesota (Cl)
University of Mississippi (Cl)
University of Montana (Cl)
University of North Carolina at Greensboro (Cl)
University of North Dakota (Cl)
University of Notre Dame (Co)
University of Oklahoma (Co)
University of Oregon (Co)
University of Ottawa (Cl)
University of Pennsylvania (Cm)
University of Rhode Island (Cl)
University of South Carolina (Cl)
University of South Dakota (Cl)
University of Southern California (Cl)
University of Texas at Austin (Cl)

University of Texas at Austin (Co)
University of Texas Southwestern Medical Center at Dallas (Cl)
University of Utah (Co)
University of Virginia—Department of Psychology (Cl)
University of Washington (Cl)
University of Wisconsin–Milwaukee (Co)
Utah State University (Cm)
Virginia Commonwealth University (Cl)
Virginia Commonwealth University (Co)
Virginia Polytechnic Institute and State University (Cl)
Wayne State University (Cl)
West Virginia University (Co)

Conduct Disorder

Antioch/New England Graduate School (Cl)
Binghamton University/State University of New York (Cl)
Forest Institute of Professional Psychology (Cl)
George Washington University (Ph.D.) (Cl)
Miami University (Cl)
Rutgers University (Ph.D.) (Cl)
Rutgers University (Psy.D.) (Cl)
University of Alabama (Cl)
University of Delaware (Cl)
University of Houston (Cl)
University of Miami (Cl)
University of Minnesota (Cl)
University of Pittsburgh (Cl)
University of Tennessee (Cl)
Virginia Polytechnic Institute and State University (Cl)
Yale University (Cl)

Consultation

George Fox University (Cl)
University of Mississippi (Cl)
University of Virginia—Department of Human Services (Cl)
Virginia Polytechnic Institute and State University (Cl)

Correctional Psychology/Prisons

Adler School of Professional Psychology (Cl)
Argosy University–Honolulu Campus (Cl)
Argosy University–Washington, DC Campus (Cl)
Brigham Young University (Cl & Co)
Chicago School of Professional Psychology (Cl)
Florida State University (Cl)
George Fox University (Cl)
Illinois School of Professional Psychology–Chicago Northwest (Cl)
Indiana State University (Co)
Indiana University–Purdue University Indianapolis (Cl)
Louisiana Tech University (Co)
Loyola College in Maryland (Cl)
Nova Southeastern University (Ph.D. & Psy.D.) (Cl)
Oklahoma State University (Co)
Southern Illinois University (Cl)
Southern Illinois University (Co)
Texas A&M University (Co)
University of Florida (Co)
University of Illinois at Urbana–Champaign (Cl)
University of Iowa (Co)

University of Kentucky (Co)
University of Louisville (Co)
University of Missouri–Columbia (Co)
University of Montana (Cl)
University of Oklahoma (Co)
University of Virginia—Department of Human Services (Cl)
University of Wisconsin–Madison (Cl)
University of Wyoming (Cl)
Virginia Commonwealth University (Cl & Co)
West Virginia University (Co)

Crisis Intervention

Argosy University–Atlanta (Cl)
Baylor University (Cl)
Georgia School of Professional Psychology (Cl)
Howard University (Cl)
Illinois School of Professional Psychology–Chicago
    Campus (Cl)
Indiana University–Purdue University Indianapolis (Cl)
Northwestern University (Cl)
Nova Southeastern University (Ph.D. & Psy.D.) (Cl)
Ohio State University (Cl)
Syracuse University (Cl)
University of Florida (Co)
University of Houston (Co)
University of Maine (Cl)
University of Minnesota (Cl)
University of South Dakota (Cl)
University of Texas at Austin (Cl)
University of Virginia—Department of Human Services (Cl)
Wright Institute (Cl)
Wright State University (Cl)

Deafness

Alliant International University–San Diego (Psy.D.) (Cl)
Gallaudet University (Cl)
Louisiana State University (Cl)
University of Iowa (Cl)
University of Texas Southwestern Medical Center at Dallas
    (Cl)
Wright State University (Cl)

Developmental Disabilities/Autism

Adler School of Professional Psychology (Cl)
Alliant International University–San Diego (Ph.D. & Psy.D.)
    (Cl)
Argosy University–Honolulu Campus (Cl)
Brigham Young University (Cl)
George Washington University (Ph.D. & Psy.D.) (Cl)
Georgia State University (Cl)
Long Island University–C.W. Post Campus (Cl)
Louisiana State University (Cl)
Miami University (Cl)
Northeastern University (Cm)
Northern Illinois University (Cl)
Northwestern University, Feinberg School of Medicine (Cl)
Ontario Institute for Studies in Education (Cm)
Purdue University (Cl) (developmental disorders)
Queen's University (Cl)
Rutgers University (Ph.D.) (Cl)
Rutgers University (Psy.D.) (Cl)
University of Alabama (Cl)

University at Albany/State University of New York (Cl)
University of California–Los Angeles (Cl)
University of California–Santa Barbara (Cm)
University of Cincinnati (Cl) (developmental disorders)
University of Connecticut (Cl)
University of Delaware (Cl)
University of Denver (Ph.D.) (Cl)
University of Georgia (Cl)
University of Hawaii at Manoa (Cl)
University of Illinois at Chicago (Cl)
University of Louisville (Co)
University of Manitoba (Cl)
University of Memphis (Cl)
University of Miami (Cl)
University of Mississippi (Cl)
University of North Carolina at Chapel Hill (Cl)
University of Pittsburgh (Cl)
University of Rochester (Cl)
University of Saskatchewan (Cl)
University of Texas Southwestern Medical Center at Dallas
    (Cl)
University of Wisconsin–Madison (Cl)
University of Wyoming (Cl)

Disabilities/Disabled Persons

Adler School of Professional Psychology (Cl)
Alliant International University–Alameda (Ph.D. & Psy.D.)
    (Cl)
Loyola College in Maryland (Cl)
Ontario Institute for Studies in Education (Cm)
University of Louisville (Cl)
Utah State University (Cm)

Disaster/Trauma/Torture

Alliant International University–San Diego (Ph.D.) (Cl)
Idaho State University (Cl)
Illinois School of Professional Psychology–Chicago
    Campus (Cl)
Nova Southeastern University (Ph.D.) (Cl)
University of Connecticut (Cl)
University of Denver (Psy.D.) (Cl)
University of Montana (Cl)
University of South Dakota (Cl)
University of South Florida (Cl)
University of Texas at Austin (Cl)
Virginia Consortium Program in Clinical Psychology
    (Cl)

Dissociative Disorder/Multiple Personality Disorder

Boston University (Cl)
George Washington University (Ph.D.) (Cl)
Rutgers University (Psy.D.) (Cl)
University of Georgia (Cl)
University of Hartford (Cl)

Divorce/Child Custody

Alliant International University–San Diego (Ph.D. & Psy.D.)
    (Cl)
University of Illinois at Urbana–Champaign (Ph.D.) (Cl)
Virginia Commonwealth University (Cl)

Dual Diagnosis Clinic

Nova Southeastern University (Ph.D. & Psy.D.) (Cl)
University of Hawaii at Manoa (Cl)
York University—Clinical-Developmental Area (Cl)

Eating Disorders/Body Image

Alliant International University–Fresno (Ph.D. & Psy.D.) (Cl)
Argosy University–Twin Cities (Cl)
Arizona State University (Cl)
Baylor University (Cl)
Boston University (Cl)
Brigham Young University (Cl & Co)
Drexel University (Cl)
Duke University (Cl)
Florida Institute of Technology (Cl)
George Washington University (Ph.D.) (Cl)
Georgia State University (Cl)
Illinois School of Professional Psychology–Chicago
	Campus (Cl)
Kent State University (Cl)
Long Island University–C.W. Post Campus (Cl)
Louisiana State University (Cl)
Loyola College in Maryland (Cl)
Loyola University–Chicago(Cl)
McGill University (Co)
Michigan State University (Cl)
Ohio State University (Cl)
Rutgers University (Ph.D. & Psy.D.) (Cl)
University at Albany/State University of New York (Cl)
University of California–Santa Barbara (Cm)
University of Central Florida (Cl)
University of Georgia (Cl)
University of Hawaii at Manoa (Cl)
University of Iowa (Cl)
University of Maine (Cl)
University of Manitoba (Cl)
University of Memphis (Cl)
University of Miami (Cl)
University of Minnesota (Cl)
University of Mississippi (Cl)
University of South Florida (Cl)
University of Vermont (Cl)
Utah State University (Cm)
West Virginia University (Cl)
Yale University (Cl)
York University—Adult Clinical Program (Cl)

Family Therapy/Systems

Adelphi University (Cl)
Alliant International University–Fresno (Ph.D. & Psy.D) (Cl)
American University (Cl)
Antioch/New England Graduate School (Cl)
Arizona State University (Cl)
Azusa Pacific University (Cl)
Baylor University (Cl)
Binghamton University/State University of New York (Cl)
Biola University (Ph.D.) (Cl)
Biola University (Psy.D.) (Cl)
Boston University (Cl)
Bowling Green State University (Cl)
Brigham Young University (Cl & Co)
Catholic University of America (Cl)

City University of New York at City College (Cl)
Clark University (Cl)
Colorado State University (Co)
Concordia University (Cl)
DePaul University (Cl)
Fairleigh Dickinson University (Cl)
Florida Institute of Technology (Psy.D.) (Cl)
Florida State University (Cl)
Fuller Theological Seminary (Ph.D. & Psy.D.) (Cl)
George Washington University (Ph.D. & Psy.D.) (Cl)
Georgia State University (Cl)
Howard University (Cl)
Idaho State University (Cl)
Illinois Institute of Technology (Cl)
Illinois School of Professional Psychology–Chicago
	Campus (Cl)
Illinois School of Professional Psychology–Chicago
	Northwest (Cl)
Indiana State University (Co)
Indiana University (Cl)
Indiana University of Pennsylvania (Cl)
Iowa State University (Co)
James Madison University (Cm)
Kent State University (Cl)
Long Island University (Cl)
Long Island University–C.W. Post Campus (Cl)
Louisiana State University (Cl)
Loyola College in Maryland (Cl)
Loyola University–Chicago (Cl)
Marquette University (Cl)
Miami University (Cl)
Michigan State University (Cl)
New Mexico State University (Co)
Northeastern University (Cm)
Northern Illinois University (Cl)
Northwestern University (Cl)
Nova Southeastern University (Ph.D. & Psy.D.) (Cl)
Ohio State University (Cl)
Ohio University (Cl)
Oklahoma State University (Cl)
Oklahoma State University (Co)
Ontario Institute for Studies in Education (Cm)
Pacific Graduate School of Psychology (Cl)
Pepperdine University (Cl)
Purdue University (Cl)
Queen's University (Cl)
Rutgers University (Ph.D.) (Cl)
Rutgers University (Psy.D.) (Cl)
St. John's University (Cl)
St. Louis University (Cl)
San Diego State University/University of California–
	San Diego (Cl)
Southern Illinois University (Cl)
Southern Illinois University (Co)
Spalding University (Psy.D.) (Cl)
Syracuse University (Cl)
Texas A&M University (Cl)
University of Akron (Co)
University of California–Los Angeles (Cl)
University of California–Santa Barbara (Cm)
University of Central Florida (Cl)
University of Colorado (Cl)
University of Delaware (Cl)

University of Denver (Ph.D.) (Cl)
University of Georgia (Cl)
University of Houston (Co)
University of Illinois at Urbana–Champaign (Cl)
University of La Verne (Cl)
University of Manitoba (Cl)
University of Maryland–Baltimore County (Cl)
University of Memphis (Cl & Co)
University of Miami (Cl)
University of Michigan (Cl)
University of Minnesota (Cl)
University of Mississippi (Cl)
University of Missouri–Columbia (Co)
University of Missouri–St. Louis (Cl)
University of Montana (Cl)
University of Nebraska–Lincoln (Co)
University of New Mexico (Cl)
University of North Carolina at Chapel Hill (Cl)
University of North Carolina at Greensboro (Cl)
University of Northern Colorado (Co)
University of Oregon (Cl)
University of Oregon (Co)
University of Ottawa (Cl)
University of Pennsylvania (Cm)
University of Pittsburgh (Cl)
University of Pittsburgh (Co)
University of Rhode Island (Cl)
University of South Carolina (Cl)
University of South Florida (Cl)
University of Southern California (Cl)
University of Tennessee (Cl)
University of Texas at Austin (Cl)
University of Texas Southwestern Medical Center at Dallas
    (Cl)
University of Toledo (Cl)
University of Utah (Cl)
University of Utah (Co)
University of Vermont (Cl)
University of Virginia—Department of Human Services (Cl)
University of Virginia—Department of Psychology (Cl)
University of Washington (Cl)
University of Wisconsin–Milwaukee (Cl)
University of Wisconsin–Milwaukee (Co)
Vanderbilt University—Department of Psychology (Cl)
Virginia Consortium Program in Clinical Psychology (Cl)
Widener University (Cl)
Wright Institute (Cl)
Wright State University (Cl)
Yeshiva University (Cl)
Yeshiva University (Cm)

Forensic

Alliant International University–Alameda (Ph.D. & Psy.D.)
    (Cl)
Alliant International University–Fresno (Ph.D. & Psy.D.) (Cl)
Alliant International University–Los Angeles (Ph.D. &
    Psy.D) (Cl)
Alliant International University–San Diego (Psy.D.) (Cl)
Antioch/New England Graduate School (Cl)
Argosy University–Atlanta (Cl)
Argosy University–Twin Cities (Cl)
Argosy University–Washington, DC Campus (Cl)
Azusa Pacific University (Cl)

Brigham Young University (Cl)
Carlos Albizu University–San Juan (Cl)
Central Michigan University (Cl)
Chicago School of Professional Psychology (Cl)
Dalhousie University (Cl)
Drexel University (Cl)
Florida Institute of Technology (Cl)
Forest Institute of Professional Psychology (Cl)
Fuller Theological Seminary (Ph.D. & Psy.D.) (Cl)
George Washington University (Ph.D.)(Cl)
Georgia School of Professional Psychology (Cl)
Georgia State University (Co)
Illinois School of Professional Psychology–Chicago
    Campus (Cl)
Illinois School of Professional Psychology–Chicago
    Northwest (Cl)
Indiana State University (Cl)
Jackson State University (Cl)
James Madison University (Cm)
Kent State University (Cl)
Long Island University (Cl)
Loyola College in Maryland (Cl)
Northern Illinois University (Cl)
Nova Southeastern University (Ph.D. & Psy.D.) (Cl)
Pepperdine University (Cl)
Queen's University (Cl)
Regent University (Cl)
Rutgers University (Psy.D.) (Cl)
Southern Illinois University (Cl)
Tennessee State University (Co)
Texas A&M University (Cl)
Uniformed Services University of Health Sciences (Cl)
University of Alabama (Cl)
University of British Columbia (Cl)
University of Florida (Cl & Co)
University of Houston (Cl)
University of Houston (Co)
University of Illinois at Urbana–Champaign (Cl)
University of Indianapolis (Cl)
University of La Verne (Cl)
University of Louisville (Cl)
University of Maryland–Baltimore County (Cl)
University of Memphis (Co)
University of Minnesota (Cl)
University of Nebraska–Lincoln (Cl)
University of Nevada–Reno (Cl)
University of North Texas (Cl)
University of Saskatchewan (Cl)
University of Texas Southwestern Medical Center at Dallas
    (Cl)
University of Utah (Cl)
University of Victoria (Cl)
University of Virginia—Department of Human Services
    (Cl)
University of Virginia—Department of Psychology (Cl)
University of Washington (Cl)
University of Western Ontario (Cl)
University of Wisconsin–Madison (Cl)
University of Wyoming (Cl)
West Virginia University (Cl)
Wright Institute (Cl)
Wright State University (Cl)
York University—Adult Clinical Program (Cl)

Gay/Lesbian/Bisexual/Transgender

Alliant International University–Alameda (Ph.D. & Psy.D.) (Cl)
Antioch/New England Graduate School (Cl)
Argosy University–Washington, DC Campus (Cl)
Chicago School of Professional Psychology (Cl)
Illinois School of Professional Psychology–Chicago Campus (Cl)
Ontario Institute for Studies in Education (Cm)
University of Pittsburgh (Cl)
Wright Institute (Cl)
York University—Clinical-Developmental Area (Cl)

Group Therapy

Adelphi University (Cl)
Antioch/New England Graduate School (Cl)
Baylor University (Cl)
Catholic University of America (Cl)
DePaul University (Cl)
Fuller Theological Seminary (Ph.D. & Psy.D.) (Cl)
George Mason University (Cl)
George Washington University (Ph.D.) (Cl)
Georgia State University (Cl)
Idaho State University (Cl)
Illinois School of Professional Psychology–Chicago Campus (Cl)
Long Island University–C.W. Post Campus (Cl)
Michigan State University (Cl)
New School University (Cl)
New Mexico State University (Co)
Nova Southeastern University (Ph.D. & Psy.D.) (Cl)
Pepperdine University (Cl)
Rutgers University (Psy.D.) (Cl)
St. John's University (Cl)
University of Colorado (Cl)
University of Denver (Psy.D.) (Cl)
University of Denver (Co)
University of Illinois at Urbana–Champaign (Cl)
University of Maryland (Co)
University of Miami (Cl)
University of Wisconsin–Madison (Cl)
Widener University (Cl)
Wright Institute (Cl)
Yeshiva University (Cl)

Hospice

Argosy University–Honolulu Campus (Cl)
Indiana University–Purdue University (Cl)
University of Florida (Co)

Humanistic/Experiential Therapy

American University (Cl)
Fielding Graduate Institute (Cl)
Illinois School of Professional Psychology–Chicago Campus (Cl)
Pepperdine University (Cl)
University of Toledo (Cl)

Hypnosis

Rutgers University (Psy.D.) (Cl)
University of Denver (Psy.D.) (Cl)

University of Northern Colorado (Co)
University of Waterloo (Cl)

Impulse Control/Aggression/Anger Control

Baylor University (Cl)
Dalhousie University (Cl)
George Washington University (Ph.D.) (Cl)
Long Island University–C.W. Post Campus (Cl)
Rutgers University (Psy.D.) (Cl)
University of Georgia (Cl)
Vanderbilt University—Department of Psychology (Cl)

Infancy/Postpartum

Chicago School of Professional Psychology (Cl)
Rutgers University (Psy.D.) (Cl)
University of Iowa (Cl)

Inpatient Psychology/Psychiatry

Alliant International University–Alameda (Ph.D. & Psy.D.) (Cl)
Argosy University–Atlanta (Cl)
Argosy University–Phoenix (Cl)
Azusa Pacific University (Cl)
Biola University (Ph.D.) (Cl)
Biola University (Psy.D.) (Cl)
Boston College (Co)
Brigham Young University (Cl)
Chicago School of Professional Psychology (Cl)
Colorado State University (Co)
Drexel University (Cl)
Florida State University (Cl)
Fordham University (Co)
Fuller Theological Seminary (Ph.D. & Psy.D.) (Cl)
George Fox University (Cl)
Georgia School of Professional Psychology (Cl)
Illinois School of Professional Psychology–Chicago Northwest (Cl)
Indiana State University (Co)
Indiana University of Pennsylvania (Cl)
Jackson State University (Cl)
James Madison University (Cm)
Long Island University (Cl)
Loyola College in Maryland (Cl)
Loyola University–Chicago(Co)
Miami University (Cl)
McGill University (Cl & Co)
New School University (Cl)
Northeastern University (Cm)
Northwestern University, Feinberg School of Medicine (Cl)
Ohio University (Cl)
Oklahoma State University (Co)
Pepperdine University (Psy.D.) (Cl)
Queen's University (Cl)
Regent University (Cl)
Southern Illinois University (Co)
Stony Brook University/State University of New York (Cl)
Suffolk University (Cl)
Tennessee State University (Co)
Texas Tech University (Co)
Texas Woman's University (Co)
Uniformed Services University of Health Sciences (Cl)

University at Albany/State University of New York (Co)
University of Denver (Ph.D.) (Cl & Co)
University of Florida (Cl & Co)
University of Hartford (Cl)
University of Houston (Co)
University of Illinois at Urbana–Champaign (Cl)
University of Iowa (Cl)
University of Iowa (Co)
University of Kentucky (Co)
University of Maryland (Cl)
University of Memphis (Co)
University of Missouri–Columbia (Cl)
University of Missouri–Columbia (Co)
University of New Mexico (Cl)
University of Oklahoma (Co)
University of Oregon (Co)
University of Pittsburgh (Cl)
University of Southern Mississippi (Cl)
University of Texas at Austin (Co)
University of Texas Southwestern Medical Center at Dallas (Cl)
University of Utah (Cl)
University of Victoria (Cl)
University of Virginia—Department of Human Services (Cl)
University of Western Ontario (Cl)
University of Wisconsin–Madison (Cl)
University of Wisconsin–Milwaukee (Cl & Co)
University of Wyoming (Cl)
Virginia Commonwealth University (Cl)
Washington State University (Cl)

Learning Disabilities

Florida State University (Cl)
George Washington University (Psy.D.) (Cm)
James Madison University (Cm)
Ontario Institute for Studies in Education (Cm)
St. Louis University (Cl)
University of Missouri–Columbia (Co)
University of Wisconsin–Milwaukee (Cl)
York University—Clinical-Developmental Area (Cl)

Marital/Couples

Arizona State University (Cl)
Binghamton University/State University of New York (Cl)
Boston University (Cl)
Catholic University of America (Cl)
Chicago School of Professional Psychology (Cl)
Clark University (Cl)
Concordia University (Cl)
Florida Institute of Technology (Cl)
Forest Institute of Professional Psychology (Cl)
Fuller Theological Seminary (Ph.D. & Psy.D.) (Cl)
George Mason University (Cl)
George Washington University (Ph.D.) (Cl)
Georgia State University (Cl)
Idaho State University (Cl)
Illinois Institute of Technology (Cl)
Illinois School of Professional Psychology–Chicago Campus (Cl)
Illinois School of Professional Psychology–Chicago Northwest (Cl)
Indiana State University (Co)

Indiana University (Cl)
Kent State University (Cl)
Long Island University–C.W. Post Campus (Cl)
Miami University (Cl)
Northwestern University (Cl)
Oklahoma State University (Cl)
Oklahoma State University (Co)
Pepperdine University (Cl)
Rutgers University (Psy.D.) (Cl)
St. Louis University (Cl)
Southern Illinois University (Co)
Stony Brook University/State University of New York (Cl)
Syracuse University (Cl)
University of Arizona (Cl)
University of British Columbia (Cl)
University of California–Los Angeles (Cl)
University of Colorado (Cl)
University of Denver (Ph.D.) (Cl)
University of Georgia (Cl)
University of Illinois at Urbana–Champaign (Cl)
University of Manitoba (Cl)
University of Maryland (Co)
University of Memphis (Co)
University of Miami (Cl)
University of Mississippi (Cl)
University of Montana (Cl)
University of Nevada–Reno (Cl)
University of New Mexico (Cl)
University of North Carolina at Chapel Hill (Cl)
University of North Dakota (Cl)
University of Northern Colorado (Co)
University of Oregon (Cl)
University of Ottawa (Cl)
University of Rhode Island (Cl)
University of Southern California (Cl)
University of Texas at Austin (Cl)
University of Virginia—Department of Human Services (Cl)
University of Virginia—Department of Psychology (Cl)
University of Washington (Cl)
University of Wisconsin–Madison (Cl)
Virginia Polytechnic Institute and State University (Cl)
Widener University (Cl)
Wright Institute (Cl)
Wright State University (Cl)
Yeshiva University (Cl)

Mental Retardation

Louisiana State University (Cl)
University of Hartford (Cl)
University of Vermont (Cl)

Minority/Cross-Cultural/Multicultural

Alliant International University–Alameda (Ph.D. & Psy.D.) (Cl)
Alliant International University–Fresno (Ph.D. & Psy.D.) (Cl)
Argosy University–Phoenix (Cl)
Biola University (Ph.D.) (Cl)
Biola University (Psy.D.) (Cl)
Catholic University of America (Cl)
Chicago School of Professional Psychology (Cl)

DePaul University (Cl)
Fairleigh Dickinson University (Cl)
Florida State University (Cl)
Forest Institute of Professional Psychology (Cl)
George Fox University (Cl)
George Washington University (Ph.D.) (Cl)
Georgia State University (Co)
Howard University (Cl)
Illinois Institute of Technology (Cl)
Illinois School of Professional Psychology–Chicago
    Campus (Cl)
Michigan State University (Cl)
New Mexico State University (Co)
Northeastern University (Cm)
Nova Southeastern University (Ph.D. & Psy.D.) (Cl)
Oklahoma State University (Co)
Ontario Institute for Studies in Education (Cm)
Our Lady of the Lake University (Co)
Pacific Graduate School of Psychology (Cl)
Rutgers University (Ph.D.) (Cl)
Rutgers University (Psy.D.) (Cl)
St. Louis University (Cl)
University at Albany/State University of New York (Cl)
University of California–Los Angeles (Cl)
University of Connecticut (Cl)
University of Denver (Co)
University of Denver (Ph.D.) (Cl)
University of Georgia (Cl)
University of Georgia (Co)
University of Hawaii at Manoa (Cl)
University of Houston (Cl)
University of Maryland (Co)
University of Massachusetts at Amherst (Cl)
University of Memphis (Cl)
University of Miami (Cl)
University of Nebraska–Lincoln (Cl)
University of Nebraska–Lincoln (Co)
University of Nevada–Reno (Cl)
University of North Dakota (Cl)
University of Oklahoma (Co)
University of South Dakota (Cl)
University of Southern California (Cl)
University of Texas at Austin (Co)
University of Utah (Cl & Co)
University of Washington (Cl)
Utah State University (Cm)
Widener University (Cl)
Wright Institute (Cl)
Wright State University (Cl)
Yeshiva University (Cl & Cm)

Neuropsychology/Clinical Neuropsychology/ Brain Injury/Stroke

Alliant International University–Alameda (Ph.D. & Psy.D.)
    (Cl)
Alliant International University–Fresno (Ph.D. & Psy.D.) (Cl)
American University (Cl)
Alliant International University–Los Angeles (Ph.D. &
    Psy.D) (Cl)
Antioch/New England Graduate School (Cl)
Argosy University–Atlanta (Cl)
Argosy University–Phoenix (Cl)
Argosy University, Washington, DC Campus (Cl)

Baylor University (Cl)
Binghamton University/State University of New York (Cl)
Boston University (Cl)
Brigham Young University (Cl)
Catholic University of America (Cl)
Central Michigan University (Cl)
Drexel University (Cl)
Duke University (Cl)
Emory University (Cl)
Fairleigh Dickinson University (Cl)
Florida Institute of Technology (Cl)
Forest Institute of Professional Psychology (Cl)
Fuller Theological Seminary (Ph.D. & Psy.D.) (Cl)
George Mason University (Cl)
George Washington University (Cl)
Georgia School of Professional Psychology (Cl)
Georgia State University (Cl)
Howard University (Cl)
Illinois Institute of Technology (Cl)
Illinois School of Professional Psychology–Chicago
    Campus (Cl)
Illinois School of Professional Psychology–Chicago
    Northwest (Cl)
Indiana University (Cl)
Indiana University–Purdue University Indianapolis (Cl)
James Madison University (Cm)
Kent State University (Cl)
Long Island University (Cl)
Long Island University–C.W. Post Campus (Cl)
Louisiana State University (Cl)
Loyola University–Chicago(Cl)
Michigan State University (Cl)
Northwestern University (Cl)
Northwestern University, Feinberg School of Medicine (Cl)
Nova Southeastern (Ph.D. & Psy.D.) (Cl)
Ohio State University (Cl)
Ohio University (Cl)
Ontario Institute for Studies in Education (Cm)
Pacific Graduate School of Psychology (Cl)
Pepperdine University (Cl)
Queen's University (Cl)
Regent University (Cl)
Rosalind Franklin University of Medicine and Science (Cl)
Rutgers University (Psy.D.) (Cl)
St. John's University (Cl)
St. Louis University (Cl)
San Diego State University/University of California–
    San Diego (Cl)
Southern Illinois University (Cl)
Suffolk University (Cl)
Syracuse University (Cl)
Texas A&M University (Cl)
Texas Tech University (Cl)
Texas Tech University (Co)
University of Alabama at Birmingham (Cl)
University at Albany/State University of New York (Cl)
University at Albany/State University of New York (Co)
University of Arizona (Cl)
University of Central Florida (Cl)
University of Cincinnati (Cl)
University of Connecticut (Cl)
University of Delaware (Cl)
University of Denver (Ph.D.) (Cl)

University of Denver (Co)
University of Florida (Cl)
University of Georgia (Cl)
University of Hawaii at Manoa (Cl)
University of Houston (Cl)
University of Illinois at Urbana–Champaign (Cl)
University of Indianapolis (Cl)
University of Iowa (Cl)
University of Kentucky (Cl)
University of Manitoba (Cl)
University of Maryland–Baltimore County (Cl)
University of Miami (Cl)
University of Minnesota (Cl)
University of Montana (Cl)
University of Nevada–Reno (Cl)
University of North Texas (Cl)
University of Northern Colorado (Co)
University of Oregon (Cl)
University of Pittsburgh (Cl)
University of Saskatchewan (Cl)
University of South Carolina (Cl)
University of South Florida (Cl)
University of Texas at Austin (Cl)
University of Texas Southwestern Medical Center at Dallas
    (Cl)
University of Toledo (Cl)
University of Vermont (Cl)
University of Victoria (Cl)
University of Virginia—Department of Human Services (Cl)
University of Virginia—Department of Psychology (Cl)
University of Washington (Cl)
University of Waterloo (Cl)
University of Wisconsin–Madison (Cl)
University of Wisconsin–Milwaukee (Cl)
Utah State University (Cm)
Vanderbilt University—Department of Psychology (Cl)
Virginia Commonwealth University (Cl)
Virginia Polytechnic Institute and State University (Cl)
Washington State University (Cl)
Wayne State University (Cl)
Widener University (Cl)
Wright Institute (Cl)
Wright State University (Cl)
York University—Adult Clinical Program (Cl)

Obsessive–Compulsive Disorder

Argosy University–Washington, DC Campus (Cl)
Case Western Reserve University (Cl)
George Washington University (Cl)
Indiana University (Cl)
Louisiana State University (Cl)
Marquette University (Co)
Rutgers University (Ph.D.) (Cl)
Rutgers University (Psy.D.) (Cl)
University of Hartford (Cl)
University of Manitoba (Cl)
University of Minnesota (Cl)
University of North Dakota (Cl)
University of Pittsburgh (Cl)
University of Texas at Austin (Cl)
University of Virginia—Department of Psychology (Cl)
University of Wisconsin–Madison (Cl)

Organizational

Chicago School of Professional Psychology (Cl)
Rutgers University (Psy.D.) (Cl)
Widener University (Cl)

Pain Management

Alliant International University–San Diego (Ph.D.) (Cl)
Argosy University–Phoenix (Cl)
Argosy University–Twin Cities (Cl)
Binghamton University/State University of New York (Cl)
Forest Institute of Professional Psychology (Cl)
George Fox University (Cl)
Illinois Institute of Technology (Cl)
Marquette University (Cl)
Nova Southeastern University (Ph.D. & Psy.D.) (Cl)
Oklahoma State University (Co)
University of Alabama (Cl)
University of Florida (Cl)
University of Indianapolis (Cl)
University of Kentucky (Cl)
University of Montana (Cl)
University of Pittsburgh (Cl)
Virginia Commonwealth University (Cl)

Parent–Child Interaction/Parent Training

Arizona State University (Cl)
Central Michigan University (Cl)
Idaho State University (Cl)
Forest Institute of Professional Psychology (Cl)
Long Island University–C.W. Post Campus (Cl)
Northern Illinois University (Cl)
Nova Southeastern University (Ph.D. & Psy.D.) (Cl)
St. Louis University (Cl)
University of Alabama (Cl)
University at Buffalo/State University of New York (Cl)
University of Florida (Cl)
University of Pittsburgh (Cl)
University of Virginia—Department of Human Services (Cl)
West Virginia University (Cl)
Yeshiva University (Cl & Cm)

Personality Disorders

Antioch/New England Graduate School (Cl)
Baylor University (Cl)
Case Western Reserve University (Cl)
Florida State University (Cl)
George Washington University (Ph.D.) (Cl)
Georgia State University (Cl)
Illinois School of Professional Psychology–Chicago
    Campus (Cl)
Loyola University–Chicago(Cl)
Miami University (Cl)
Purdue University (Cl)
Rutgers University (Ph.D.) (Cl)
Rutgers University (Psy.D.) (Cl)
St. Louis University (Cl)
Southern Illinois University (Cl)
University of Arkansas (Cl)
University of Georgia (Cl)
University of Minnesota (Cl)

University of Montana (Cl)
University of Nevada–Reno (Cl)
University of North Dakota (Cl)
University of Northern Colorado (Co)
University of Pittsburgh (Cl)
University of South Florida (Cl)
University of Tennessee (Cl)
University of Texas at Austin (Cl)
University of Texas Southwestern Medical Center at Dallas (Cl)
University of Utah (Cl)
University of Washington (Cl)
Vanderbilt University—Department of Psychology (Cl)
Virginia Consortium Program in Clinical Psychology (Cl)
Wright Institute (Cl)

Posttraumatic Stress Disorder/Trauma

Alliant International University–San Diego (Psy.D.) (Cl)
Argosy University–Washington, DC Campus (Cl)
Auburn University (Cl)
Duke University (Cl)
Florida Institute of Technology (Cl)
Pepperdine University (Cl)
University of Houston (Cl)
University of Houston (Co)
University of Mississippi (Cl)
University of Nevada–Reno (Cl)
University of North Texas (Cl)
University of Ottawa (Cl)
University of Pittsburgh (Cl)
Western Michigan University (Cl)

Prevention

Arizona State University (Cl)
Boston College (Co)
Clark University (Cl)
Illinois School of Professional Psychology–Chicago Campus (Cl)
University of Maryland–Baltimore County (Cl)
University of Missouri–Columbia (Cl)
University of Vermont (Cl)

Private Practice

Brigham Young University (Cl)
Chicago School of Professional Psychology (Cl)
Iowa State University (Co)
James Madison University (Cm)
Loyola College in Maryland (Cl)

Psychiatric Emergency Care

University of Maryland–Baltimore County (Cl)
University of Pittsburgh (Cl)
University of Texas Southwestern Medical Center at Dallas (Cl)

Psychoanalytic/Psychodynamic Therapy

American University (Cl)
Antioch/New England Graduate School (Cl)
Arizona State University (Cl)

Brigham Young University (Cl)
Catholic University of America (Cl)
Central Michigan University (Cl)
Columbia University, Teachers College (Cl)
Concordia University (Cl)
Emory University (Cl)
Fielding Graduate Institute (Cl)
Fuller Theological Seminary (Ph.D. & Psy.D.) (Cl)
George Mason University (Cl)
George Washington University (Ph.D.) (Cl)
Illinois School of Professional Psychology–Chicago Campus (Cl)
Kent State University (Cl)
Long Island University–C.W. Post Campus (Cl)
Nova Southeastern University (Ph.D. & Psy.D.) (Cl)
Pepperdine University (Cl)
Rutgers University (Psy.D.) (Cl)
St. John's University (Cl)
St. Louis University (Cl)
University of Colorado (Cl)
University of Denver (Psy.D.) (Cl)
University of Louisville (Cl)
University of Massachusetts at Amherst (Cl)
University of Minnesota (Cl)
University of Montana (Cl)
University of North Carolina at Chapel Hill (Cl)
University of North Dakota (Cl)
University of Rochester (Cl)
University of Utah (Cl)
University of Wisconsin–Madison (Cl)
Virginia Consortium Program in Clinical Psychology (Cl)
Widener University (Cl)
Wright Institute (Cl)
Yale University (Cl)
Yeshiva University (Cl)

Psychotherapy Integration

Adelphi University (Cl)
Alliant International University–San Diego (Ph.D.) (Cl)
Brigham Young University (Cl)
McGill University (Co)
University of Wyoming (Cl)
Wright Institute (Cl)

Rational-Emotive Therapy

Rutgers University (Ph.D.) (Cl)
Rutgers University (Psy.D.) (Cl)
St. John's University (Cl)
University of Utah (Cl)

Rehabilitation

Antioch/New England Graduate School (Cl)
Argosy University–Atlanta (Cl)
Brigham Young University (Cl)
Georgia School of Professional Psychology (Cl)
Georgia State University (Cl)
Illinois School of Professional Psychology–Chicago Campus (Psy.D. & Ph.D.) (Cl)
Illinois School of Professional Psychology–Chicago
Indiana University–Purdue University Indianapolis (Cl)

Jackson State University (Cl)
Northwest (Psy.D. & Ph.D.) (Cl)
Ohio State University (Co)
Ohio University (Cl)
Pepperdine University (Cl)
Queen's University (Cl)
Southern Illinois University (Cl)
Southern Illinois University (Co)
University of Hawaii at Manoa (Cl)
University of Houston (Cl)
University of Illinois at Urbana–Champaign (Co)
University of Maryland–Baltimore County (Cl)
University of Missouri–Columbia (Cl)
University of Missouri–Columbia (Co)
University of Oklahoma (Co)
University of Texas Southwestern Medical Center at Dallas (Cl)
University of Victoria (Cl)
University of Washington (Cl)
University of Western Ontario (Cl)
Virginia Commonwealth University (Co)
Wright Institute (Cl)
York University—Adult Clinical Program (Cl)
York University—Clinical-Developmental Area (Cl)

Religion/Spirituality

Biola University (Ph.D.) (Cl)
Biola University (Psy.D.) (Cl)
Forest Institute of Professional Psychology (Cl)
George Fox University (Cl)
Illinois School of Professional Psychology–Chicago
    Campus (Cl)
Pepperdine University (Cl)
Regent University (Cl)

Rural Mental Health/Psychology

Antioch/New England Graduate School (Cl)
Baylor University (Cl)
Chicago School of Professional Psychology (Cl)
George Fox University (Cl)
Indiana State University (Cl)
Miami University (Cl)
New Mexico State University (Co)
Oklahoma State University (Co)
Southern Illinois University (Co)
Texas A&M University (Cl)
Texas Tech University (Co)
University at Buffalo/State University of New York (Cm)
University of Florida (Co)
University of Kentucky (Co)
University of Missouri–Columbia (Co)
University of Montana (Cl)
University of New York (Cm)
University of North Dakota (Cl)
University of South Dakota (Cl)
University of Southern Mississippi (Co)
University of Wyoming (Cl)

Schizophrenia/Psychosis/Serious Mental Illness

Baylor University (Cl)
Binghamton University/State University of New York (Cl)

Boston University (Cl)
Case Western Reserve University (Cl)
George Washington University (Ph.D. & Psy.D.) (Cl)
Howard University (Cl)
Illinois Institute of Technology (Cl)
Indiana University (Cl)
Kent State University (Cl)
Louisiana State University (Cl)
Michigan State University (Cl)
Northeastern University (Cm)
Northwestern University (Cl)
Pepperdine University (Cl)
Rutgers University (Psy.D.) (Cl)
University of California–Los Angeles (Cl)
University of Florida (Cl)
University of Houston (Cl)
University of Illinois at Urbana–Champaign (Cl)
University of Kansas (Cl)
University of Louisville (Cl)
University of Minnesota (Cl)
University of Montana (Cl)
University of Pittsburgh (Cl)
University of Texas at Austin (Cl)
University of Virginia—Department of Psychology (Cl)
University of Wisconsin–Madison (Cl)
Vanderbilt University—Department of Psychology (Cl)
Wayne State University (Cl)
Wright Institute (Cl)

School/Educational

Adler School of Professional Psychology (Cl)
Alliant International University–Fresno (Ph.D. & Psy.D.) (Cl)
Alliant International University–Los Angeles (Ph.D. &
    Psy.D) (Cl)
Argosy University–Atlanta (Cl)
Argosy University–Honolulu Campus (Cl)
Argosy University–Phoenix (Cl)
Argosy University–Washington, DC Campus (Cl)
Arizona State University (Cl)
Azusa Pacific University (Cl)
Baylor University (Cl)
Binghamton University/State University of New York (Cl)
Boston College (Co)
Bowling Green State University (Cl)
Brigham Young University (Cl)
Central Michigan University (Cl)
Chicago School of Professional Psychology (Cl)
Clark University (Cl)
Concordia University (Cl)
Duke University (Cl)
Florida State University (Cm)
George Fox University (Cl)
Georgia State University (Co)
Georgia School of Professional Psychology (Cl)
Illinois School of Professional Psychology–Chicago
    Campus (Cl)
Illinois School of Professional Psychology–Chicago
    Northwest (Cl)
Indiana University (Cl)
Indiana University–Purdue University Indianapolis (Cl)
Long Island University–C.W. Post Campus (Cl)
Louisiana State University (Cl)
James Madison University (Cm)

Miami University (Cl)
Ohio State University (Cl)
Ontario Institute for Studies in Education (Cm)
Our Lady of the Lake University (Co)
Purdue University (Cl)
Queen's University (Cl)
Rutgers University (Psy.D.) (Cl)
Suffolk University (Cl)
Syracuse University (Cl)
Texas Tech University (Co)
University at Buffalo/State University of New York (Cm)
University of California–Los Angeles (Cl)
University of California–Santa Barbara (Cm)
University of Central Florida (Cl)
University of Georgia (Co)
University of Houston (Cl)
University of Houston (Co)
University of Illinois at Urbana–Champaign (Cl)
University of Illinois at Urbana–Champaign (Co)
University of Iowa (Co)
University of Maine (Cl)
University of Maryland–Baltimore County (Cl)
University of Memphis (Cl)
University of New Mexico (Cl)
University of North Carolina at Greensboro (Cl)
University of Oklahoma (Co)
University of South Florida (Cl)
University of Virginia–Department of Human Services (Cl)
University of Washington (Cl)
University of Waterloo (Cl)
Utah State University (Cm)
Virginia Commonwealth University (Cl)
West Virginia University (Cl)
Western Michigan University (Co)
Widener University (Cl)
Xavier University (Cl)
Yeshiva University (Cl & Cm)
York University—Clinical-Developmental Area (Cl)

Sex Therapy/Deviation and Dysfunction

Alliant International University–Fresno (Ph.D. & Psy.D) (Cl)
Argosy University–Twin Cities (Cl)
Carlos Albizu University (Cl)
Indiana University (Cl)
Ohio State University (Cl)
Rutgers University (Ph.D.) (Cl)
Rutgers University (Psy.D.) (Cl)
Southern Illinois University (Co)
University of Florida (Co)
University of Georgia (Cl)
University of Louisville (Co)
University of Rhode Island (Cl)
University of Tennessee (Cl)
University of Utah (Cl)
Widener University (Cl)

Sleep Disorders

Southern Illinois University (Cl)
University of Arizona (Cl)
University of Memphis (Cl)

University of Texas Southwestern Medical Center at Dallas (Cl)
University of Wisconsin–Madison (Cl)

Smoking Cessation

Indiana University (Cl)
University of Illinois at Chicago (Cl)
University of Mississippi (Cl)
University of Pittsburgh (Cl)
University of Rochester (Cl)
University of Texas at Austin (Cl)

Sports Psychology

Carlos Albizu University–San Juan (Cl)
Illinois School of Professional Psychology–Chicago Campus (Cl)
University of Manitoba (Cl)
University of Washington (Cl)

Stress

Georgia State University (Co)
Indiana University of Pennsylvania (Cl)
Long Island University–C.W. Post Campus (Cl)
Loyola College in Maryland (Cl)
Loyola University–Chicago(Cl)
Nova Southeastern University (Ph.D. & Psy.D.) (Cl)
Southern Illinois University (Co)
University of Connecticut (Cl)
University of Florida (Cl)
University of Georgia (Cl)
University of Wisconsin–Milwaukee (Cl)

Substance Abuse/Addiction

Adelphi University (Cl)
Alliant International University–Los Angeles (Ph.D. & Psy.D.) (Cl)
Antioch/New England Graduate School (Cl)
Argosy University–Atlanta (Cl)
Argosy University–Honolulu Campus (Cl)
Argosy University–Phoenix (Cl)
Argosy University–Washington, DC Campus (Cl)
Auburn University (Co)
Azusa Pacific University (Cl)
Baylor University (Cl)
Binghamton University/State University of New York (Cl)
Brigham Young University (Cl)
Fairleigh Dickinson University (Cl)
Duke University (Cl)
George Fox University (Cl)
George Washington University (Ph.D. (Cl)
Georgia School of Professional Psychology (Cl)
Howard University (Cl)
Illinois School of Professional Psychology–Chicago Campus (Cl)
Illinois School of Professional Psychology–Chicago Northwest (Cl)
Long Island University (Cl)
Loyola University–Chicago(Cl)
Marquette University (Co)
New Mexico State University (Co)

Nova Southeastern University (Ph.D. & Psy.D.) (Cl)
Ohio University (Cl)
Pepperdine University ((Cl)
Rutgers University (Ph.D.) (Cl)
Rutgers University (Psy.D.) (Cl)
Southern Illinois University (Cl)
Southern Illinois University (Co)
University at Albany/State University of New York (Cl)
University at Albany/State University of New York (Co)
Syracuse University (Cl)
Texas A&M University (Cl)
Uniformed Services University of Health Sciences (Cl)
University of Central Florida (Cl)
University of Cincinnati (Cl)
University of Colorado (Cl)
University of Florida (Co)
University of Georgia (Cl)
University of Hawaii at Manoa (Cl)
University of Houston (Co)
University of La Verne (Cl)
University of Manitoba (Cl)
University of Maryland–Baltimore County (Cl)
University of Memphis (Cl)
University of Memphis (Co)
University of Miami (Cl)
University of Minnesota (Cl)
University of Mississippi (Cl)
University of Montana (Cl)
University of Nebraska–Lincoln (Cl)
University of Nevada–Reno (Cl)
University of North Dakota (Cl)
University of Pittsburgh (Cl)
University of South Florida (Cl)
University of Southern Mississippi (Co)
University of Utah (Cl & Co)
University of Vermont (Cl)
University of Washington (Cl)
University of Wisconsin–Madison (Cl)
Virginia Commonwealth University (Cl & Co)
Virginia Polytechnic Institute and State University (Cl)
Wright Institute (Cl)
Yale University (Cl)
York University—Adult Clinical Program (Cl)

Suicide/Prevention

Baylor University (Cl)
University of Houston (Cl)
University of Pittsburgh (Cl)

Supervision

Antioch/New England Graduate School (Cl)
Binghamton University/State University of New York (Cl)
Fuller Theological Seminary (Ph.D. & Psy.D.) (Cl)
Georgia State University (Cl)
James Madison University (Cm)
University of California–Los Angeles (Cl)
University of Denver (Psy.D.) (Cl)
University of Georgia (Cl)
University of Georgia (Co)
University of Manitoba (Cl)
University of Maryland (Co)
University of Massachusetts at Amherst (Cl)

University of Northern Colorado (Co)
University of Southern Mississippi (Co)
Wright State University (Cl)

Veterans Hospital/Medical Center

Argosy University–Honolulu Campus (Cl)
Argosy University–Phoenix (Cl)
Brigham Young University (Cl)
Chicago School of Professional Psychology (Cl)
Indiana State University (Co)
Iowa State University (Co)
Louisiana Tech University (Co)
New School University (Cl)
Ohio State University (Co)
Oklahoma State University (Co)
Regent University (Cl)
Southern Illinois University (Co)
Stony Brook University/State University of New York (Cl)
Texas A&M University (Co)
Uniformed Services University of Health Sciences (Cl)
University of Akron (Co)
University at Albany/State University of New York (Co)
University of British Columbia (Cl)
University of Denver (Co)
University of Houston (Co)
University of Illinois at Urbana–Champaign (Co)
University of Indianapolis (Cl)
University of Iowa (Co)
University of Kentucky (Co)
University of Missouri–Columbia (Cl)
University of Missouri–Columbia (Co)
University of Oklahoma (Co)
University of Oregon (Co)
University of Southern Mississippi (Co)
University of Texas at Austin (Co)
University of Utah (Co)
University of Wisconsin–Milwaukee (Co)
Virginia Commonwealth University (Co)
West Virginia University (Co)

Victim/Violence/Sexual Abuse

Alliant International University–Fresno (Ph.D. & Psy.D)
    (Cl)
Alliant International University–San Diego (Psy.D.) (Cl)
Antioch/New England Graduate School (Cl)
Argosy University–Phoenix (Cl)
Baylor University (Cl)
Boston College (Co)
Boston University (Cl)
Carlos Albizu University–San Juan (Psy.D.) (Cl)
Carlos Albizu University–San Juan (Ph.D.) (Cl)
Clark University (Cl)
Duke University (Cl)
Florida Institute of Technology (Cl)
Fuller Theological Seminary (Ph.D. & Psy.D.) (Cl)
George Washington University (Ph.D.) (Cl)
Georgia State University (Cl)
Howard University (Cl)
Illinois School of Professional Psychology–Chicago
    Campus (Cl)
Indiana University (Cl)
Long Island University–C.W. Post Campus (Cl)

Loyola University–Chicago(Cl)
Michigan State University (Cl)
Northern Illinois University (Cl)
Oklahoma State University (Co)
Rutgers University (Psy.D.) (Cl)
St. Louis University (Cl)
Southern Illinois University (Cl)
Texas Woman's University (Co)
University of California–Santa Barbara (Cm)
University of Delaware (Cl)
University of Florida (Co)
University of Georgia (Cl)
University of Houston (Cl)
University of Iowa (Cl)
University of Manitoba (Cl)
University of Maryland–Baltimore County (Cl)
University of Memphis (Co)
University of Miami (Cl)
University of Mississippi (Cl)
University of Missouri–St. Louis (Cl)
University of Montana (Cl)
University of Nebraska–Lincoln (Cl)
University of Nevada–Reno (Cl)
University of North Carolina at Chapel Hill (Cl)
University of North Dakota (Cl)
University of Oklahoma (Co)
University of Pennsylvania (Cm)
University of Pittsburgh (Cl)
University of Rochester (Cl)
University of Toledo (Cl)
University of Utah (Co)
University of Virginia—Department of Psychology (Cl)
University of Wisconsin–Milwaukee (Cl)
West Virginia University (Cl)
Wright State University (Cl)

Vocational/Career Development

Florida State University (Cm)
New Mexico State University (Co)
Southern Illinois University (Co)
Temple University (Co)
Uniformed Services University of Health Sciences (Cl)
University of California–Santa Barbara (Cm)
University of Florida (Co)
University of Georgia (Co)
University of Maryland (Co)
University of Missouri–Columbia (Co)
University of Nebraska–Lincoln (Co)
University of Texas Southwestern Medical Center at Dallas (Cl)
University of Western Ontario (Cl)
Virginia Commonwealth University (Co)
Virginia Consortium Program in Clinical Psychology (Cl)

Weight Management

Allegheny University of the Health Sciences (Cl)
Oklahoma State University (Cl)
University at Buffalo/State University of New York (Cl)
University of Florida (Cl)
University of Illinois at Chicago (Cl)
University of Pittsburgh (Cl)
University of South Florida (Cl)

Women's Studies/Issues

Alliant International University–Alameda (Ph.D. & Psy.D.) (Cl)
Northeastern University (Cm)
Oklahoma State University (Co)
Southern Illinois University (Co)
Texas A&M University (Co)
University of Illinois at Urbana–Champaign (Cl)
University of Iowa (Co)
University of Missouri–Columbia (Co)
University of Missouri–St. Louis (Cl)
University of Utah (Co)
Wright Institute (Cl)

Miscellaneous

adjustment reactions—University of Illinois at Chicago (Cl)
adoption—University of California–Los Angeles (Cl)
Alzheimer's/dementia—University of Houston (Cl)
attachment disorder—University of Montana (Cl)
behavior genetics—University of Oregon (Cl)
behavioral dentistry—West Virginia University (Cl)
bereavement—University of Wyoming (Cl)
child custody evaluation—Alliant International University–San Diego (Ph.D.) (Cl); University of Houston (Cl)
clinical outcome studies—George Washington University (Psy.D.) (Cl)
creative & expressive arts—Chicago School of Professional Psychology (Cl)
data management systems—Virginia Polytechnic Institute and State University (Cl)
day treatment—Nova Southeastern University (Ph.D. & Psy.D) (Cl); Argosy University–Honolulu Campus (Cl)
diabetes—University of Miami (Cl)
dialectical behavior therapy—University of Kentucky (Cl)
intervention—Utah State University (Cm); Widener University (Cl)
epilepsy clinic—Argosy University–Twin Cities (Cl)
fire setting—Ontario Institute for Studies in Education (Cm)
gambling—University of Memphis (Cl)
homeless shelters—University of Georgia (Co); University of Utah (Cl)
individualized specialty settings—University of Iowa (Co)
interpersonal therapy—Yale University (Cl); Emory University (Cl)
life-span—University of Georgia (Co)
long-term care—University of Miami (Cl)
low income—New Mexico State University (Co)
media and psychology—University of Massachusetts at Boston (Cl); Alliant International University–San Diego (Psy.D.) (Cl)
motivational interviewing—University of Montana (Cl)
peer relationships—Dalhousie University (Cl)
personal injury—Brigham Young University (Cl)
play therapy—University of Northern Colorado (Co); Michigan State University (Cl)
primary/interdisciplinary care—University of Wyoming (Cl), University of Arkansas (Cl)
program evaluation—Wright Institute (Cl)
psychoneuroimmunology—Howard University (Cl)
psychopharmacology/medication management—Forest Institute of Professional Psychology (Psy.D.) (Cl); Nova Southeastern University (Ph.D. & Psy.D.) (Cl)

public policy/advocacy—Wright Institute (Cl)

public sector impairment treatment—Duke University (Cl)

selective mutism—University of South Florida (Cl)

short-term psychotherapy—Adelphi University (Cl)

skills treatment and enhancement program (STEP)—Nova Southeastern University (Ph.D. & Psy.D.) (Cl)

social stereotypes—University of Massachusetts at Boston (Cl)

somatization disorders—Rutgers University (Ph.D.) (Cl); University of Alabama (Cl)

systems management—Virginia Polytechnic Institute and State University (Cl)

teaching—Chicago School of Professional Psychology (Cl)

third world placements—Brigham Young University (Cl)

REFERENCES

Accredited doctoral programs in professional psychology: 2002. (2002). *American Psychologist, 57,* 1096–1109.

Accredited doctoral programs in professional psychology: 2004. (2004). *American Psychologist, 59,* 930–944.

Actkinson, T. R. (2000, Winter). Master's and myth. *Eye on Psi Chi, 4,* 19–25.

American Psychological Association. (1986). *Careers in psychology.* Washington, DC: Author.

American Psychological Association. (2000). *Graduate study in psychology.* Washington, DC: Author.

American Psychological Association. (2002). Ethical principles of psychologists and code of conduct. *American Psychologist, 57,* 1060–1073.

American Psychological Association Research Office. (1999). *Demographic characteristics of Division 12 and Division 17 members: 1997.* Washington, DC: Author.

American Psychological Association Research Office. (2000). *1998–1999 Survey of Graduate Departments of Psychology.* Washington, DC: Author.

American Psychological Association Research Office. (2003). *2001 doctorate employment survey.* Washington, DC: Author.

Anderson, N., & Shackleton, V. (1990). Decision making in the graduate selection interview: A field study. *Journal of Occupational Psychology, 63,* 63–76.

APA Practice Directorate. (1991). *Summary of psychology licensing or certification laws.* Washington, DC: Author.

Appleby, D. C., & Appleby, K. M. (2003, August). *The "kisses of death" in the graduate school applications process.* Poster presented at the annual convention of the American Psychological Association, Toronto.

Appleby, D., Keenan, J., & Mauer, B. (1999, Spring). Applicant characteristics valued by graduate programs in psychology. *Eye on Psi Chi, 3,* 39.

Association of State and Provincial Psychology Boards and National Register of Health Service Providers in Psychology. (2005). *Doctoral psychology programs meeting designation criteria.* Washington, DC: National Register.

Astin, A. W., Green, K. C., & Korn, W. S. (1987). *The American freshman: Twenty-year trends 1966–85.* University of California, Cooperative Institutional Research Program, American Council on Education.

Ault, R. L. (1993). To waive or not to waive? Students' misconceptions about the confidentiality choice for letters of recommendation. *Teaching of Psychology, 20,* 44–45.

Barron, J. (1986). Search for survival and identity—and power. *The Clinical Psychologist, 39,* 61–63.

Bartsch, R. A., Warren, T. D., Sharp, A. D., & Green, M. A. (2003). Assessment of psychology graduate program information on the Web. *Teaching of Psychology, 30,* 167–170.

Bechtoldt, H., Norcross, J. C., Wyckoff, L. A., Pokrywa, M. L., & Campbell, L. F. (2001). Theoretical orientations and employment settings of clinical and counseling psychologists: A comparative study. *The Clinical Psychologist, 54*(1), 3–6.

Bernal, M. E., Sirolli, A. A., Weisser, S. K., Ruiz, J. A., Chamberlain, V. J., & Knight, G. P. (1999). Relevance of multicultural training to students' applications to clinical psychology programs. *Cultural Diversity and Ethnic Minority Psychology, 5,* 43–55.

Bernstein, B. L., & Kerr, B. (1993). Counseling psychology and the scientist–practitioner model: Implementation and implications. *The Counseling Psychologist, 21,* 136–151.

Bersoff, D. N., Goodman-Delahunty, J., Grisso, J. T., Hans, V. P., Poythress, N. G., & Roesch, R. G. (1997). Training in law and psychology: Models from the Villanova Conference. *American Psychologist, 52,* 1301–1310.

Beutler, L. E., & Fisher, D. (1994). Combined specialty training in counseling, clinical, and school psychology: An idea whose time has returned. *Professional Psychology: Research and Practice, 25,* 62–69.

Biaggio, M., Orchard, S., Larson, J., Petrino, K., & Mihara, R. (2003). Guidelines for gay/lesbian/bisexual-affirmative educational practices in graduate psychology programs. *Professional Psychology: Research & Practice, 34,* 548–554.

Boitano, J. J. (1999, August). *Graduate training in neuroscience.* Paper presented at the 107th annual convention of the American Psychological Association, Boston, MA.

Bonifzi, D. Z., Crespy, S. D., & Reiker, P. (1997). Value of a master's degree for gaining admission to doctoral programs in psychology. *Teaching of Psychology, 24,* 176–182.

REFERENCES

Bottoms, B. L., & Nysse, K. L. (1999, Fall). Applying to graduate school: Writing a compelling personal statement. *Eye on Psi Chi, 4,* 20–22.

Boudreau, R. A., Killip, S. M., MacInnis, S. H., Milloy, D. G., & Rogers, T. B. (1983). An evaluation of Graduate Record Examinations as predictors of graduate success in a Canadian context. *Canadian Psychology, 24,* 191–199.

Brems, C., & Johnson, M. E. (1997). Comparison of recent graduates of clinical versus counseling psychology programs. *Journal of Psychology, 131,* 91–99.

Briihl, D. S., & Wasieleski, D. T. (2004). A survey of master's-level psychology programs: Admissions criteria and program policies. *Teaching of Psychology, 31,* 252–256.

Bullock, M. (1997, July/August). Federal funding is available for psychology graduate students. *Psychological Science Agenda,* p. 4.

Buskist, W., & Mixon, A. (1998). *Master's programs in psychology and counseling psychology.* Needham Heights, MA: Allyn & Bacon.

Cashin, J. R., & Landrum, R. E. (1991). Undergraduate students' perceptions of graduate admissions in psychology. *Psychological Reports, 69,* 1107–1110.

Castle, P. H., & Norcross, J. C. (2002, August). *Empirical data and integrative perspectives on combined doctoral programs.* Paper presented at the 110th annual convention of the American Psychological Association, Chicago, IL.

Ceci, S. J., & Peters, D. (1984). Letters of reference: A naturalistic study of the effects of confidentiality. *American Psychologist, 39,* 29–31.

Chapman, C. P., & Lane, H. C. (1997). Perceptions about the use of letters of recommendation. *The Advisor, 17,* 31–36.

Chernyshenko, O. S., & Ones, D. S. (1999). How selective are psychology graduate programs? The effect of the selection ration on GRE score validity. *Educational and Psychological Measurement, 59,* 951–961.

Collins, L. H. (2001, Winter). Does research experience make a significant difference in graduate admissions? *Eye on Psi Chi, 5,* 26–28.

Conway, J. B. (1988). Differences among clinical psychologists: Scientists, practitioners, and scientist–practitioners. *Professional Psychology: Research and Practice, 19,* 642–655.

Corcoran, K. J., Michels, J. L., & Ahina, L. K. (1999, August). *Clinical surfing: Clinical psychology doctoral programs on the web.* Paper presented at the 107th annual convention of the American Psychological Association, Boston, MA.

Coyle, S. L., & Bae, Y. (1987). *Summary report 1986: Doctorate recipients from United States universities.* Washington, DC: National Academy Press.

Crowe, M. B., Grogan, J. M., Jacobs, R. R., Lindsay, C. A., & Mack, M. M. (1985). Delineation of the roles of clinical psychology: A survey of practice in psychology. *Professional Psychology: Research and Practice, 16,* 124–137.

Dattilio, F. (1992). Doctoral studies for master's level licensed psychologists. *The Pennsylvania Psychologist Quarterly, 52*(2), 7, 11.

Dollinger, S. J. (1989). Predictive validity of the Graduate Record Examination in a clinical psychology program. *Professional Psychology: Research and Practice, 20,* 56–58.

Drummond, F., Rodolfa, E., & Smith, D. (1981). A survey of APA- and non-APA-approved internship programs. *American Psychologist, 36,* 411–414.

Eddy, B., Lloyd, P. J., & Lubin, B. (1987). Enhancing the application to doctoral professional programs: Suggestions from a national survey. *Teaching of Psychology, 14,* 160–163.

Educational Testing Service (ETS). (1984). *Analysis of score change patterns of examinees repeating the GRE General test.* Princeton, NJ: Educational testing Service.

Educational Testing Service. (1995). *Practicing to take the GRE Psychology Test* (3rd ed.). Princeton, NJ: Author.

Elam, C. L., et al. (1998). Letters of recommendation: Medical school admission committee members' recommendations. *The Advisor, 18,* 4–6.

Farry, J., Norcross, J. C., Mayne, T. J., & Sayette, M. A. (1995, August). *Acceptance rates and financial aid in clinical psychology: An update.* Poster presented at the 103rd annual convention of the American Psychological Association, New York, NY.

Fennell, K., & Kohout, J. (2002). *Characteristics of graduate departments of psychology: 1999–2000.* Washington, DC: American Psychological Association.

Ferrari, J. R., & Hemovich, V. B. (2004). Student-based psychology journals: Perceptions by graduate program directors. *Teaching of Psychology, 31,* 272–275.

Fitzgerald, L. F., & Osipow, S. H. (1986). An occupational analysis of counseling psychology. How special is the specialty? *American Psychologist, 41,* 535–544.

Fretz, B. R. (1976, Spring). Finding careers with a bachelor's degree in psychology. *Psi Chi Newsletter, 2,* 5–13.

Fretz, B. R., & Stang, D. J. (1980). *Preparing for graduate study in psychology: Not for seniors only!* Washington, DC: American Psychological Association.

Gaddy, C. D., Charlot-Swilley, D., Nelson, P. D., & Reich, J. N. (1995). Selected outcomes of accredited programs. *Professional Psychology: Research and Practice, 26,* 507–513.

Gartner, J. D. (1986). Antireligious prejudice in admissions to doctoral programs in clinical psychology. *Professional Psychology: Research and Practice, 17,* 473–475.

Gehlman, S., Wicherski, M., & Kohout, J. (1995). *Characteristics of graduate departments of psychology: 1993–1994.* Washington, DC: American Psychological Association Research Office.

Goldberg, E. L., & Alliger, G. M. (1992). Assessing the validity of the GRE for students in psychology: A validity generalization approach. *Educational and Psychological Measurement, 52,* 1019–1027.

Golding, J. M., Lang, K., Eymard, L. A., & Shadish, W. R. (1988). The buck stops here: A survey of the financial status of Ph.D. graduate students in psychology, 1966–1987. *American Psychologist, 43,* 1089–1091.

Goliszek, A. (2000). *The complete medical school preparation and admissions guide.* New York: Healthnet Press.

Gordon, R. A. (1990). Research productivity in master's-level psychology programs. *Professional Psychology: Research and Practice, 21,* 33–36.

Graduate Record Examinations. (2001). *2001–2002 GRE information and registration bulletin.* Princeton, NJ: Educational Testing Service.

Grote, C. L., Robiner, W. N., & Haut, A. (2001). Disclosure of negative information in letters of recommendation: Writers' intentions and readers' experiences. *Professional Psychology: Research and Practice, 32,* 655–661.

Halgin, R. P. (1986). Advising undergraduates who wish to become clinicians. *Teaching of Psychology, 13,* 7–12.

Hayes, S. C., & Hayes, L. J. (1989). Writing your vitae. *APS Observor, 2*(3), 15–17.

Heppner, P. P., & Downing, N. E. (1982). Job interviewing for new psychologists: Riding the emotional rollercoaster. *Professional Psychology, 13,* 334–341.

Hersh, J. B., & Poey, K. (1984). A proposed interviewing guide for intern applicants. *Professional Psychology, 15,* 3–5.

Hershey, J. M., Kopplin, D. A., & Cornell, J. E. (1991). Doctors of psychology: Their career experiences and attitudes toward degree and training. *Professional Psychology: Research and Practice, 22,* 351–356.

Hines, D. (1985). Admissions criteria for ranking master's-level applicants to clinical doctoral programs. *Teaching of Psychology, 13,* 64–66.

Holmes, C. B., & Beishline, M. J. (1996, August). *Doctoral admission rates for students with GRE scores below 1000.* Poster presented at the 104th annual meeting of the American Psychological Association, Toronto.

Huss, M. T., Randall, B. A., Patry, M., Davis, S. F., & Hansen, D. J. (2002). Factors influencing self-rated preparedness for graduate school: A survey of graduate schools. *Teaching of Psychology, 29,* 275–281.

Ilardi, S. S., Rodriguez-Hanley, A., Roberts, M. G., & Seigel, J. (2000). On the origins of clinical psychology faculty: Who is training the trainers? *Clinical Psychology: Science and Practice, 7,* 346–354.

Ingram, R. E. (1983). The GRE in the graduate admissions process: Is how it is used justified by the evidence of its validity? *Professional Psychology: Research and Practice, 14,* 711–714.

Jacob, M. C. (1987). Managing the internship application experience: Advice from an exhausted but content survivor. *The Counseling Psychologist, 15,* 146–155.

Jay, M. (1999). *Cracking the GRE Psychology* (5th ed.). Princeton: The Princeton Review.

Jensen, A. R. (1998). *The g factor: The science of mental ability.* Westport, CT: Praeger.

Kalat, J. W., & Matlin, M. W. (2000). The GRE Psychology Test: A useful but poorly understood test. *Teaching of Psychology, 27,* 24–27.

Keith-Spiegel, P. (1991). *The complete guide to graduate school admission.* Hillsdale, NJ: Lawrence Erlbaum.

Keith-Spiegel, P., Tabachnick, B. G., & Spiegel, G. B. (1994). When demand exceeds supply: Second-order criteria used by graduate school selection committees. *Teaching of Psychology, 21,* 79–81.

Keith-Spiegel, P., & Wiederman, M. W. (2000). *The complete guide to graduate school admission* (2nd ed.). Mahwah, NJ: Lawrence Erlbaum.

Keller, J. W., Beam, K. J., Maier, K. A., & Pietrowski, C. (1995, April). *Research or clinical experience: What doctoral applicants need to know.* Paper presented at the annual meeting of the Southeastern Psychological Association, Savannah, GA.

Kellogg, R. T. (2000). *Best preparation for the GRE in psychology.* Piscataway, NJ: Research & Education Association.

Khubchandani, A. (2002). To disclose or not to disclose: That is the question. *The APAGS Newsletter, 14*(4), 24–26.

King, D. W., Beehr, T. A., & King, L. A. (1986). Doctoral student selection in one professional psychology program. *Journal of Clinical Psychology, 42,* 399–407.

Kluger, J. (2002, June 10). Pumping up your past. *Time,* p. 45.

Kohout, J. L., & Wicherski, M. M. (1992). *1991 salaries in psychology.* Washington, DC: American Psychological Association.

Kohout, J., & Wicherski, M. (1993). *1991–1992 characteristics of graduate departments of psychology.* Washington, DC: American Psychological Association.

Kohout, J. & Wicherski, M. (1999). *1997 doctorate employment survey.* Washington, DC: American Psychological Association Research Office.

Kohout, J., Wicherski, M., & Pion, G. (1991). *Characteristics of graduate departments of psychology: 1988–89.* Washington, DC: American Psychological Association.

Kopala, M., Keitel, M. A., Suzuki, L. A., Alexander, C. M., Ponterotto, J. G., Reynolds, A. L., & Hennessy, J. J. (1995). Doctoral admissions in counseling psychology at Fordham University. *Teaching of Psychology, 22,* 133–135.

Korn, J. H. (1984). New odds on acceptance into Ph.D. programs in psychology. *American Psychologist, 39,* 179–180.

Kuncel, N. R., Hezlett, S. A., & Ones, D. S. (2001). A comprehensive meta-analysis of the predictive validity of the graduate record examinations: Implications for graduate student selection and performance. *Psychological Bulletin, 127,* 162–181.

Kupfersmid, J., & Fiola, M. (1991). Comparison of EPPP scores among graduates of varying psychology programs. *American Psychologist, 46,* 534–535.

Kyle, T. M. (2000, July/August). Investigating and choosing: The decision-making process among first-year graduate students. *APA Monitor,* p. 19.

Landrum, R. E. (2003). Graduate admissions in psychology: Transcripts and the effect of withdrawals. *Teaching of Psychology, 30,* 323–325.

Landrum, R. E., & Nelson, L. R. (2002). The undergraduate research assistantship: An analysis of benefits. *Teaching of Psychology, 29,* 15–19.

Lark, J. S., & Croteau, J. M. (1998). Lesbian, gay, and bisexual doctoral students' mentoring relationships with faculty in counseling psychology: A qualitative study. *The Counseling Psychologist, 26,* 754–776.

Lovitts, B. E., & Nelson, C. (2000, November–December). Attrition from Ph.D. programs. *Academe,* pp. 44–50.

Lubin, B. (1993, Winter). Message of the president. *Psi Chi Newsletter, 19,* 1.

Maher, B. A. (1999). Changing trends in doctoral training programs in psychology: A comparative analysis of research-oriented versus professional-applied programs. *Psychological Sciences, 10,* 475–481.

Mayne, T. J., Norcross, J. C., & Sayette, M. A. (1994). Admission requirements, acceptance rates, and financial assistance in clinical psychology programs: Diversity across the practice–research continuum. *American Psychologist, 49,* 605–611.

McWade, P. (1996). *Financing graduate school.* Princeton, NJ: Peterson's Guides.

Megargee, E. I. (1990). *A guide to obtaining a psychology internship.* Muncie, IN: Accelerated Development.

Megargee, E. I. (2001). *Megargee's guide to obtaining a psychology internship* (4th ed.). New York: Taylor & Francis.

Minke, K. M., & Brown, D. T. (1996). Preparing psychologists to work with children: A comparison of curricula in child-clinical and school psychology programs. *Professional Psychology: Research and Practice, 27,* 631–634.

Mitchell, S. L. (1996). Getting a foot in the door: The written internship application. *Professional Psychology: Research and Practice, 27,* 90–92.

Morgan, R. D., & Cohen, L. M. (2003, August). *Counseling and clinical psychology: Are we training students differently?* Poster presented at the annual convention of the American Psychological Association, Toronto.

Morrison, T., & Morrison, M. (1995). A meta-analytic assessment of the predictive validity of the quantitative and verbal components of the Graduate Record Examination with graduate grade point average representing the criterion of graduate success. *Educational and Psychological Measurement, 55,* 309–316.

Munoz-Dunbar, R., & Stanton, A. L. (1999). Ethnic diversity in clinical psychology: Recruitment and admission practices among doctoral programs. *Teaching of Psychology, 26,* 259–263.

Murray, B. (1996). Psychology remains top college major. *APA Monitor, 27,* 1, 42.

Murray, T. M., & Williams, S. (1999). *Analyses of data from graduate study in psychology: 1997–98.* Washington, DC: American Psychological Association Research Office.

Nauta, M. M. (2000). Assessing the accuracy of psychology undergraduates' perceptions of graduate admissions criteria. *Teaching of Psychology, 27,* 277–280.

Nevid, J. S., & Gildea, T. J. (1984). The admissions process in clinical training: The role of the personal interview. *Professional Psychology: Research and Practice, 15,* 18–25.

Norcross, J. C., Castle, P. H., Sayette, M. A. & Mayne, T. J. (2004). The Psy.D.: Heterogeneity in practitioner training. *Professional Psychology: Research and Practice, 35,* 412–419.

Norcross, J. C., Gallagher, K. M., & Prochaska, J. O. (1989). The Boulder and/or the Vail model: Training preferences of clinical psychologists. *Journal of Clinical Psychology, 45,* 822–828.

Norcross, J. C., & Goldfried, M. R. (Eds.). (2005). *Handbook of psychotherapy integration.* New York: Oxford University Press.

Norcross, J. C., Hanych, J. M., & Terranova, R. D. (1996). Graduate study in psychology: 1992–1993. *American Psychologist, 51,* 631–643.

Norcross, J. C., Hedges, M., & Prochaska, J. O. (2002). The face of 2010: A Delphi poll on the future of psychotherapy. *Professional Psychology: Research and Practice, 33,* 316–322.

Norcross, J. C., & Kaplan, K. J. (1995). Training in psychotherapy integration. Integrative/eclectic programs. *Journal of Psychotherapy Integration, 5*(3).

Norcross, J. C., Karg, R. S., & Prochaska, J. O. (1997a). Clinical psychologists in the 1990s: Part I. *The Clinical Psychologist, 50*(2), 4–9.

Norcross, J. C., Karg, R. S., & Prochaska, J. O. (1997b). Clinical psychologists in the 1990s: Part II. *The Clinical Psychologist, 50*(3), 4–11.

Norcross, J. C., Karpiak, C. P., & Santoro, S. O. (2005). Clinical psychologists across the years: The Division of Clinical Psychology from 1960 to 2003. *Journal of Clinical Psychology, 61*(11).

Norcross, J. C., Kohout, J. L., & Wicherski, M. (in press). Graduate study in psychology, 1971–2004. *American Psychologist.*

Norcross, J. C., & Oliver, J. M. (2005, March). *An update on PsyD programs; Acceptance rates, financial assistance, and selected outcomes by program setting.* Poster presented at the 76th annual meeting of the Eastern Psychological Association, Boston, MA.

Norcross, J. C., Sayette, M. A., Mayne, T. J., Karg, R. S., & Turkson, M. A. (1998). Selecting a doctoral program in professional psychology: Some comparisons among Ph.D. counseling, Ph.D. clinical, and Psy.D. clinical psychology programs. *Professional Psychology: Research and Practice, 29,* 609–614.

O'Donohue, W., Plaud, J. J., Mowatt, A. M., & Fearon, J. R. (1989). Current status of curricula of doctoral training programs in clinical psychology. *Professional Psychology: Research and Practice, 20,* 196–197.

Oliver, J. M., Norcross, J. C., Sayette, M. A., Griffin, K., & Mayne, T. J. (2005, March). *Doctoral study in clinical, counseling, and combined psychology: Admission requirements and student characteristics.* Poster presented at the 76th annual meeting of the Eastern Psychological Association, Boston, MA.

O'Neill, J. V. (2001, September). Image seen as key to social work's future. *NASW News,* p. 3.

Osborne, R. E. (1996, Fall). The "personal" side of graduate school personal statements. *Eye on Psi Chi, 1,* 14–15.

Otto, R. K., & Heilbrun, K. (2002). The practice of forensic psychology: A look toward the future in light of the past. *American Psychologist, 57,* 5–18.

Pate, W. E. II. (2001). *Analyses of data from Graduate Study in Psychology: 1999–2000.* Washington, DC: American Psychological Association Research Office.

Peterson, D. R. (1976). Need for the doctor of psychology degree in professional psychology. *American Psychologist, 31,* 792–798.

Peterson, D. R. (1982). Origins and development of the Doctor of Psychology concept. In G. R. Caddy, D. C. Rimm, H. Watson, & J. H. Johnson (Eds.), *Educating professional psychologists* (pp. 19–38). New Brunswick, NJ: Transaction Books.

Peterson, D. R., Eaton, M. M., Levine, A. R., & Snepp, F. P. (1982). Career experiences of doctors of psychology. *Professional Psychology, 13,* 268–277.

Peterson's grants for graduate and postdoctoral study (5th ed.). (1998). Princeton, NJ: Peterson's.

Piotrowski, C., & Keller, J. W. (1996). Research or clinical experience: What doctoral applicants need to know. *Journal of Instructional Psychology, 23,* 126–127.

Prevoznak, M. A., & Bubka, A. (1999, April). *Word-a-day method in preparation for the GRE.* Poster presented at the annual meeting of the Eastern Psychological Association, Providence, RI.

Psychological Corporation. (1994). *Miller Analogies Test: Technical manual.* San Antonio, TX: Author.

Purdy, J. E., Reinehr, R. C., & Swartz, J. D. (1989). Graduate admissions criteria of leading psychology departments. *American Psychologist, 44,* 960–961.

Rader, J. (2000). Disclosing a lesbian, gay, or bisexual identity in graduate psychology programs: Risk and rewards. *APAGS, 12*(2).

Raphael, S., & Halpert, L. H. (1999). *Graduate Record Examination—Psychology* (3rd ed.). New York: Prentice Hall.

Rem, R., Oren, E. M., & Childrey, G. (1987). Selection of graduate students in clinical psychology: Use of cutoff scores and interviews. *Professional Psychology: Research and Practice, 18*, 485–488.

Resnick, J. H. (1991). Finally, a definition of clinical psychology: A message from the President, Division 12. *The Clinical Psychologist, 44*(1), 3–4.

Rheingold, H. L. (1994). *The psychologist's guide to an academic career.* Washington, DC: American Psychological Association.

Robyak, J. E., & Goodyear, R. K. (1984). Graduate school origins of diplomates and fellows in professional psychology. *Professional Psychology: Research and Practice, 15*, 379–387.

Sachs, M. L., Burke, K. L., & Schrader, D. C. (2001). *Directory of graduate programs in applied sport psychology* (6th ed.). Morgantown, WV: Fitness Information Technology.

Salzinger, K. (Chair). (1998, August). *Combined professional–scientific psychology: Greater than the sum of its parts?* Symposium presented at the 106th annual convention of the American Psychological Association, San Francisco, CA.

Sayette, M. A., & Mayne, T. J. (1990). Survey of current clinical and research trends in clinical psychology. *American Psychologist, 45*, 1263–1267.

Sayette, M. A., Mayne, T. J., Norcross, J. C., & Giuffre, D. E. (1999, June). *Letting a hundred flowers bloom? Ph.D. clinical psychology training in the 1990s.* Paper presented at annual meeting of the Academy of Psychological Clinical Science, Denver, CO.

Schaefer, S. E. (1995). Stigmatization of psychology doctoral program applicants who have a history of psychological counseling. *Dissertation Abstracts, 57*(02B), 1427.

Scott, W. C., & Silka, L. D. (1974). Applying to graduate school in psychology: A perspective and guide. *Journal Supplement Abstract Service,* MS. 597.

Shaffer, D. R., & Tomarelli, M. (1981). Bias in the ivory tower: An unintended consequence of the Buckley Amendment for graduate admissions. *Journal of Applied Psychology, 66*, 7–11.

Smith, R. A. (1985). Advising beginning psychology majors for graduate school. *Teaching of Psychology, 12*, 194–198.

Snepp, F. P., & Peterson, D. R. (1988). Evaluative comparison of Psy.D. and Ph.D. students by clinical internship supervisors. *Professional Psychology: Research and Practice, 19*, 180–183.

Society for Industrial and Organizational Psychology. (2003). *Graduate training in industrial/organizational psychology and related fields.* Bowling Green, OH: Author.

Stapp, J., Tucker, A. M., & VandenBos, G. R. (1985). Census of psychological personnel: 1983. *American Psychologist, 40*, 1317–1351.

Steinpreis, R., Queen, L., & Tennen, H. (1992). The education of clinical psychologists: A survey of training directors. *The Clinical Psychologist, 45*, 87–94.

Sternberg, R. J. (Ed.). (1997). *Career paths in psychology: Where your degree can take you.* Washington, DC: American Psychological Association.

Sternberg, R. J., & Williams, W. M. (1997). Does the graduate record examination predict meaningful success in the graduate training of psychologists? *American Psychologist, 52*, 630–641.

Stewart, A. E., & Stewart, E. A. (1996). A decision-making technique for choosing a psychology internship. *Professional Psychology: Research and Practice, 27*, 521–526.

Stewart, D. W., & Spille, H. A. (1988). *Diploma mills: Degrees of fraud.* New York: Macmillan.

Strickland, B. R. (1985). Over the Boulder(s) and through the Vail. *The Clinical Psychologist, 38*, 52–56.

Terry, R. L. (1996, December). Characteristics of psychology departments at primarily undergraduate institutions. *Council on Undergraduate Research Quarterly,* pp. 86–90.

Tibbits-Kleber, A. L., & Howell, R. J. (1987). Doctoral training in clinical psychology: A students' perspective. *Professional Psychology: Research and Practice, 18*, 634–639.

Tipton, R. M. (1983). Clinical and counseling psychology: A study of roles and functions. *Professional Psychology: Research and Practice, 14*, 837–846.

Titus, J. B., & Buxman, N. J. (1999, Spring). Is Psi Chi meeting its mission statement? *Eye on Psi Chi, 3*, 16–18.

Todd, D. M., & Farinato, D. (1992). A local resource for advising applicants to clinical psychology graduate programs. *Teaching of Psychology, 19*, 52–54.

Toia, A., Herron, W. G., Primavera, L. H., & Javier, R. A. (1997). Ethnic diversification in clinical psychology training. *Cultural Diversity and Mental Health, 3*, 193–206.

Toma, J. D., & Cross, M. E. (1998). Intercollegiate athletics and student college choice: Exploring the impact of championship seasons on undergraduate applications. *Research in Higher Education, 39*, 633–661.

Tryon, G. S. (1985). What can our students learn from regional psychology conventions? *Teaching of Psychology, 12*, 227–228.

Tryon, G. S. (2000). Doctoral training issues in school and clinical child psychology. *Professional Psychology: Research and Practice, 31*, 85–87.

Turkington, C. (1986). Practitioner training. *APA Monitor, 17*(1), 14, 17.

Turkson, M. A., & Norcross, J. C. (1996, March). *Doctoral training in counseling psychology: Admission statistics, student characteristics, and financial assistance.* Paper presented at the annual conference of the Eastern Psychological Association, Philadelphia, PA.

VandeCreek, L., & Fleisher, M. (1984). The role of practicum in the undergraduate psychology curriculum. *Teaching of Psychology, 11*, 9–14.

VandenBos, G. E., Stapp, J., & Kilburg, R. R. (1981). Health service providers in psychology. *American Psychologist, 36*, 1395–1418.

Walfish, S. (2004). An eye-opening experience: Taking an online practice Graduate Record Examination. *Eye on Psi Chi, Winter 2004*, 18, 19, 69.

Walfish, S., Stenmark, D. E., Shealy, J. S., & Shealy, S. E. (1989). Reasons why applicants select clinical psychology graduate programs. *Professional Psychology: Research and Practice, 20*, 350–354.

Walfish, S., & Sumprer, G. F. (1984). Employment opportunities for graduates of APA-approved and non-APA-approved training programs. *American Psychologist, 39*, 1199–1200.

Waters, J., Drew, B., & Ayers, J. (1988). Integrating conflicting needs in curriculum planning: Advice to faculty. In P. J. Woods (Ed.), *Is psychology for them?* Washington, DC: American Psychological Association.

Watkins, C. E., Lopez, F. G., Campbell, V. L., & Himmell, C. D. (1986a). Contemporary counseling psychology: Results of a national survey. *Journal of Counseling Psychology, 33,* 301–309.

Watkins, C. E., Lopez, F. G., Campbell, V. L., & Himmell, C. D. (1986b). Counseling psychology and clinical psychology: Some preliminary comparative data. *American Psychologist, 41,* 581–582.

Whitbourne, S. K. (1999, April). *A guide to personal statements.* Paper presented at the 70th annual meeting of the Eastern Psychological Association, Boston, MA.

Wicherski, M., & Kohout, J. (1992). *Characteristics of graduate departments of psychology: 1990–1991.* Washington, DC: American Psychological Association.

Young, K. S., & VandeCreek, L. (1996, March). *Ethnic minority selection procedures in clinical training graduate admissions.* Paper presented at the 67th annual meeting of the Eastern Psychological Association, Philadelphia, PA.

Zebala, J. A., Jones, D. B., & Jones, S. B. (1999). *Medical school admissions: The insider's guide.* New Haven, CT: Mustang.